Management
of
Rheumatic
Disorders

MANAGEMENT OF RHEUMATIC DISORDERS

J.M.H. Moll

BSc, DM, PhD, FRCP

Consultant Physician in Rheumatology,
Nether Edge Hospital, Sheffield;
Head, Sheffield Centre for Rheumatic Diseases;
Honorary Clinical Lecturer in Rheumatic Diseases,
University of Sheffield

LONDON
Chapman and Hall

First published 1983
by Chapman and Hall Ltd,
11 New Fetter Lane, London EC4P 4EE

© 1983 J.M.H. Moll

Printed in Great Britain at the
University Press, Cambridge

ISBN 0 412 15790 X

British Library Cataloguing in Publication Data

Moll, J.M.H.
  Management of rheumatic disorders.
  1. Arthritis   2. Rheumatism
  I. Title
  616.7′206   RC933
  ISBN 0-412-15790-X

To my family

THE PATIENT

Health and an able body are two jewels.

Francis Beaumont (1584–1616)
and John Fletcher (1579–1625)
The Wild-Goose Chase, Act II, sc. I

But pain is perfect miserie, the worst
Of evils, and excessive, overturnes
All patience.

John Milton (1608–74)
Paradise Lost, Bk. VI

There is a great wonder in regard to them (arthritis
and gout); there is not the slightest pain in them,
although you cut and squeeze them; but if pained of
themselves, no other pain is stronger than this.

Aretaeus of Cappadocia (AD 81–138?)
On the Causes and Symptoms of Chronic Diseases,
II. 12 (translated by Francis Adams)

THE DOCTOR

The treatment of a disease may be entirely impersonal; the care of a patient must be completely personal.

Francis Weld Peabody (1881–1927)
The Care of the Patient

It is by poultices, not by words, that pain is ended,
although pain is by words both eased and diminished.

Petrarch (1304–74)
Letter to Guido Sette, 1359

Would you not think his cunning to be great that
could restore this cripple to his legs again?

William Shakespeare (1564–1616)
Henry VI, Part II, II. i. 133

Contents

Preface

In general, existing texts concerned with rheumatic therapy have either been addressed to specific aspects of treatment or have formed only part of more general textbooks. This book has therefore been written to fulfil a need for a convenient and comprehensive distillation of material covering the various treatment entities, the interrelationships between them, and the wide potential for their application.

A further need for such a book stems from the fact that approaches to treatment and their associated research reports have continued to grow at a high rate in recent years. This is particularly so in relation to drug therapy, and the task of reviewing this massive literature in sufficient breadth and depth to do justice to these advances is mirrored in Chapters 5 and 6.

Although each country and indeed each practitioner may favour a particular blend of therapies, this book is based primarily on the findings of what might be termed the international research community. The approach is therefore a combination of review and personal opinion. Furthermore, an attempt has been made to redress international differences, and this applies particularly to variations in drug nomenclature between the UK, USA, and other countries.

In the opening chapters of the book the historical background to rheumatic therapy and the general principles of management are covered, with particular emphasis on the team approach and the concept of therapeutic spectra.

An additional chapter on heterodox procedures has been provided. Neither a recommendation nor a condemnation, this is aimed at providing doctors with a critical appraisal of facts to satisfy the growing number of patients seeking such information.

Chapters concerning individual methods of treatment form the core of the book and discuss communication, drugs, local injection therapy, radiotherapy, surgery, and rehabilitation.

With regard to the general plan of the book, the chapters are largely self-contained and can be read in any order. However, it is recommended that the 'introductory' chapters (Chapters 1, 2, and 4) should be read before those succeeding them. If a more circuitous route is preferred each chapter is supplied with a list of contents and a summary to aid swift appraisal. A generous system of cross-references and some repetition of salient points are also intended to help the reader who uses the book as a reference source. A summary of the whole book is given in the last chapter (Section 12.10) and contains conclusions about the present status of the various approaches to therapy, together with suggestions about the future.

Bibliographies are listed for convenience at the end of each chapter. No attempt has been made to separate textual citations (the large majority) from suggestions for further reading as it has been assumed that the significance of each entity will be evident from the text. In most chapters clear-cut subdivisions of the subject matter have enabled corresponding subdivisions of the biographical lists.

The preparation of any medical book involves an inexorable fight against time. In the field of therapeutics generally, and of drugs in particular, where new data are published daily, this fight can never be won. However, perhaps the deliberate act of writing the fastest-moving subjects last will guard against the more gross symptoms of premature senility.

This book is intended primarily for physicians responsible for patients with rheumatic disorders, but it should also be of value to clinicians whose domain overlaps with rheumatology, such as orthopaedic surgeons, rehabilitationists, and clinical investigators.

J.M.H. Moll
Nether Edge Hospital
Sheffield

Acknowledgements

I gratefully acknowledge the kindness and help of Mrs Pat Drake, who took the manuscript through its various stages and who so often combined this *tour de force* with the role of research assistant and librarian.

I have received much assistance from colleagues at Nether Edge Hospital and elsewhere, and I especially wish to thank the following: Dr R.S. Amos; Dr M.S. Derini; Mr R.E. Elson, FRCS; Dr R.E.S. Gray; Dr G.R. Newns; Professor V. Wright; Mrs Angela Garstang, SRN; Mrs Margaret Lee, SRN; Mrs M. Gunton, BSc, CQSW; Mrs M. Harris, Dip COT; Mrs M. Sellars, MCSP, SRP; Mrs Joan Weatherington, MCSP, SRP; Mr R. Giles, BPharm, MPS; Mrs H. Hebron, BPharm, MPS; and Mrs Edna Dawson and Mrs Pat Large (Medical Secretaries).

Staff of the Department of Medical Illustration, Northern General Hospital, Sheffield have enduringly rendered my preliminary designs into formal images, and I am particularly indebted to Miss Carol Tim and Mr J.B. Williamson (Medical Artists), and Messrs R.E. Brooks and A.J. Emery, and Miss Cecilia McKenzie-Pratt (Medical Photographers).

Finally, I am most grateful to Dr Barry Shurlock of Chapman and Hall, whose editorial collaboration has been productive and stimulating throughout.

Note on referencing

1. As is usual practice, text citations for references have been placed next to statements associated with them. The exception to this chiefly concerns the two drug chapters, Chapters 5 and 6. Here, in view of the often large number of important references for sections containing a lot of detail these citations have been grouped at the end of these sections. This has been done to avoid overburdening the text and to avoid unnecessary repetition.

2. References to the tables in the appendices appear in the main bibliographies but are marked with* for an appendix reference, and† for a reference that appears both in the main text and in the appendix.

1
Historical background

1.1 INTRODUCTORY COMMENT

The term 'rheumatism' (a term dating from 1601 in the English language) is derived from the Greek word *rheumatismos*, which designated mucus (catarrh) as an evil humour which was thought to flow from the brain to the joints and other portions of the body, producing pain. As recent studies have shown that a change in a constituent of joint mucin–the mucopolysaccharide, hyaluronic acid–occurs in at least some of the rheumatic diseases, the basis of the term 'rheumatism' has some, although probably fortuitous, relevance.

Arthritis (a term dating from 1544 in the English language) is one of the oldest known, yet most neglected diseases. The earliest known example of multiple arthritis in a fossil vertebrate is in a skeleton of a platycarpus (a large swimming reptile), which lived about 100 000 000 years ago. This now resides in the Museum of Natural History in the University of Kansas. Chronic arthritis of the spine was present in the Ape Man of 2 000 000 years ago, as well as in our ancestors, the Java and the Lansing men of 500 000 years ago, and in Egyptian mummies dating from 8000 BC. The Romans built extensive baths throughout their empire because of this disease.

The literature concerning historical aspects of rheumatic disorders is often difficult to interpret due to confusion in terminology over past years. In bygone centuries 'rheumatology' was essentially a division between 'the gout' and 'rheumatism'. As awareness of further differentiations developed added confusions arose from the opaque distinction between osteoarthritis and rheumatoid arthritis. In more recent years a similar problem of identification has arisen from a blurring between rheumatoid arthritis and disorders which are now classified as and with ankylosing spondylitis.

Much of the following account has been derived from classical works concerning general aspects of arthritis (mainly gout) and rheumatism (e.g. Baillou, 1642; Dumoulin, 1710; Latham, 1796; Mitchell, 1831; MacLagan, 1881; Delpeuch, 1900; Poynton and Paine, 1913; Poynton and Schlesinger, 1937). For further details the reader is referred either to these original sources or to the valuable monograph on rheumatological history by Copeman (1964).

More specific historical sources covering individual disease entities are less abundant, as might be expected from the fact that sophistication of rheumatological classification has developed only relatively recently. However, the following sources have been used as reference material in this chapter: gout (Talbott, 1942; Graham and Graham, 1955; Bywaters, 1962; Copeman, 1964); rheumatoid arthritis (Goldthwait, 1904; Copeman, 1964); osteoarthritis (Spender, 1889); rheumatic fever (West, 1878); juvenile joint disease

(Still, 1896–97); ankylosing spondylitis (Marie, 1898; Léri, 1899; O'Connell, 1956; Copeman, 1964; Moll, 1978; Bywaters, 1980); the spondarthritides (Wright and Moll, 1976). Further references can be found in relation to specific points made in subsequent sections.

Apart from the literature mentioned here, I wish to acknowledge at this point the additional perspective that has been gleaned from visits to various libraries containing historical works of rheumatological interest, notably; the Heberden Society Library, the library of the Royal College of Physicians of London, the library of the Royal Society of Medicine, and the Wellcome Historical Medical Library.

1.2 DEVELOPMENT OF MODERN RHEUMATOLOGY

1.2.1 Development of a professional framework for the specialty

In view of the fact that many of the rheumatic diseases are chronic, painful disorders without, until recently, satisfactory methods of prevention and treatment, patients have tended to comfort themselves with palliative and symptomatic treatment, usually physical therapies offered by spas and similar centres.

Such forms of treatment had a strong influence on the early growth of rheumatology. For example, in 1931 the Section of Balneology and Climatology of the Royal Society of Medicine joined with the Section of Electrotherapeutics to form the Section of Physical Medicine. In 1973 this became the Section of Rheumatology and Rehabilitation.

In 1944 the Minister of Health appointed a subcommittee, under the chairmanship of Sir Henry Cohen, to advise him on this discipline. Seven years later the special committee of the Royal College of Physicians concluded that the rheumatic diseases should be considered as a subspecialty within the field of general medicine. It was also felt that certain special centres should be developed in the Hospital Regions to promote research and teaching in this subject. Desiderata for the training of the specialist physicians who should take charge of such centres were laid down. In 1953 the University of Manchester appointed the first Professor of Rheumatology within the British Commonwealth. At this time the World Health Organization interested itself in this subject and published a Report (No. 78).

Within the boundaries of modern rheumatology have developed many of the advances in clinical immunology and epidemiology. Concepts of scientific clinical techniques, such as the design of therapeutic trials and establishment of diagnostic criteria, have also been closely linked with the specialty.

In parallel with these developments in the clinical field, national and international organizations have been established to co-ordinate the fight against the rheumatic diseases. Glover's Report on Chronic Rheumatism to the British Ministry of Health in 1927 and the formation of the Committee on Chronic Rheumatic Diseases by the Royal College of Physicians in 1935 helped to lay the foundation stone of this cohesive effort in the United Kingdom and formed the nucleus of the Empire Rheumatism Council (now the Arthritis and Rheumatism Council for Research in Great Britain and the Commonwealth). The Council today supports most of the research and education in rheumatic diseases in this country and also provided the initiative for making the Government and profession aware of the importance of this group of diseases in Great Britain.

The British League against Rheumatism consists of scientific and community sections, representing the medical and other health professions, patients, and voluntary bodies. It is affiliated to the Arthritis and Rheumatism Council, the British Rheumatism and Arthritis Association (primarily concerned with patient welfare), and the British Council for Rehabilitation of the Disabled.

The International League Against Rheumatism (ILAR) was formed in 1927, several years before the present constituent regional leagues EULAR (European League Against Rheumatism), PANLAR (Pan American League Against Rheumatism), and SEAPAL (South-East Asia and Pacific Area League Against Rheumatism). The original function of ILAR and the regional leagues was to organize international scientific congresses every 4 years, but as part of the new constitution of 1974 six co-ordinated standing committees were set up ('International and National Agencies', 'Education', 'Publications', 'Epidemiology', 'International Clinical Studies', and 'Social and Community Agencies').

Coinciding with the fiftieth anniversary of its foundation, ILAR, together with its regional leagues, and with the support of the World Health Organization, designated 1977 as World Rheumatism Year. This was aimed at, and actually achieved, increasing our knowledge of the rheumatic diseases, improving availability and quality of care and developing research policies.

The advancement of modern rheumatology has undoubtedly been enhanced since the start of World War II by the founding of the *Annals of the Rheumatic Diseases* in 1941 by the Empire Rheumatism Council, and of the American equivalent *Arthritis and Rheumatism* (official Journal of the American Rheumatism Association) somewhat later, in 1958.

The Americans, however, were first to publish an extensive rheumatological textbook – *Arthritis and Allied Conditions. A Textbook of Rheumatology* appearing under B.I. Comroe's editorship in 1940 (Comroe, 1940). This work is now in its ninth edition. The British counterpart *Textbook of Rheumatic Diseases*, now in its fifth edition, was first published in 1948 under the editorship of W.S.C. Copeman (Copeman, 1948). Over the past 10 years the extent of the rheumatological library has burgeoned together with that of other specialties, and several new rheumatological textbooks and monographs are now appearing every year.

1.2.2 Development in terms of changing nomenclature and classification of rheumatic disorders

Even into the early years of this century, knowledge of rheumatic disorders was limited to division of clinical entities into 'arthritis deformans', 'chronic rheumatism', 'muscular rheumatism' and 'gout'. Arthritis deformans or 'osteo-arthritis', as it became known, was used in a much wider sense than is applied nowadays, and encompassed rheumatoid arthritis, Still's disease, generalized osteo-arthritis, localized osteo-arthritis, Heberden's nodes, and spondylitis deformans (ankylosing spondylitis) (Osler, 1910; Monro, 1911; Taylor, 1911).

Childhood arthritis was classified principally according to infective influences as follows: 'rheumatic', 'gonorrhoeal', 'pneumococcal', 'suppurative with pneumonia', 'with specific fevers', 'with empyema', and 'with syphilis' (Still, 1909). However, Still had described the disease now known by his name 12 years previously (Still, 1897).

It was not until the early 1920s that a more clear distinction was made between common rheumatic entities, particularly between rheumatoid arthritis and osteoarthritis*, and the Ministry of Health Classification of 1924 makes this clear. Further clarification (discussed by Hill and Ellman, 1938) developed in the 1930s (British Medical Association in 1933; Royal College of Physicians of London in 1934; International League Against Rheumatism in 1934). The classification used nowadays is based either on that proposed by the ILAR in 1957, or the more extensive one recommended by the American Rheumatism Association in 1963. The details of these classifications can be found in Appendix 1.7.1.

The whole question of classification and nomenclature is rapidly becoming changed (Ropes *et al.*, 1956; CIOMS, 1966; Bennett and Wood, 1968; Kellgren, 1968; Wood, 1970a, b, 1974; Feldman *et al.*, 1972; de Dombal *et al.*, 1974). For example, one new approach

---

* The term osteoarthrosis (used throughout this book) has replaced 'osteoarthritis' in recent years, although the latter term is re-emerging in view of current emphasis on inflammatory aspects of the disease.

has been to adopt principles used in botanical identification. As Wood (1978) has pointed out, this is accomplished by means of a flora or key, and application of this to a system for classifying inflammatory arthropathies could be useful. Such a system, although still only experimental, is shown in Appendix 1.7.2. Although Wood is quick to point out that problems in medicine are much more changeable and immediate, and that they are related to processes rather than to objects like a plant, such a system highlights that diagnostic decision making may be explored more productively by using a series of discriminators in sequence rather than by matching the patient to a model profile, which is currently the method involved in the application of diagnostic criteria.

1.3 HISTORICAL ASPECTS OF TREATMENT OF SPECIFIC RHEUMATIC DISORDERS

For much of the material contained in the following sections the author is indebted to Copeman's *A Short History of the Gout and the Rheumatic Diseases* (1964), to which the reader is referred for further details.

1.3.1 Gout

The ancients, basing their treatment on the humoral theory of disease, remained remarkably constant in their therapeutic approach throughout the Greek, Roman, Byzantine, Moslem, and Medieval periods. The aim was to eliminate offending matter from the system by all available routes, and when this had been achieved it was assumed that the body would act as its own physician. The methods employed were, therefore, bleeding and blistering, sweating, purging with scammony, white hellebore, or other herbal cathartics, and the administration of emetics and diuretics.

The Greeks' frequent use of hermodactyl, a close relation of *Colchicum autumnale*, was probably not recognized by them as specific therapy, this plant being normally administered merely as a drastic purge. It was only later noticed by some physicians, notably by Alexander of Tralles (AD 525–605), that its effect was of a more direct nature.

From earliest times, and throughout the Middle Ages, great importance was attached to abstinence from diet and wine, especially at the start of an attack. Healthy sleep and moderate regular exercise were fervently encouraged and excess in 'venery in all its forms' was to be avoided. All these therapeutic practices were brought together by the nineteenth century in the combined regimen at 'watering places' such as Bath, Wiesbaden and Aix which sprang up throughout

Europe. These became very fashionable and 'to take the cure' became a new way of life, particularly for the gentry.

Many famous physicians throughout the ages had their own special mixtures, cordials, elixirs, or 'specifics'. However, most of these appear to have been simple and harmless herbal concoctions whose efficacy doubtless had more to do with the personality and reputation of the prescriber than with the ingredients.

Thus, the medicinal treatment of gout remained static until the reintroduction of colchicum towards the beginning of the nineteenth century, after which a host of 'secret' remedies containing this drug appeared in the markets of Europe. The uricosuric drugs were introduced during the present century and marked a great step forwards.

Local treatments have been varied: hot and cold fermentations, emollient ointments, counter-irritation by means of cautery or burning flax, scarification by knife and blister, hot sand, saline and mineral-water baths, and sometimes light friction of the affected joints with salt and oil. There was, however, always a school of thought that considered it to be dangerous to employ local measures of any sort, especially during the acute attack, lest they interfere with nature's own efforts to expel the 'peccant humour'.

Apart from Sydenham, who revived the Greek's philosophy of moderation, most physicians during the seventeenth and eighteenth centuries greatly overtreated their patients with the severe methods at their disposal.

Views on bleeding varied greatly through the ages. Until the time of Sydenham it had been widely advocated and extensively used. The main point of dispute concerned the site at which it should be carried out: on the side of the body opposite the lesion (according to Moslem fashion), on the side near the joint, or even in another limb. There was also controversy about whether the lancet or the leech was the preferable instrument. 'Wet cupping' was introduced as a further refinement towards the end of the eighteenth century. Although Sydenham was in general opposed to bleeding, well into the nineteenth century Gairdner (1849) wrote in favour of small, repeated bleedings, and Garrod used the remedy occasionally in early arthritis in patients who were otherwise healthy. However, Garrod was against the local use of leeches or blisters in affected joints because of problems of slow healing. Therapeutic bleeding has been used in the treatment of many gouty patients who are still living – a vivid reminder of the recentness of this bygone era.

With regard to purging, a similar variation of opinion existed as it did concerning bleeding, and much variety and ingenuity in the compounding of purgative prescriptions was manifest from Roman times onwards.

Sydenham and both Richard Mead and Boerhaave shared a reluctance to purge, although they would sometimes prescribe small doses of Glauber's Salt, a recent introduction from the continent. Purgation was restored to fashionable favour by Sir Charles Scudamore in the 1820s.

The clyster, a refinement that was popular before and during the eighteenth century, was a large form of enema syringe made out of a pig's bladder, with which various mixtures – which generally contained honey – were injected for the purpose of clearing the lower bowel of its 'excrementous residuum'.

These somewhat fierce methods of treatment temporarily diminished in popularity when Dr William

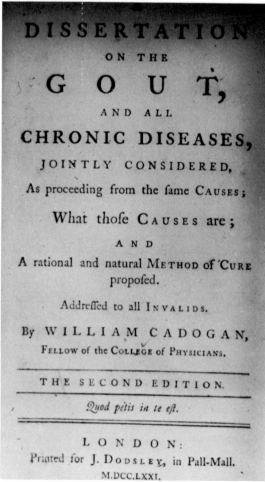

Fig. 1.1 Title page of Cadogan's *A Dissertation on the Gout and on All Chronic Diseases* (1771). (Courtesy of the Heberden Society.)

Cadogan (1711–99) published his best-selling book, *A Dissertation on the Gout and on All Chronic Diseases* (1771) (see Fig. 1.1). In it, he refuted specific treatment and, with great originality as was then thought, advocated a permanently temperate way of life.

Regarding the use of anodynes (drugs that allay pain), Hippocrates had warned against them, and Sydenham avoided their use when he could. Cullen wrote: 'Whilst opiates give the most certain relief from pain, yet when given in the beginning of a gouty paroxysm they cause it to return later with even greater volume'. Garrod himself withheld them if possible, owing to 'their baneful influence upon the secreting organs', but if pressed he would prescribe a little Dover's Powder, or occasionally some henbane or belladonna.

About 1780 a French regimental officer, M. Nicholas Husson, discovered a method of extracting and standardizing the potency of the autumn crocus (*Colchicum autumnale*), a therapy whose value had earlier been rediscovered by Anton von Störck in Vienna (see Fig. 1.2). Husson was able to preserve its effectiveness for long periods and patented and advertised it extensively with success as the secret 'specific', L'Eau d'Husson. Its active principle was identified as colchicum in 1814, and this had the important effect of attracting the attention of the new medical chemists not only to study colchicum, but also to examine the pathology and biochemistry of gout generally.

Tophi—'Those little chalky excrescences not unlike crabs' eyes' – as Sydenham had called them, were well recognized and described as a feature of gout by all the ancient writers. However, it is a curious fact that their well-observed occurrence in the ears of gouty patients received no published notice until the sixteenth century. Soranus of Ephesus, writing during the second century AD, said in the course of his excellent description of the gout: 'Then stones develop that disorganise the joints and distend the skin. These may burst through and jut out. They can be removed surgically, or upon their early appearance may be merely lifted out with a spoon-shaped instrument, though later they will grow again.' His colleague, Rufus of Ephesus, mentioned that he had occasionally seen them dissolve during the course of treatment. Most other Greek writers preferred to leave them *in situ* if they did not respond to simple heat and poultices. Occasionally they would try to dissolve them away with a paste of quicklime and nitre in lard.

With the beginnings of chemistry in the eighteenth century it was proposed by Boerhaave, who believed tophi to be composed of true chalk, that they should be dissolved away by the frequent application of hydrochloric acid in turpentine. His pupil, Van Swieten, used a compound made by heating crude tartar with a solution of quicklime in water, and reported that they would often disappear within a few days.

In the nineteenth century, Sir Charles Sudamore attempted to dissolve them with a solution of potash, whilst his successor, Sir Alfred Garrod, tried to achieve the same effect with the use of lithia (lithium oxide).

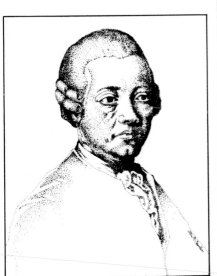
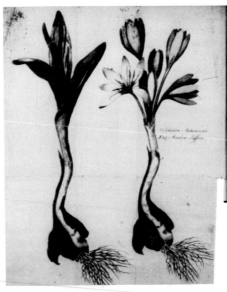
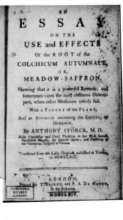

(a)   (b)

Fig. 1.2 (*a*) Anton Frei herr von Störck (1731–1803). (*b*) Title page and frontispiece of Storck's book *An Essay on the Use and Effects of the Root of the Colchicum Autumnale or, Meadow-Saffron* (1761). (Courtesy of the Heberden Society.)

It is only during the last few years that efficient agents – uricosuric drugs and xanthine oxidase inhibitors – have been devised by which, if the level of uric acid in the blood can be controlled, the tophi will dissolve and often disappear completely in time.

1.3.2 Rheumatic fever and chorea

(a) Treatment of rheumatic fever

P.M. Latham (1845) said: 'No disease has been treated by such various and opposite methods. Venesection and opium have wrought their cures, so has calomel. And so has colchicum, and so have drastic purgatives.' Baillou had written that: 'If pain and swelling of the joints remain after the fever is abated by means of frequent bleedings, apply 3 to 4 leeches to the parts, and let the blood ooze until it stops of itself.' Bleeding remained the mainstay until the middle of the nineteenth century.

Once the significance of cardiac disease had been understood in the nineteenth century, rest was firmly advocated by Sir Thomas Watson and others. The alkaline treatment phase followed. This was based on the belief that chilling could inhibit the normal working of the sweat glands in the skin. These would therefore be unable to excrete lactic acid, which would accumulate in the bloodstream and cause the manifestations of acute rheumatism. An 'acid-free diet' designed to combat this disorder was devised by Alexander Haig and was very fashionable for a time.

The Peruvian bark (quinine) had been, from Sydenham's time, the favourite drug; but therapeutic scepticism existed in academic circles, although its antipyretic action was recognized. Dr Thomas MacLagan of Glasgow, like Haygarth at the beginning of the century, erroneously believed acute rheumatism to be akin to malaria – the result of a minute parasitic organism which lived in the marshy country where the disease flourished best. The diseases being similar, he thought that 'there might – nay, there ought–to be some drug capable of exercising over its course the same controlling influence that quinine exercises over the course of ague'. Being a devout man, and believing that God had arranged that natural remedies often lie not far from their causes, he noticed the willow. This led to trying the effect of salicin, the glucoside that had been extracted from its bark by Piria in 1839. The drug was found to be successful in its effects although it was very expensive, the natural finished product costing 12 guineas per pound.

Unknown to him this effect of salicin had been discovered in similar fashion a century previously by the Reverend Edward (Edmund) Stone (Appendix 1.7.3). This clinically orientated cleric tried it on about 50 sufferers with rheumatic fever during a period of 5 years, and found that it almost never failed to be beneficial.

In 1876 MacLagan published his results, a milestone in the establishment of the specific action of the salicylate group of drugs in rheumatic fever. Sodium salicylate, which a short time before (1874) had been synthesized (by allowing carbon dioxide to act upon carbolic acid in the presence of an alkali) was now on the market, and, being less toxic, was soon substituted for salicin at the suggestion of the German Professor, Hermann Senator. From 1899 onwards sodium acetyl-salicylate (aspirin) became generally adopted. It was easier to take, as it was in tablet form, was of less unpleasant taste, and caused less gastric irritation. Furthermore, its price was now only 12 shillings a pound.

During the second and third decades of the present century, it became common practice to administer salicylates together with large doses of sodium bicarbonate in order to increase tolerance and reduce side effects. After the introduction of plasma-level estimations, however, it was soon noted that alkalis greatly increased the rate of excretion of the salicylates, with consequent reduction of therapeutic effect.

In 1949, after the discovery of the therapeutic anti-inflammatory effect of the corticosteroid hormones by Philip Hench and E.C. Kendall, it was thought that these drugs might substitute for the salicylates. Subsequent clinical trials, however, failed to confirm the value of such a substitution, as both groups of drugs were shown to have a satisfactory effect in controlling acute rheumatism.

Sir Henry Souttar was the first surgeon intentionally to open the living human heart. He paved the way for the surgical treatment of chronic rheumatic heart disease when, in 1925 at the London Hospital, he operated on a girl of 16 suffering with mitral stenosis and regurgitation, and attempted to stretch the contracted valve. For various reasons no further development occurred in this sphere until Sir Russell Brock in London and Professor Alfred Blalock at Johns Hopkins later succeeded in establishing cardiac surgery as a safe and helpful procedure.

The development of methods of inducing hypothermia, and the development of machines enabling extracorporeal circulation of the bloodstream, led to continued growth in this type of surgery.

In the preventive field, the main advance was the introduction of so-called 'interval treatment' with sulphonamides, or with antibiotics such as penicillin, with the intention of preventing re-infection with haemolytic streptococci. This has led to a significant reduction in the prevalence of chronic rheumatic heart disease.

The other main advance was the provision of help for the sufferers with disabling heart disease, as well as the promotion of further research by social organizations and government authorities.

(b)   Treatment of chorea

Chorea, which is now regarded as a curious variant of acute rheumatism, was first described by Thomas Sydenham, after whom it is often named 'Sydenham's chorea'. St. Vitus, a Roman missionary who was boiled in oil by the citizens of Ulm in AD 303, has been the reputed patron of chorea through the ages. Sufferers with all types of 'the dancing malady' could be cured by a visit to St. Vitus' shrine. Thus, he became associated with this disorder in the popular mind. Sydenham advocated small doses of laudanum to calm the paroxysms of this malady.

Drs F.J. Poynton and A. Paine of Great Ormond Street Children's Hospital reported in 1901 that they believed that they had proved, both microscopically and experimentally, that chorea was a rheumatic meningoencephalitis.

The treatment used by Poynton was modern. He stressed the importance of procuring for the child prolonged mental as well as physical rest. His insistence on this often incurred the wrath of parents and visitors, as they were excluded from his ward until the patient was convalescent. He would also exert his authority against sending them for convalescence at the seaside, as he thought that the restlessness of the waves produced an undesirable effect. He prescribed aspirin in large doses to reduce the tendency to rheumatic carditis; sedatives for the period during which they were required; and an ample and nutritious diet, supplemented with cod-liver oil. He opposed the then popular view that arsenic in large dosage should be prescribed for this disorder. He believed that, if this had any effect, it was to produce a peripheral neuritis.

This disease is seen less often today, but its treatment is still much as it was in Dr Poynton's time, and the results are similar. More modern embellishments to the traditional approach include: lessons in hospital to avoid educational deprivation and psychological difficulties later, and 'play-therapy' to help regain muscular co-ordination of the finer movements and to restore the child's self-confidence.

1.3.3   Treatment of rheumatoid arthritis

The treatment of rheumatoid arthritis has, until relatively recently, been empirical. This has been largely due to the complete ignorance of its nature and origins, coupled with a belief that the nervous system appeared to be involved, which often led to a preference for dramatic methods.

Folklore remedies which have remained popular through the ages include: the juice of a lemon in hot water on waking; fresh fruit juice with Epsom salts; barley water; spiritual healing; washing soda in the bath water; sulphur in the socks; honey and cider vinegar; bicarbonate of soda in milk; mud and foam baths; acupuncture; whisky and camphor massage; bicycling; and horseback riding – to mention only a few. (Further comments on folklore remedies are to be found in Chapter 11.)

(a)   Physical exercise

Both exercise and rest in varying degrees and forms have always been advocated. Hippocrates gave up-to-date advice for the use of chronic arthritics whose hands were affected: 'In such cases of arthritis it is well to give the patients wax to knead with the fingers....' He also stressed the advantage of active as opposed to passive exercises: 'For lack of exercise, when the patient has been immobile a long while, the joints become weak ... the joints are affected for the reason that the sinews and muscles have become weakend.'

Sydenham was a firm believer in physical exercise for the chronic arthritic, as well as for the sufferer with gout. Soon several ingenious machines were introduced whereby the action of horseback riding could be simulated without the patient needing to leave the house. In 1704 Dr Francis Fuller introduced the idea of remedial exercises much as we know them today, in a book entitled *Medicina Gymnastica*.

Cullen said, in *First Lines of the Practice of Physic* (1776): 'The chief cure of the chronic rheumatism is to be expected of external remedies. Of these heat is the chief, being that which sets the whole processes of the body going... but this may be hurtful if improperly applied.' He also wrote at length on the use of movements and of friction; the latter he considered could most conveniently be produced with the aid of the flesh-brush. This was a type of large scrubbing brush with bristles of light whalebone, to be used either by itself or in conjunction with a hot bath. He also advocated an occasional course of sulphur baths, such as were to be found in the nearby Scottish spa of Strathpeffer.

(b)   Rest

It took until 1863 for an intelligent appraisal of the use of rest. In that year John Hilton, surgeon to Guy's Hospital, published his celebrated book, *Rest and Pain*. In this he stressed the need to rest joints inflamed with arthritis, this being nature's method of cure, and pain her method of securing that rest.

Dr Robert Bridges, a physician at St. Bartholomew's Hospital who afterwards became the Poet Laureate of England, reported his success with multiple splinting in

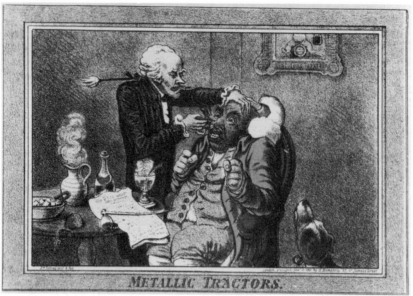

Fig. 1.3 A caricature by James Gillray showing the use of metallic tractors (1801). (Author's collection.)

acute and chronic arthritis, and drew the attention of his colleagues to the work of Otto Heubner of Leipzig (1871) who had popularized this method in Germany, and to the work of his predecessor in the same field, Professor Concato of Bologna. In the USA, the credit of pioneering the use of light plaster splintage to relieve pain and prevent deformity in rheumatoid arthritis must go to Loring Swain of Boston (1934).

The sole early reference to the nursing care of patients who are crippled with this disease appears to be that of S.A. Tissot, professor of physic in Lausanne, who said in his little book, *Advice with Regard to Health* (translation 1793): 'We may save these sick a good deal of pain by putting one strong towel always under their back, and another under their thighs, in order to move them the more easily. Later, when their hands are without pain, a third towel hung upon a cord which is fastened across the bed will assist them in moving themselves.'

(c) Electricity

This therapy is certainly far from being a modern innovation. As an early example, we may consider the report of the Roman physician, Scribonius Largus, who treated his patients by advising them to place their feet on a torpedo fish which is capable of generating a considerable shock of static electricity.

The first modern reference to the use of electricity for arthritis is contained in a lecture delivered by William Cullen in Edinburgh in 1766. Cullen said that 'it appeared to be a very powerful stimulus to the sanguinous system, as also to the nerves... hence I have ordered it in many cases of chronic rheumatism'.

On the lay side, the enthusiastic Reverend John Wesley, founder of Methodism, wrote a small book, *The Desideratum, or Electricity Made Plain and Useful* (1759), in which he mentioned, amongst many other diseases suitable for this new method, several examples of gout and arthritis which were cured 'by setting them on Rosin* while one drew sparks from the diseased parts'. This may have led to a static therapeutic electrical machine being installed in the Middlesex Hospital in 1797 (at a cost of less than 5 guineas), and a larger one in St. Bartholomew's Hospital 10 years later.

(d) Quacks (see Chapter 11)

The introduction of such mysterious forces as magnetism and electricity were naturally seized upon avidly by the quacks. The most celebrated of these was Elisha Perkins, born in 1741 in Connecticut. There he patented his 'Celebrated Metallic Tractors' (see Fig. 1.3) and made an easy fortune. His tractors consisted of a pair of metal compasses whose points were of different metals and about the size and shape of a pencil. The cure

---

* A resin, e.g. when turpentine is prepared from dead pine wood – also called colophony.

resulted from the 'affinity they have with the offending matter which will be drawn out'. This method was 'effective for all arthritic, gouty and rheumatic pains, both acute and chronic, including the toothache (which at this time was regarded as arthritis of the dental socket), as well as paralysis – either in men or horses'. Ultimately, Perkins was discredited by Dr John Haygarth, who reported (1810) exactly similar results obtained in Bath Hospital with 'a pair of painted wooden tractors and a sufficiency of verbal mumbo-jumbo'.

Through the next 100 years, electricity still seemed to the quacks a productive field. Electric belts and corsets were sold for high prices, and 'magnetic' rings and amulets came into fashion again.

(e) Other non-medicinal therapeutic approaches

The belief that untreated rheumatoid arthritis will eventually 'burn itself out' dies hard, and it was no doubt this which led Sir William Osler, who had no great interest in this field of medicine, to say that his favourite prescription for this disease was: 'Time and hope in equal and divided doses.' During the post-war period, 1920–35, many remedies for rheumatoid arthritis were introduced amid popular acclaim. Today they are mostly forgotten. Of these may be recalled the removal of hypothetical foci of infection; treatment by protein shock; vaccines controlled with the 'opsonic index'; bee venom; fever therapy; sulphur injections in many forms; and Professor Bier's method of passive congestion of the joints with a rubber bandage.

(f) Medicinal remedies

Effective medicinal remedies, other than salicylates, have only been available since Forestier introduced in 1929 the use of intramuscular injections of gold salts. Next came the eventful introduction of the corticosteroid drugs by Philip Hench of the Mayo Clinic. The rapid, although brief effect, of large doses upon patients crippled with rheumatoid arthritis was dramatically shown in 1949 in New York before a large international medical audience. In the next year, with his collaborator E.C. Kendall, he received the Nobel Prize.

The introduction of corticosteroids was followed by the manufacture of other types of synthetic anti-inflammatory drugs, unconnected with cortisone, notably phenylbutazone and later indomethacin (for further details see Section 1.4.1), although the search for a truly curative agent for this disease continues.

1.3.4 Treatment of ankylosing spondylitis

John Hilton refers to this disease in his *Rest and Pain* (1863) and says that complete rest 'will generally result in a complete cure... but ankylosis will generally be found to be complete'.

Sir Richard Quain, in his *Dictionary of Medicine* (1882), a standard work, had little further to add except that: 'If anchylosis has taken place in an incomplete degree an attempt may be made to restore mobility by forceful or gradual extension, by passive motion, or by massage.'

Spa treatment (hydrotherapy) became deservedly popular towards the beginning of the present century, and in the late 1920s deep X-ray treatment was introduced by Gilbert Scott and others. Such treatment was found to be effective in suppressing the activity of the disease and in relieving its pain, but has fallen under a cloud in recent years for reasons to be discussed later in this section (see also Chapter 8).

Modern treatment avoids immobilization and depends largely upon the use of analgesic/anti-inflammatory drugs. It is rare now to see patients with ankylosing spondylitis who have progressed to severe deformity, such as were common 50 years ago. The failures of earlier times, visible on the streets today, were due to the lack of education both of patient and of doctor about the value of maintaining posture and movement during the active period of the disease, and often to a failure to recognize and diagnose the disease and its insidious nature.

The use of therapeutic irradiation with X-rays is almost a thing of the past. Even more so does this apply to treatment with thorium X (Léri and Thomas, 1922), advocated for the later stages of ankylosing spondylitis by Weil and Bach as late as 1938, and to treatment with radon (D'Arsonval, 1932).

X-rays were employed therapeutically in rheumatic disease as early as 1899 (Sokolow), and for ankylosing spondylitis by Kohler in 1926 and by Kahlmeter 4 years later (Kahlmeter, 1930). Scott (1936) popularized radiation treatment which spread widely and was enthusiastically followed (Smythe, Freyberg and Lampe, 1941; Freyberg, 1946). Despite only one controlled trial (Desmarais, 1953), there was widespread evidence for the immediate benefits obtained (Sharp and Easson, 1954; Howard, 1957; Hart, 1958), although Wilkinson and Bywaters (1958) were not impressed by this in relation to the natural history of the disease. It was not until 1955 that Court-Brown and Abbatt, after observations by van Swaay (1955), drew attention to the high incidence of leukaemia in people who had received high doses of radiation for ankylosing spondylitis; Court-Brown and Doll (1965) pointed out the high incidence of aplastic anaemia in these people. Since that time, radiation has been employed very much less, greatly limited in extent and dosage, and reserved only for severely affected patients, unresponsive to other forms of treatment.

1.3.5 Treatment of osteoarthrosis (osteoarthritis)

Until quite recently, treatment was no different from that considered suitable for arthritis due to chronic gout.

R.B. Todd (1843) believed that 'it will never be found to be curable owing to the organic changes which take place in the bone itself'. However, he listed the following as possibly effective therapies: warm baths, leeches applied locally, small doses of potassium iodide, cod-liver oil both internally and externally, and 'Chelsea Pensioner Electuary' (a nauseous concoction containing quaiacum, rhubarb, and sulphur mixed with honey or the like). Rest in the early stages he thought important, and in the later phases exercises were encouraged. He was sceptical regarding the efficacy of spa treatment. The use of leeches locally was universal, although Pringle had warned that benefit would only be obtained if the joints to which they were applied were inflamed and swollen.

Sir Thomas Watson, the author of the most celebrated textbook of his time, stated (1848) that pain may often be alleviated by applying warmth and light friction to the joints. He recommended flannel underwear and hot brine or vapour baths. Guaiacum (a greenish medicinal resin from the tropical American genus of trees of the bean-caper family, also the source of lignum-vitae), he thought, should constitute routine medication, with the addition of Dover's powder for pain. For those who could afford it he advised moving to a warm, dry climate during cold weather.

Until the era of modern analgesics the prescription of drugs was generally thought to be less helpful in 'chronic osteoarthritis' than in other 'rheumatisms'.

However, electuaries continued to be popular, as well as another even more curious remedy of the seventeenth and eighteenth centuries – 'Oleum Philosophorum', described in the European pharmacopoeias, and more prosaically and accurately called 'Oil of Bricks' in English editions. This was made by heating building bricks to red heat, then quenching them rapidly to saturation point with olive oil. They were then ground up and the powder heated in a retort 'until a distillate of oil and spirit is obtained'. This final product could be used either internally or externally for the 'cure' of chronic arthritis and other complaints.

About 1850 E.C. Lasegue of Paris introduced tincture of iodine for the treatment of osteoarthritis, both by mouth and externally. Orally he recommended one drop to be taken in wine three times daily, increasing this by the same amount each day to a maximum of 15 drops, and then down the scale again in the same way. This often appeared to help, and not surprisingly remained popular.

However, it was the introduction of aspirin in 1899 that opened the way to the modern therapeutic approach to osteoarthrosis.

(a) Spa treatment

It had been known from early times that a stiff joint could be moved more easily below water than above it, and it is notable that warm bathing had been prescribed for arthritic patients by the Egyptians, the Greeks, and the Romans.

At Salerno, where the first medical school was established in Europe, physicians continued in the twelfth century to recommend spa treatment. The places selected were those where natural mineral and sulphur or brine waters abounded, such as at Acqui and Abano in Italy, and at La Bourboulle in France, places that are still used for a similar purpose. The first authoritative publication on this subject was a collection of works entitled *De Balneis*, which appeared in Venice in 1553.

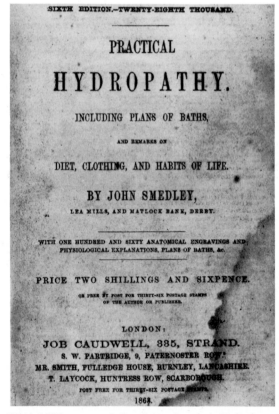

SIXTH EDITION.—TWENTY-EIGHTH THOUSAND.

PRACTICAL

HYDROPATHY.

INCLUDING PLANS OF BATHS,

AND REMARKS ON

DIET, CLOTHING, AND HABITS OF LIFE.

BY JOHN SMEDLEY,

LEA MILLS, AND MATLOCK BANK, DERBY.

WITH ONE HUNDRED AND SIXTY ANATOMICAL ENGRAVINGS AND PHYSIOLOGICAL EXPLANATIONS, PLANS OF BATHS, &c.

PRICE TWO SHILLINGS AND SIXPENCE.

OR FREE BY POST FOR THIRTY-SIX POSTAGE STAMPS OF THE AUTHOR OR PUBLISHER.

LONDON:

JOB CAUDWELL, 335, STRAND.

S. W. PARTRIDGE, 9, PATERNOSTER ROW.

MR. SMITH, FULLEDGE HOUSE, BURNLEY, LANCASHIRE.

T. LAYCOCK, HUNTRESS ROW, SCARBOROUGH.

POST FREE FOR THIRTY-SIX POSTAGE STAMPS.

1863.

Fig. 1.4 Title page of Smedley's *Practical Hydrotherapy* (1863)—an account of two Derbyshire spas. (Author's collection.)

At this time the waters were generally taken internally, as well as being administered externally.

During the eighteenth century, spa treatment became highly organized in England, notably at Bath, and arthritis sufferers as well as those seeking general improvement in their health flocked there.

During the next century spas opened all over Europe, and the wealthy and the rheumatic flocked to them annually. At places such as Aix, Baden-Baden, Vichy, Wiesbaden and Homberg, as well as in this country (see Fig. 1.4), hydrotherapy facilities became particularly well developed, and other ingenious methods of additional physical therapy were added to the original regime of bathing and 'taking the waters'. It was in the wake of this latter objective that physiotherapy and medical electrical therapy developed towards the end of the century, both in the spas and in the town centres.

(b) Surgery

Until the turn of the century, orthopaedic surgery was little more than a name and an aspiration. Pioneers such as Sir Robert Jones of Liverpool, J.E. Goldthwait of Boston, and later Reginald Watson-Jones of London started to adapt its principles to the treatment of osteoarthrotic joints. These principles, in historical order, were: the correction of deformity, redistribution of body weight with the help of various types of apparatus and shoes, arthrodesis, and arthroplasty.

The last term implies the formation of an artificial joint to replace the defective one. Early developments in this field include Jean Judet's idea to substitute the head of the femur with a plastic surrogate and M.N. Smith-Petersen's experiments in 1925 with a cup-arthroplasty, whereby the socket of the hip joint is replaced by a metallic cup within which the head of the femur can articulate.

1.3.6 Treatment of non-articular rheumatism ('fibrositis')

In medieval times, St. Gregory was decreed the patron of all rheumatic victims, and rings and medallions bearing his effigy, and blessed by some suitably holy man, were much used both for prophylactic and therapeutic purposes. So-called 'cramp rings' were also worn for the relief of rheumatic pains – much as are copper bangles today. These were said to have been devised by King Edward the Confessor, who gave them to those in need of such relief 'without money or petition'. This practice was continued by later monarchs, including Henry VIII. With the development of the scientific approach in the seventeenth century, iodine, sulphur, and other chemical lockets came into favour for similar use.

Conventional medical treatment did not clearly distinguish between articular and non-articular types of rheumatism until modern times. In the eighteenth century, Cullen and others advocated a hot bath, 'with the plentiful application of the flesh-brush to the afflicted area'. The cold-water cure of Dr Cheshire was also popular, and as a possible alternative in more humble circles, 'flogging with weeds of stinging nettle'. During the eighteenth and nineteenth centuries, and even before, affluent patients would flock to the 'spaws' for thermal water or mud treatment to be 'boiled for the rheumatism'. It was for the purpose of taking patients from their lodgings to the medicinal baths that the 'bath chair' (also 'Bath chair') was designed.

Varying degrees of 'sophistication' were added. These included vapour baths (see Fig. 1.5) and replacing deficient blood elements by adding them to the steam 'which would carry it into the innermost recesses of the body'.

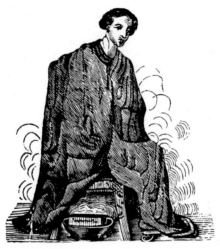

Fig. 1.5 Page from Fox's *The Model Botanic Guide to Health* (1897) showing a vapour bath. (Author's collection.)

Spa treatment has always consisted of 'taking the waters' as well as their external application. Indeed, eventually a visit in person was considered by some to be an unnecessary imposition on the rheumatic sufferer. Consequently, bottles of spa water were sent by carriers all over the country. Dr Johnson of Malvern, for instance, advertised the advantages of his local bottled water over the prescriptions of ordinary doctors and advocated a graduated course of hydrotherapeutic home treatment. The bottled 'Natural Medicated Spring-water Cure for Home Use' also became profit making in the USA throughout the last century.

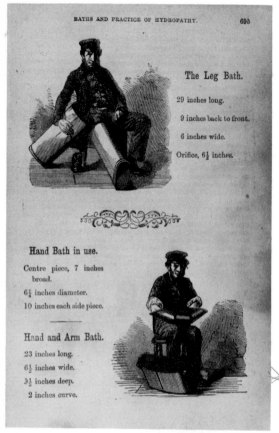

BATHS AND PRACTICE OF HYDROPATHY. 69b

The Leg Bath.

29 inches long.

9 inches back to front.

6 inches wide.

Orifice, 6¼ inches.

Hand Bath in use.

Centre piece, 7 inches broad.

6¼ inches diameter.

10 inches each side piece.

Hand and Arm Bath.

23 inches long.

6½ inches wide.

9½ inches deep.

2 inches curve.

Fig. 1.6 Page from Fox's *The Model Botanic Guide to Health* (1897) showing leg and hand baths and instructions on how to use them ('rheumatic armour'). (Author's collection.)

Rational do-it-yourself therapy seems to have reached its zenith in the hands of the Reverend Sydney Smith, the celebrated political writer and wit, in his 'rheumatic armour'. This (a similar version of which is shown in Fig. 1.6) he kept in a large bag in his study and would demonstrate it to all his callers, one of whom wrote:

> You must fancy him in a fit of his rheumatism: his legs in two narrow buckets which he calls his Jack boots; round the throat a hollow tin collar: over each shoulder a large tin thing like a leg of mutton; on his head a hollow tin helmet and a breast place and stomacher, all filled with hot water. He says that the stomach-tin is the greatest comfort in life.

Massage was introduced for the treatment of non-articular rheumatism towards the middle of the nineteenth century, largely as a result of Robert Froriep's

conception of its cause being the development of 'fibroid patches, or indurations, in the muscles or in the fibrous tissues overlying them'. This Berlin surgeon thought that in the early phase of the disease these could be dispersed by deep friction. His ideas were published in 1843 in *De Rheumatische Schwielen*.

Before the present-day era, came the phase in which hidden foci of infection were postulated and removed. This era was cynically encapsulated by an American sufferer in 1920:

> Sometimes we yank the tonsils, and sometimes we yank the teeth,
> (In hope that there are foci of infection there beneath).
> Sometimes we wash the sinus; and sometimes that helps it too;
> But sometimes we merely wonder what the devil we can do.

The present therapeutic approach, usually a combination of analgesics and physical therapy, is unfortunately only a marginal improvement on Osler's favourite regime for 'fibrositis': 'Hope and Nux Vomica in moderate dosage.'

1.4 HISTORICAL ASPECTS OF SPECIFIC THERAPEUTIC APPROACHES

1.4.1 Drugs

Sections 1.4.1 (a) – (i) cover drugs used in the treatment of rheumatoid arthritis. The last section (1.4.1 (j)) reports historical aspects of anti-gout drugs.

(a) Aspirin

As indicated earlier, apart from the ancients – Hippocrates, Pliny, Celsus, Dioscorides and Galen – it was really the Reverend Edward Stone who drew the attention of the new scientific world to the willow in his communication to the Royal Society in 1763.

In 1878 an apothecary in Bath, Mr William White, was able to save at least £20 a year for charity by substituting willow bark for Peruvian bark, and Wilkinson, a hard-headed business man from Sunderland, though rather apprehensive of its commercial value, endorsed its efficacy. Wilkinson, Stone, White and others used willow bark mainly for agues, fevers, abscesses, and fluxes – chiefly as an antipyretic. Only rarely, and almost by accident, was it used in a patient with rheumatism.

MacLagan, just over 100 years later, took the powder himself before giving it to his first patient, William R., aged 48, seen on the fourth day of his second attack of rheumatic fever – and the powder worked.

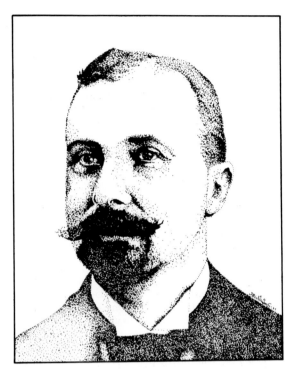

Fig. 1.7 Felix Hofmann (1868–1946).

Since the time of MacLagan (1876) salicylates have never looked back. Stricker and Reiss both introduced salicylic acid in 1876, and aspirin was produced some 20 years later.

In 1897 Felix Hofmann (Fig. 1.7), in search of a gastrically innocuous preparation to soothe his father's arthritic pains, discovered acetylated salicylate in the Bayer Laboratories. Aspirin (acetyl salicylic acid) was first produced commercially in 1899.

The development of aspirin is summarized in the following chronology (after Bywaters, 1963).

Ancient history
Hippocrates, Celsus, Pliny, Dioscorides, Galen, down to Boerhaave in 1751

The bark

Salix alba	1763	Reverend Edward Stone, of Chipping Norton
Salix latifolia	1792	Samuel James, Surgeon, of Hoddesdon, Hertfordshire
	1798	William White, Apothecary, of Bath
	1803	G. Wilkinson, of Sunderland

Pharmacological properties

Antipyretic	1763	Stone
Antirheumatic	1874–76	MacLagan and Stricker
Uricosuric	1877	See

Chemical structure

Salicin	1826–29	Leroux
Salicylic acid	1835–38	Löwing and Piria
Salicylic acid synthesized	1860	Kolbe and Lautemann
Acetylated salicylate discovered	1897	Hofmann
Aspirin introduced	1899	Bayer Laboratories

(b) Phenylbutazone

Phenylbutazone (1, 2-diphenyl-3, 5-diketo-4-n-butyl-pyrazolidine) was first synthesized in 1946 by H. Stenzl (Fig. 1.8) in the course of investigations into pyrazolone and pyrazolidine derivatives. It was something of a gamble on his part to have another look at these compounds as they had been the subject of many investigations within the previous 50 years. However, the fact that a compound with novel pharmacological properties and of clinical value turned up is clear

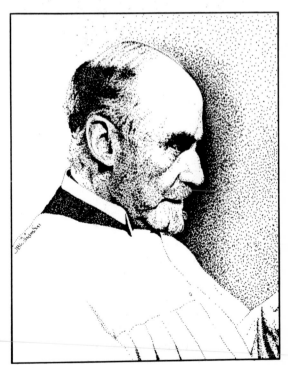

Fig. 1.8 H. Stenzl (1880–1980).

evidence that a field that seems to have been thoroughly explored may still reward persistence and skilful modification of the basic structure. In 1948 Gsell and Rechenberg first carried out clinical trials with phenylbutazone. The results were published in 1950 (Gsell and Müller, 1950).

(c) Indomethacin

Indomethacin was chosen as an anti-inflammatory agent from a systematic study of 300 indole acetic acid compounds, due to the antagonistic effect of these compounds on 5-hydroxytryptamine (serotonin) in inflammation (Healey, 1967; Shen *et al.*, 1963).

Clinical testing of indomethacin began in 1961, and in 1965 it was made aviailable on prescription in the USA and in the UK as a new antirheumatic agent.

(d) Proprionic acid derivatives

The substituted phenylalkanoic acids, a major group of non-steroidal anti-inflammatory agents, were first developed in the Research Department of the Boots Company Ltd., Nottingham, England, and were found to be active in the rheumatic diseases in the early 1960s. Ibuprofen, the first of the 'proprionic' subseries, was introduced into medicine in 1969. Its clinical efficacy, although generally regarded as being less effective than salicylates or indomethacin, was well established in the early 1970s (Mitchell and MacDonald, 1974; Godfrey and de la Cruz, 1974; Cardoe, 1970).

The development of other antirheumatic agents in the proprionic acid series such as flurbiprofen, ketoprofen, fenoprofen, and naproxen occupied the remaining years of the 1970s, and these products now serve as useful additions to the non-steroidal anti-inflammatory armamentarium.

(e) Corticosteroids and ACTH

Original conceptions of the adrenal glands
More than a hundred years ago Thomas Addison (1855), physician at Guy's Hospital, drew attention to the clinical importance of the suprarenal gland. He is still chiefly remembered for his clear description of the disease which is called after him, but it may be that in the future he will be remembered for the fact that in 1855 he suggested that the adrenal gland is essential to life.

This idea was supported by the French physician Brown-Séquard from a number of animal experiments. At that time, the idea of a secretion or hormone from the suprarenal, or any gland for that matter, was contrary to contemporary thought that regarded the nervous system as the main controlling system.

A further milestone was reached in 1924 when Stewart wrote: 'The cortex is the part of the adrenal essential to life. How it exercises its function is utterly unknown.' Many of the conclusions drawn from physiological experiments at that time were conflicting, and this was due in part to inexpert animal surgery which usually resulted in quick death after adrenalectomy. Because of this only animals in a state of acute collapse were available for study.

Discovery of steroid hormones
In the late 1920s the intimate connection between the pituitary gland and the adrenal cortex was demonstrated.

The active principle governing the intimate contact between the two glands was later named adrenocorticotropic hormone (ACTH; referred to as corticotrophin in subsequent chapters). Another important landmark was the demonstration that pituitary extracts could also bring about adrenal repair in the hypophysectomized rat.

In 1926 Rogoff and Stewart had prepared aqueous extracts of adrenal glands which produced rather uncertain results in experimental animals, but soon afterwards Swingle and Pfiffner (1930) showed that lipid extraction yielded a substance that would keep both adrenalectomized animals and patients with Addison's disease alive indefinitely.

In the early 1930s energetic study was applied to the chemical constituents of the adrenal cortex by three different groups of investigators led by Reichstein in Basle, Kendall at the Mayo Foundation, and Wintersteiner and Pfiffner at Columbia University. By 1940, 28 crystalline steroids had been isolated. At this stage it was not envisaged that the steroids would have much application in clinical medicine, apart from substitution therapy in Addison's disease, and this at first discouraged attempts at commercial production.

However, as so often in the history of medicine, the outbreak of a war furnished a stimulus, for it was rumoured that the German pilots were being given adrenal extracts to increase their fighting efficiency.

Commercial production of cortisone and ACTH
The National Research Council of the USA called together a group of steroid chemists to consider the production of these substances on a commercial scale. This work led to the preparation of cortisone (compound E) by Merck and Co. Inc. The method was initially worked out in Kendall's laboratory, and later Sarett (1948) devised a method to increase the yield a hundred fold. In 1948 there still seemed little prospect of cortisone having much application to clinical medicine, either for research or treatment. Philip Hench (Fig. 1.9), an important pioneer in the rheumatological application of corticosteroids, had studied rheumatoid ar-

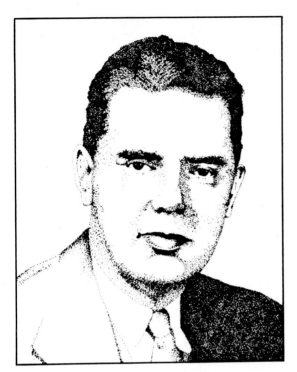

Fig. 1.9 Philip Showalter Hench (1896–1965).

thritis for many years, and had been particularly impressed with the suppression of the disease in pregnancy and after jaundice. In 1941 he discussed with Kendall the possibility of trying cortisone in rheumatoid arthritis.

Meanwhile further work was proceeding with ACTH. In 1943 Li, Simpson and Evans working in California with sheep pituitaries, and Sayers and his colleagues (1943) at Yale working with pig pituitaries, independently isolated proteins with high adrenocorticotropic properties. The Armour Company subsequently prepared pig protein ACTH on a commercial scale, and other companies in the USA and in Great Britain and elsewhere followed suit.

First clinical application
On September 21, 1948, at the Mayo Clinic, the first injection of 100 mg cortisone was administered to a woman with active long-standing rheumatoid arthritis, with dramatic results. During that winter 15 more patients received the hormone, and in the spring it was given to five patients with rheumatic fever. In 1949 Hench *et al.* published their first account of the effects of cortisone and ACTH in these diseases. The results were soon confirmed, notably by Freyberg (1950) and Boland (1950) in the USA, and by Copeman and his colleagues

(1950) in Great Britain. As referred to previously, in 1950, Hench, Kendall and Reichstein were awarded the Nobel Prize in Medicine for their work in this field. Since then many long- and short-term studies have been published and further developments achieved concerning both corticosteroids and ACTH.

(f) Gold therapy

The first reported use of gold for the treatment of rheumatoid arthritis was that of Lande who, in 1927, reported benefit from the use of gold thioglucose in 14 patients. In the same year, Pick reported two failures with gold in the treatment of arthritis. The greatest boost in the development of chrysotherapy for rheumatoid arthritis was the report by Forestier (Fig. 1.10) in 1929 that gold therapy benefited many patients. His use of this form of treatment was based on the knowledge that gold could inhibit growth of tubercle bacilli *in vitro* and that benefit had been reported in tuberculous patients treated with gold. Because of some clinical similarities between rheumatoid arthritis and tuberculosis, it seemed reasonable to Forestier that gold might help rheumatoid patients. In 1934 Forestier discussed this subject at several treatment centres in the USA, and a year later a summary of Forestier's 6 years'

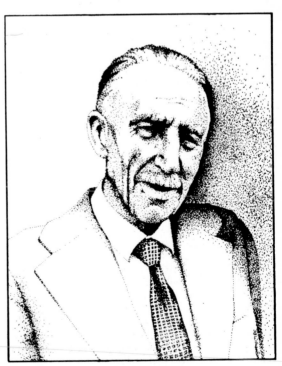

Fig. 1.10 Jacques Forestier (1890–1978).

experience with gold therapy for rheumatoid arthritis appeared. The earliest American reports on chryso-therapy appeared in 1936. In 1937 Hartfall *et al.* from Leeds published impressive results from a series of 900 patients, 750 of whom had rheumatoid arthritis. Since then many investigations of gold therapy have been reported across the world, most of them indicating benefit in rheumatoid arthritis.

(g) D-*penicillamine*

D-penicillamine, an amino acid analogue of cysteine and valine, and a crystalline degradation product of penicillin, was first isolated by Sir Ernest Chain in 1942.

The efficacy of penicillamine in the treatment of rheumatoid arthritis was first demonstrated in sequential studies in which patients served as their own historical controls (Jaffe, 1965, 1970). These observations were later confirmed in a double-blind controlled trial which demonstrated the effectiveness of penicillamine compared with placebo in the treatment of severe rheumatoid arthritis (Multicentre Trial Group, 1973). Further trials have shown the drug to be comparable in efficacy with gold (Huskisson *et al.*, 1974) and with azathioprine (Berry *et al.*, 1976) in suppressing the signs, symptoms and laboratory manifestations of rheumatoid arthritis.

(h) *Antimalarials*

There have been almost 30 years of experience with chloroquine since Page's original report (Page, 1951) on the use of antimalarial drugs in rheumatoid arthritis. The continued use of the 4-amino-quinolone drugs in rheumatoid arthritis rests mainly on the controlled studies by Popert *et al.* (1961) and by Hamilton and Scott (1962), the first trial showing significant clinical improvement in a prolonged study lasting 2 years. A fall in erythrocyte sedimentation rate (ESR) and in rheumatoid factor were also demonstrated. In the second study a therapeutic effect was demonstrated over a shorter period.

(i) *Cytotoxic agents*

Although cytotoxic drugs were developed for cancer chemotherapy, they were evaluated for the management of renal disease, including that due to systemic lupus erythematosus, and in rheumatoid arthritis (Diaz *et al.*, 1951; Baldwin *et al.*, 1953; Dubois, 1954) over 30 years ago. This early interest in cytotoxic drug therapy diminished when corticosteroids became available, but a rebound of interest in these drugs is now developing with the aim of controlling patients with potentially life-threatening or serious disease not controlled by more

conservative means. There is yet no firm evidence that they alter the natural history of rheumatoid arthritis.

(j) *Anti-gout drugs*

The history of colchicine parallels the history of gout in that its discovery was followed by a wane of interest and then rediscovery. The provenance of the name of this drug is probably from an ancient district in Asia Minor called Colchis. A drug probably identical with colchicine had been described in the Ebers papyrus (1500 BC), probably used as a purgative. White hellebore, a cousin of colchicum, was recommended by Hippocrates and his followers as a 'sovereign purge' for the gout. In the second century AD, Aretaeus the Cappadocian noted that hellebore was more specific for gout than its mere purgative effect would explain and could restore the patient to health even with limited purging and wretching. However, it is not until the writings of Alexander of Tralles (AD 525–605) that we learn about its selective and specific properties for the first time. Its specific use in gout continued into the thirteenth century and then ceased, to remain in disrepute until its rediscovery in 1763 by Baron Anton von Störck, who advocated its use mainly in the treatment of dropsy. Its rediscovery as a specific treatment for gout followed the formulation of a patent medicine containing colchicum (among other ingredients) by Nicolas Husson (see also Section 1.3.1). L'Eau d'Husson was subsequently introduced into the USA in 1798 by Benjamin Franklin for the treatment of his own gout. However, it was not until 1814 that the alkaloid colchicum, obtained from the corm of *Colchicum autumnale*, was identified by Dr James Want as the active substance in Husson's concoction responsible for the specific effect in acute gout. Led by Scudamore, most nineteenth century physicians enthusiastically adopted the use of colchicine in gout.

1.4.2 Physical therapy and rehabilitation (see also Section 1.2.1 and Chapter 11)

The sun, the air, water, exercises and manipulation have been Medicine's therapeutic servants since earliest times. Each one has been claimed as the panacea for man's ills – or for their prevention – and it is this faith that continues in various systems of therapy to this day.

Some 50 years ago the large teaching hospitals in the country began to set up special departments in which physical methods in diagnosis and treatment were used. It is worth noting that diagnosis was as central a feature as treatment in the early years of physical medicine. In the early 'Electrical Departments', for example, the discoveries of Erb and Duchenne (Fig. 1.11) were followed and developed, providing considerable help in differential diagnosis. As the various forms of 'ray

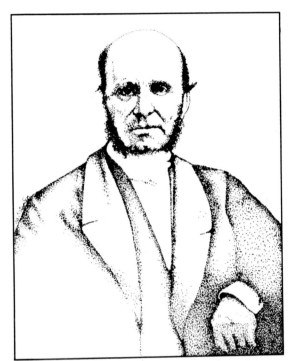

Fig. 1.11 Guillaume-Benjamin-Amand   Duchenne   (1806–1875).

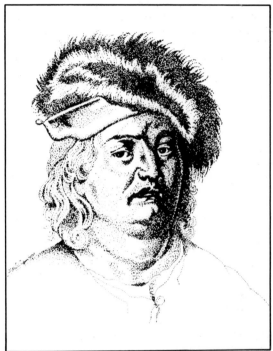

Fig. 1.12 Paracelsus   (Philippus   Theophrastus   Aureolus Bombastus von Hohenheim) (1493–1541).

therapy' were introduced these were added to the 'electrical' service. Similarly, departments were set up for massage and gymnastics. These were usually supervised by an orthopaedic surgeon.

These 'departments' were often tucked away in obscure corners of hospitals and it was the clinical cast-offs of his medical and surgical colleagues with which the chief had to deal. Water, reintroduced by Paracelsus (Fig. 1.12) as a therapeutic agent, was in the hands of the 'balneologist' at the spas, and air and sunlight were restricted to the tuberculous patient. X-ray therapy had, both for diagnosis and treatment, grown so rapidly in demand that it soon became a specialty in itself.

It was by an amalgamation of these early departments some two decades ago that the first integration took place leading to the special hospital service that became known as 'physical medicine'. As referred to earlier (Section 1.2.1), a particular landmark in the formation of this specialty occurred in 1931 when the Section of Balneology and Climatology of the Royal Society of Medicine fused with the section of Electrotherapeutics and formed the Section of Physical Medicine.

Then came the powerful addition of a relatively new element – diagnostic and therapeutic measures, both preventive and curative, resulting from experience gained in 'physical training' during World War II. So short was fit manpower in the early phase of the war that those responsible for the fighting personnel decided to devote particular attention to the substantial number of unfit men who had enlisted. They sought the help of key medical men in an effort to up-grade a large proportion of these unfit recruits. The experience thus gained was carried over into peacetime and rapidly became a central feature in the new idea of physical medicine.

With the development of physical training another advance was taking place – the Chartered Society of Physiotherapists was becoming a body of highly trained women and men available for skilled service in physical medicine.

The congeries resulting from the union between these disciplines resulted in furthering the basis of the specialty of physical medicine. The consolidation of this specialty was not without some acrimony between the founding factions, but the formation of the British Association of Physical Medicine in 1943 went far to establish a reasonable and mutually beneficial equilibrium.

Partly because of the inexactness of diagnosis and

treatment, and partly because physical therapy represents only a segment of the total management of patients, the term 'physical medicine' has fallen into disrepute. 'Rehabilitation' has replaced it and embraces the many physical, social and organizational aspects of the after-care of most patients who require more than acute, short-term definitive care. This trend is reflected in a change of nomenclature concerning the societies and journals associated with the specialty. For example, the British Association for Physical Medicine is now the British Association for Rheumatology and Rehabilitation, and its journal, *The Annals of Physical Medicine*, is now *Rheumatology and Rehabilitation*. Similarly, the Section of Physical Medicine of the Royal Society of Medicine is now the Section of Rheumatology and Rehabilitation.

Although these changes also indicate a firm link between physical medicine (rehabilitation) and rheumatology, at the time of writing there are signs in the UK of a dichotomy based on two main considerations: (1) that rehabilitation is of at least equal relevance to certain other specialties (e.g. orthopaedics, neurology); and (2) that the importance of the discipline merits its consideration as a specialty in its own right. Despite moves towards a 'split' between rheumatology and rehabilitation, current opinion continues to be somewhat divided on this issue. However, whatever the ultimate outcome of current professional and political machinations in this complex matter, there can be little doubt that at the practical level rheumatologists will, in general, continue to be responsible for supervising the rehabilitation of their own patients (in a fashion no different from their involvement in drug therapy and other integral aspects of management).

1.4.3 Splinting

(a) Origins of splinting

Although in about 1600 BC the Egyptians were using coatings for walls derived from gypsum, their obvious knowledge of plastering does not seem to have been applied to the making of bandages or splints for the treatment of the injured until the last few centuries BC. Instead, they used self-setting bandages, probably derived from the type used by embalmers.

In 350 BC Hippocrates wrote of the use of bandages containing waxes, resins and similar ingredients. Throughout history many other substances and mixtures have been used, including a mixture of lime and egg albumen employed by Arabian practitioners during the Middle Ages.

According to Ballingall, a military surgeon, writing in 1852, some sort of clay was used in India for casting fractured limbs.

A more ingenious method was devised by Hubenthal, who prepared a cast from equal parts of plaster of Paris and minced blotting paper. Having greased the damaged limb to prevent sticking, he applied the cast as anterior and posterior shells with interlocking serrated edges. These were also greased to prevent them sticking together.

In Berlin, in 1828, casts were being made by pouring a creamy mixture of plaster into a box surrounding the damaged limb; when the cast had set, the box was removed.

(b) Early plaster bandages

It was Mathijsen, the Dutch military surgeon, who first made casts using plaster bandages consisting of strips of coarse cotton cloth into which finely powdered plaster had been rubbed. By Mathijsen's method, which was popular between 1852 and 1930, and survives in some places even today, patients suffering lower limb injuries were, for the first time, able to get about on crutches.

Plastering by the use of bandages owes both its origins and its development to military surgery. During World War I, Sir Robert Jones formed the first Surgical Orthopaedic Unit at Hammersmith Hospital, and this led to substantial progress in improving the quality of bandages and in developing the technique generally. Before commercially made bandages became available, all plaster of Paris bandages were made by rubbing plaster powder into stiffened muslin by hand; a method that produced much variation in quality.

(c) Modern plaster bandages

In 1931 the first successful commercially prepared plaster bandages became available in Germany. They were made by spreading plaster, mixed with volatile liquids, onto soft cloth. After evaporation only minute quantities of the volatile solvents remained in the bandages, and these were non-irritant.

Only a short time was to pass before bandages prepared by a similar process were being produced in Great Britain. These bandages (later to be known as 'Gypsona') contained a generous proportion (90%) of superfine quality plaster, and the special interlock weave cloth, known as 'leno' did away with the need for artificial stiffening, and had the additional advantage that it moulded more easily.

1.4.4 Radiotherapy

The historical development of radiation therapy stems from the discovery of the X-ray by Wilhelm Conrad Röntgen (1845–1923) on November 8, 1895. This important finding was quickly followed by the classic observation by Becquerel and Curie in 1896 that certain substances were naturally radioactive, a revelation that led the Curies*, jointly, to name a new element 'radium' in 1898. This new element was isolated as one decigram of pure radium chloride in 1902 (Kaplan, 1949).

Another landmark in the history of radiotherapy includes the work of Bergonie and Tribondeau who in 1906 formulated their law concerning the increased radiosensitivity of less differentiated cells and proliferating cells.

The biological effects of radiation were initially explained by the 'direct effect' or 'target' theory of Dessaur in 1922, and later by a more satisfactory 'indirect effect' theory by Dale *et al.* (cited by Prasad, 1974). The latter theory postulated that biological molecules in aqueous solution are inactivated by free radicals which are formed when radiation interacts with water (as opposed to a direct 'hit effect' in inactivating molecules as postulated by the target theory).

The hazards of radiation were suspected as far back as 1902, but were not given prominence until nine deaths due to bone cancer were recorded between 1922 and 1924 among Swiss watch industry workers who painted dials with radium.

In 1935 Coutard introduced the concept of using fractional doses of X-rays or gamma rays in order to provide maximal impact on the tumour and minimal damage to the skin and other normal tissues.

Early clinical applications are discussed in Section 8.3.1.

1.4.5 Surgery

Orthopaedics, as part of medicine, depends to a great extent on basic discoveries, such as the understanding of anatomy and physiology, antisepsis, anaesthesia and so on.

Operations on bones and joints have been carried out for centuries, reaching a sophisticated level by the early nineteenth century. Osteotomy, arthroplasty and major amputations featured in the repertoire of surgeons of this time, although anaesthesia, antiseptics and blood transfusion had not been introduced. Synovectomy was introduced somewhat later and was first used in rheumatoid arthritis in 1887 by Schiller after its beneficial effect in tuberculosis had been demonstrated (cited by Mowat, 1978). Despite the technical expertise available, the mortality from these procedures was alarming; lack of suitable materials, lack of means to control infection and other factors hampered the progress of the specialty for a time. Typical problems prevalent in these early days of 'modern' surgery abound in the literature. For example, Langenbeck nailed a hip fracture in 1775 but

the metal corroded. A fractured humerus was wired together in 1775 but infection killed the patient.

The techniques and disciplines that advanced surgery to its present-day standards are best discussed in chronological order.

(a) Anaesthesia

This was introduced in the 1840s in the USA. The early history and claims for priority are debatable, but it was certainly William T.G. Morton, a Boston dentist, who realized its tremendous worth at the end of 1846. Within 2 months it was used in London, and very soon anaesthesia, based on nitrous oxide, ether, and chloroform, was being widely administered.

(b) Aseptic surgery

In 1865 Lord Lister performed his first operation using *anti*septic surgery, and 2 years later he described this technique at the annual meeting of the British Medical Association.

Despite Lister's claim, antiseptic surgery took many years to establish itself. Most of the younger surgeons readily accepted his ideas, but many of the more senior surgeons carried on as before.

(c) Radiology

The origin of radiology, like that of radiotherapy, stems from Röntgen's discovery of the X-ray (see Section 1.4.4). Röntgen found that when he passed a high voltage current through a Crookes' vacuum tube, a ray was generated which would pass through cardboard, wood and limbs. He demonstrated this at a meeting at Würzburg and proposed that the rays should be called 'X-rays'. The president of the meeting suggested 'Röntgen rays'.

Within weeks of the discovery of X-rays they came into medical use. At first they were used for discovering metallic foreign bodies, but as the equipment improved over the next 10 years they came into wider use.

(d) Metallurgy

It was only about 30 years ago that electrolytic corrosion was realized to be a major problem affecting metallic implants, in addition to the original drawback – the risk of infection.

The use of materials was empirical until Charles Venables and Walter Stuck began studying the problem of corrosion in the 1930s. One of the better materials was stainless steel. This was first invented by Harry Breasley in 1913. Later in 1926 one of the many variants, 18–8 S. Mo. Stainless Steel was introduced. It consisted

---

* Mme Curie died in 1934 from aplastic anaemia, probably due to prolonged exposure to radiation (Prasad, 1974).

of 18% chromium, 8–10% nickel and 2–4% molybdenum. Venables and Stuck found that this material, which was fairly popular, was better than most, but still corroded to a small extent.

A dental friend introduced them to vitallium while they were carrying out this study, because it did not corrode in the mouth. Vitallium, a non-ferrous alloy composed of 65% cobalt, 30% chromium, and 3% molybdenum, had been developed in 1929. On chemical and animal tests they found it more inert than stainless steel and started to use it clinically in 1936.

Since then stainless steel and vitallium have become the standard, and corrosion is now hardly ever a problem.

(e) *Antibiotics*

Sulphonamides paved the way in 1935, but were unfortunately not particularly active against the organisms of orthopaedic significance. Penicillin was a wartime development. The antituberculous and wide-spectrum drugs were introduced after the war.

The reduction of chronic infection is largely due to the antibiotics, though better nutrition, and better conditions of living have contributed.

(f) *Vaccines*

These have changed the face of orthopaedics. In World War I tetanus vaccine came into use and drastically cut this complication of trauma. In the 1950s Salk and then Sabin polio vaccine were used and have almost eradicated this problem.

(g) *Development of 'rheumatological orthopaedics'*

The development of orthopaedic surgery in the context of rheumatological management began to emerge in the early 1950s. However, earlier historical milestones can be traced, particularly to do with surgical treatment of hip disease.

As long ago as 1770 Charles White (Fig. 1.13) proposed excision of the head and neck of the femur, but did not carry it out except on cadavers.

In 1827 Barton introduced the concept of restoring movement to an ankylosed joint. In 1885 an interposition material was used by Ollier. In 1923 Smith-Petersen (Fig. 1.14) carried out pioneer work concerning prosthetic replacement of the hip (Smith-Petersen, 1925). He first used glass in 1923, and in 1925 tried viscaloid. In 1933 he returned to Pyrex glass, and in 1933 he used a

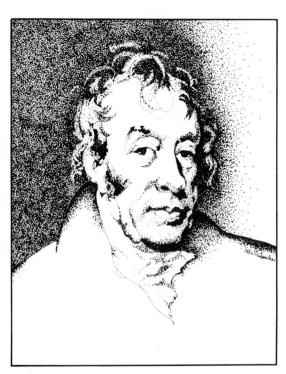

Fig. 1.13 Charles White (1728–1813).

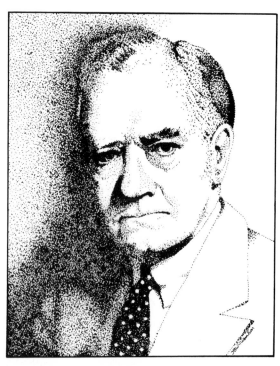

Fig. 1.14 M.N. Smith-Petersen (1886–1953).

Bakelite interposition mould (Smith-Petersen, 1939). In 1938 the first vitallium hip cup was inserted. Moore and Bohlman advanced prosthetic arthroplasty in 1942 by developing a fixed metallic hip replacement. Acetabular cups were also developed by Urist (1957) and by McBride (1960).

The current phase of hip arthroplasty centres on the use of total hip joint prostheses. In this regard it is noteworthy that in 1891 Gluck described an ivory ball and socket total hip joint which was fixed to bone by cement composed of colophony, pumice powder and plaster of Paris.

Wiles (1958) designed stainless steel component parts and placed them in six patients with Still's disease. McKee developed a series of prosthetic models for total hip replacement in 1941, and started to use them in patients in 1951 (McKee and Watson-Farrar, 1966).

In 1958 Charnley (Charnley, 1960a) first reported his clinical experience with total hip replacement in humans. In 1960 he described the acrylic fixation of the component parts to bone, and by 1962 he had begun to use high-density polyethylene as a substance for the acetabular component (Charnley, 1960b). Charnley has pioneered the development of low-friction arthroplasty and has studied extensively the wear patterns of the component parts of the hip prosthesis.

1.4.6 Heterodox therapy

The pattern of medical practice, and in particular its relationship to the balance between 'orthodoxy' and 'unorthodoxy', shows a widely varying picture through the ages.

The medicine of early man depended heavily on folklore and superstition in an attempt to identify the factors that were causing their afflictions. These 'causative' factors included: sorcery or witchcraft, the breaking of taboos, the intrusion of disease-objects, the action of disease-spirits, and loss of soul (Camp, 1973). Eradication of these evil forces was often done through wise or 'witch' men who acted as a channel of communication between their fellows and the gods they worshipped.

Eventually the idea that diseases were caused by biological factors rather than by gods or evil spirits developed. Hippocrates was pre-eminent in this new philosophy, and thus sowed the seeds of modern medical science.

The popularity of medical practice waxed and waned over the centuries and was met with particular hostility by the early Christian Church, as it was the belief that God alone had the power of healing. Even when this was overcome, for another 1500 years medical progress was shackled by the 'humoral theory'. According to this all ills were attributed to the malfunction of one of the four

'humours' of which the body was thought to be composed – black bile, yellow bile, blood and phlegm.

Further developments within medicine include a declaration in 1130 by the Council of Clermont to force clerics to treat the poor free of charge, as hitherto they were denying medical treatment to all who could not afford their high fees. By the end of the thirteenth century the Vatican forbade all priests to practice medicine. This opened the way to many amateurs and quacks. In England, Henry VIII made it illegal for anyone to diagnose disease or cure the sick without a licence from the Bishop of London or the Dean of St. Paul's. In 1504, 5 years before Henry came to the throne, the ancient association of barbers and surgeons had formed their own professional company and insisted that only their own members could practise 'barbery, shavery, surgery and the letting of blood' within the City of London. In 1518 Henry VIII granted a charter to the College of Physicians which made it illegal for any but college members to deal in 'physick' within 7 miles of London.

In the same way that surgeons and barbers were united, so were the apothecaries and the grocers.

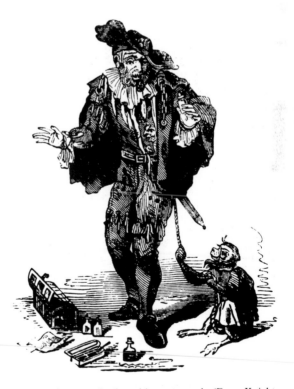

Fig. 1.15 A mountebank or itinerant quack. (From Knight, 1864.)

However, the apothecaries, like the physicians and the surgeons, wanted to become a company in their own right, but it was not until 1617 that James I granted them their charter, despite well-founded opposition from the physicians who feared the apothecaries would encroach upon their own function.

This fear materialized not only in the form of professional encroachment by the apothecaries but also, after the Restoration of Charles II in 1660, by an invasion of mountebanks* (Fig. 1.15), quacks and swindlers who flocked to England in his wake, many of them claiming royal patronage.

This paved the way to the era of mid-eighteenth century charlatanry, otherwise known as 'the golden age of quackery'. The word quack, meaning a charlatan, is an abbreviation of quack-salver (as in *Volpone*, Act II, sc. 2, by Ben Johnson: 'They are Quack-salvers, Fellows that live by senting oyles and drugs'). To *quack* is to utter a harsh, croaking sound, like a duck, which is what these practitioners sounded like when they talked noisily to make vain and loud pretensions. The term *salver* means one who undertakes to perform cures by the application of ointments and cerates. Hence the term 'quack-salver' was commonly used to signify an ignorant person who was wont to extol the curative virtues of his salves. Another interpretation of quack is derived from an ancient Saxon word signifying small, slender and trifling. It has also been maintained that quack is a corruption of quake, the name given to the intermittent fevers of patients living in marshy districts which were often treated by ignorant persons – quake-doctors – who professed to be able to charm away the disease (Lawrence, 1910). The term charlatan, often used synonymously with quack, has an origin that also alludes to the vocal characteristics of these itinerant pedlars and is thought to originate from the Italian word *cialatano* meaning babbler.

In order to put the place of the quack practitioners of this bygone era in perspective with regard to the present-day unorthodox–orthodox spectrum, it should be stressed that they were usually ignorant practitioners, *pretending* to have medical skill. They boasted about having a knowledge of wonderful remedies and boasted about their ability to cure diseases with them. Most of them were medical imposters in the fullest sense. William Hogarth's satirical print 'Consultation of Physicians' (Fig. 1.16) (also titled 'The Company of Under-takers') represents a visual pun on eighteenth century quackery in heraldic form.

One such quack was Thomas Saffold, who obtained

his licence from the Bishop of London in 1674 and advertised in a verse beginning:

> It's Saffold's Pills, much better than the rest,
> Deservedly have got the name of Best.

Dr Case was another seventeenth century quack who claimed to cure:

> The Croup, the Stitch,
> The Squirt, the Itch,
> The Gout, the Stone, the Pox;
> The Mulligrubs,
> The Bonny Scrubs
> And all Pandora's Box.

Another dubious medical personality of this time advertised as follows: Doctor Frederick lately come from Germany begs to acquaint the Publick, that he undertakes to Cure the Gout, and Rheumatism.

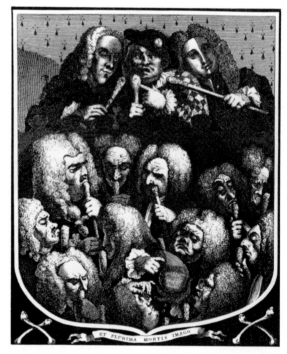

Fig. 1.16 This engraving by William Hogarth entitled *Consultation of Physicians* (1736/7) was originally intended to be called *A Consultation of Quacks*. The satirical elements of the design, which represents a visual pun on the coat-of-arms of the medical profession, include the ominous crossbones, the motto meaning 'And many an image of death', and the depiction of three well-known quacks of the era—Sarah Mapp (centre), Joshua Ward (right), and probably John Taylor (left)—in the upper portion of the shield, which, traditionally, is the most honourable portion. (Author's collection.)

---

* A mountebank (lit. mount-on-bench) was an itinerant quack who from a platform appealed to his audience by means of stories, tricks, juggling, and the like, often with the assistance of a professional clown.

Quackery of this kind continued by means of potions, lotions, and gadgetry of the most imaginative construction and effect until late Victorian times which paved the way to more respectable medical therapies whether orthodox or unorthodox. The use of the term 'quack' in modern times has taken on a new significance and often implies derision, either aimed at a heterodox practitioner by an orthodox practitioner, or at an orthodox practitioner by one of his own kind.

1.5 SUMMARY AND CONCLUSIONS

This chapter has considered historical aspects in two ways. First, from the standpoint of treatment of specific rheumatic disorders through the ages, and second from the development of each therapeutic approach.

It is particularly striking that so many parallels can be drawn between rheumatological practice hundreds of years ago and that practised today. For example, modern drug therapy has its origins in willow bark (salicylate) and the autumn crocus (colchicine); physical therapy; particularly the use of bathing, splinting and the application of heat, has been practised for centuries. Surgery on bone and joints, albeit crude in early times, had been performed many hundreds of years before the development of the sophisticated techniques of joint replacement and reconstruction so well established today. To extend these parallels to the present day, it could be claimed that even plasma exchange (see Section 12.4) had an early counterpart in bleeding, so popularly practised by our Georgian forebears.

1.6 REFERENCES AND FURTHER READING

In some of the publications from the last century, and in earlier works, the intials of the author(s) were not cited in the original publication.

Where no publisher's name is included in some of these older references this signifies that it has not been possible to obtain the original work, and it has been necessary to quote the literature from a secondary source.

Introductory comment

Baillou, G. de (1642) *Liber de Rhumatismo*. Translated into English by C.C. Barnard (1940) Quesnel, Paris; reproduced in *Br. J. Rheum.* **2**, 141.
Bywaters, E.G.L. (1962) Gout in the time and person of George IV. *Ann. Rheum. Dis.*, **21**, 325.
Bywaters, E.G.L. (1980) in *Ankylosing Spondylitis* (ed. J.M.H. Moll), Churchill Livingstone, Edinburgh, pp. 1–15.
Copeman, W.S.C. (1964) *A Short History of the Gout and the Rheumatic Diseases*, University of California Press, Berkeley and Los Angeles.
Delpeuch, A. (1900) *La Goutte et le Rheumatisme*, Carré and C. Naud, Paris.
Dumoulin, M. (1710) *Nouveau Traité du Rhumatisme et des Vapeurs*, L. d'Houry, Paris.
Goldthwait, J.E. (1904) The differential diagnosis and treatment of the so-called rheumatoid disease. *Boston Med. Surg. J.*, **151**, 529.
Graham, W. and Graham, K.M. (1955) Our gouty past. *Can. Med. Assoc. J.*, **73**, 485.
Hollander, J.L. (1960) in *Arthritis and Allied Conditions. A Textbook of Rheumatology* (ed. J.L. Hollander), 6th edn, Kimpton, London, p. 19.

Latham, J. (1796) *On Rheumatism and Gout*, Longman, London.
Léri, A. (1899) La spondylose rhizomélique. *Rev. Méd.*, **19**, 597.
MacLagan, T.J. (1881) *Rheumatism: Its Nature, Its Pathology, and Its Successful Treatment*, Pickering, London.
Marie, P. (1898) Sur la spondylose rhizomélique. *Rev. Méd.*, **18**, 285.
Mitchell, J.K. (1831) On a new practice in acute and chronic rheumatism. *Am. J. Med. Sci.*, **15**, 55.
Moll, J.M.H. (1978) in *Copeman's Textbook of the Rheumatic Diseases* (ed. J.T. Scott), 5th edn, Churchill Livingstone, Edinburgh, p. 512.
O'Connell, D. (1956) Ankylosing spondylitis. The literature up to the close of the nineteenth century. *Ann. Rheum. Dis.*, **15**, 119.
Poynton, F.J. and Paine, A. (1913) *Researches on Rheumatism*, Churchill, London.
Poynton, F.J. and Schlesinger, B.E. (1937) *Recent Advances in the Study of Rheumatism*, Churchill, London.
Spender, J.K. (1889) *The Early Symptoms and the Early Treatment of Osteo-Arthritis (Commonly Called Rheumatoid Arthritis)*, Lewis, London.
Still, G.F. (1896–1897) On a form of chronic joint disease in children. *Medico-Chir. Trans.*, **80**, 47.
Talbott, J.H. (1942) The treatment of gout. *Bull. N. Y. Acad. Med.*, **18**, 318.
West, S. (1878) Analysis of forty cases of rheumatic fever. *St. Bartholomew's Hosp. Rep.*, **14**, 221.
Wright, V. and Moll, J.M.H. (1976) *Seronegative Polyarthritis*, North Holland, Amsterdam.

Development of modern rheumatology

Comroe, B.I. (ed.) (1940) *Arthritis and Allied Conditions. A Textbook of Rheumatology*, Kimpton, London.
Copeman, W.S.C. (ed.) (1948) *Textbook of the Rheumatic Diseases*, Livingstone, Edinburgh and London.

Development in terms of changing nomenclature and classification of rheumatic disorders

Bennett, P.H. and Wood, P.H.N. (eds) (1968) *Population Studies of the Rheumatic Diseases*, International Congress Series No. 148, Excerpta Medica, Amsterdam, pp. 453, 477.

CIOMS (Council for International Organizations of Medical Sciences) (1966) *Medical Terminology and Lexicography*, Karger, Basle.

de Dombal, F.T., Leaper, D.J., Horrocks, J.C. *et al.* (1974) Human and computer-aided diagnosis of abdominal pain: further report with emphasis on performance of clinicians. *Br. Med. J.*, i, 376.

Feldman, S., Klein, D.F. and Honigfeld, G. (1972) The reliability of a decision tree technique applied to psychiatric diagnosis. *Biometrics*, **28**, 831.

Hill, L. and Ellman, P. (eds) (1938) *The Rheumatic Diseases*, Arnold, London, p. 33.

Kellgren, J.H. (1968) in *Rheumatic Diseases* (eds J.J.R. Duthie and W.R.M. Alexander), University Press, Edinburgh, p. 8.

Monro, T.K. (1911) *Manual of Medicine*, 3rd edn, Ballière, Tindall and Cox, London, p. 228.

Osler, W. (1910) *The Principles and Practice of Medicine*, 7th edn, Appleton, New York.

Ropes, M.W., Bennet, G.A., Cobb, S. *et al.* (1956) Proposed criteria for rheumatoid arthritis. *Bull. Rheum. Dis.*, **7**, 121.

Still, G.F. (1897) On a form of chronic joint disease in children. *Medico-Chir. Trans.*, **80**, 47.

Still, G.F. (1909) *Common Disorders and Diseases of Childhood*, Frowde (Oxford University Press) and Hodder and Stoughton, London.

Taylor, F. (1911) *The Practice of Medicine*, 9th edn, Churchill Livingstone, London, p. 996.

Wood, P.H.N. (1970a) Peculiarities of medical characters for taxonomic purposes. *Classification Soc. Bull.*, **2**, 23.

Wood, P.H.N. (1970b) Epidemiology of rheumatic disorders: problems in classification. *Proc. R. Soc. Med.*, **63**, 189.

Wood, P.H.N. (1974) An international nomenclature for rheumatology. *European League against Rheumatism (EULAR) Information Bulletin*, **3**, 138.

Wood, P.H.N. (1978) in *Copeman's Textbook of Rheumatic Diseases* (ed. J.T. Scott), 5th edn, Churchill Livingstone, Edinburgh, p. 14.

Historical aspects of treatment of specific rheumatic disorders

Collegii Regalis Medicorum Londinensis (1809) *Pharmacopoeia*. Longman, Hirst, Rees and Orme, London.

Copeman, W.S.C. (1964) *A Short History of the Gout and the Rheumatic Diseases*, University of California Press, Berkeley and Los Angeles.

Court-Brown, W.M. and Abbatt, J.D. (1955) The incidence of leukaemia in ankylosing spondylitis with X-ray treatment. *Lancet*, i, 1283.

Court-Brown, W.M. and Doll, R. (1965) Mortality from cancer and other causes after radiotherapy for ankylosing spondylitis. *Br. Med. J.*, ii, 1327.

D'Arsonval, A. (1932) *Applications Médicales des Emanations Radioactives*, Compte rendu de l'Academie des Sciences, Paris.

Desmarais, M.H.L. (1953) Radiotherapy in arthritis. *Ann. Rheum. Dis.*, **12**, 25.

Forestier, J., Jacqueline, F. and Rotés-Querol, J. (1956) *Ankylosing Spondylitis* (translation of the 1951 Paris edition), Thomas, Springfield.

Freyberg, R.H. (1946) Roentgen therapy for rheumatic diseases. *Med. Clin. N. Am.*, **30**, 603.

Hart, F.D. (1958) A critical survey of the value of radiotherapy in the treatment of ankylosing spondylitis. *Br. Med. J.*, ii, 1082.

Howard, N. (1957) Value of irradiation in ankylosing spondylitis. *Br. J. Radiol.*, **30**, 371.

Kahlmeter, G. (1930) The Roentgen treatment of arthritis. *Br. J. Actino-therapy*, **9**, 371.

Kohler, A. (1926) Uber die roentgen Behandlung der Arthritis deformans und Spondylitis deformans. *Klin. Wochenschr.*, **5**, 204.

Léri, A. and Thomas (1922) Le thorium X dans le traitement des rheumatismes chroniques. *Bull. Med.*, **36**, 348.

Scott, S.G. (1936) Chronic infection of the sacroiliac joints as a possible cause of spondylitis adolescens. *Br. J. Radiol.*,**9**, 126.

Sharp, J. and Easson, E.C. (1954) Deep X-ray therapy in spondylitis. *Br. Med. J.*, i, 619.

Smythe, C.J., Freyberg, R.H. and Lampe, I. (1941) Roentgen therapy and rheumatoid arthritis of the spine. *J. Am. Med. Assoc.*, **117**, 826.

Sokolow (1899) Roentgenstrahlen gegen gelenkrheumatismus. *Fortschritte auf dem Gebiete der Rontgenstrahlen*, **1**, 209.

Swaay, van H. (1955) Aplastic anaemia and myeloid leukaemia after irradiation of the vertebral column. *Lancet*, ii, 225.

Weil, M.P. and Bach, F. (1938) Radioactive substances and the treatment of rheumatism. *Rep. Chron. Rheum. Dis.*, No. 4, 70.

Wilkinson, M. and Bywaters, E.G.L. (1958) Clinical features and course of ankylosing spondylitis. *Ann. Rheum. Dis.*, **17**, 209.

Historical aspects of specific therapeutic approaches

Drugs

Aspirin

Bywaters, E.G.L. (1963) in *Salicylates* (eds A. St. J. Dixon, B.K. Martin, M.J.H. Smith and P.H.N. Wood), Churchill Livingstone, London, p. 3.

Stone, E. (1763) An account of the success of the bark of the willow in the cure of agues. In a Letter to the Right Honourable George, Earl of Macclesfield, President of the Royal Society from the Rev. Mr Edmund Stone, of Chipping Norton in Oxfordshire. *Phil. Trans.*, **53**, 195.

Phenylbutazone

Gsell, O. and Müller, W. (1950) Parenterale Pyramidon-Pyrazolidin-Therapie von Rheumatismus und Infekten mittels Irgapyrin. *Sch. Med. Wochenschr.*, **12**, 1950.

Rechenberg, von H.K. (1962) *Phenylbutazone (Butazolidin)*, Arnold, London, p. 1.

Indomethacin

Healey, L.A. (1967) An appraisal of indomethacin. *Bull. Rheum. Dis.*, **18**, 483.

Shen, T.Y., Windholz, T.B., Rosegay, A. *et al.* (1963) Non-steroidal anti-inflammatory agents. *J. Am. Chem. Soc.*, **85**, 488.

Proprionic acid derivatives

Cardoe, N. (1970) A review of long term experience with ibuprofen with special reference to gastric intolerance. *Rheumatol. Phys. Med.*, Suppl. 10, 28.

Godfrey, R. and Cruz, de la S. (1974) Effect of ibuprofen dosage on patient response in rheumatoid arthritis. *J. Rheumatol.*, **1**, Suppl. 1, 58.

Mitchell, D.M. and MacDonald, G. (1974) Controlled trial of ibuprofen in rheumatoid arthritis. *J. Rheumatol.*, **1**, Suppl. 1, 59.

Corticosteroids and ACTH

Addison, T. (1855) *On the Constitutional and Local Effects of Diseases of the Supra-renal Capsules*, Highley, London.

Boland, E.W. (1950) Relation of the adrenal cortex to rheumatic disease. *Ann. Rheum. Dis.*, **9**, 1.

Copeman, W.S.C. (1953) *Rheumatic and Collagen Diseases in Cortisone and ACTH in Clinical Practice* (ed. W.S.C. Copeman), Butterworth, London, p. 1.

Freyberg, R.H. (1950) Effects of cortisone and ACTH in rheumatoid arthritis. *Bull. N. Acad. Med.*, **26**, 206.

Hench, P.S., Kendall, E.C., Slocumb, C.H. and Polley, H.F. (1949) The effect of a hormone of the adrenal cortex (17-hydroxy-11-dehydrocortisterone: compound E) and of pituitary adrenocorticotropic hormone on rheumatoid arthritis. *Proc. Mayo Clin.*, **24**, 181.

Li, C.H., Simpson, M.E. and Evans, H.M. (1943) Adreno-corticotropic hormone. *J. Biol. Chem.*, 1949, 413.

Rogoff, J.M. and Stewart, G.N. (1926) Studies on adrenal insufficiency in dogs. *Am. J. Physiol.*, **78**, 711.

Sarett, L.H. (1948) A new method for the preparation of 17(α)-hydroxy-20-ketopregnanes. *J. Am. Chem. Soc.*, **70**, 1454.

Sayers, G., Sayers, M.A., White, A. and Long, C.N.H. (1943) Preparation of pituitary adrenotropic hormone. *Proc. Soc. Exp. Biol.*, **52**, 199.

Steward, G.N. (1924) Adrenalectomy and the relation of the adrenal bodies to metabolism. *Physiol. Rev.*, **4**, 163.

Swingle, W.W. and Pfiffner, J.J. (1930) An aqueous extract of the suprarenal cortex which maintains the life of bilaterally adrenalectomized cats. *Science*, **71**, 321.

Walton, J.N. (cited by) (1977) in *Brain's Diseases of the Nervous System*, 8th edn, Oxford University Press, Oxford, p. 45.

Gold therapy

Cooperating Clinics of the American Rheumatism Association (1973) A controlled trial of gold salt therapy in the treatment of rheumatoid arthritis. *Arthr. Rheum.*, **16**, 353.

Empire Rheumatism Council (1961) Gold therapy in rheumatoid arthritis: final report of a multicentre controlled trial. *Ann. Rheum. Dis.*, **20**, 315.

Forestier, J. (1929) L'aurothérapie dans les rheumatismes chroniques. *Bull. Mém. Soc. Méd. Hôpitaux de Paris*, **8**, 23.

Forestier, J. (1935) Rheumatoid arthritis and its treatment by gold salts: the results of six years' experience. *J. Lab. Clin. Med.*, **20**, 827.

Fraser, T.N. (1945) Gold therapy in rheumatoid arthritis. *Ann. Rheum. Dis.*, **4**, 71.

Hartfall, S.J., Garland, H.F. and Goldie, W. (1937) Gold treatment of arthritis. A review of 900 cases. *Lancet*, **ii**, 784, 838.

Holbrook, W.P. and Hill, D.F. (1936) Treatment of atrophic arthritis. *J. Am. Med. Assoc.*, **107**, 34.

Lande, K. (1927) Die günstige Beeinflussung schleichender Dauerinfekte durch Solganal. *Münchener Med. Wochenschr.*, **74**, 1132.

Phillips, R.T. (1936) The treatment of arthritis with gold salts. *N. Engl. J. Med.*, **214**, 114.

Pick, E. (1927) Verusche einer Goldbehandlung des Rheumatismus. *Wiener Klin. Wochenschr.*, **40**, 1175.

Sigler, J.W., Bluhm, G.B., Duncan, H. *et al.* (1974) Gold salts in the treatment of rheumatoid arthritis. *Ann. Int. Med.*, **80**, 21.

Penicillamine

Berry, H., Liyanage, S.P., Durance, R.A. *et al.* (1976) Azathioprine and penicillamine in treatment of rheumatoid arthritis: a controlled trial. *Br. Med. J.*, **i**, 1052.

Day, A.T., Golding, J.R., Lee, P.N. and Butterworth, A.D. (1974) Penicillamine in rheumatoid disease: a long-term study. *Br. Med. J.*, **i**, 180.

Dixon, A. St. J., Davies, J., Dormandy, T.L. *et al.* (1975) Synthetic D(−)penicillamine in rheumatoid arthritis. *Ann. Rheum. Dis.*, **34**, 416.

Huskisson, E.C., Gibson, T.J., Balme, H.W. *et al.* (1974) Trial comparing D-penicillamine and gold in rheumatoid arthritis. *Ann. Rheum. Dis.*, **33**, 532.

Jaffe, I.A. (1965) The effect of penicillamine on the laboratory parameters in rheumatoid arthritis. *Arthr. Rheum.*, **8**, 1064.

Jaffe, I.A. (1970) The treatment of rheumatoid arthritis and necrotizing vasculitis with penicillamine. *Arthr. Rheum.*, **13**, 436.

Jaffe, I.A. (1975) The technique of penicillamine administration in rheumatoid arthritis. *Arthr. Rheum.*, **18**, 513.

Antimalarials

Hamilton, E.B.D. and Scott, J.T. (1962) Hydroxychloroquine sulphate ('plaquenil') in treatment of rheumatoid arthritis. *Arthr. Rheum.*, **5**, 502.

Page, F. (1951) Treatment of lupus erythematosus with mepacrine. *Lancet*, **ii**, 755.

Popert, A.J., Meijers, K.A.E., Sharp, J. and Bier, F. (1961) Chloroquine diphosphonate in rheumatoid arthritis: a controlled trial. *Ann. Rheum. Dis.*, **20**, 18.

Cytotoxic agents

Baldwin, D.S., McLean, P.G., Chasis, H. and Goldring, W. (1953) Effect of nitrogen mustard on clinical course of glomerulonephritis. *Arch. Int. Med.*, **92**, 162.

Diaz, C.J., Garcia, E.L. and Merchante, A. (1951) Treatment of rheumatoid arthritis with nitrogen mustard. *J. Am. Med. Assoc.*, **147**, 1418.

Dubois, E.L. (1954) Nitrogen mustard in treatment of systemic lupus erythematosus. *Arch. Int. Med.*, **93**, 667.

Hahn, B.H., Kantor, O.S. and Osterland, C.K. (1975) Azathioprine plus prednisone compared with prednisone alone in the treatment of systemic lupus erythematosus. *Ann. Int. Med.*, **53**, 597.

Rothfield, N.F. (1975) Immunosuppressive therapy in lupus erythematosus. *Ann. Int. Med.*, **83**, 727.

Anti-gout drugs

Cohen, A., (1936) Gout. *Am. J. Med. Sci.*, **192**, 488.

Copeman, W.S.C. (1964) *A Short History of the Gout and the Rheumatic Diseases*, University of California Press, Berkeley.

Gutman, A.B. and Yu, T-F (1951) Benemid p-(di-n-propylsulfamyl)benzoic acid uricosuric agent in chronic gouty arthritis. *Trans. Assoc. Am. Phys.*, **64**, 279.

Hartung, E.F. (1954) History of the use of colchicum and related medicaments in gout. *Ann. Rheum. Dis.*, **13**, 190.

Rundles, R.W., Wyngaarden, J.B., Hitchings, C.H. *et al.* (1963) Effects of a xanthine oxidase inhibitor on thiopurine metabolism, hyperuricemia and gout. *Trans. Assoc. Am. Phys.*, **76**, 126.

Störck, A. de (1764) *An Essay on the Use and Effects of the Root of the Colchicum autumnale, or Meadow Saffron*, Translated from the Latin by T. Becket and P.A. de Honet, London.

Talbott, J.H., Bishop, C., Norcross, B.M. and Lockie, L.M. (1951) The clinical and metabolic effects of Benemid in patients with gout. *Trans. Assoc. Am. Phys.*, **64**, 372.

Want, J. (1814) The use of *Colchicum autumnale* in rheumatism. *Med. Physiol. J.*, **32**, 312.

Wyngaarden, J.B. and Kelley, W.N. (1976) *Gout and Hyperuricaemia*, Grune and Stratton, New York, p. 3.

Yu, T.-F. and Gutman, A.B. (1961) Efficacy of colchicine prophylaxis in gout. Prevention of recurrent gouty arthritis over a mean period of five years in 208 gouty subjects. *Ann. Int. Med.*, **55**, 179.

Physical therapy

Lord Horder (1953) in *Physical Medicine and Rehabilitation* (ed. B. Kiernander), Blackwell Scientific Publications, Oxford.

Nichols, P.J.R. (ed.) (1980) *Rehabilitation Medicine. The Management of Physical Disabilities*, Butterworths, London, p. 1.

Splinting

Plaster of Paris Technique: A Handbook for Students (Undated), Smith and Nephew, Welwyn Garden City.

Radiotherapy

Coutard, H. (1935) Conception of periodicity as a possible directing factor in roentgen therapy of cancer. *Proc. Inst. Med., Chicago*, **10**, 310.

Kaplan, I.I. (1949) *Clinical Radiation Therapy*, 2nd edn, Hoeber, New York, pp. 2–6.

Prasad, K.N. (1974) *Human Radiation Biology*, Harper and Row, Hagerstown, p. 4.

Surgery

Barton, J.R. (1827) On the treatment of ankylosis by the formation of artificial joints. *N. Am. Med. Sci. J.*, **3**, 279.

Charnley, J. (1960a) Surgery of the hip joint: present and future development. *Br. Med. J.*, **i**, 821.

Charnley, J. (1960b) Anchorage of the femoral head prosthesis to the shaft of the femur. *J. Bone Joint Surg.*, **42B**, 28.

Gluck, T. (1891) Referat uber die Durch des moderne chirurgische Experiment gewonnenen positiven Resultate, betrefend die naht und den Ersatz von Defected Nohrer Gewebe, Sowie uber die Verwerthung resorbisbander und Lebendiger Tampons in der Chirurgie. *Arch. Klin. Chir.*, **41**, 186.

McBridge, E.D. (1960) The shackled acetabular replacement prosthesis. *J. Bone Joint Surg.*, **42A**, 901.

McKee, G.K. and Watson-Farrar, J. (1966) Replacement of arthritic hips by the McKee-Farrar prosthesis. *J. Bone Joint Surg.*, **48B**, 245.

Moore, A.T. and Bohlman, H.R. (1943) Metal hip joint. A case report. *J. Bone Joint Surg.*, **25**, 688.

Mowat, A.G. (1978) in *Copeman's Textbook of Rheumatology* (ed. J.T. Scott), 5th edn, Churchill Livingstone, Edinburgh, p. 464.

Ollier, L. (1885) *Traite des Resections et des Operations Conservatrices qu'on peut Pratiquer sur le Systeme Osseux*, Paris.

Rang, M. (1968) *Anthology of Orthopaedics*, Livingstone, Edinburgh, p. 2.

Smith-Petersen, M.N. (1925) Joint ankylosis. *Trans. Interstate Post-Grad. Med. Assembly, N. Am.*

Smith-Petersen, M.N. (1939) Arthroplasty of the hip: a new method. *J. Bone Joint Surg.*, **21**, 269.

Speed, J.S. (1924) Synovectomy of the knee joint. *J. Am. Med. Assoc.*, **83**, 1814.

Urist, M.R. (1957) The principles of hip-socket arthroplasty. *J. Bone Joint Repl.*, **39A**, 786.

Wiles, P. (1958) The surgery of the osteoarthritic hip. *Br. J. Surg.*, **45**, 488.

Heterodox therapy

Camp, J. (1973) *Magic, Myth and Medicine*, Priory, London.

Knight, C. (ed.) (1864) *Old England: A Pictorial Museum of Regal, Ecclesiastical, Municipal, Baronial and Popular Antiquities*. Vol II, Sangiter and Co., London, p. 208.

Lawrence, R.M. (1910) *Primitive Psycho-therapy and Quackery*, Constable, London.

1.7 APPENDICES

1.7.1 Development of schemata for classifying rheumatic disorders

(a) Ministry of Health, 1924

A (1) Rheumatic fever.
   (2) Subacute rheumatism.

B (*Non-articular manifestations.*)
   (1) Muscular rheumatism (myalgia) including fibrositis, pleurodynia and torticollis.
   (2) Lumbago. (Classified alone on account of its occupational interest.)
   (3) Sciatica and brachial neuritis.

C (*Chronic joint changes.*)
   (1) Rheumatoid arthritis. (Infective peri-arthritis.)
   (2) Osteo-arthritis.
   (3) Gout, acute and chronic.
   (4) Chronic joint changes, unclassifiable.

(b) British Medical Association, 1933

	Synonyms	
Rheumatoid arthritis	Chronic polyarthritis (continental nomenclature) Atrophic (Goldthwait) Proliferative (Nichols and Richardson) (American nomenclature)	Primary cause unknown, this as knowledge increases may merge into Secondary associated with focal or general infection.
Chronic villous arthritis		Mainly occurring in women at or about the menopause.
Osteo-arthritis	Hypertrophic (Goldthwait) Degenerative (Nichols and Richardson)	Primary, no definite association with infection. Secondary, associated with infection.
Spondylitis	Ankylopoietica Osteo-arthritica	Arthritis of spinal joints with bony ankylosis, spreading centrifugally to adjacent large joints. Osteo-arthritis of the spine (the labourer's spine).
Fibrositis	Intramuscular Periarticular Bursal and tenosynovial Subcutaneous (panniculitis) Perineuritic	

(c) Royal College of Physicians of London, 1934

Group 1. Rheumatic fever, acute (synonym: acute rheumatism) or subacute.
Group 2. Acute gout.
Group 3. Chronic arthritis.
    A. *Rheumatoid* type ('atrophic, proliferative').
      (1) Specific causation. Known ætiology.
        (*a*) Gonococcal arthritis.
        (*b*) Tuberculous arthritis.
        (*c*) Syphilitic arthritis.
        (*d*) Arthritis following other specific infections such as dysentery, scarlet fever, rheumatic fever.

(2) Non-specific causation. Unknown ætiology.
  (*a*) With known associated factors.
  (i) Metastatic or 'focal' arthritis, including the so-called 'multiple infective arthritis.'
  (ii) Associated with disordered metabolism (e.g. gout).
  (iii) Climacteric arthritis (villous type).
  (*b*) With no known associated factors.
  (i) Classical type of rheumatoid arthritis of women usually of child-bearing period.
  (ii) Rheumatoid arthritis in children, including Still's disease.
  The term 'rheumatoid arthritis' when utilized should be confined to the above two conditions, all other forms being designated 'rheumatoid type.'
B. *Osteo-arthritic* type ('hypertrophic, degenerative').
  (1) Known ætiology.
    (*a*) Secondary to trauma.
    (*b*) Secondary to arthritis of rheumatoid type.
    (*c*) Associated with disordered metabolism (climacteric, gouty, scurvy, hæmophilia).
    (*d*) Associated with organic disease of the nervous system (e.g. Charcot's joints and syringomyelia).
  (2) Unknown ætiology.
    So-called 'senile variety' (e.g. morbus coxæ senilis).
Group 4. Non-articular affections.

(*d*) *International League Against Rheumatism, 1934*

A. *Articular.*

(English)	(1)	Subchronic rheumatic arthritis (following on rheumatic fever).
(German)		Secondar sub-chronische gelenkrheumatismus.
(French)		Polyarthrite secondaire.
(English)	(2)	Rheumatoid arthritis (arthritis variously described as focal, chronic infective, non-specific, multiple infective, of unknown origin, non-suppurative).
(German)		Primar progressive polyarthritis (arthritis deformans generalis).
(French)		Polyarthrites deformante (polyarthrites symetriques progressives, rheumatisme noueux, rheumatoid tuberculeux, polyarthrites post-influenzale).
(English)	(3)	Climacteric arthritis (endocrine, metabolic hypoglandular rheumatism, villous arthritis, rheumatic gout, gout in women).
(German)		Arthropathica climacterica (deformans endocrina).
(French)		Rheumatisme de la menopause (rheumatoid goutteux, Trissier, lipoarthrite bilaterale et symétrique des genoux – Francon, rheumatisme hyperthyroidien).
(English)	(4)	Osteo-arthritis (hypertrophic arthritis, arthritis senile, mon-arthritis).
(German)		Arthrosis deformans.
(French)		Arthrite deformante.
(English)	(5)	Spondylitis (spondylosis rhizomelica, ankylosing spondylitis).
(German)		Spondyarthritis ankylopoetica (spondylosis deformans).
(French)		Spondylose rhizomélique (spondylite deformante, kyphose heredo-traumatique–Leri.

B. *Non-articular.*
(English)   Fibrositis, myositis, cellulitis, panniculitis (lumbago, sciatica, perineuritis, adiposalgia, etc.).

(*e*) *International League Against Rheumatism, 1957*

I. A proposed classification of the diseases and disorders of connective tissue commonly accepted as rheumatic

A. Articular
  1. Inflammatory
  Idiopathic:
    (*a*) Rheumatic fever.
    (*b*) Rheumatoid arthritis.
    (*c*) Atypical forms:
Arthritis with psoriasis, psoriasic arthropathy.
Juvenile rheumatoid arthritis (Chauffard–Still's disease).
Rheumatoid arthritis with spleno-adenomegaly and leucopenia (Felty's syndrome).
Polyarthritis with keratoconjunctivitis sicca (Sjögren's syndrome).
Polyarthritis with non-specific urethritis (Reiter's syndrome).
    (*d*) Special forms:
Ankylosing spondylitis.

Intermittent hydrarthrosis.
Palindromic rheumatism.
Infectional:
   Arthritis due to specific infection.
2. Degenerative
Osteoarthritis, degenerative joint diseases or osteo-arthrosis.
Intervertebral disc lesions.
Osteochondrosis.

B. Non-articular
   Bursitis.
   Fasciitis.
   Fibrositis.
   Myositis, myalgia.
   Neuritis, neuropathy, neuralgia.
   Disorders of fatty tissue, panniculitis.
   Periarthritis.
   Tendovaginitis, tenosynovitis.
   Tendinitis, tendinosis, peritendinitis.

II. Diseases and disorders with rheumatic features

A. Traumatic and mechanical disorders
   Traumatic arthropathy.
   Postural syndromes.

B. Inflammatory, idiopathic
   Dermatomyositis,
   Periarteritis nodosa and arteritis.
   Scleroderma.
   Systemic lupus erythematosus.

C. Hypersensitivity states with musculoarticular reactions to serum, drugs etc.
   Erythema multiforme.
   Erythema nodosum.

Purpura (various types).
Purpura rheumatica.
Serum sickness.
Reiter's syndrome.

D. Metabolic disturbances
   Gout
   Alcaptonuria.

E. Endocrine disturbances
   Hyperparathyroidism.
   Acromegaly.
   Myxoedema and others.
   Osteoporosis (menopausal, senile, others).

F. Blood diseases
   Leukaemia.
   Haemophilia etc.

G. Pulmonary diseases
   Sarcoidosis.
   Hypertrophic pulmonary osteo-arthropathy.

H. Diseases or disorders of the nervous system
   Neuroarthropathy.
   Reflex dystrophy.

I. Psychiatric states and psychological syndromes

J. Neoplastic diseases
   Neoplasms of articular or periarticular tissues.

K. Osteochondrodystrophies

(*f*) *American Rheumatism Association, 1963*

A. Polyarthritis of unknown aetiology
   Rheumatoid arthritis.
   Rheumatoid arthritis of the juvenile type (Still's disease).
   Ankylosing spondylitis.
   Psoriatic arthritis.
   Reiter's syndrome.
   Others.

B. 'Connective tissue' disorders ('collagen diseases')
   Systemic lupus erythematosus.
   Polyarteritis nodosa.
   Scleroderma (progressive systemic sclerosis).
   Polymyositis and dermatomyositis.
   Others.

C. Rheumatic fever (acute rheumatism)

D. Degenerative joint disease (osteo-arthritis or -osis)
   Primary.
   Secondary.

E. Non-articular rheumatism
   Fibrositis.

Intervertebral disc and low back syndromes.
Myositis and myalgia.
Tendinitis and peritendinitis (bursitis).
Tenosynovitis.
Fasciitis.
Carpal-tunnel syndrome.
Others.

F. Diseases with which arthritis is frequently associated
   Sarcoidosis
   Relapsing polychondritis
   Henoch–Schönlein syndrome.
   Ulcerative colitis.
   Regional ileitis.
   Whipple's disease.
   Sjögren's syndrome.
   Familial Mediterranean fever.
   Others.

G. Associated with known infectious agents
   (1) Bacterial
      Brucella.
      Gonococcus.

Mycobacterium tuberculosis.
Pneumococcus.
Salmonella.
Staphylococcus.
Streptobacillus moniliformus (Haverhill fever).
Treponema pallidum (Syphilis).
Treponema pertenue (Yaws).
Others.
(2) Rickettsial
(3) Viral.
(4) Fungal.
(5) Parasitic.

H. Traumatic and/or neurogenic disorders
Traumatic arthritis.
Lues (tertiary syphilis).
Diabetes.
Syringomyelia.
Shoulder–hand syndrome.
Mechanical derangements of joints.
Others.

I. Associated with known biochemical or endocrine abnormalities
Gout
Ochronosis.
Hæmophilia.
Hæmoglobinopathies (e.g. sickle cell disease).
Agammaglobulinæmia.
Gaucher's disease.
Hyperparathyroidism.
Acromegaly.
Hypothyroidism.
Scurvy (hypovitaminosis C).
Xanthoma tuberosum.
Others.

J. Tumour and tumour-like conditions
Synovioma.
Pigmented villonodular synovitis.
Giant-cell tumour of tendon sheath.
Primary juxta-articular bone tumours.
Metastatic.
Leukæmia.
Multiple myeloma.
Benign tumours of articular tissue.
Others.

K. Allergy and drug reactions
Arthritis due to specific allergens (e.g. serum sickness).
Arthritis due to drugs (e.g. hydralazine syndrome).
Others.

L. Inherited and congenital disorders
Marfan's syndrome.
Ehlers–Danlos syndrome.
Hurler's syndrome.
Congenital hip dysplasia.
Morquio's disease.
Others.

M. Miscellaneous disorders
Amyloidosis.
Aseptic necrosis of bone.
Behçet's syndrome.
Chondrocalcinosis ('pseudo gout').
Erythema multiforme (Stevens–Johnson syndrome).
Erythema nodosum.
Hypertrophic osteoarthropathy.
Juvenile osteochondritis.
Osteochondritis dissecans.
Reticulohistocytosis of joints (lipoid dermatoarthritis).
Tietze's disease.
Others.

1.7.2 A proposed outline assignment key for inflammatory arthropathies (Wood, 1978)

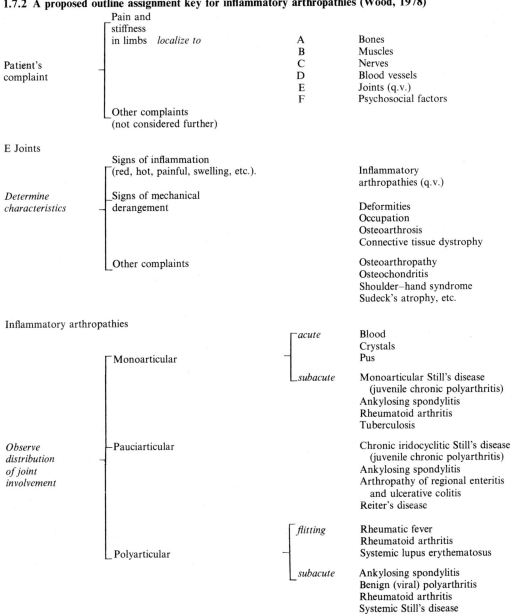

Patient's complaint

Pain and stiffness in limbs *localize to*

A	Bones
B	Muscles
C	Nerves
D	Blood vessels
E	Joints (q.v.)
F	Psychosocial factors

Other complaints (not considered further)

E Joints

Determine characteristics

Signs of inflammation (red, hot, painful, swelling, etc.).
Inflammatory arthropathies (q.v.)

Signs of mechanical derangement
Deformities
Occupation
Osteoarthrosis
Connective tissue dystrophy

Other complaints
Osteoarthropathy
Osteochondritis
Shoulder–hand syndrome
Sudeck's atrophy, etc.

Inflammatory arthropathies

Observe distribution of joint involvement

Monoarticular
- *acute*
  Blood
  Crystals
  Pus
- *subacute*
  Monoarticular Still's disease (juvenile chronic polyarthritis)
  Ankylosing spondylitis
  Rheumatoid arthritis
  Tuberculosis

Pauciarticular
Chronic iridocyclitic Still's disease (juvenile chronic polyarthritis)
Ankylosing spondylitis
Arthropathy of regional enteritis and ulcerative colitis
Reiter's disease

Polyarticular
- *flitting*
  Rheumatic fever
  Rheumatoid arthritis
  Systemic lupus erythematosus
- *subacute*
  Ankylosing spondylitis
  Benign (viral) polyarthritis
  Rheumatoid arthritis
  Systemic Still's disease (juvenile chronic polyarthritis)
  Other

1.7.3 Early reference to the efficacy of willow bark in a paper to the Royal Society by the Reverend E.* Stone (1763)

XXXII. *An Account of the succefs of the Bark of the Willow in the Cure of Agues. In a Letter to the Right Honourable George Earl of* Macclesfield, *Prefident of R.S. from the Rev. Mr.* Edmund Stone, *of* Chipping-Norton *in* Oxfordfhire.

My Lord,   Read June 2d. 1763

Among the many ufeful difcoveries, which this age hath made, there are very few which, better deferve the attention of the public than what I am going to lay before your Lordfhip.

There is a bark of an Englifh tree, which I have found by experience to be a powerful aftringent, and very efficacious in curing aguifh and intermitting diforders.

About fix years ago, I accidentally tafted it, and was furprifed at its extraordinary bitternefs; which immediately raifed me a fufpicion of its having the properties of the Peruvian bark. As this tree delights in a moift or wet foil,

---

* Note the discrepancy concerning his first name – Edmund in the title and Edward (probably correct) at the end of the letter.

where agues chiefly abound, the general maxim, that many natural maladies carry their cures along with them, or that their remedies lie not far from their caufes, was fo very appofite to this particular cafe, that I could not help applying it

And this is how it ended:

...cinnamon or lateritious colour, which I believe is the cafe with the Peruvian bark and powders.

I have no other motives for publifhing this valuable fpecific, than that it may have a fair and full trial in all its variety of circumftances and fituations, and that the world may reap the benefits accruing from it. For thefe purpofes I have given this long and minute account of it, and which I would not have troubled your Lordfhip with, was I not fully perfuaded of the wonderful efficacy of this Cortex Salignus in agues and intermitting cafes, and did I not think, that this perfuafion was fufficiently fupported by the manifold experience, which I have had of it.

I am, my Lord
with the profoundeft fubmiffion and refpect,

Chipping-Norton,	your Lordfhip's moft obedient
Oxfordshire,	humble Servant
April 25, 1763	Edward Stone

2

General therapeutic factors and principles

2.1 GENERAL COMMENT

The major part of this book is concerned with details covering the various therapeutic approaches currently available to treat rheumatic disorders. Thus, there are individual chapters on drugs, local injection therapy, radiotherapy, surgery, and rehabilitation. However, to provide a perspective idea of how these are interrelated in the process of overall management it is necessary to discuss certain general aspects. This chapter has been written with this intention, and it is hoped that the following sections will enable a rational approach to emerge from the wealth of detail which it has been necessary to document under specific therapies.

2.2. SIZE AND SCOPE OF THE RHEUMATIC PROBLEM

The different forms of rheumatic disorders are the most widespread, crippling, and usually painful conditions to which our population is subject. The scope of rheumat-

ology includes not only the many disorders involving the locomotor or musculoskeletal system (bones, joints and related structures – Fig. 2.1), but also involvement of systems beyond the locomotor system. Involvement of other systems not only increases the overall morbidity of rheumatic problems but may even result in death.

Arthritis and rheumatism affect people of all ages – infants and children, adolescents, adults, and the elderly – their incidence increasing quite significantly with age. In fact, it is unlikely that anyone escapes some form of rheumatic problem during the course of his or her life. Different forms have a predilection for men and women variously, and life style, occupation, and leisure activities may also exert an influence.

In the USA there are about 20 million persons suffering from some form of arthritis or related disease (Arthritis Foundation, 1976), and more than one million are impaired by 'rheumatic disorders' in the UK. More than one fifth of the latter are severely or very severely disabled – 51 000 confined to bed, chair or wheelchair, and 143 000 housebound (Wood, 1977). In the UK about 20 million people experience some form

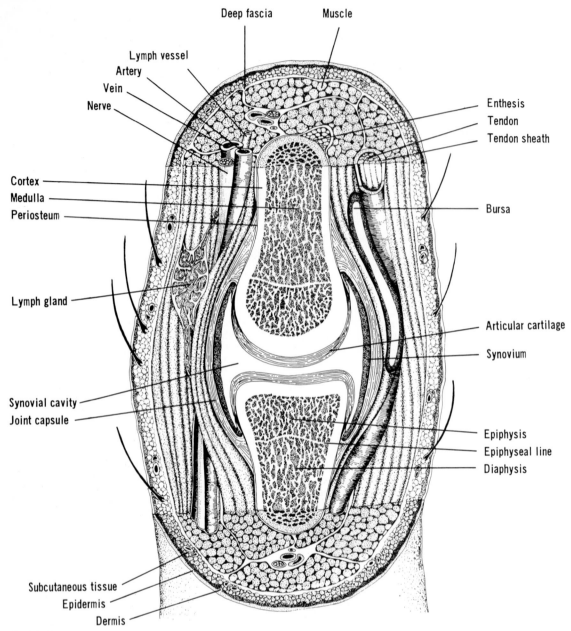

Fig. 2.1 Musculoskeletal structures – bones, joints and related soft-tissue structures – which may be involved in rheumatic disorders.

of rheumatic complaint during the course of one year. More than a million spells of incapacity occur, leading to the loss of 44 million days from work – a burden exceeding that due to industrial disputes. Most of these conditions are difficult to diagnose in their early stages.

Some are rare, while others affect millions; many last a lifetime, while a few lead inexorably to death. It is difficult to estimate the prevalence of many of these disorders, although more than 10 000 children are affected by Still's disease, at least half a million have

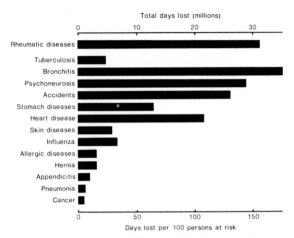

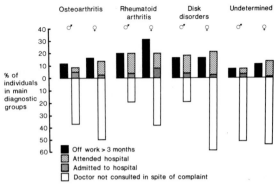

Fig. 2.2 The size of the problem posed by rheumatic diseases compared with other diseases (redrawn from Lawrence, 1977).

Fig. 2.4 Incapacity due to various rheumatic disorders. Note extent of incapacity due to rheumatoid arthritis – particularly in women (redrawn from Lawrence, 1977).

rheumatoid arthritis and something like 5 million have osteoarthrosis.

The economic cost of these ailments is equal to an important function of the gross national product. Thus, the loss in productivity in a year amounts to at least £420 millions, a figure taking no account of losses attributable to premature death and to the inability of housewives to sustain their home-making and related activities.

As Lawrence has clearly indicated (Lawrence, 1977), the size of the problem posed by rheumatic diseases generally, compared with other diseases, is substantial and is summarized in Fig. 2.2. From this it will be seen that second to bronchitis, in terms of days lost from work, it is the largest cause of incapacity caused by medical disorders. As with chronic disorders affecting non-locomotor disease systems, the size of the burden

imposed by rheumatic diseases increases with age (Fig. 2.3). When the rheumatic disorders are sub-classified, rheumatoid arthritis, particularly in women, represents the most potent cause of prolonged incapacity (off work more than 3 months), although other identifiable rheumatic states give a substantial contribution to rheumatic-induced incapacity as a whole (Fig. 2.4).

2.3 INDICATIONS FOR REFERRAL TO A RHEUMATOLOGIST

Guidelines for referral to a rheumatologist or similar specialist in rheumatic diseases may be summarized as follows:

1. When the patient requires a further opinion.
2. When the diagnosis is unclear or when an established diagnosis requires confirmation.
3. For specialized diagnostic studies (e.g. joint aspiration for synovial fluid analysis and synovial biopsy).
4. When a rheumatic disease is persistent, especially when symptoms are severe.
5. When the disease is running a downhill course or when the patient is rapidly becoming disabled.
6. When a systemic illness presents puzzling rheumatic features.
7. For recommendation of a total management programme.
8. For follow-up care of patients with complicated problems.
9. For therapeutic monitoring when the family doctor 'inherits' a patient taking potentially dangerous drugs (e.g. gold, penicillamine, antimalarials, cytotoxic agents).

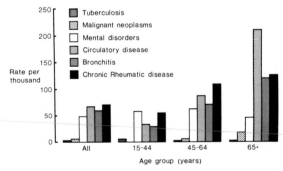

Fig. 2.3 Increased frequency of rheumatic and non-rheumatic illnesses with age (redrawn from Lawrence, 1977).

2.4 CLINICAL ASSESSMENT AND EVALUATION SCHEMES

2.4.1 General comment

Assessment and evaluation of rheumatic patients is essential for the clinician attempting to arrest or reverse lifelong, often naturally progressive, diseases. In therapeutic trials, often involving more than one observer, the grading of activity must be precise and uniform. The basic principles of, and the indices useful for, the clinical evaluation of arthritis are the subjects of this section.

It is almost always possible for an arthritic patient to state whether his condition is better or worse compared with the previous encounter with the physician. However, if 'Better or worse?' questions are asked, when no baseline has been established, no meaningful answer can be expected.

The problem of assessment of activity in rheumatoid arthritis will be discussed in greatest detail, but many of the measurements and problems are common to other inflammatory forms of arthritis.

Requisites for items of evaluation are as follows:

1. Economy – ease of performance, short time needed.
2. Validity – does the measurement really measure the attribute it is supposed to measure?
3. Objectivity – degree of interobserver agreement.
4. Reliability – degree of agreement between different but comparable measurements.
5. Sensitivity – responsiveness of test to alterations in attributes being measured.

2.4.2 Assessment of specific features

Clinical and laboratory observations used to measure rheumatoid arthritis and other inflammatory arthritides fall into three main categories:

1. Inflammatory manifestations. These may be either articular or systemic and, collectively, constitute 'activity' of the disease.
2. Structural manifestations, such as cartilage or bone erosion, which at best are only partly reversible.
3. Functional changes which may be due to a combination of (1) and (2).

(a) Measurement of inflammatory manifestations

Joint inflammation

It might be thought that grading inflammation by such obvious variables as tenderness, pain, swelling, warmth, redness, and range of motion should be easy and highly objective. However, this is not so in general experience, and the consensus view is that *tenderness* is the most sensitive feature.

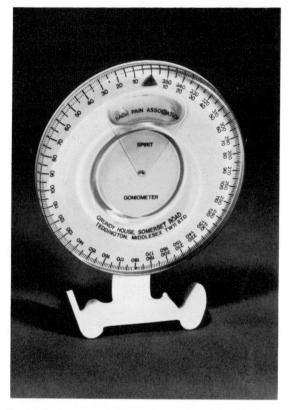

Fig. 2.5 Inclinometer (spirit goniometer) used by the Back Pain Association.

The value of measuring peripheral and spinal joint *motion* is now well established. Numerical data for normal thoracolumbar spinal joint motion (Moll and Wright, 1971, 1972), and simple objective methods using a tape measure to measure the various directions of spinal motion (Macrae and Wright, 1969; Moll *et al.*, 1972a, b), have originated from the Leeds group. More complicated, but useful, tools to measure spinal motion include the spondylometer (Dunham, 1949; Sturrock *et al.*, 1973; Hart *et al.*, 1974) and the inclinometer (Loebl, 1967) (Fig. 2.5). The classic fingertips-to-floor method, even using special instrumentation, is no longer recommended in view of the fact that it measures not only spinal mobility but also hip flexion (some patients with established spondylitis can touch their toes with ease). Objective methodology has also been introduced to measure movements of the cervical spine, such as the device shown in Fig. 2.6 to measure rotation. Various other forms of instrumentation exist to measure spinal mobility and thoracospinal mobility (chest expansion), and for further information the

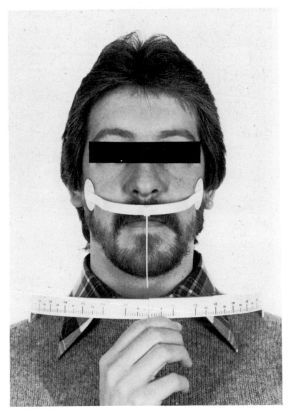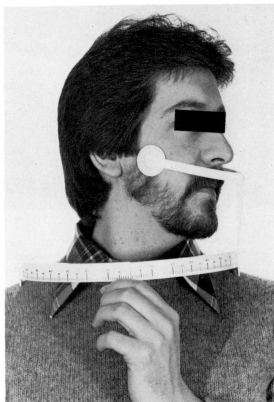

Fig. 2.6 A device for measuring rotation of the cervical spine.

reader is referred to more detailed sources (Moll and Wright, 1976, 1980).

Stress has been placed on the importance of allowing for the effects of age and sex when questioning whether a particular measurement lies within the normal range. Concerning peripheral joint motion, no normal ranges of mobility have yet been delineated, and all that is available at present are average figures for such movements. In view of the breadth of the normal range, such information is clearly of limited value. However, in paired joints in which only one joint is affected, the most meaningful assessment is a comparison with the opposite side. Of course, this is not possible in the spine.

For reasonably accurate measurement of many joint movements, such as at the knee, the goniometer (Fig. 2.7) is of considerable value. The neutral zero method of the American Academy of Orthopaedic Surgeons (1966) is recommended. It stresses the importance of measuring joint motion from defined zero

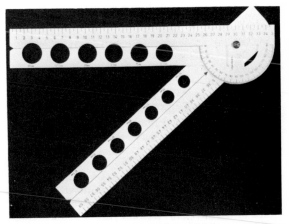

Fig. 2.7 Goniometer. In this particular model the arms of the device are provided with perforations of different sizes to measure small joint circumference (see Fig. 2.8).

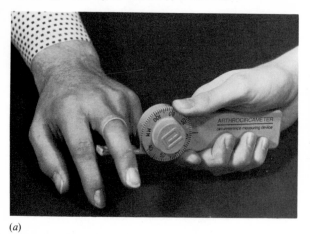

(a)

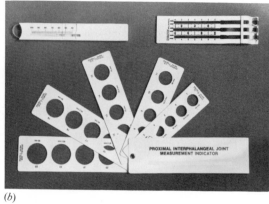

(b)

Fig. 2.8 (*a*) Arthrocircameter (based on jeweller's tape principle) to measure small-joint swelling. (*b*) Other devices to measure small joint circumference.

starting positions; movement is then recorded in degrees.

Goniometric determination of peripheral joint motion is of limited value in reflecting small or moderate changes of synovial activity, with the exception of finger joint motion. However, goniometry of peripheral joints is particularly useful in assessing the results of surgery and other therapeutic procedures.

Measurements of spinal and chest motion are more useful as indices of therapy and prognosis than as diagnostic indices. Studies of the place of spinal movement and of chest expansion as accurate indices of ankylosing spondylitis, for example, have shown these attributes to be too insensitive and too specific (Moll and Wright, 1973a, b).

Joint *swelling* is the most specific index. A jeweller's tape or rings affords a precise, rapid way to measure swelling of small joints (± 1 mm reproducibility). A jeweller's tape adapted for this purpose (an 'arthrocircameter') has been standardized (Willkens *et al.*, 1973). This and other devices to measure peripheral joint circumference are shown in Fig. 2.8. A standardized method for measuring the circumference of the knee joint has also appeared (Nicholas *et al.*, 1976). Smyth *et al.*, (1963) have shown that measures of hand and foot volume by water displacement are highly reproducible (the error is about 1%). Variations in skin temperature over inflamed joints (which can be 6–8°C above that of the surrounding skin) have been quantified with a thermocouple (Steele and McCarty, 1966), and Haberman *et al.* (1977) have quantified infra-red irradiation by thermography. Differences of 0.5°C can be detected with the back of the examiner's fingers when

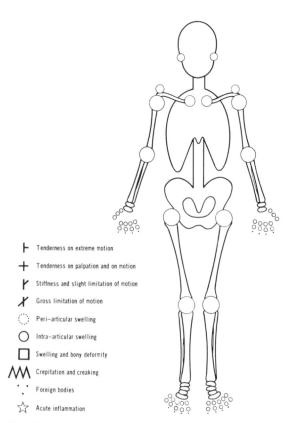

⊢	Tenderness on extreme motion
+	Tenderness on palpation and on motion
⊬	Stiffness and slight limitation of motion
✗	Gross limitation of motion
⁞⋯	Peri–articular swelling
○	Intra–articular swelling
□	Swelling and bony deformity
⋀⋀	Crepitation and creaking
⋯	Foreign bodies
☆	Acute inflammation

Fig. 2.9 Schema for documenting components of inflammatory joint disease (redrawn from McCarty, 1972).

comparing skin over affected joints with surrounding normal skin.

The importance of documenting the components of inflammatory joint disease cannot be over stressed. A useful general scheme even though lacking objectivity is that used by McCarty (1972). The components and symbol equivalents of this system are shown in Fig. 2.9.

Joint dysfunction

The American Rheumatism Association functional classification (Steinbrocker *et al.*, 1949) represents a more sharply defined system of categories than Taylor's original system of overall functional impairment (Taylor, 1937). The components of the American Rhematism Association classification are as follows:

Class I – *Complete*. (Ability to carry on all usual duties without handicaps.)

Class II – *Adequate for normal activities* (despite handicap of discomfort or limited motion at one or more joints).

Class III – *Limited* (only to little or none of duties of usual occupation or self-care).

Class IV – *Incapacitated, largely or wholly.* (Bedridden or confined to wheelchair; little or no self-care.)

Muscle weakness

This may be measured by the patient's ability to compress an inflated sphygmomanometer cuff under standard conditions. This and other devices to measure hand function are shown in Fig. 2.10.

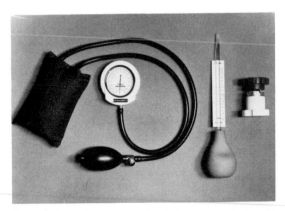

Fig. 2.10 Devices to measure hand function. Left to right: Inflated sphygmomanometer cuff and pressure gauge; fluid-filled compressible rubber bulb attached to calibrated tube; 'torque-meter' – device measuring counter-rotation of the two notched grips.

Morning stiffness

The duration of morning stiffness is a good non-specific indicator of local inflammation and is quantitatively proportional to its severity. It can be measured largely objectively by the arthrograph of Wright and Johns (1960).

Pain

Quantification of pain has been approached in many ways – direct questioning as to its severity, distinction between pain felt on motion and pain felt at rest, pain severe enough to prevent sleep, and pain that is or is not controlled by salicylates. The daily aspirin count is a reasonably useful index of the degree of pain, but has its pitfalls. A count of inflamed joints (the Articular Index) is another measure of pain in terms of elicited pain (tenderness). Other methods to assess pain include visual analogue scales and the dolorimeter – a standardized instrument designed to apply pressure to the joint.

Fatigue

This, like morning stiffness, is expressed as the time elapsed from rising in the morning to the onset of fatigue.

Body weight

A change in body weight is not recommended as an index of inflammatory activity in view of the many other factors affecting it. These include weight loss due to drug-induced anorexia and weight gain due to corticosteroid administration.

Fever

Because of the low incidence of fever in rheumatoid arthritis it is of little or no value as a criterion of disease activity.

Erythrocyte sedimentation rate (ESR)

The ESR is accepted by nearly all observers as one of the most reliable and objective criteria of disease activity, but in short-term drug trials it has not always provided statistically significant information. In some instances it may remain very rapid despite clinical evidence of relative disease inactivity. The Westegren is less laborious than the Wintrobe and is the most widely accepted method.

Anaemia

The value of anaemia as a measure of rheumatoid activity is lessened by its presence in less than half of those with active disease. However, if present (and not aggravated by the water-retention effect of certain drugs, e.g. corticosteroids, phenylbutazone, or by silent intermittent bleeding due to chronic ingestion of aspirin or other antirheumatic agents), the haemoglobin level gradually returns to normal as patients go into remission.

Leukocyte count

The leukocyte count has not been well studied in relation to disease activity. Leukocytes may diminish as the patient improves, but not with sufficient regularity as to be useful as a measure of activity.

Serum proteins

Falls in serum albumin and/or rises in serum globulin levels are intimately associated with the activity and possibly with the stage of the disease. However, little work has been done to clarify this relationship.

Role of other laboratory tests

The C-reactive protein, tests to measure rheumatoid factor titre, the mucopolysaccharide–protein ratio, and the sialic acid test may be useful. Responses of some of them may be helpful in assessing drug therapy, e.g. the fall in rheumatoid factor titre in patients with rheumatoid arthritis treated with long-term suppressants such as gold. Serial measurement of total haemolytic complement, or of antinuclear antibody, or of circulating immune complexes may help in evaluating systemic lupus. No similar helpful laboratory tests, except the acute-phase reactants and rheumatoid factor tests, exist for the assessment of disease activity in rheumatoid arthritis.

Serum glycosaminoglycan levels have been advocated as a guide both to the diagnosis of gout and to the monitoring of the prophylactic use of colchicine but are not in general use.

(b) Measurement of structural manifestations

Serial radiographs

Although radiographs are often not helpful in early diagnosis of rheumatoid arthritis, they are easily obtainable and easily standardized, and provide a permanent record of joint changes. Retardation or reversal of bony erosions and of joint space narrowing is good evidence that a given therapeutic agent is effective.

Radionuclide evaluation

The objectivity of radionuclear methods of evaluating arthritis makes them inherently appealing, but several studies of scintigraphic imagery usually using technetium-99^m as the pertechnetate ($^{99m}TCO_4$) have shown effects equally or less sensitive than clinical measurements (McCarty *et al.*, 1970; Green and Hays, 1972; Hays and Green, 1972; Deodhar *et al.*, 1973).

Thermographic methods

Measurement of infra-red irradiation from the skin over involved joints provides opportunities for objectivity.

The subject has recently been reviewed by Bacon *et al.* (1976), who concluded that the technique represents a useful tool both in therapeutic assessment and in the study of joint pathophysiology. It is safe, reproducible and acceptable to the patient. It is also totally objective.

2.4.3 Global systems of evaluation

(a) General

Concerning the number of measurable facets of rheumatoid disease used as indices of activity, several ways have been proposed to combine them in an attempt to identify the intensity of the process as a whole. These will be outlined shortly in subsequent sections.

The uses of a general system of evaluation include the following:

1. To indicate and identify for other clinicians the degree of rheumatoid activity in a given patient.
2. To follow the response of patients to treatment. There is little doubt as to the value of selected criteria for this purpose. A formal summation of data, as suggested by Lansbury (see Section 2.4.3(*b*)), is sometimes, but not always, helpful clinically in the detection and documentation of either an early flare or the beginning of improvement.
3. To follow the course of patients in drug trials. In drug trials each item should also be separately recorded and evaluated, since drug treatment often affects certain items more than others.

(b) Clinically based systems

Some clinically based systems to express overall rheumatoid activity are shown in Table 2.1, one of the most extensively used and widely accepted being that of Lansbury and colleagues (Lansbury, 1958; Lansbury *et al.*, 1962).

I have recently devised a 'spondylitic index' based on measurements of chest expansion (reduced in spondylitis), abdominal protrusion (increased), and diaphragm excursion (increased) in order to improve diagnostic accuracy in ankylosing spondylitis (Moll, 1975). The expression:

$$\frac{\text{Chest expansion}}{\text{Abdominal protrusion} + \text{diaphragm excursion}}$$

has been found to effect useful separation between spondylitics and controls. Thus, 92% of 56 spondylitics had an index less than 0·7 (the best dividing line between patients and controls), contrasted with controls in whom 80% had an index greater than 0·7.

Table 2.1 Selected systems used to sum rheumatoid activity – 'indices'*

Author	Method	Description
Lansbury (Lansbury, 1958; Lansbury *et al.*, 1962)	Systemic index	5 fixed criteria with empirical weighting of each. (Criteria: morning stiffness, fatigue onset, grip strength, aspirin (or other salicylate) tablet count, and ESR)
	Articular index	Sum of active joints (tenderness and pain on passive motion) corrected for joint size
	Activity index	Articular index treated as a sixth criterion or substituted for one of the systemic index criteria
Cooperating Clinics Committee of the American Rheumatism Association (ARA) (1965)	Joint count	Number of joints tender, painful on passive movement, or that show non-bony swelling
Ritchie *et al.* (1958)	Articular index	Weighted summation of active joints using a 4-point tenderness scale as weighting factor
Lee *et al.* (1973)	Pain rating method	Subjective pain rating by daily pain chart

* From McCarty (1979).

(c) Statistically based systems

In addition to the simple scoring methods applied to various measurements mentioned above, several sophisticated statistical methods for analysis of data from clinical trials have appeared. For example, McQuire and Wright (1971) found that the Lansbury system index failed to distinguish between either of two drugs (indomethacin and phenylbutazone) and placebo, whereas several of the individual components of the system did. An index using these factors, weighted by a technique similar to discriminant function analysis, provided maximal difference between patient groups. The method was called 'maximization of statistical significance'. A second statistical approach, factor analysis, was also applied to these data. This approach is based on an assumption that variables showing a high mutual correlation may share a common underlying factor. Thus, in this study the decreased aspirin consumption, used as an index of pain, and the subjective relief of pain noted with indomethacin treatment, were isolated as independent variables from factors reflecting inflammation *per se*. It was concluded that, in rheumatoid arthritis, the drug was an effective analgesic, but had no direct anti-inflammatory effect.

Another method of value has been described by Smythe *et al.* (1977). In this, treatment differences in the various indices in the entire population sample (treated and control groups) are converted into derived units (normalized) by dividing them by their standard deviations. Such derived measures have a common initial value of zero, a common standard deviation of 1, and a similar range and mean. The grand mean of all the measurements is the 'pooled index' in derived units.

Another method, used by Eberl and colleagues (1976), is the 'components of variance' analysis of variance performed for each variable measured clinically. This technique provides insight into the reasons for variability and is a reasonable measure of the reliability of a clinical measurement. The latter – the 'coefficient of generalizability' – has been calculated for morning stiffness, the ARA joint count, the Ritchie articular index, and other systems of evaluation. All were found to be acceptably reliable, having coefficient values of at least 0·88 (ideal value 1·00).

Detailed methods for evaluating the structural and functional status of the rheumatoid hand have been proposed by Flatt (1963) and by Swanson *et al.* (1968), and a less detailed, rapid method with standardization by a vigorous item-by-item statistical analysis has been described by Trenhaft *et al.* (1971).

2.4.4 Clinical trials

The general principles of clinical trial design apply not only to drugs but to other modes of therapy such as physical treatment and surgery. It will be appreciated, however, that the approach to assessing a therapy may not follow optimal criteria for ethical and practical reasons. For example, the 'counsel of perfection' that it may be possible to apply to assessing 'simple' drug therapy will not be possible when assessing surgery, radiotherapy, or cancer chemotherapy. In these cases, clinical trials based on random selection would be unacceptable and resort would have to be made to historical comparisons.

There are many reasons for starting a clinical trial and, particularly concerning drugs, it may be intended to answer one or more of the following questions:

1. Does the proposed treatment have any benefit at all?

2. What is the optimal dosage range?
3. How does it compare with standard therapy?
4. Is it safe?

These questions are also appropriate to non-drug forms of treatment, such as radiotherapy and physical treatment, and with the exception of (2), to surgery.

Concerning drug trials, question (1) may be subdivided:

(a) Is the drug of symptomatic value?
(b) Does it have a controlling or a curative effect?

Further general points to emphasize in planning a clinical trial are that there is no 'right' or 'wrong' way to design a trial. The definitive plan will represent a distillation of the type of therapy to be assessed, the therapeutic questions to be answered, and the demographic/diagnostic details of the patients to be studied. Regarding the questions to be answered, it is preferable that in any one trial attention be focused on answering only one main question. It is a common mistake to try to answer questions about subgroups of the disease in a general trial. For example, when comparing the effectiveness of drug A with drug B on spinal symptoms in ankylosing spondylitis, one should avoid comparing their effect on say, uveitis or other often 'after-thought' comparisons. (If this type of information is required, patients specially selected for this clinical feature should be studied.)

With regard to the nature of the patient population to be studied the following factors should be clearly defined:

1. Diagnosis.
2. Age.
3. Sex.
4. Severity of symptoms.
5. Stage of disease.
6. Activity of disease.
7. Previous treatment.
8. Complications of the disease.
9. Additional diseases.
10. Drug history.
11. Patient individuality.

Clinical trials may be classified as follows:

1. Open studies.
2. Single-blind studies.
3. Double-blind studies.

All of the above may compare placebo with one or two active treatments, or compare two or more active treatments.

Trials may be further subdivided:

(a) Between-patient studies in which separate groups of patients each receive a different treatment.

(b) Crossover (within-patient) studies in which the patient receives more than one treatment.

For further details the reader is referred to Fowler (1980).

The methods of therapeutic assessment for drug trial purposes have been discussed in Sections 2.4.2 and 2.4.3 and will only be summarized here:

1. Pain.
2. Morning stiffness.
3. Range of movement.
4. Function.
5. Radiological changes.
6. Laboratory investigations.
7. Overall assessment.

The main three methods of overall assessment (7) are:

(a) Comparison with pre-trial condition of treatment.
(b) Description of general condition.
(c) Preference for one or other treatment in a crossover study.

2.5 DIAGNOSTIC CRITERIA

2.5.1 General comment

There are three main uses for diagnostic criteria:

1. As a *guide* to clinical diagnosis of individual patients.
2. In population surveys to measure the size of a disease problem.
3. In the field of drug assessment and in other therapeutic trials.

In (2) and (3) homogeneity of diagnosis is of the essence. The last listed need for diagnostic criteria is clearly of particular relevance to the subject of this book.

2.5.2 Diagnostic criteria for certain rheumatic disorders

Diagnostic criteria have been established for a number of rheumatological entities, and these are summarized in Table 2.2. For some rheumatic disorders, no more than loose definitions exist, and further study is required to establish generally agreed criteria for these conditions. Perhaps it should be noted that the setting up of criteria does not necessarily prove their worth; this can only be achieved by subsequent evaluation, preferably using objective methodology and comparisons with control data obtained from normal populations (Moll, 1980).

Table 2.2 Literature relating to diagnostic criteria and definitions of some rheumatic and allied disorders

Rheumatic disorder	Reference(s)
Rheumatoid arthritis	Kellgren *et al.* (1963)
	Bennett and Wood (1968)
Systemic lupus erythematosus	Mustakallio *et al.* (1966)
	Barnett (1969)
Systemic sclerosis	Masi *et al.* (1978)
Ankylosing spondylitis	Kellgren *et al.* (1963)
	Bennett and Wood (1968)
	Moll and Wright (1973a)
	Moll (1980)
Psoriatic arthritis	Hench (1927)
	Jeghers and Robinson (1937)
	Dawson and Tyson (1938)
	Epstein (1939)
	Bauer *et al.* (1941)
	Fawcitt (1950)
	Sterne and Schneider (1953)
	Pillsbury *et al.* (1956)
	Wright (1956)
	Meaney and Hays (1957)
	Short *et al.* (1957)
	Carrier (1958)
	Moll (1971)
	Moll and Wright (1973b)
Reiter's disease	Paronen (1948)
	Czonka (1958)
	Maddocks (1967)
	Dunlop *et al.* (1968)
	Ford (1968)
Juvenile chronic polyarthritis	Ansell and Bywaters (1959)
Rheumatic fever	WHO (1966)
	Bisno and Ofek (1974)
Gout	Kellgren *et al.* (1963)
	Bennett and Wood (1968)
	Chalmers *et al.* (1970)
Osteoarthrosis	Bennett and Wood (1968)
Disc degeneration	Kellgren (1963)
Chondrocalcinosis	Lawrence (1977)
Ankylosing hyperostosis	Lawrence (1977)
Osteoporosis	Cameron and Sorenson (1963)
	Horsman (1976)
Paget's disease of bone	Collins (1956)

2.6 TEAM APPROACH IN MANAGEMENT

2.6.1 General comment

Some rheumatic disorders respond to a simple regimen of therapy. Subdeltoid bursitis, for example, usually responds to a local injection of corticosteroids and basic range-of-motion exercises. Most arthritic disorders, however, require rather complex, comprehensive programmes to achieve the goals of pain relief, improved function, prevention of deformity, and, when possible, cosmesis or even cure. The team concept of management is a *sine qua non* in the care of patients with anything more than simple, isolated problems that can be remedied by simple, isolated treatments. In fact, team management may be regarded as a modality in its own right. The team approach requires not only doctors and therapists, but a concerted, well-timed programme which should be regularly reassessed and modified if necessary. Without this, it is apt to fail and will produce results no better than those obtained by team members working in isolation.

The rheumatology centre is a relatively recent concept underlying organized team care and originated in specialised treatment centres, many of which began as spas. While most centres are now hospital based, this is not essential. Nor must they necessarily be in-patient orientated. However, it is important that the centres serve as referral organizations committed first to complete assessment and diagnosis, and then to the total management of the rheumatic patient.

It is a reasonable expectation that an institution housing the centre for rheumatic diseases (whether a general or special hospital) should contain full diagnostic and therapeutic services, including the availability of professional expertise in specialities other than rheumatology. Furthermore, the centre should be responsible for clinical and basic research and medical and paramedical training.

The structure of the rheumatology team and the interrelationships between its members might vary from centre to centre, but in general it follows a pattern as charted in Fig. 2.11, which represents the system operable in the author's unit. The basic roles of the individual members of the team are defined in the next section, with the caveat that the patient is also a member of the team.

2.6.2 Responsibilities of individual members of the team

Any scheme of suggestions (and they are no more than this) relating to individual roles within the rheumatology team should be interpreted against the backcloth of local, national, and international factors prevailing. Another modifying factor concerns the system of medical care, i.e. whether it is largely associated with private medical insurance schemes, as in the USA, or whether it is based largely on a national health service, as in the UK. It is therefore impossible to delineate a universal approach, or even a 'mid-Atlantic' one, although the following recommendations perhaps represent a workable compromise.

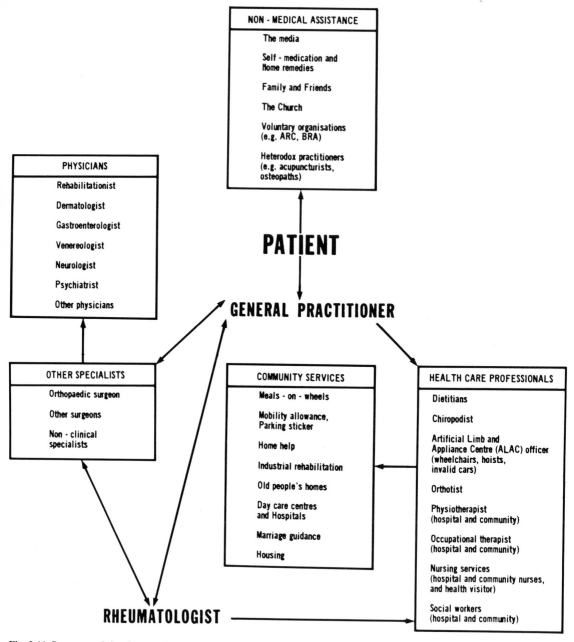

Fig. 2.11 Structure of the rheumatology team and some interrelationships within it.

The responsibilities of the various members of the rheumatology team have been well summarized by others, particularly by Katz (1977), and one can do no better than to quote extensively from this source (Appendix 2.1) with some modifications to allow for USA–UK differences. For additional details the reader is referred to Ehrlich (1973), Hill (1978), and Nichols (1980).

Table 2.3 Matrix showing large variety in therapeutic scope between clinical entities (listed vertically) and between treatment procedures (listed horizontally)

Relevant chapter for further therapeutic detail:	Communication	Simple analgesics	Analgesic anti-inflammatories	Corticosteroids and corticotrophins	Long-term suppressants	Other specific antirheumatics	Adjuvant drugs	Local injection therapy	Radiotherapy	Surgery	Physiotherapy	Occupational therapy	Other supportive measures
	3	5	5	6	6	6	6	7	8	9	10	10	10
Rheumatoid arthritis and variants	+++	+++	+++	+	++	++	++	+++	−	+++	+++	+++	+++
The spondarthritides	+++	+++	+++	(+)	+	+	+	++	(+)	+++	+++	+++	+++
Degenerative joint disease	+++	+++	++	−	−	−	−	++	−	++	+++	+++	+++
Crystal-induced joint disease	+++	+++	++	−	−	+	+	+	−	−	−	−	+
Inflammatory disorders of connective tissue	+++	+++	++	++	++	++	++	+	−	−	+++	++	++
Vasculitic syndromes	+++	++	++	++	+	++	++	−	−	++	++	+	+
Infective arthritis	+	+	−	−	−	−	−	−	−	++	+	−	−
Joint disease of systemic disorders	+++	+++	+	−	−	−	++	−	−	+++	+++	+++	−
Heritable disorders	+++	+++	−	−	−	++	+	−	−	++	+++	+++	+++
Disorders of bone and cartilage	+++	+++	−	−	−	++	+	−	+	+++	+++	+++	+++
Neoplastic disorders	+++	+++	+++	−	−	+	+	++	+	+++	+++	+++	+++
'Medical orthopaedic' problems	+++	+++	+++	(+)	+	−	+	+	−	+	+++	+++	+++
Childhood disorders	+++	+	+	−	+	+	−	−	−	−	+++	−	+
Psychogenic syndromes	+++	++	+	−	−	−	+	−	−	−	+	+	+
Iatrogenic syndromes	+	(+)	−	−	−	−	−	−	−	−	−	+	+
Non-disease	+	−	−	−	−	−	−	−	−	−	−	−	−

2.7 SPECTRA OF THERAPEUTIC APPROACHES

Although it has not been the intention in this book to delineate individual therapeutic regimens for individual rheumatic entities, it is important to include a note on what may be termed 'principles of therapeutic spectra'. The principles to be outlined are applicable to all rheumatic problems – from the most trivial to the most complex.

2.7.1 General scope of therapy in rheumatology

The various therapeutic methods available to treat rheumatological disorders and the main categories of rheumatic conditions involved can be represented as a matrix (Table 2.3). This is intended to show, both vertically and horizontally, the large variety in therapeutic scope between clinical entities and between treatment procedures. It should be stressed that neither the list of clinical disorder categories nor the list of therapies is all-embracing, nor are the symbols indicating treatment/no treatment necessarily definitive. (For further details of individual treatment methods the reader is referred to the relevant chapters indicated at the top of the table.)

2.7.2 Breadth of the therapeutic spectrum

The fact that patients presenting to the rheumatologist, as to other specialists, only infrequently manifest isolated problems raises the principle of the *breadth* of the therapeutic spectrum. This is illustrated in Fig. 2.12, using psoriatic arthritis with attendant problems as an example. The figure emphasizes the 'lateral' scope posed by such a clinical 'full house', with its consequent need to consider in addition treatment of general features, 'co-diseases', 'complications', and fortuitously occurring 'coexisting disorders'. As will be reiterated elsewhere, the somewhat extravagant nature of this example is meant to underline the constantly recurring theme within rheumatology – a theme based on the fact that so often clinical problems involve more than isolated bone, joint and related structures.

Table 2.4 is intended to develop this theme, and shows the wide variation in spectral breadth between minor and major, and mild and severe conditions.

The telegraphic style of representing therapeutic components shown in Table 2.4 can be extended to what could be termed 'clinicotherapeutic formulae' with clinical problems on one side of the 'equation' and therapeutic 'solutions' on the other. Such a system of clinical shorthand could be used to document individual therapeutic problems or data for clinical studies. Using

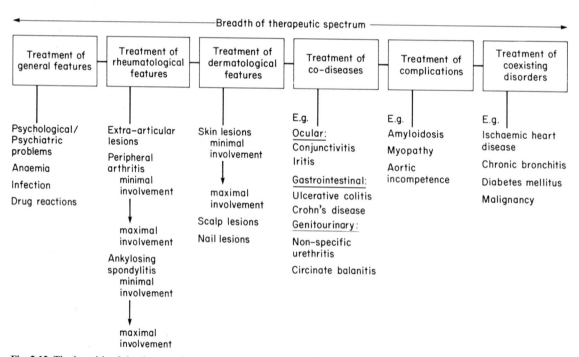

Fig. 2.12 The breadth of the therapeutic spectrum, using psoriatic arthritis and attendant problems as an example.

Table 2.4 Examples showing the variation in breadth of the therapeutic spectrum

Rheumatic problem	Breadth of various therapeutic spectra with components*
Minor aches and pains not reaching doctor	N
Infective arthritis	SD
De Quervain's tenosynovitis	C + LIT
Recurrent gout	C + AAD + SD
Moderate osteoarthrosis (with inflammatory component)	C + AAD + LIT + PT
Mild/moderate juvenile chronic polyarthritis	C + AAD + LIT + PT + OT
Moderate rheumatoid arthritis	C + AAD + SA + LIT + PT + OT
Severe osteoarthrosis	C + AAD + SA + LIT + PT + OT + S
Severe juvenile chronic polyarthritis	C + AAD + SA + SD + LIT + PT + OT + S
Severe juvenile chronic polyarthritis + eye disease	C + AAD + SA + SD + CS + LIT + PT + OT + S
Severe rheumatoid arthritis + anaemia	C + AAD + SA + SD + CS + AD + LIT + PT + OT + S
Severe ankylosing spondylitis + peripheral arthritis + co-disease	C + AAD + SA + SD + CS + AD + LIT + PT + OT + R† + S
Severe ankylosing spondylitis + peripheral arthritis + co-disease + psychiatric problem	C + AAD + SA + SD + CS + AD + LIT + PT + OT + R + S + PS

* Not necessarily in the order in which treatment is given.
† Treatment of peripheral joint, not spine or sacroiliac joints.
N = No treatment; C = Communication (advice/instruction); PS = psychotherapy; SA = simple analgesic; AAD = analgesic/anti-inflammatory drug; SC = corticosteroid or corticotrophin; SD = specific drug; AD = adjuvant drug; LIT = local injection therapy; R = radiotherapy; S = surgery; PT = physiotherapy; OT = occupational therapy.

symbols to denote clinical disorders (e.g. peripheral arthritis = *PA*; spondylitis = *S*; extra-articular involvement = *E*; co-disease = *CD*; complication = *C*; coexisting disease = *CE*), the range of clinicotherapeutic complexity can be expressed using the following examples from Table 2.4.

Treatment of infective arthritis:

$$PA = SD$$

Treatment of moderate rheumatoid arthritis:

$$PA + E = C + AAD + SA + LIT + PT + OT$$

Treatment of 'complicated' ankylosing spondylitis:

$$S + PA + E + CD + C + CE = C + AAD + SA + SD + CS + AD + LIT + PT + OT + R + S + PS$$

2.7.3 Depth of therapeutic spectra

Within patients bearing a single diagnostic label (e.g. uncomplicated rheumatoid arthritis) the therapeutic approach will vary according to the severity of the problem. 'Severity' may be taken to imply intensity and/or duration of clinical features.

Figs 2.13–2.16 provide examples, in terms of flow charts, of increasingly complicated therapeutic schemata which may be necessary in certain rheumatic conditions ('uncomplicated' lateral humeral epicondylitis, lumbar disc disease, ankylosing spondylitis, and rheumatoid arthritis, respectively) chosen to make this point. In each example, a progression in depth of

therapeutic penetration may be needed to manage refractory problems. With regard to the first three examples (Figs 2.13–2.15) all forms of therapy have been included in the spectrum. In the last example (Fig. 2.16) only drug therapy has been used to illustrate the principle. Further details about the principles involved in the more global management of rheumatoid arthritis are discussed in the next section.

2.8 APPLICATION OF THE TEAM APPROACH AND SPECTRAL SCOPE TO THE MANAGEMENT OF RHEUMATOID ARTHRITIS AND OTHER CHRONIC RHEUMATOSES

2.8.1 General comment

The following comments are applicable in varying degree to chronic inflammatory arthritides generally. However, the main focus will be on rheumatoid arthritis.

Many rheumatoid patients do not require the full complement of therapeutic modalities. The type of therapeutic approach will be governed by the type of disease, the duration of illness, its severity, the response or lack of response to previous therapy, the presence of coexisting disorders, concurrent drugs, and the potential for harmful side effects. Generally, the more aggressive the therapy, the greater the frequency and variety of iatrogenic disorders. In most instances it is

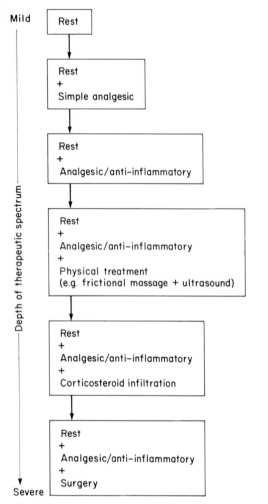

Fig. 2.13 Depth of therapeutic spectrum relating to lateral humeral epicondylitis (tennis elbow). The order and content of these therapeutic stages will vary between clinicians and according to clinical circumstances.

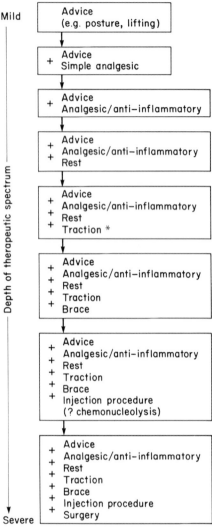

Fig. 2.14 Depth of therapeutic spectrum relating to lumbar disc disease. The order and content of these therapeutic stages will vary between clinicians and according to clinical circumstances. *Some patients respond to other manipulative techniques.

wise to start with a simple programme and advance to more sophisticated treatments if necessary. Usually, only the early phases of the multi-tiered management programme are required to effect a favourable outcome. In severe, rapidly progressing disease, some treatment phases have to be breached. Each previous phase may be continued together with the next one. Rheumatological management of rheumatoid arthritis and other chronic inflammatory arthritides is therefore based on an *additive* policy, rather than involving the replacement of a simple form of treatment by a more 'complicated' one.

2.8.2 Specific plans of management phasing

These therapeutic plans appertain to chronic rheumatoses such as rheumatoid arthritis and ankylosing spondylitis and have no place in the treatment of acute transient disorders (e.g. tennis elbow) or disorders with acute phases (e.g. gout).

There is no universally accepted 'ideal' scheme for management phasing in rheumatoid arthritis and other

Mild

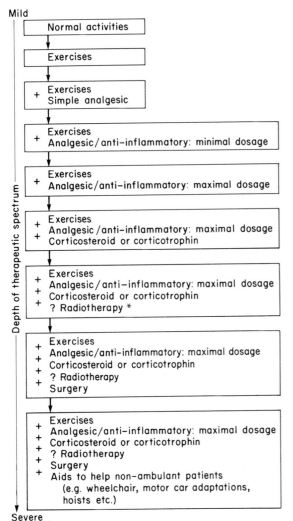

Fig. 2.15 Depth of therapeutic spectrum relating to ankylosing spondylitis; spinal involvement only (i.e. no peripheral joint involvement and no 'co-disease'). The order and content of these therapeutic stages will vary between clinicians and according to clinical circumstances. *This form of therapy for irradiation of the spine has fallen into disrepute. Occasionally it may be indicated for isolated peripheral joints where there is minimal danger of exposure to large areas of normal tissue.

Mild

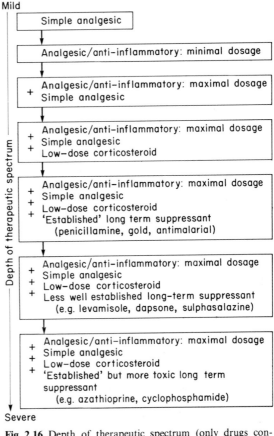

Fig. 2.16 Depth of therapeutic spectrum (only drugs considered) in rheumatoid arthritis. The order and content of these therapeutic stages will vary between clinicians and according to clinical circumstances.

rest; (3) maintain the team approach to management throughout.

The similarities, and certain differences, between management phasing schemes will perhaps be clarified by considering the following schedules advocated by Engleman (1960), Katz (1977), and Lightfoot (1979). These are listed in their original form, with the exception of some minor details. As mentioned previously the emphasis is on the management of rheumatoid arthritis.

(a) Engleman (1960)

Basic programme

1. *Systemic rest*: Daily rest, e.g. 2–4 hours in mild disease, allowing patient to continue at work by restricting only his avocational pursuits.
2. *Emotional rest*: Regular psychological support,

chronic rheumatoses, although common threads between different schemes are clearly discernible. The essential guiding principles to observe (in addition to the fundamental importance of establishing satisfactory doctor–patient rapport) are: (1) start with simple therapies, and progress to more complex treatment only if firmly indicated; (2) recognize the therapeutic value of though formal psychiatric intervention is rarely necessary.

3. *Articular rest*: This is accomplished by rest in bed and may be enhanced by appropriate supports and splints.
4. *Physical therapy*: The most important item being exercises.
5. *Drugs*: This category implies 'simple' analgesic/anti-inflammatory drugs such as aspirin, supplemented if necessary by plain analgesics such as dextropropoxyphene.
6. *Adequate nutrition.*

Additional programme

The above basic programme is recommended for *all* patients with rheumatoid arthritis. If these measures should prove inadequate, other measures such as corticosteroids, gold therapy and surgery are recommended.

(b) Katz (1977)

Phase I (Basic Programme)

Patient education and reassurance. The nature of the illness, plans for therapy, and outlook are described to the patient in sufficient detail. The patient is encouraged to ask questions and express himself freely.

Rest. Avoidance of weight bearing and partial or complete rest in bed is advised, depending upon the nature and course of the illness. Involved joints are put to rest by avoiding activity, splinting, or simple orthopaedic devices.

Analgesia. Relief of pain may be afforded by drugs, splinting, ice or heat, or by injections of local anaesthetic.

Specific therapy. Underlying diseases accounting for rheumatic symptoms are treated with 'specific' therapy if available (e.g. antibiotics for infectious arthritis, uric acid-lowering drugs for gout, long-term suppressants for rheumatoid arthritis). In this phase of treatment, life-saving measures are instituted if indicated.

Phase II

Drugs. Anti-inflammatory agents such as aspirin, phenylbutazone, indomethacin, naproxen, tolmetin, fenoprofen and ibuprofen are introduced. Local corticosteroids are administered as needed.

Physical therapy. Range-of-motion exercises to prevent contractures, muscle strengthening exercises, casting, and other simple physical modalities are added in this phase.

Phase III

Drugs. Oral corticosteroids are administered if indicated and if no other anti-inflammatory agent is effective. Remittive agents such as gold for rheumatoid arthritis and hydroxychloroquine for systemic lupus erythematosus or rheumatoid arthritis are prescribed.

Physical therapy. Therapy becomes more aggressive. Gait training and assistive devices to aid in activities of daily living are used.

Surgery. Preventive surgery such as early synovectomy is performed. Manipulation under anaesthesia is sometimes required.

Miscellaneous modalities. Hospitalization at this phase is often required. Family counselling and long-term planning for an established chronic rheumatic disease may be necessary. Special procedures and minor changes in job description are sometimes needed.

Phase IV

Drugs. Immunosuppressive agents, if indicated, may be introduced by experienced physicians at this stage.

Physical therapy. The programme is advanced, usually requiring a total rehabilitation effort. Devices to aid in activities of daily living are usually essential. Transfer and gait training techniques are applicable.

Surgery. Surgical intervention is usually for purposes of reconstruction and arthroplasty, including total joint replacements.

Miscellaneous. Occupational changes are usually required. Professional psychosocial support greatly aids the long-term management programme. Hospitalization in a rehabilitation centre is beneficial in this phase.

Phase V

Experimental drugs such as penicillamine, experimental surgery such as new types of total joint replacement, and long-term hospitalization are required for those few patients who fail to respond to the other phases of medical and surgical management.

(c) Lightfoot (1979)

Lightfoot's approach is expressed in terms of a treatment pyramid depicting relationships between the various therapies used in rheumatoid arthritis (Fig. 2.17).

My approach follows the general lines of the above schemes and, in terms of Lightfoot's pyramid for

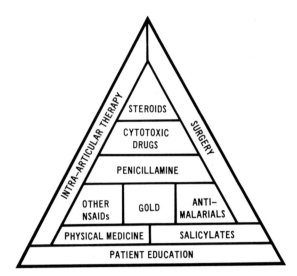

Fig. 2.17 Lightfoot's treatment pyramid to express the content of, and relationships between, treatments in the management plan for rheumatoid arthritis (redrawn from Lightfoot, 1979).

managing rheumatoid arthritis, can be summarized as in Fig. 2.18. It will be seen from this that the main difference between my approach and that of Lightfoot, for example, lies in the classification of first-, second- and other-line drugs, particularly the stage at which corticosteroids are used. The specific question of phasing drug therapy, as opposed to the total approaches used in the management armamentarium, will be discussed in Chapter 4.

2.9 WHEN IS THE PATIENT 'BETTER'?

Few patients with rheumatic disorders can be completely cured, although there are some dramatic examples of response to treatment, e.g. the response of both early rheumatoid arthritis and polymyalgia rheumatica to corticosteroids, the response of acute gout to colchicine, the response of infective arthropathies to antimicrobial agents, and the response of various soft-tissue syndromes to local corticosteroid injection. In these instances, the amelioration of the particular rheumatic crisis concerned will often be clear-cut enough to regard the patient as being 'better', even if not cured, and from the rheumatologist's point of view may signify the time to refer patients back to their family doctor.

In many instances, however, decisions of 'better' versus 'not better' are much less obvious, particularly in patients with established rheumatoid arthritis and other chronic rheumatoses such as ankylosing spondylitis. Patients needing long-term suppressant drugs are usual-

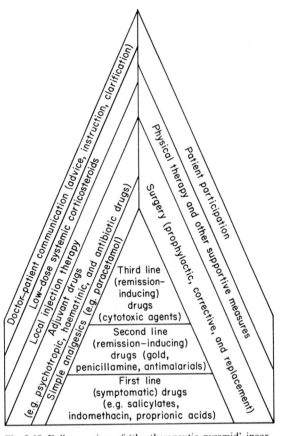

Fig. 2.18 Fuller version of 'the therapeutic pyramid' incorporating modifications based on personal preferences.

ly followed up routinely in the rheumatology clinic, but patients not requiring such supervision may be referred back to their family doctor during times of remission, with the emphasis that such decisions are based largely on clinical rather than on laboratory features. For example, it would seem unreasonable to keep a rheumatoid patient, who is otherwise well, on the hospital books solely because of a persistently raised ESR. Further appointments can always be made if especially indicated, such as problems with drug side effects, lack of therapeutic response, the need for local corticosteroid injections, or the need for other specialist aspects of treatment such as physical therapy or surgical referral. Such a system obviously depends on a satisfactory rapport between the hospital and family doctor.

Having made these comments, rheumatologists in fact vary considerably in their preparedness to refer patients back to their family doctor, and some of these differences will depend on the interest of individual family doctors in managing rheumatic disorders. In my view, patients should be returned to primary care as soon as this is clinically sensible, both for the patient's sake, to boost their sense of personal freedom, and for the sake of preventing inordinate build-up of hospital waiting lists.

However, a common problem is the patient with long-established rheumatoid disease who has become 'hospitalized'. These patients, often elderly, seem to come to rely on their hospital attendances, not so much for specific therapeutic measures, but for the sociodomestic comfort they provide. Such long-established relationships between patient and hospital can be difficult to break. The back-log of patients attending hospital unnecessarily is easier to control if the specialist follows up his own patients. Where this responsibility is deputed to constantly changing junior members of staff, positive decisions to refer patients back to their family doctor are less readily made.

2.11 REFERENCES AND FURTHER READING

General comment

Arthritis Foundation (1976) *Annual Report*, Arthritis Foundation, New York.
Wood, P.H.N. (1977) *The Challenge of Arthritis and Rheumatism*, British League Against Rheumatism, London, p. 2.

Size and scope of the rheumatic problem

Lawrence, J.S. (1977) *Rheumatism in Populations*, Heinemann, London, pp. 32–67.

Indications for referral to a rheumatologist

Katz, W.A. (1977) in *Rheumatic Diseases: Diagnosis and Management* (ed. W.A. Katz), Lippincott, Philadelphia, p. 7.

Clinical assessment and evaluation schemes

American Academy of Orthopaedic Surgeons (1966) *Joint Motion: Method of Measuring and Recording*, Churchill Livingstone, Edinburgh, p. 50.
Bacon, P.A., Collins, A.J., Ring, F.J. and Cosh, J.A. (1976) In *Clinics in Rheumatic Diseases*, Vol. 2, No. 1, *Diagnosis and Assessment* (ed. M.I.V. Jayson), Saunders, London, p. 51.
Cooperating Clinics Committee of the American Rheumatism Association (1965) A seven-day variability study of 499 patients with peripheral rheumatoid arthritis. *Arthr. Rheum.*, **8**, 302.
Deodhar, S.D., Dick, W.C., Hodgkinson, R. and Buchanan, W.W. (1973) Measurement of clinical response to anti-inflammatory drug therapy in rheumatoid arthritis. *Q. J. Med.* (*New Series*), **42**, 387.

2.10 SUMMARY AND CONCLUSIONS

This chapter has been intended to provide a perspective prelude to subsequent chapters – a bird's eye view on rheumatological management.

The chapter has emphasized that rheumatological management must involve a team approach. It also discusses such subjects as the size of the rheumatic problem, indications for referral to a rheumatologist, methods of assessment, diagnostic criteria, the team approach to management, phases of therapy, spectra of therapeutic approaches, and factors involved in deciding when the patient is 'better'.

Provided that management of the patient with a chronic rheumatosis is based on a cohesive approach, with management viewed as a stage-wise procedure, there is much to offer rheumatic patients, even if most of them cannot be cured.

Dunham, W.F. (1949) Ankylosing spondylitis: measurement of hip and spine movement. *Br. J. Phys. Med.*, **12**, 126.
Eberl, D.R., Fasching, V., Rahlfs, V. *et al.* (1976) Repeatability and objectivity of various measurements in rheumatoid arthritis. *Arthr. Rheum.*, **19**, 1278.
Flatt, A.E. (1963) *Rheumatoid Hand Research Project* (Booklets), Department of Orthopaedics, University of Iowa, Iowa City.
Fowler, P.D. (1980) in *Ankylosing Spondylitis* (ed. J.M.H. Moll), Churchill Livingstone, Edinburgh, p. 176.
Green, F.A. and Hays, M.T. (1972) The pertechnetate joint scan: II. Clinical correlations. *Ann. Rheum. Dis.*, **31**, 278.
Haberman, J.A., Sisk, C.W., Tourtellotte, C.D. *et al.* (1971) Thermography in arthritis. *Arthr. Rheum.*, **14**, 387.
Hart, F.D., Strickland, D. and Cliffe, P. (1974) Measurement of spinal mobility. *Ann. Rheum. Dis.*, **33**, 136.
Hays, M.T. and Green, F.A. (1972) The pertechnetate joint scan. I. Timing. *Ann. Rheum. Dis.*, **31**, 272.
Lansbury, J. (1958) Report of a three-year study on the systemic and articular indexes in rheumatoid arthritis: theoretical and clinical considerations. *Arthr. Rheum.*, **1**, 505.
Lansbury, J., Baier, H.N. and McCracken, S. (1962) Statistical study of variation in systemic and articular indexes. *Arthr. Rheum.*, **5**, 445.
Lee, P., Jasani, M.K., Dick, W.C. and Buchanan, W.W. (1973) Evaluation of a functional index in rheumatoid arthritis. *Scand. J. Rheumatol.*, **2**, 71.
Loebl, W.Y. (1967) Measurement of spinal posture and range of spinal movement. *Ann. Phys. Med.*, **9**, 103.
Macrae, I.F. and Wright, V. (1968) Measurement of back movement. *Ann. Rheum. Dis.*, **28**, 584.
McCarty, D.J. (1972) in *Arthritis and Allied Conditions. A Textbook of Rheumatology* (eds. J.L. Hollander and D.J. McCarty), 8th edn, Lea and Febiger, Philadelphia, p. 420.
McCarty, D.J. (1979) in *Arthritis and Allied Conditions. A Textbook of Rheumatology* (ed. D.J. McCarty), 9th edn, Lea and Febiger, Philadelphia, p. 142.
McCarty, D.J., Poleyn, R.E. and Collins, P.A. (1970) 99^{m}

Technetium scintiphotography in arthritis. II. Its nonspecificity and clinical and roentgenographic correlation in rheumatoid arthritis. *Arthr. Rheum.*, **13**, 21.

McQuire, R.J. and Wright, V. (1971) Statistical approach to indices of disease activity in rheumatoid arthritis. *Ann. Rheum. Dis.*, **30**, 574.

Moll, J.M.H. (1975) A diagnostic feature of spondylitis. *Scand. J. Rheumatol.*, **4**, Suppl. 1, Abstract 2017.

Moll, J.M.H. and Wright, V. (1971) Normal range of spinal mobility: an objective clinical study. *Ann. Rheum. Dis.*, **30**, 381.

Moll, J.M.H. and Wright, V. (1972) An objective clinical study of chest expansion. *Ann. Rheum. Dis.*, **31**, 1.

Moll, J.M.H. and Wright, V. (1973a) New York clinical criteria for ankylosing spondylitis – a statistical evaluation. *Ann. Rheum. Dis.*, **32**, 354.

Moll, J.M.H. and Wright, V. (1973b) The pattern of chest and spinal mobility in ankylosing spondylitis – an objective clinical study of 106 patients. *Rheumatol. Rehabil.*, **12**, 115.

Moll, J.M.H. and Wright, V. (1976) In *Clinics in Rheumatic Diseases*, Vol. 2, No. 1. *Diagnosis and Assessment* (ed. M.I.V. Jayson), Saunders, London, p. 3.

Moll, J. and Wright, V. (1980) in *The Lumbar Spine and Back Pain* (ed. M.I.V. Jayson), 2nd edn, Pitman, Tunbridge Wells, p. 157.

Moll, J.M.H., Liyanage, S.P. and Wright, V. (1972a) An objective clinical method to measure lateral spinal flexion. *Rheumatol. Phys. Med.*, **11**, 293.

Moll, J.M.H., Liyanage, S.P. and Wright, V. (1972b) An objective clinical method to measure spinal extension. *Rheumatol. Phys. Med.*, **11**, 293.

Nicholas, J.J., Taylor, F.H., Buckingham, R.B. and Ottonello, D. (1976) Measurement of circumference of the knee with ordinary tape measure. *Ann. Rheum. Dis.*, **35**, 282.

Ritchie, D.M., Boyle, J.A., McInnes, J.M. *et al.* (1958) Clinical studies with an articular index for the assessment of joint tenderness in patients with rheumatoid arthritis. *Q. J. Med. (New Series)*, **37**, 393.

Smythe, H., Helewa, A. and Goldsmith, C.A. (1977) 'Independent assessor' and 'Pooled index' as techniques for measuring treatment effects in rheumatoid arthritis. *J. Rheumatol.*, **4**, 144.

Smyth, C.J., Velayos, E.E. and Hlad, C.J. (1963) A method for measuring swelling of hands and feet, Part I: Normal variations and applications in inflammatory joint diseases. *Acta Rheumatol. Scand.*, **9**, 293.

Steele, A.D. and McCarty, D.J. (1966) An experimental model of acute inflammation in man. *Arthr. Rheum.*, **9**, 430.

Steinbrocker, O., Traeger, C.H. and Batterman, R.C. (1949) Therapeutic criteria in rheumatoid arthritis. *J. Am. Med. Assoc.*, **140**, 659.

Sturrock, R.D., Wojtulewski, J.A. and Hart, F.D. (1973) Spondylometry in a normal population and in ankylosing spondylitics. *Rheumatol. Rehab.*, **12**, 135.

Swanson, A.B., Mays, J.D. and Yamuchi, Y. (1968) A rheumatoid arthritis evaluation record for the upper extremity. *Surg. Clin. N. Am.*, **48**, 1003.

Taylor, D. (1937) A table for the degree of involvement in chronic arthritis. *Can. Med. Assoc. J.*, **36**, 608.

Trenhaft, P.S., Lewis, M.R. and McCarty, D.J. (1971) A rapid method for evaluating the structure and function of the rheumatoid hand. *Arthr. Rheum.*, **14**, 75.

Willkens, R.F., Gleichert, J.E. and Gade, E.T. (1973) Proximal interphalangeal joint measurement by arthrocircameter. *Ann. Rheum. Dis.*, **32**, 585.

Wright, V. and Johns, R.J. (1960) Observations on the measurement of joint stiffness. *Arthr. Rheum.*, **3**, 328.

Diagnostic criteria

Ansell, B.M. and Bywaters, E.G.L. (1959) Prognosis in Still's disease. *Bull. Rheum. Dis.*, **9**, 189.

Barnett, E.V. (1969) Diagnostic aspects of LE cells and antinuclear factor. *Proc. Mayo Clin.*, **44**, 645.

Bauer, W., Bennett, G.A. and Zeller, J.W. (1941) Pathology of joint lesions in patients with psoriasis and arthritis. *Trans. Assoc. Am. Phys.*, **56**, 349.

Bennett, P.H. and Wood, P.H.N. (1968) *Population Studies of the Rheumatic Diseases*. Excerpta Medica, Amsterdam.

Bisno, A.L. and Ofek, I. (1974) Serologic diagnosis of streptococcal infection. *Am. J. Dis. Child.*, **127**, 676.

Cameron, J.R. and Sorenson, J. (1963) Measurement of bone mineral in vivo: an improved method. *Science*, **142**, 230.

Carrier, J.W. (1958) Psoriatic arthritis. *Am. J. Roentgenol.*, **74**, 612.

Chalmers, T.M., Danchot, J., Kellgren, J.H. *et al.* (1970) Test of diagnostic criteria – experience in England and Wales, *Ann. Rheum. Dis.*, **29**, 200.

Collins, D.H. (1956) Paget's disease of bone: incidence and subclinical forms. *Lancet*, **ii**, 51.

Csonka, G.W. (1958) The course of Reiter's syndrome. *Br. Med. J.*, **i**, 1088.

Dawson, M.H. and Tyson, T.L. (1938) Psoriasis arthropathia with observations on certain features common to psoriasis and rheumatoid arthritis. *Trans. Assoc. Am. Phys.*, **53**, 303.

Dunlop, E.M.C., Harper, I.A. and Jones, B.R. (1968) Seronegative polyarthritis. The bedsonia group of agents and Reiter's disease. *Ann. Rheum. Dis.*, **27**, 334.

Epstein, E. (1939) Differential diagnosis of keratosis blenorrhagica and psoriatic arthropathy. *Arch. Dermatol. Syphilis*, **40**, 547.

Fawcitt, J. (1950) Bone and joint changes associated with psoriasis. *Br. J. Radiol.*, **23**, 440.

Ford, D.K. (1968) Non-gonococcal urethritis and Reiter's syndrome. *Can. Med. Assoc. J.*, **99**, 900.

Hench, P.S. (1927) Arthropathia psoriatica – presentation of a case. *Proc. Mayo Clin.*, **2**, 89.

Horsman, A. (1976) In *Calcium, Phosphate and Magnesium Metabolism* (ed. B.E.C. Nordin), Churchill Livingstone, Edinburgh, p. 357.

Jeghers, H. and Robinson, L.J. (1937) Arthropathica psoriatica – report of a case and discussion of the pathogenesis, diagnosis and treatment. *J. Am. Med. Assoc.*, **108**, 949.

Kellgren, J.H. (1963) *The Epidemiology of Chronic Rheumatism*, Vol. 2, *Atlas of Standard Radiographs of Arthritis*, Blackwell, Oxford.

Kellgren, J.H., Jeffrey, M.R. and Ball, J. (1963) *Epidemiology of Chronic Rheumatism*, Vol. 1, Blackwell, Oxford.

Lawrence, J.S. (1977) *Rheumatism in Populations*, Heinemann, London.

Maddocks, I. (1967) Reiter's disease in Port Moresby, Papua. *Br. J. Ven. Dis.*, **43**, 280.

Masi, A.T., Rodnan, G.P., Medsger, T.A., *et al.* (1978) Clinical criteria for early diagnosed systemic sclerosis: preliminary results of the ARA Multicenter Cooperative Study. *Arthr. Rheum.*, **21**, 576.

Meaney, T.F. and Hays, R.A. (1957) Roentgen manifestations of psoriatic arthritis. *Radiology*, **68**, 403.

Moll, J.M.H. (1971) *A Family Study of Psoriatic Arthritis.* D.M. thesis, University of Oxford.

Moll, J.M.H. (1980) in *Ankylosing Spondylitis* (ed. J.M.H. Moll), Churchill Livingstone, Edinburgh, p. 137.

Moll, J.M.H. and Wright, V. (1973a) New York clinical criteria for ankylosing spondylitis: A statistical evaluation. *Ann. Rheum. Dis.*, **32**. 354.

Moll, J.M.H. and Wright, V. (1973b) Psoriatic arthritis. *Sem. Arthr. Rheum.*, **3**, 55.

Mustakallio, K.K., Lassus, A. and Putkonen, T. (1966) Factor analysis in the evaluation of criteria and variants of SLE. *Meth. Inf. Med. (Bielefeld)*, **5**, 184.

Paronen, I. (1948) Reiter's disease. A study of 344 cases observed in Finland. *Acta Med. Scand.*, **131**, Suppl., 212.

Pillsbury, D.M., Shelley, W.B. and Kligman, A.M. (1956) *Dermatology*, Saunders, Philadelphia, p. 728.

Schurman, D., Calin, A., Fries, J. and Porta, J. (1977) in *Proceedings of the XIV International Congress of Rheumatology*, San Francisco, 1977, Abstract 770, Arthritis Foundation, New York, p. 181.

Short, L.C., Bauer, W. and Reynolds, W.E. (1957) *Rheumatoid Arthritis*, Harvard University Press, Cambridge, Mass., p. 38.

Sterne, E.H. and Schneider, B. (1953) Psoriatic arthritis. *Ann. Int. Med.*, **38**, 512.

Wallace, S.L., Robinson, H., Masi, A.T. *et al.* (1977) Preliminary criteria for the classification of the acute arthritis of primary gout. *Arthr. Rheum.*, **2**, 895.

Waller, M. and Toone, E.C. (1968) Normal individuals with positive tests for rheumatoid factor. *Arthr. Rheum.*, **11**, 50.

WHO Expert Committee (1966) Preventing rheumatic fever. *WHO Tech. Rep. Ser.*, Geneva, No. 342.

Wright, V. (1956) Psoriasis and arthritis. *Ann. Rheum. Dis.*, **15**, 348.

Team approach in management

Ehrlich, G.E. (1973) in *Total Management of the Arthritic Patient* (ed. G.E. Ehrlich), Lippincott, Philadelphia, pp. 211–13.

Hill, A.G.S. (1978) in *Copeman's Textbook of the Rheumatic Diseases* (ed. J.T. Scott), 5th edn, Churchill Livingstone, Edinburgh, p. 400.

Katz, W.A. (1977) in *Rheumatic Diseases: Diagnosis and Management* (ed. W.A. Katz), Lippincott, Philadelphia, p. 865.

Nichols, P.J.R. (ed.) (1980) *Rehabilitation Medicine. The Management of Physical Disabilities*, 2nd edn, Butterworths, London.

Specific plans of management phasing

Engleman, E.P. (1960) in *Arthritis and Allied Conditions: A Textbook of Rheumatology* (ed. J.L. Hollander), 6th edn, Krimpton, London, p. 275.

Katz, W.A. (1977) in *Rheumatic Diseases: Diagnosis and Management* (ed. W.A. Katz), Lippincott, Philadelphia, pp. 866–7.

Lightfoot, R.W. (1979) in *Arthritis and Allied Conditions: A Textbook of Rheumatology* (ed. D.J. McCarty), 9th edn, Lea and Febiger, Philadelphia, p. 513.

2.12 APPENDIX: ROLES OF INDIVIDUAL MEMBERS OF THE MANAGEMENT TEAM (AFTER KATZ, 1977)

Patients

1. Openly relate symptoms and problems to the physician and paramedical personnel.
2. Gain an understanding of the nature of their disease.
3. Report untoward effects of medication or other forms of therapy.
4. Maximally co-operate in all aspects of the programme.

Family doctor (general practitioner)

1. Gain a knowledge of rheumatic diseases sufficient to recognize at least the nature of his patient's complaints and to initiate the basic programme.
2. Refer to the rheumatologist and/or rheumatology centre problems in diagnosis and management.

3. Co-operate with rheumatology team members and take part, when possible, in conferences and discussions relevant to his patient.
4. Continue the daily long-term care of the patient, seeking consultation regularly with the team when necessary.

Rheumatologist

1. Obtain a thorough assessment, clinical and ancillary, of his patient and establish as precise a diagnosis as possible.
2. Co-ordinate the activities of the total team.
3. Recommend short- and long-term medical management.
4. Prescribe analgesic, anti-inflammatory, and long-term suppressant drugs.
5. Carry out specialized in-patient and out-patient procedures.
6. Arrange team and family conferences periodically.
7. Communicate and co-operate closely with the referring family doctor.
8. Inform the patient of his illness and prepare him for any new investigations and therapies that may be necessary.
9. Consult with the surgeon before and after surgery, and

provide close patient observation and management after surgical procedures.
10. Consult with other specialists relevant to the patient.
11. Provide reassurance and psychological support to the patient and family members.
12. Rectify any breakdowns in the overall team management approach.
13. Train other physicians in the diagnostic and management aspects of rheumatic diseases.
14. Check regularly, and update if necessary, the ancillary facilities of the rheumatology centre.
15. Conduct basic and clinical rheumatological research.

Other physicians may assume in part the role of the rheumatologist but have specific responsibilities as well.

Rehabilitationist

1. Appraise the patient regarding the nature of the functional disability.
2. Be aware of medical problems that will interfere with the total rehabilitation programme.
3. Prescribe physical and occupational therapy.
4. Assess the need for and prescribe braces, splints, and other supportive devices. Recommend training in transportation.
5. Monitor the progression of walking re-training.
6. Supervise occupational and physical therapists.
7. Prepare the patient for vocational re-training and communicate with vocational rehabilitation personnel, if available.
8. Continually reassess rehabilitation goals.

Other physicians

This category includes dermatologists, ophthalmologists, gastroenterologists, cardiologists, venereologists, nephrologists, endocrinologists, haematologists, pulmonary specialists, psychiatrists, dentists, and radiologists who may be called upon to work with team members when appropriate problems arise.

Orthopaedic surgeon

1. Evaluate certain patients admitted to the rheumatology centre even if surgery is not considered imminent.
2. Recommend manipulative or orthopaedic devices that may benefit the patient.
3. Recommend surgery and explain both short- and long-term goals to the patient and to other members of the team.
4. Set up a schedule of staged procedures when multiple joints are involved.
5. Provide close postoperative follow-up.
6. Work closely with the rheumatologist on special problems of anticoagulation, corticosteroid coverage, etc.
7. Keep abreast of, and if possible undertake research in, new procedures for relieving pain and preventing deformity.

Hospital nurse

Occupational therapist

Physiotherapist

Social worker

see Chapter 10

3
Communication: the basis of management

There is virtually no medical activity in which communication is unimportant.

Fletcher, 1973

3.1 INTRODUCTORY COMMENT

Perhaps the best way to express the meaning of medical education generally and doctor–patient communication in particular is to put the following questions: Do my patients really understand the information I have given them? Do I listen to them if they have any doubts? Does the information I give them lead to their following my instructions? Clearly these questions involve overlap between 'pure' communication and related aspects such as feedback and compliance. Fig. 3.1 illustrates these relationships.

Patients derive information from many sources (Fig. 3.2), and confusion may arise through conflict between such advice. Satisfactory communication between medical personnel and patients should, therefore, involve not only effective and reliable explanation of the facts but also clarification where there is confusion. The justification for devoting a separate chapter in this book to the subject of communication rests on the belief that in rheumatology, as in many other medical specialties, the standard of medical care depends largely on satisfactory communication between medical personnel and patients. On the positive side, there is evidence that good communication can result in psychological and even physical improvement of patients; and on the negative side bad communication can be detrimental and even fatal. These general aspects of communication both in hospital and community practice have been discussed in depth elsewhere (Cartwright, 1964, 1967; Ley and Spelman, 1967; Fletcher, 1973, 1979; Harlem, 1977; Moll and Wright, 1978; Moll, 1982).

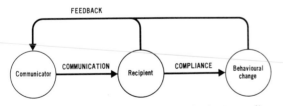

Fig. 3.1 Relationship between communication, compliance and feedback (from Moll, 1981).

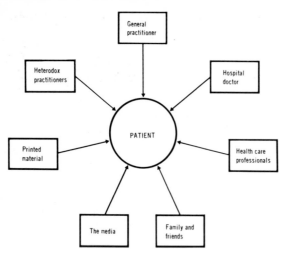

Fig. 3.2 Some sources from which patients derive information.

3.2 GENERAL PRINCIPLES OF COMMUNICATION

Fletcher (1973) has outlined some general principles of communication. These may be summarized as follows:

1. The purpose of communication is not just to deliver a message but to effect a change in the recipient in respect of his knowledge, his attitude and, eventually, his behaviour (compliance).
2. The value of a communication is to be judged not on its purpose or content, but on its effect on the recipient. An elegant or witty communication may satisfy the communicator but leave the recipient uninformed and unmoved.
3. Good communication is difficult. Few can master it without special tuition and without constant attention to its effectiveness.
4. Communication must be matched against a back-cloth embodying the recipient's knowledge, social background, interests, purposes, and needs. To this may be added the recipient's personality.
5. Communication is transmitted not only by words, which must have the same meaning for giver and receiver, but also by attitudes, expressions, and gestures. This is especially relevant in the consultation, where patient and doctor are both givers and receivers.
6. If communication is to change behaviour, the required change in the recipient must be seen by him to have more advantages than drawbacks. Otherwise a change will not ensue or, if it does, will not persist.
7. To ensure that a communication has been successful,

information about its effects (feedback), both immediate or subsequent, is needed. In the consultation setting the doctor sometimes fails to utilize the feedback information by not listening to the patient.
8. Communication demands effort, thought, time, and often money.

3.3 IMPORTANCE OF COMMUNICATION IN RHEUMATOLOGY

The particular relevance of satisfactory communication in rheumatology has already been emphasized by the late Dr Michael Mason (Joyce *et al.*, 1969), who pointed out that in some rheumatic patients self-help is the most that can be offered. For example, controlling weight, carrying out regular exercises, and protecting certain joints are all aspects of management that the patient can do for himself, if properly instructed.

At a more specific level, adequate communication regarding drug therapy is especially important in rheumatology not only to ensure that patients understand how and when to take their drugs to achieve maximal symptom relief, but also how to avoid the misuse of more potent therapy such as corticosteroids and long-term rheumatoid suppressants.

With regard to advice both on physical therapy and drug treatment there is a relationship (albeit a complex one) between what the patient is advised to do and the degree to which this advice is followed. As will be shown later, however, some patients are poor compliers even if they have understood what they have been told.

In a negative sense, telling patients that they do not have an illness that they had feared can often produce much peace of mind and amelioration or disappearance of symptoms. Indeed, one of the common problems in rheumatology concerns reassuring patients who have been falsely labelled as having a potentially crippling rheumatic illness; one example being the diagnosis of rheumatoid arthritis based on a combination of minor aches and pains and a false-positive test for rheumatoid factor.

Communication extends beyond that involving the doctor–patient axis. The art of listening to patients (feedback) represents an equally important aspect of the communication process, without which the relationship between medical adviser and patient cannot function optimally (Moll, 1978). Another important element in the communications network involves interplay between the various members of the rheumatology/rehabilitation team. At all levels the individual members of the team should be made aware of details beyond but relevant to their own special functioning. For example, clearly written letters from the family doctor to the rheumatologist (including the reasons for referral and details of current drug therapy) and equally clear reports from the specialist to referring practitioner (including details of hospital treatment and likely prognosis) are mandatory to ensure the best possible care for the patient. 'Lateral' communication between specialists is also important. For example, proper liaison between rheumatologist, orthopaedic surgeon and anaesthetist will reduce errors arising from incomplete knowledge of the patient's medication or unawareness of potentially fatal complications of a disease (e.g. atlantoaxial subluxation in rheumatoid arthritis) should the patient need surgery.

Often the communication process involves 'sociodomestic' matters rather than 'harder' aspects of management to do with drugs, physical therapy and surgery. The patients' work and home life often loom larger than the immediate physical aspects of the disease. Such anxieties include those to do with occupational insecurity, erosion of the role as breadwinner, interrupted marital relations, and fears concerning menstruation, contraception, pregnancy, childbirth and child-rearing, as well as fears that the disease may be transmitted to offspring. These 'troubled waters' often remain hidden unless close contact is established between medical personnel and the patient's family and friends. In this way much of rheumatological communication is in fact 'counselling'.

Of all that has been written on the subject of communication, and on the closely related subject, compliance, the salient fact remains that its efficacy will always depend more on 'medicine the art' than on 'medicine the science'. An interested doctor who is prepared to listen to his patient and express his comments in a sympathetic and empathetic way, coupled with a congeniality and a little humour, will always achieve more success than the practitioner who relies on a more 'mechanical' approach characterized by an aloof, dogmatic manner and advice phrased in medical jargon.

3.4 METHODS OF COMMUNICATION

3.4.1 General comment

Various methods are available to enable medical personnel to communicate information to patients, and these are summarized in Fig. 3.3. The most important is the classic method embodied in the consultation. Other communicational means are available but it should be emphasized that these should supplement but not replace the consultation.

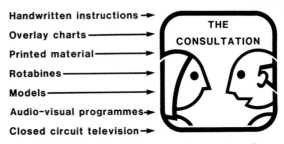

Fig. 3.3 Some means by which doctors convey information to patients.

(a) The consultation

Of the many communicational approaches the consultation is the crucial method on which doctor–patient communication depends. Its success depends on the extent to which doctors *and* patients communicate in both its components – the interview ('taking the history') and the exposition (explaining diagnosis, prognosis and treatment). After a few years of clinical practice most doctors become confident that they are reasonably competent at interviewing and explaining things to their patients. However, recent studies have shown that this is by no means always true. These

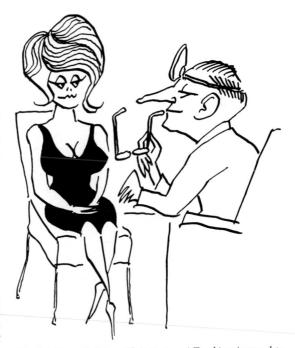

Fig. 3.4 From *Talking with Patients – A Teaching Approach* to stress the importance of rapport (illustration by the author, courtesy of the Nuffield Provincial Hospitals Trust).

revelations have been drawn together in an illustrated booklet, '*Talking with Patients – a Teaching Approach*', by a working party of the Nuffield Provincial Hospitals Trust. This most insightful publication summarizes the general skills and aims needed by the doctor in order to conduct an effective and efficient interview:

1. Create the right atmosphere to establish rapport (Fig. 3.4).
2. Encourage the patient to volunteer information and to feel involved in his own case.
3. Identify and share with the patient the goals of the interview.
4. Tolerate emotionally disturbing things that the patient may say.
5. Interview logically and systematically.
6. Use a style that is appropriate to each particular patient at each stage of the interview.
7. Recognize when an interview is going wrong and make appropriate adjustments (any mistake in communication can be put right so long as the patient is sure of the doctor's concern for him).
8. Avoid jargon and explain the meaning of medical terms.
9. Understand and use non-verbal communication.
10. Get the patient to accept the doctor's recommendations.

Of the above, rapport with the patient is obviously of particular importance. Regrettably this has not been the subject of detailed study in the past, perhaps because it has always been assumed that doctors are not lacking in this area. However, there can be little doubt that some doctors have a better 'bedside manner' than others, and it is surprising that this important clinical attribute is not tested in either undergraduate or postgraduate qualifying examinations. What social characteristics help to establish good rapport are difficult to define but kindness, empathy, sympathy, humour and 'professionalism' are expectations often mentioned by patients.

Some rather more specific additional techniques to be considered in establishing a successful interview include:

1. Ask open-ended questions.
2. Ask closed questions.
3. Handle sensitively or avoid painful, 'private', or embarrassing issues.
4. Listen and *be seen* to be listening.
5. Remember what you have said and heard.
6. Clarify inconsistencies.
7. Insist on precision.
8. Explain purposes.
9. Interrupt the patient whilst still maintaining the flow of the interview.

10. Challenge denial when appropriate.
11. Avoid commenting adversely on treatment given by others.
12. Summarize.

For further details concerning problems and pitfalls of the consultation the reader is referred to several recent papers – Meadow and Hewitt (1972), Hampton *et al.* (1975), Shaw and Gath (1975), Browne and Freeling (1976), Byrne and Long (1976), Fraser (1976), Butt (1977), Davis and Horobin (1977), Maguire and Rutter (1976a,b), Fletcher (1979), Kessel (1979).

Ley and his colleagues have made a particular study over the years of specific ways in which communicational efficiency can be boosted (Ley, 1974, 1976, 1977, 1979; Ley and Spelman, 1965, 1967; Ley *et al.* 1972, 1973, 1976a,b). Some of their suggestions for improving communications are as follows: whenever possible present instructions and advice at the *start* of the information, as patients remember best what they have read first; when providing patients with instructions and advice, stress their *importance*; use *short words* and *short sentences*; use explicit *categorization* where possible; *repeat* things where feasible; when giving advice make it as *specific*, *detailed* and *concrete* as possible; try to provide a calm and relaxed atmosphere in the clinic or surgery.

3.4.2 Other means of communication

(a) Printed material

Books, pamphlets, leaflets, brochures, and magazines are useful to patients in some circumstances. Various drug companies, the Government Printing Office, national health organizations such as the Cancer Society, the Muscular Dystrophy Association, and the American Heart Association supply a wealth of material for teaching. If not free, the cost is usually minimal.

Printed material has some advantages over other types of teaching aids. It is highly mobile and can be taken home or given to other patients. It is either free, or costs very little. Printed material can be updated at nominal expense, and is therefore likely to be current. Several pieces of literature can be used to complement each other and get a point across. Booklets and brochures can be partially read, or re-read without requiring help from others.

However, printed material often presents a particular view or practice, say of one medical school. The language may not be suited to the patient who needs the teaching, thus the patient might be confused rather than helped by the information. These disadvantages can be minimized if discussion periods are held in which the patient is encouraged to ask questions.

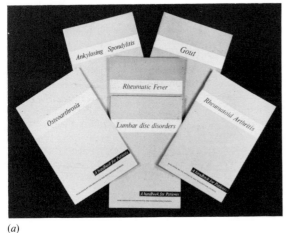

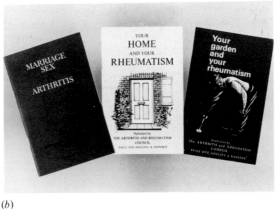

(a)   (b)

Fig. 3.5 Booklets published by the Arthritis and Rheumatism Council (London) on: (*a*) various rheumatic disorders; (*b*) various sociodomestic subjects.

Printed information is now readily available for patients with various rheumatic disorders. These have been written either by fellow sufferers, such as Eve Orme's '*My Fight Against Osteo-Arthritis*' (Orme, 1955), or by professionals of varying degrees of orthodoxy. One of the first instructional books written for patients by a medical practitioner was A.E. Phelps' '*Arthritis: What Can Be Done About It*' (Phelps, 1945). The Arthritis and Rheumatism Council (then the Empire Rheumatism Council) has also contributed early literature in this field. One of the first booklets, written by a team of rheumatologists, was '*Osteo-arthritis*' published in April 1956. Since then many more excellent booklets have been printed on many forms of rheumatic illness, and on ways of helping patients to live a better life (Fig. 3.5). In the USA the Arthritis Foundation provides a similar service. Many of these booklets are illustrated (Fig. 3.6), and I have shown in a recent study (Moll, 1981) that, as has been suspected on subjective grounds, pictorial material enhances the communicational value of these booklets.

Not all rheumatological literature written by 'professionals' is written by orthodox practitioners. Many of these books written by unorthodox authors contain emotive medical language, uncontrolled 'research facts', and much emphasis – without valid evidence – on the near-magical effects of diet. Some authors 'prove' their discoveries by experimenting on themselves to produce rheumatic-like symptoms, and then 'defeat' the illness with 'special' diets. Such books also contain other unsubstantiated comments such as claims that sugar destroys lubricating oils needed to fight arthritis and that eating oil-bearing foods helps back stiffness due to gelling of tissue fluids.

It is difficult to know how these heterodox publications influence the general population, but judging from the frequency and seriousness with which they are quoted by patients, there can be little doubt that they command a wide and dedicated readership.

However, to offset this, there are many orthodox

Table 3.1 Some books for patients on rheumatic subjects. For details of this literature, see References*

Author	Date	Subject
Phelps	1945	General
Orme	1955	Osteoarthritis (autobiographical)
Crain	1971	General
Tucker	1973	Home treatment and posture
Jayson and Dixon	1974	General
Lettvin	1976	Back pain
MacFarlane	1976	Self-help (autobiographical)
Fairley	1978	Pain
Freese	1978	General
Rule	1978	Back pain
Fries	1979	General
Berson	1980	General/Self-help (semi-autobiographical)
Robinson	1980	Rheumatoid arthritis (autobiographical)
Scott	1980	General
Moll	In press	General

* From Moll (1981).

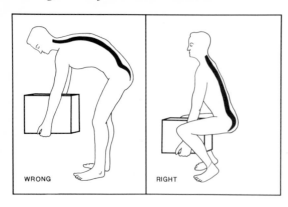

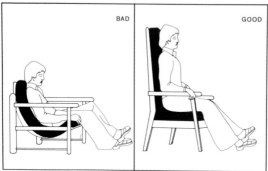

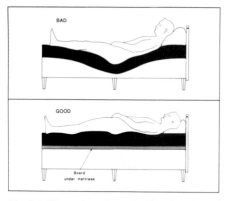

Fig. 3.6 Illustrations from *Lumbar Disc Disorders* (1980) to communicate simple facts to do with posture in patients with disc problems (courtesy of the Arthritis and Rheumatism Council).

publications available either in booklet or book form. Most of these state the basic health facts to do with rheumatic disorders in a cogent, coherent way, and often the publications are illustrated.

Some of the books and booklets which have been written for rheumatic sufferers are summarized in Tables 3.1 and 3.2, respectively.

INSTRUCTIONS

1 DO NOT STOP taking the steroid drug except on medical advice. Always have a supply in reserve.

2 In case of feverish illness, accident, operation (emergency or otherwise), diarrhoea or vomiting the steroid treatment MUST be continued. Your doctor may wish you to have a LARGER DOSE or an INJECTION at such times.

3 If the tablets cause indigestion consult your doctor AT ONCE.

4 Always carry this card while receiving steroid treatment and show it to any doctor, dentist, nurse or midwife whom you may consult.

5 After your treatment has finished you must still tell any new doctor, dentist, nurse or midwife that you have had steroid treatment.

10251 191229 200m (5) 10/73 WPLtd Gp709

I am a patient on—

STEROID
TREATMENT
which must not be
stopped abruptly

and in the case of intercurrent illness
may have to be increased

full details are available
from the hospital or general→
practitioners shown overleaf

	Name and Address	Tel No.	Treatment was commenced on_____		
			DRUG	DATE	DOSE
Patient					
General Practitioner					
Hospital					
Consultant or Specialist		Hospital No			

Fig. 3.7 Written instructions for patients regarding corticosteroid therapy.

In addition to written material about rheumatic illness, useful information about specific aspects of the patient's management (e.g. corticosteroid therapy) is also available (Fig. 3.7).

(b) Other communicational devices

In addition to books, booklets and leaflets other communicational devices include overlay charts, moulded and real models, Rotabines (rotating illuminated drawings displaying information in poster format), closed circuit television, and audiovisual presentations. Many pharmaceutical companies now cater for the patient's need for prescribing information on drug packages, and often this material is illustrated (Fig. 3.8).

To this list may be added the useful ploy of drawing simple sketches to reinforce what has been said. Doctors do not need to be artists to make a success of this. In addition to their communication value at the time of the consultation such pictorial material can be taken away by the patient to serve as a reminder of what infor-

Table 3.2 Some booklets for patients on various rheumatic subjects*

Title	Publisher	Place
Osteoarthrosis	Arthritis and Rheumatism Council	London
Rheumatoid Arthritis	Arthritis and Rheumatism Council	London
Gout	Arthritis and Rheumatism Council	London
Ankylosing Spondylitis	Arthritis and Rheumatism Council	London
Pain in the Neck	Arthritis and Rheumatism Council	London
Lumbar Disc Disorders	Arthritis and Rheumatism Council	London
Rheumatic Fever	Arthritis and Rheumatism Council	London
Your Home and Your Rheumatism	Arthritis and Rheumatism Council	London
Your Garden and Your Rheumatism	Arthritis and Rheumatism Council	London
Marriage, Sex and Arthritis	Arthritis and Rheumatism Council	London
About Your Gouty Arthritis	Wellcome Foundation	Berkamstead
Gout	Merck, Sharp and Dohme International	New York
Aches, Pains and Rheumatism	British Medical Association	London
Understanding Rheumatism	British Medical Association	London
The Patient Questions the Doctor on Arthritis and Rheumatism	Greater Glasgow Health Board	Glasgow
Rheumatoid Arthritis	Leeds Area Health Authority	Leeds
Arthritis – the Basic Facts	Arthritis Foundation	New York
Home Care Programme in Arthritis	Arthritis Foundation	New York
Osteoarthritis	Arthritis Foundation	New York
Rheumatoid Arthritis	Arthritis Foundation	New York
Conseils à un Ami Goutteux	Libraire le François	Paris
Die Gicht	Verlag für Medizin	Heidelberg
Die häusliche Pflege des Rheumakranken	Schweizerische Rheumaliga	Zurich
Bewegungsübungen für Rheumakranke	Schweizerische Rheumaliga	Zurich
Arthrosis Deformans	Nederlands Huis artsen Institut	Utrecht
De Ziekte van Bechterew	Nederlands Huis artsen Institut	Utrecht
Rheumatoide Arthritis	Nederlands Huis artsen Institut	Utrecht
Rheumatoide Arthritis	Aesopus Verlag	Wiesbaden
Das Rheumatische Fieber	Aesopus Verlag	Wiesbaden
Weichteilreheumatismus	Aesopus Verlag	Wiesbaden

Most of the publications are undated and are the result of a committee of authors.
*From Moll (1981).

mation was given. In addition to this, patients may find it useful to make their own notes.

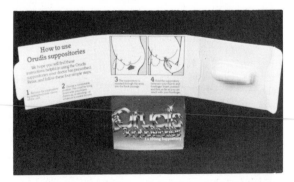

Fig. 3.8 Medicine package carrying illustrated instructions.

3.5 PSYCHOLOGICAL ASPECTS OF COMMUNICATION AND COMPLIANCE: SOME RECENT STUDIES

3.5.1 Communication studies

One of the first investigations of doctor–patient communication in a rheumatological setting was that of Joyce *et al.* (1969). These workers observed marked differences in the kind and amount of information retained by patients. They also found that there was a large difference between interviewers in the amount of information they elicited, and between physicians in the kind (but not the total) of information they imparted. In general, patients remembered about half of the 10 facts they were told, and as has been shown in another study (see Wright and Hopkins, 1978) most of the forgetting appeared to occur immediately. Patients forgot more facts to do with diagnosis or treatment than to do with instructional statements.

Surprisingly little work has been done to test the value of printed material. Of that which has been done, much has come from Leeds and Sheffield.

Moll and Wright (1972) studied a sample of 53 consecutive patients with gout and used a multiple-choice knowledge-testing questionnaire to evaluate the communication value of the Arthritis and Rheumatism Council's '*Handbook on Gout*'. The authors found that long-term recall of information was well maintained (mean questionnaire score 70%), and that a single reading of the booklet was sufficient in most patients. Details of management and treatment were recalled less well than information about the general nature of the disease. Significant positive correlations were found between questionnaire score and social status, educational level, and order of learning (facts mentioned first were remembered best). No relationship was found between questionnaire score and factors such as duration of illness, time interval between learning and test, and number of times booklet read.

Moll and Wright extended this study (Moll *et al.*, 1977) to see whether or not increasing the number of illustrations in the gout handbook would increase its communication value. Patients were divided into two groups: one group was given a profusely illustrated booklet (especially designed for the study) containing one cartoon for every item of information in the booklet (total 89 illustrations); the other group was given a booklet without illustrations. Surprisingly, no significant difference in communication value was found between the illustrated and unillustrated booklets. The subjective reaction of patients to these booklets, as well as previous evidence to support the value of pictures versus words in learning, led me to pursue attempts to enhance medical communications pictorially. This latest study has in fact shown the superiority of cartoons over other graphic images (pinmen, symbols, representational drawings, photographs) when used to illustrate instructional handbooks. A further aspect of this study has revealed, rather surprisingly, no difference between patients' understanding of a 'simple' text compared with 'hard' text. However, it was felt that an 'interaction' existed between text and picture in that an 'easy' pictorial style (e.g. cartoon) tended to work better with 'hard' text in relation to instructional effect, and vice versa (Moll, 1981).

Communication work at Leeds has recently been redirected to examine the meanings attached to words by patients and by doctors (Wright and Hopkins, 1977). Among rheumatic patients, good agreement was only reached for the terms 'rheumatism' and 'hereditary'. Non-rheumatic patients showed better agreement than

rheumatic patients, although it was felt this may have been due to there being more in the professional classes among the former group. The poorest agreement among rheumatic patients was for 'numbness', 'sciatica', 'slipped disc', 'vertebra', 'cervical', 'spinal cord', 'arthritis', 'deformity', 'anaemia', 'ligaments', 'osteoarthritis', 'lumbar', 'sacrum' and 'back'. Poor concordance was obtained for 'back' among rheumatologists and hospital doctors and for 'arthritis' among general practitioners. The word 'sciatica' meant very different things to different doctors. A difference of more than 40% was found between patients' and rheumatologists' understanding of 'numbness', 'spinal cord', 'cervical', 'sacrum', 'loin', 'slipped disc', 'arthritis', 'osteoarthritis' and 'steroids'. The study therefore revealed much doctor–patient disagreement, not to speak of disagreement between doctors. Apart from its general value, the investigation emphasized areas where reassurance (e.g. about the nature and prognosis of arthritis) is important.

Tring and Hayes-Allen (1973) carried out a similar study in Sheffield to evaluate differences of interpretation of some commonly used medical terms (including the term 'arthritis') among preclinical medical students and non-medical graduates. There was close agreement between all students at a high level of accuracy (over 80%) for the terms 'arthritis', 'a medicine', 'constipation' and 'least starchy food', but less close agreement about 'heartburn', 'good appetite', 'piles' and 'bronchitis'. These results agree with those of Boyle (1970) who tested doctors and patients with common medical terms. 'Arthritis' was defined correctly by 100% of doctors and almost 86% of patients.

Wright and Hopkins (1978) have studied seven different lecturing techniques in 14 groups of nurses at two hospitals. The authors showed that although a significant amount of knowledge was imparted by the lecturer, as much as a third was forgotten by the end of the lecture, and a half to two-thirds was forgotten within 3 months. The three teaching approaches that scored best were: giving questionnaires before lecture; giving hand-outs; using the blackboard. (The other teaching techniques were: note-taking encouraged; note-taking forbidden; structured handouts; told beforehand that test would follow.)

Anderson *et al.* (1979) have investigated recall among 151 patients (diagnoses not specified) attending a rheumatology clinic. Total recall (assessed from a written rather than a sound recording) of information was 40%. Recall of 'treatment' facts was higher than for facts to do with diagnosis. (The meaning of 'treatment' was unclear, but presumably referred to general advice and/or physical therapy, as there was a separate category 'medication'.) Patients over the age of 70 years remembered less information. Anxious patients recalled more than those who were relaxed. However, the reliability of patients rating their own anxiety level (more relaxed than usual, normal, slight anxiety, moderate–severe anxiety) is to be doubted, and the fact that less than 10% classed themselves in the moderate–severe anxiety group under these test conditions might support this. Patients misconstrued 48% of what they thought they recalled. The more facts given, the lower the proportion correctly remembered.

The recall of 40% is comparable with the figure obtained by Joyce *et al.* (1969) who found a 47% recall among their rheumatic patients, but lower than that of Moll and others (Moll and Wright, 1972; Moll *et al.*, 1977) who reported recall of between 65.5% and 70%, depending on the type of instructional booklet the patients had read. The results of the last studies are comparable with those of Ley and Spelman, who found a recall of 63% among general medical patients.

3.5.2 Compliance studies

> One problem has always been that giving people information about health doesn't necessarily change their behaviour.
>
> Jessop, 1979

Getting patients to follow medical advice is a major problem in many types of long-term disease. Levels of compliance are often low and may be associated with poor therapeutic effect (Porter, 1969; Marston, 1970; Capell *et al.*, 1979). This problem is particularly so in chronic rheumatoses such as osteoarthrosis and rheumatoid arthritis for which there is no known cure and which persist for a long time with intermittent exacerbations and remissions. An exercise regimen, involving changes in patient behaviour, often without marked improvement may be difficult to maintain. The problem is further complicated by the tendency of many medical practitioners to over-estimate compliance among their patients, and by their failure to take precautionary steps to increase the likelihood of patients following advice (Carpenter and Davis, 1976).

Joyce (1962, 1968) has drawn attention to non-compliance in pill-taking in rheumatic patients. In his first communication (Joyce, 1962) the author used phenylbutazone (20410 (Ciba) (1-phenyl-2 methyl-4, dimethylamino-3, 6-dioxo-1, 2, 3, 6-tetra hydropyridazine) and lactose placebo containing 10 mg of phenol red to act as a urine marker; the presence of marker in the urine thus provided an indication of patient co-operation. Only 38 out of the 108 urine samples that should have contained marker gave positive results.

Studies have suggested a number of factors that may be associated with compliance. Among these are: the expectations and social support received by the patient from others, educational attainment and socioeconomic status (Elling *et al.*, 1960; Davis and Eichlorn, 1963), and perceived seriousness or threat of disease (Rosenstock, 1966; Backer *et al.*, 1972).

A more recent study by Carpenter and Davis (1976) has examined further factors involved in compliance. These workers found in arthritic patients that housewives were more likely to be represented in the complying group. This was thought to be related to family support rather than to the patients' sex, the latter having been suggested by Ludwig and Adams (1968). The family support hypothesis receives additional support from the finding that compliers are more likely than non-compliers to be married.

Carpenter and Davis (1976) also found that non-compliers were significantly more likely to be taking drugs. An explanation for this is not yet established, but it could be that the complacency engendered by the pain-relieving effects of drugs lessens patients' motivation to carry out exercises. Alternatively, it could be argued that compliers may feel less need for drugs because of the benefits of the exercise regimen.

The above workers have also shown that instructional pamphlets, together with personal, in-hospital instruction in the exercise programme may be more useful than personal instruction alone. In this regard, it has been shown that patients retain limited knowledge after receiving verbal instructions from their physician (Davis, 1966, 1968).

Similar findings have been obtained by Glossop *et al.* (personal communication). These workers studied a small mixed group of patients with rheumatoid arthritis and ankylosing spondylitis and found that the combination of verbal instruction and a booklet resulted in better exercise compliance than verbal instruction alone or booklet alone.

Professional home visits from the visiting nurse, physiotherapist and/or social worker have not been found to increase compliance (Carpenter and Davis, 1976).

Although non-rheumatological, a recent study by Sackett *et al.* (1975) is of interest. Over 200 Canadian steelworkers with hypertension took part in a randomized trial to test whether or not compliance with antihypertensive drugs could be improved. Arrangements were made for them either to see their family doctor outside working hours or the industrial physician during working hours. The same men were randomly given instructions on hypertension and its treatment (slide–audiotape plus booklet). Surprisingly, the convenience of follow-up at work had no effect on compliance. Similarly, although men receiving health education learned more about hypertension they were not more likely to take their medicine.

The above studies confirm a long-suspected view that

the relationship between communication and compliance is by no means a simple one, and clearly further studies are required to add to our understanding of this relationship and to highlight, if possible, ways in which compliance can be improved.

3.6 SUMMARIZING CONCEPT – 'WHEELS OF COMMUNICATION'

Doctor–patient communication may be regarded as a process involving the interaction of three main groups of factors – 'the wheels of communication' (Moll, 1982). This concept is summarized in Fig. 3.9. Many of these factors have already been discussed, but others have been added to fill gaps not detailed previously. As this diagram implies, adequate communication rests not

Ability to communicate
Interest
Kindness
Empathy
Sympathy
Humour
Professionalism

Wish to learn
Educational level
Social background
Anxiety level
Feedback motivation
Pleasantness/Hostility
Clinical problems
Language barrier
Compliance potential

Effectiveness of the communication
Environmental distractions
Presence of other people

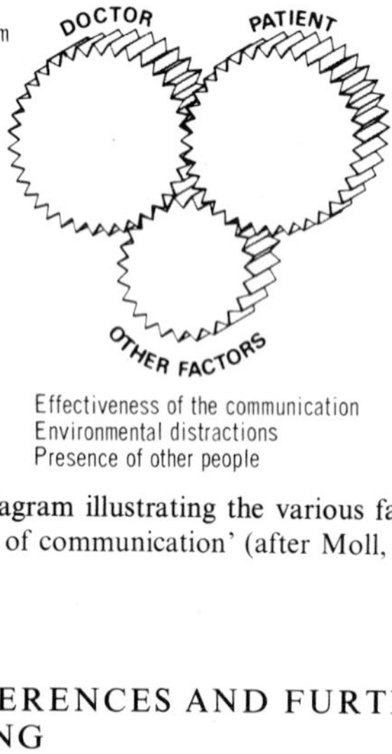

Fig. 3.9 Diagram illustrating the various factors involved in 'the wheels of communication' (after Moll, 1982).

only on factors to do with doctor and patient, but also on 'external' factors such as the effectiveness of the communication. Optimal directional 'pull' and harmonious interaction between these factors may be looked upon as the oil needed to lubricate the wheels of communication.

3.7 SUMMARY AND CONCLUSIONS

This chapter has considered various aspects of communication in its application to rheumatology, including general principles, methods and psychological aspects. The related subject, compliance, has also been discussed and this, together with other factors, has been embodied in the concept of 'the wheels of communication'.

The reasons for the neglect of communication in medicine for so long are difficult to understand, but perhaps our previous efforts have been too much in the direction of diagnosis and treatment. However, as Harlem (1977) has indicated, this is perhaps understandable as it was not so long ago that many diseases (e.g. 'traditional' infectious diseases), now controllable, were life threatening and needed absolute priority in their control.

The medical profession has at last begun to recognize the value of satisfactory communication with patients, as well as the importance of communication between medical personnel. In general, the value of satisfactory communication arises from the psychological and physical benefits that spring from it, and from the importance of avoiding the consequences of inadequate communication which may be detrimental or even fatal. The particular value of communication in rheumatology lies in the fact that in this specialty advice is often the only thing of value that can be offered to the patient.

3.8 REFERENCES AND FURTHER READING

Anderson, J.L., Dodman, S., Kopelman, M. and Fleming, A. (1979) Patient information recall in a rheumatology clinic. *Rheumatol. Rehabil.*, **18**, 18.
Arthritis and Rheumatism Council (1956) *Osteoarthritis*, Arthritis and Rheumatism Council, London.
Arthritis and Rheumatism Council (1980) *Lumbar Disc Disorders*, Arthritis and Rheumatism Council, London.
Bain, D.J.G. (1977) Patient knowledge and the content of the consultation in general practice. *J. Med. Educ.*, **11**, 347.
Balint, M. (1964) *The Doctor, his Patient and the Illness*, 2nd edn, Pitman Medical, London.

Barlund, D.C. (1976) The mystification of meaning: doctor–patient encounters. *J. Med. Educ.*, **51**, 716.
Becker, M.H., Drachman, R.H. and Kirscht, J.T. (1972) Predicting mothers' compliance with pediatric regimens. *J. Pediatr.*, **81**, 843.
Berson, D. (1980) *Pain-free Arthritis*, New English Library, London.
Boyle, C.M. (1970) Difference between patients' and doctors' interpretation of some common medical terms. *Br. Med. J.*, **ii**, 286.
Bradshaw, P.W., Ley, P., Kincey, J.A. and Bradshaw, J. (1975) Recall of medical advice. *Br. J. Soc. Clin. Psychol.*, **14**, 55.
Brooke, B.N. (1960) The clinical approach. *Lancet*, **ii**, 810.
Browne, K. and Freeling, P. (1976) *The Doctor–Patient Relationship*, 2nd edn, Churchill Livingstone, London.

Butt, H.R. (1977) A method for better physician–patient communication. *Ann. Int. Med.*, **86**, 478.

Byrne, P.S. and Long, E.L. (1976) *Doctors Talking to Patients: A Study of Verbal Behaviour of General Practitioners Consulting in their Surgeries*, HMSO, London.

Capell, H.A., Rennie, J.A.N., Rooney, P.J., *et al.* (1979) Patient compliance: a novel method of testing non-steroidal anti-inflammatory analgesics in rheumatoid arthritis. *J. Rheumatol.*, **6**, 584.

Carpenter, J.O. and Davis, L.J. (1976) Medical recommendations – followed or ignored? Factors influencing compliance in arthritis. *Arch. Phys. Med. Rehabil.*, **57**, 241.

Cartwright, A. (1964) *Human Relations and Hospital Care*, Routledge and Kegan Paul, London.

Cartwright, A. (1967) *Patients and their Doctors. A Study of General Practice*, Routledge and Kegan Paul, London.

Crain, D.C. (1972) *The Arthritis Handbook: A Patient's Handbook on Arthritis, Rheumatism and Gout*, Arlington, London.

Davis, M.S. (1966) Variations in patients' compliance with doctors' orders: analysis of congruence between survey responses and results of empirical investigations. *J. Med. Educ.*, **41**, 1037.

Davis, M.S. (1968) Variations in patients' compliance with doctors' advice: empirical analysis of patterns of communication. *Am. J. Pub. Hlth.*, **58**, 274.

Davis, M.S. and Eichlorn, R.L. (1963) Compliance with medical regimens: panel study. *J. Hlth. Hum. Behav.*, **4**, 240.

Davis, A. and Horobin, G. (eds) (1977) *Medical Encounters: The Experience of Illness and Treatment*, Croom Helm, London.

Dunkelman, H. (1979) Patients' knowledge of their conditions and treatment and how it might be improved. *Br. Med. J.* **ii**, 311.

Elling, R., Whittemore, R. and Green, M. (1960) Patient participation in a pediatric program. *J. Hlth. Hum. Behav.*, **1**, 183.

Enelow, A.J. and Swisher, S.N. (eds) (1979) *Interviewing and Patient Care*, 2nd edn, Oxford University Press, New York.

Enzer, N.B., Weil, W.B. and Ryan, M. (1979) in *Interviewing and Patient Care* (eds A.J. Enelow and S.N. Swisher), 2nd edn, Oxford University Press, New York, pp. 111–37.

Fairley, P. (1978) *The Conquest of Pain*, Michael Joseph, London.

Fishbein, M. (1976) in *Communication between Doctors and Patients* (ed. A.E. Bennett), Oxford University Press, for the Nuffield Provincial Hospitals Trust, London, pp. 101–27.

Fleckenstein, L. (1977) Attitudes towards patient package inserts. *Drug Inf. J.*, **11**, 23.

Fletcher, C. (1979) in *Mixed Communications* (ed. G. McLachlan), Oxford University Press, for the Nuffield Provincial Hospitals Trust, London, p. 3.

Fletcher, C.M. (1973) *Communication in Medicine*, Rock Carling Monograph, Nuffield Provincial Hospitals Trust, London.

Fraser, C. (1976) in *Communication Between Doctors and Patients* (ed. A. Bennett), Oxford University Press, for the Nuffield Provincial Hospitals Trust, London, pp. 5–28.

Freese, A. (1978) *Help for Your Arthritis and Rheumatism: All the Facts your Doctor Doesn't Have Time to Tell You*, New American Library, New York.

Fries, J.F. (1980) *Arthritis and How to Cope with it*, Granada, London.

Glossop, E.S., Goldenberg, E., Smith, D.S. and Williams, I.M. (in preparation) A patient compliance study of instruction by physiotherapists.

Grennan, D.M., Taylor, S. and Palmer, D.G. (1978) Doctor–patient communication in patients with arthritis. *N. Z. Med. J.*, **88**, 431.

Hampton, J.R., Harrison, M.J.G., Mitchell, J.R.A., *et al.* (1975) Relative contribution of history-taking, physical examination, and laboratory investigation to diagnosis and management of medical outpatients. *Br. Med. J.*, **ii**, 486.

Harlem, O.K. (1977) *Communication in Medicine – A Challenge to the Profession*, Karger, Basel.

Hawkins, C. (1979) Patients' reactions to their investigations: A study of 504 in-patients. *Br. Med. J.*, **ii**, 638.

Helfer, R.E. (1970) An objective comparison of the paediatric interviewing skills of freshmen and senior medical students. *Paediatrics*, **45**, 623.

Helfer, R.E. and Ealy, K.F. (1972) Observations of paediatric interviewing skills. *Am. J. Dis. Child.*, **123**, 556.

Hulka, B.S., Kupper, L.L., Cassel, J.C. and Mayo, F. (1975) Doctor–patient communication and outcomes among diabetic patients. *J. Commun. Hlth.*, **1**, 15.

Jayson, M.I.V. and Dixon, A. St J. (1974) *Rheumatism and Arthritis. What They Are and What You Should Know About Them*, Pan, London.

Jessop, J. (1979) The future of preventive medicine in Britain. *On Call*, April 26th, p. 5.

Johnston, M. (1976) in *Communication between Doctors and Patients* (ed. A.E. Bennett), Oxford University Press, for the Nuffield Provincial Hospitals Trust, London, pp. 29–44.

Joubert, P. and Lasagna, L. (1975) Patient package inserts: 1. Nature, notions and needs. *Clin. Pharmacol. Ther.*; **18**, 507.

Joyce, C.R.B. (1962) Patient co-operation and the sensitivity of clinical trials. *J. Chron. Dis.*, **15**, 1025.

Joyce, C.R.B. (1968) in *Psychopharmacology. Dimensions and Perspectives* (ed. C.R.B. Joyce), Tavistock, London, pp. 229–30.

Joyce, C.R.B., Caple, G., Mason, M., *et al.* (1969) Quantitative study of doctor–patient communication. *Q. J. Med.* (*New Series*), **38**, 183.

Kessel, N. (1979) Reassurance. *Lancet*, **i**, 1128.

Kincey, J.A., Bradshaw, P.W. and Ley, P. (1975) Patients' satisfaction and reported acceptance of advice in general practice. *J. R. Coll. Gen. Pract.*, **25**, 558.

Korsch, B.M. and Negrete, V.F. (1972) Doctor–patient communication. *Sci. Am.*, August, p. 66.

Leading Article (1978) Patient package inserts. *Br. Med. J.*, **iii**, 586.

Ley, P. (1972a) Primacy, rated importance and recall of medical information. *J. Hlth. Soc. Behav.*, **13**, 311.

Ley, P. (1972b) Complaints made by hospital staff and patients: a review of the literature. *Bull. Psychol. Soc.*, **25**, 115.

Ley, P. (1974) Communication in the clinical setting, *Br. J. Orthodont.*, **1**, 173.

Ley, P. (1976) in *Communications between Doctors and Patients* (ed. A.E. Bennett), Nuffield Provincial Hospitals Trust, London.

Ley, P. (1977) in *Contributions to Medical Psychology* (ed. S. Rachman), Pergamon Press, Oxford, pp. 9–42.

Ley, P. (1979) Memory for medical information. *Br. J. Soc. Clin. Psychol.*, **18**, 245.

Ley, P. and Spelman, M.S. (1965) Communications in an outpatient setting. *Br. J. Soc. Clin. Psychol.*, **4**, 114.

Ley, P. and Spelman, M.S. (1967) *Communicating with the Patient*, Staples Press, London.

Ley, P., Goldman, M., Bradshaw, *et al.* (1972) The comprehensibility of some X-ray leaflets. *J. Inst. Hlth. Educ.*, **10**, 47.

Ley, P., Bradshaw, P.W., Eaves, D. and Walker, C.M. (1973) A method for increasing patients' recall of information presented by doctors. *Psychol. Med.*, **3**, 217.

Ley, P., Skilbeck, C.E. and Tulips, J.G. (1975) Correlates of reported satisfaction and compliance in general practice. Unpublished manuscript.

Ley, P., Bradshaw, P.W., Kincey, J.A. and Atherton, S.T. (1976a) Increasing patients' satisfaction with communications. *Br. J. Soc. Clin. Psychol.*, **15**, 403.

Ley, P., Whitworth, M.A., Skilbeck, C.E., *et al.* (1976b) Improving doctor patient communications in general practice. *J. R. Coll. Gen. Pract.*, **26**, 720.

Lettvin, M. (1976) *The Back Book. Healing the Hurt in Your Lower Back*, Souvenir Press, London.

Lindeman, C.A. and Van Aernam, B. (1971) Nursing intervention with the pre-surgical patient – effects of structured and unstructured preoperative teaching. *Nurs. Res.*, **20**, 319.

Ludwig, E.G. and Adams, S.D. (1968) Patient cooperation in rehabilitation center: assumption of client role. *J. Hlth. Soc. Behav.*, **9**, 328.

MacFarlane, H.B. (1976) *Arthritis. Help in Your Own Hands*, Thorsons, Wellingborough.

MacNamara, M. (1974) Talking with patients: some problems met by medical students. *Br. J. Med. Educ.*, **8**, 17.

Maguire, G.P. and Rutter, D.R. (1976a) History taking for medical students. 1. Deficiencies in performance; 2. Evaluation of a training programme. *Lancet*, **ii**, 556.

Maguire, G.P. and Rutter, D.R. (1976b) In *Communication Between Doctors and Patients* (ed. A.E. Bennett), Oxford University Press, for the Nuffield Provincial Hospitals Trust, London, pp. 47–74.

Maguire, G.P., Pritchard, C.A. and Silvo, F. (1977) An experimental comparison of three courses in history-taking skills for medical students. *Med. Educ.*, **11**, 175.

Maguire, G.P., Roe, P., Goldberg, D., *et al.* (1978) The value of feedback in teaching interviewing skills to medical students. *Psychol. Med.*, **8**, 695.

Marston, M.V. (1970) Compliance with medical regimens: review of literature. *Nurs. Res.*, **19**, 312.

McIntosh, J. (1974) Processes of communication: Information seeking and control associated with cancer. *Soc. Sci. Med.*, **8**, 167.

Meadow, R. and Hewitt, C. (1972) Teaching communication skills with the help of actresses and video-tape simulation. *Br. J. Med. Educ.*, **6**, 317.

Midgley, J.M. and Macrea, A.W. (1971) Audio-visual media in general practice. *J. R. Coll. Gen. Pract.*, **21**, 346.

Moll, J.M.H. (1978) In *Proceedings of the 3rd World Congress of the International Rehabilitation Medicine Association*, Basle, Switzerland, 1978, Internationale Vereinigung für Rehabilitations – Medizin, Basel, Abstract 13–8, p. 175.

Moll, J.M.H. (1981) *Studies of Visual Perception in Medical Communication*, Ph.D. thesis, University of Leeds.

Moll, J.M.H. (1982) in *Topical Reviews in Rheumatic Disorders* (ed. V. Wright), Vol. 2, Wright, Bristol.

Moll, J.M.H. (in press) *Arthritis and Rheumatism*, Churchill Livingstone, London.

Moll, J.M.H. and Wright, V. (1972) Evaluation of the Arthritis and Rheumatism Council handbook on gout. An objective study of doctor–patient communication. *Ann. Rheum. Dis.*, **31**, 405.

Moll, J.M.H. and Wright, V. (1978) in *Reports on Rheumatic Diseases*, No. 64 (eds. C. Hawkins and H.L.F. Currey), Arthritis and Rheumatism Council, London.

Moll, J.M.H., Wright, V., Jeffrey, M.R., *et al.* (1977) The cartoon in doctor–patient communication. Further study of the Arthritis and Rheumatism Council handbook on gout. *Ann. Rheum. Dis.*, **36**, 225.

Morris, L.A. and Halperin, J. (1979) Effects of written drug information on patient knowledge and compliance: A literature review. *Am. J. Publ. Hlth.*, **69**, 47.

Novack, D.H., Plumer, R., Smith, R.L. *et al.* (1979) Changes in physicians' attitude toward telling the cancer patient. *J. Am. Med. Assoc.*, **241**, 897.

Nuffield Provincial Hospitals Trust (undated), Talking with patients. A teaching approach. *Observations of a Nuffield Working Party on Communicating with Patients* (Chairman Sir John Walton). Nuffield Provincial Hospitals Trust, London.

Orme, E. (1955) *My Fight Against Osteo-Arthritis*, Faber, London.

Parkin, D.M. (1976) Survey of the success of communications between hospital staff and patients. *Publ. Hlth.*, **90**, 203.

Phelps, A.E. (1945) *Arthritis: What Can Be Done About It*, Medical Publications, London.

Porter, A.M. (1969) Drug defaulting in general practice. *Br. Med. J.*, **i**, 218.

Reynolds, M. (1978) No news is bad news: Patients' views about communication in hospital. *Br. Med. J.*, **i**, 1973.

Riley, C.S. (1966) Patients' understanding of doctors' instructions. *Med. Case*, **4**, 34.

Robinson, M. (1980) *Arthritis and You*, Ian Henry, Hornchurch.

Rosenstock, I.M. (1966) Why people use health services. *Milbank Mem. Fund Q.*, **44**, 94.

Rule, L.G. (1978) *Understanding Back Pain: Today's Plague on Young People*, Heinemann, London.

Sackett, D.L., Haynes, R.B., Gibson, E.S., *et al.* (1975) Randomised clinical trial of strategies for improving medication compliance in primary hypertension. *Lancet*, **i**, 1205.

Scott, J. Bodley (1965) The bedside manner. *Trans. Med. Soc. Lond.*, 193rd Session, pp. 1–12.

Scott, J.T. (1980) *Arthritis and Rheumatism – The Facts*, Oxford University Press, Oxford.

Shaw, P.M. and Gath, D.H. (1975) Teaching the doctor–patient relation to medical students. *Br. J. Med. Educ.*, **9**, 176.

Spence, J. (1949) The need for understanding the individual as part of the training and function of doctors and nurses. National Association for Mental Health. Reprinted in: *The Purpose and Practice of Medicine*, Oxford University Press, London, 1960, pp. 271–80.

Stillman, P.L., Darrell, L.S. and Redfield, D.L. (1971) Use of trained mothers to teach interviewing skills to first-year medical students. *Paediatrics*, **60**, 165.

Storlie, F. (1975) *Patient Teaching in Critical Care*, Appleton-Century-Crofts, New York.

Svarstad, B.L. (1974) *The Doctor–Patient Encounter*, Unpublished Ph.D. Thesis, University of Wisconsin.

Tamer, B. (ed.) (1976) *Language and Communication in General Practice*, Hodder and Stoughton, London.

Tring, F.C. and Hayes-Allen, M.C. (1973) Understanding and misunderstanding of some medical terms. *Br. J. Med. Educ.*, **7**, 53.

Tucker, W.E. (1973) *Home Treatment and Posture in Injury, Rheumatism and Osteoarthritis*, Churchill Livingstone, Edinburgh.

Waitzkin, M. and Stoeckle, J.D. (1972) The communication of information about illness. *Adv. Psychol. Med.*, **8**, 180.

Welford, W. (1975) Closing the communication gap. *Nursing Times*, 16 January.

Worby, C.M. (1979) in *Interviewing and Patient Care*, (eds A.J. Enelow and S.N. Swisher), 2nd edn, Oxford University Press, New York, pp. 138–63.

Wright, V. (1978) in *Proceedings of the 3rd World Congress of the International Rehabilitation Medicine Association*, Basle, Switzerland, Internationale Vereinigung für Rehabilitations – Medizin, Basel, Abstract 13.3, p. 169.

Wright, V. and Hopkins, R. (1977) Communicating with the rheumatic patient. *Rheumatol. Rehabil.*, **16**, 107.

Wright, V. and Hopkins, R. (1978) Teaching rheumatology to nurses. *Ann. Rheum. Dis.*, **37**, 385.

4

Drug therapy (1): general aspects

4.1 INTRODUCTORY COMMENT

Few patients need so many drugs so regularly as patients with chronic rheumatic disorders. Arthritis sufferers not only have to contend with the 'long pain', but often also the added distress of disablement and the effects of associated diseases.

Anti-rheumatic drugs are featuring more and more prominently in rheumatological therapy, and the ultimate solution to the control of the various rheumatic disorders is more likely to come from drug therapy than from other therapeutic approaches.

This brief chapter is intended to provide an outline of general facts, principles, and cautions relevant to rheumatological prescribing.

Most prescriptions will be orientated towards relieving pain directly or indirectly. However, it is sometimes not appreciated that the rheumatic 'pain', particularly in chronic inflammatory disorders, is an infernal combination of localized pain and general aching, coupled with a feeling of 'unwellness', fever, weakness and fatiguability, depression and anxiety, and symptoms derived from systemic illness. Added to this the patient may have to contend with the discomfort and inconvenience induced by adverse reactions to drug therapy.

It is the chronicity and degree of discomfort of many of these disorders that set the rheumatic sufferer apart from many other medical disorders, and it is this that demands particular therapeutic skill and perseverance from clinicians involved in their management. The challenges and complexities of rheumatological drug therapy are preferably handled on a 'one physician – one patient' basis if optimal disease control and confidence of the patient is to be established and maintained.

Despite the undoubted value of drugs in easing the burden of the rheumatic patient, it should be stressed that drug therapy represents only one item in the total management approach. The prescribing of systemic drugs should always be combined with adequate instruction (see 'doctor–patient communication', Chapter 3) and will often be associated with the involvement of other therapeutic 'modalities', such as physical treatment, local injection therapy, and surgery.

4.2 GENERAL FACTORS IN PRESCRIBING DRUGS

4.2.1 Considerations before prescribing drugs

(a) General clinical considerations

Before treating any patient with drugs the doctor should have considered several points:

72 *Management of Rheumatic Disorders*

1. Whether he should intervene at all.
2. What alteration in the patient's condition he hopes to achieve.
3. That the drug he intends to use is capable of bringing this about.
4. What other effects the drug may have, and whether these may be harmful (e.g. interactions with other drugs or other diseases).
5. Whether the likelihood of benefit outweighs the likelihood of risk.

If there is significant doubt about any of the above factors it is preferable to withold prescribing the drug.

(b) Special considerations in children

The number of drugs available for treating juvenile chronic arthritis is smaller than that available for treating adults. This is party because most studies, particularly those concerning non-steroidal anti-inflammatory agents, have been conducted only in adult patients. Second, as there are much fewer children with juvenile arthritis, there is probably less commercial motivation to study this field.

The following facts, general rules, and ethical principles concerning drug therapy in children have been outlined by Baum (1982).

1. It is prudent to remember that children are not small adults, and proper dosage levels and side effects cannot be deduced from data obtained from adult studies.
2. In general, there seem to be fewer side effects with non-steroidal anti-inflammatories used in children.
3. As a general rule, no drug should be used in a child until it has been tested and used in adults, preferably for at least a year in order to provide an adequate opportunity to examine long-term as well as short-term side effects.
4. Are new drugs needed? The newer non-steroidal anti-inflammatory drugs do have the advantage of longer half lives, and thus can be given less often – a distinct advantage in the treatment of children.
5. Which disease-modifying drug? Disease-modifying drugs have been incompletely evaluated in children. The US–USSR collaborative clinics intend to study penicillamine and hydroxychloroquine for efficacy and toxicity, and these results will be awaited with interest. Gold has been accepted for use in children for some time, although there are no well-controlled studies in this field. Penicillamine has been used in children for about 7 years, but the optimal dose is still not known. Chloroquine and hydroxychloroquine have been used extensively in Scandinavia, but there have been few formal studies to examine their place in chronic arthritis of childhood.

6. What are the risks of a drug to be tested? The risks of any drug to be used for childhood therapy should have been previously established in adults. When testing in children is undertaken, careful follow-up with white blood counts, urinalysis, liver function tests, and examination for occult blood in the stools should be carried out. A recent example of drug unacceptibility in children has concerned levamisole which appeared to be associated with unduly high mortality and morbidity risks.
7. Which patients should be involved in the studies? Juvenile chronic polyarthritis appears to be a collection of diseases, the pauci-articular type being the most common presentation, with a high natural remission rate. Studies with disease-modifying drugs should therefore not include such patients, and should be confined only to those with the more severe and potentially crippling polyarticular disease.
8. What age should a patient be for consent to participate in a drug trial? In Baum's view, in children below the age of 12 the parent or guardian should be responsible for providing consent. From the age of 12 upwards, informed consent should be from the children themselves as well as from the legal guardian. This approach is supported by recent work by Bibace and Walsh (1980), who found that children in the USA have a beginning realization and understanding of disease in terms of disordered physiology at the age of 11. Below this age, concepts of disease are essentially non-physiological.

(c) Financial considerations

In order to gain a perspective view of the financial implications of prescribing, and of the factors upon which the relationship between the medical profession and the pharmaceutical industry depend, the reader is referred to two trenchant critiques covering this field – *There's Gold in Them Thar Pills* (Klass, 1975) and *The Medicine Men* (Coleman, 1977). The first is 'an enquiry into the medical–industrial complex' and the second 'a shattering analysis of the drugs industry'. These writers commendably draw attention to certain iniquities such as the wide differences in the cost of identical or near-identical products, the marked differences between East and West prices (e.g. in India the cost of prednisone was quoted as being 357% higher than the average European price), and the overzealous wording of pharmaceutical advertisements. Also highlighted is the universal power of the drug industry, whose overall profits in the United States, for example, have for many years been twice the average for all other industries (Klass, 1975).

Nowadays, hospital doctors and general practitioners are inundated by pharmaceutical literature, often presented in a pictorially sophisticated and persuasive form (see Appendix 4.11.1). Considerable judgement is therefore required to achieve a balance between personal preference, genuine advancements in therapy, and the colourful lure of modern advertising, particularly among clinicians whose special interests do not lie within rheumatology.

Table 4.1 gives examples of the difference in cost between some proprietary and non-proprietary preparations. It should be pointed out that the actual cost of these drugs is often substantially less than the figures quoted due to hospital discounts.

Table 4.1 Comparison of cost* of some commonly prescribed proprietary and non-proprietary (BP) preparations

Drugs	Cost (£) per 100 tablets
Paracetamol BP	0·39
Panadol	0·82
Soluble aspirin BP	0·24
Solprin	0·45
Phenylbutazone BP	0·32
Butazolidin	1·34
Indomethacin BP	3·23
Indocid	5·53

* Data from local wholesalers' lists (September 1981), and the Chemist and Druggist Price List (April, 1982).

Appendix 4.11.2 shows cost comparisons of some proprietary preparations of comparable effect. Substantial differences will be noted.

In both Table 4.1 and Appendix 4.11.2 the prices will have doubtless changed by the time of publication, but the main reason for documenting them here is for their comparative rather than for their absolute values.

Guides to the pricing of drugs in the UK include the *Chemist and Druggist Price List* (Benn Publications Ltd), MIMS (Monthly Index of Medical Specialities; Haymarket Publishing Company), and the *National Health Service (England and Wales) Drug Tariff* (DHSS). Another useful source is the *British National Formulary* (*BNF*) (British Medical Association and The Pharmaceutical Society of Great Britain) which also provides a comparison between the basic cost of proprietary and non-proprietary preparations in terms of a coding system to show relative price bands (A = up to 20p; B = 21–50p; C = 51–100p; D = 101–180p; E = 181–300p; F = 301–450p; G = 451–650p; H = 651–900p; I = 901–1200p; J = over 1200p per preparation. 'Preparation' in this context refers to a specific quantity of the drug (e.g. 20 tablets, 100 ml, etc.). Although a valuable guide for comparison, because of other elements involved in determining the price of drugs these figures bear no direct relationship to the actual cost of the dispensed medicine which is always greater than that stated.

It is recommended that where non-proprietary drugs are available, these should be used in prescribing. This will enable any suitable product to be dispensed, thereby saving delay to the patient, and sometimes expense. In exceptional circumstances, particularly where bio-availability properties are especially important, it may be in the patient's interests to be given the product of a particular manufacturer. In such instances, the brand name or the manufacturer should be clearly stated when prescribing.

4.2.2 Considerations after prescribing a drug

Having decided to use a particular drug the following should be borne in mind:

1. Ensure that the patient *understands* what, when and how the drug(s) should be taken.
2. Use the *minimal number* of drugs – avoid 'polypharmacy'.
3. Prescribe the *minimal amount* of any single drug consistent with adequate control of the disease.
4. Start with the *least toxic* drug.
5. *Monitor* drug therapy regularly for therapeutic response, and for toxicity and interactions with other drugs.
6. Regard *new drugs* with particular suspicion.

4.3 CLASSIFICATION OF DRUGS USED IN RHEUMATIC THERAPY

Classification of drugs used in rheumatic therapy is an essential preliminary to understanding and applying the wide range of pharmacological agents available to the clinician. This has become all the more important in recent years in view of the large number of new preparations that have been introduced. The extensive spillover of rheumatic symptomatology into other sectors of medicine makes it necessary to consider not only anti-rheumatic drugs but also adjuvant drugs which are used to treat co-diseases, complications and coexisting disorders. Imperfect agreement still exists regarding an ideal classification of anti-rheumatic drugs, the main point of argument being concerned with the appropriateness of dividing non-steroidal anti-inflammatory agents into 'minor' and 'major' drugs. Another point of variance concerns divisions based on generic characteristics and those based on similarity of clinical effect. This, again, applies particularly to the non-steroidal anti-inflammatory group of drugs.

The following classification scheme is suggested, though individual clinicians will doubtless have their own preference.

1. *Non-specific (or symptomatic) anti-rheumatic drugs*
(a) Simple analgesics (e.g. paracetamol).
(b) Analgesic/anti-inflammatory drugs (or non-steroid anti-inflammatory drugs (NSAIDs)), (e.g. salicylates, indomethacin, phenylbutazone, proprionic acid derivatives).
(c) Non-analgesic/anti-inflammatory drugs (or pure anti-inflammatory drugs) (e.g. corticosteroids, corticotrophin).

2. *Specific anti-rheumatic drugs*
(a) For rheumatoid arthritis ('long-term suppressants', 'disease-modifying', 'disease-modulating', or 'remission-inducing agents', e.g. gold, penicillamine, antimalarials, cytotoxic agents).
(b) For gout (anti-hyperuricaemic agents, e.g. probenecid (uricosuric), allopurinol (xanthineoxidase inhibitor)).
(c) For other musculoskeletal disorders (e.g. calcitonin etidronate for Paget's disease of bone; antibiotics for infective arthritis).

3. *Adjuvant drugs*
(a) For 'complications' and other intimately associated problems: muscle relaxants; psychotropic drugs (hypnotics, tranquillizers, antidepressants); haematinics; and antibiotics.
(b) For 'co-diseases' (e.g. psoriasis, ulcerative colitis, genitourinary disease).
(c) For disorders coexisting fortuitously (e.g. ischaemic heart disease, diabetes mellitus, chronic bronchitis, alcoholism).

4. *New drugs*
For example: orgotein (pure anti-inflammatory); levamisole, dapsone, sulphasalazine (long-term rheumatoid suppressants).

For descriptive convenience analgesic/anti-inflammatory (non-steroidal anti-inflammatory) drugs have been sub-classified according to their generic origin, as follows.
Carboxylic acids: salicylic acids and esters (aspirin, salicylsalicylic acid, benorylate, diflunisal); acetic acids; indole acetic acids (indomethacin, sulindac, tolmetin); phenylacetic acids (diclofenac, fenclofenac); proprionic acids (ibuprofen, naproxen, fenoprofen, ketoprofen, flurbiprofen, fenbufen, benoxaprofen, indoprofen); fenamic acids (flufenamic acid, mefenamic acid).
Enolic acids: Pyrazolones (phenylbutazone, oxyphenbutazone, azapropazone, feprazone); oxicams (piroxicam).
As has been pointed out elsewhere, grouping of drugs according to the above generic scheme is not always consistent with comparability of therapeutic and toxic effects.

The author's avoidance of sub-classifying drugs under 1(b) into minor and major analgesic/anti-inflammatory drugs stems from the paucity of appropriate comparative trials to justify fully such a division. It is conceded, however, that such a scheme probably has some justification in practice. Clinicians basing anti-rheumatic therapy on such a division generally allocate proprionic acid derivatives and drugs with clinical effects resembling them (e.g. sulindac, tolmetin, azapropazone, diflunisal, flufenamic acid, mefenamic acid, diclofenac) to the 'minor' group, and salicylates, indomethacin and phenylbutazone (and oxyphenbutazone) to the 'major' group.
The term 'non-steroidal' analgesic anti-inflammatory drugs is often used to describe drugs of group 1(b). However, since the introduction of orgotein – a pure anti-inflammatory drug of non-steroidal origin – the term may soon become obsolete.
The use of the term 'specific' in drugs of group 2 should not be taken too literally. This particularly concerns drugs used for long-term suppression of rheumatoid arthritis as they are also used in other inflammatory disorders such as systemic lupus erythematosus.
It will be noted that antibiotics feature twice in the classification (groups 2(c) and 3(a). In group 2(c) the implication is antibiotic usage to treat primary infective arthropathies (e.g. gonococcal, tuberculous). In group 3(a) antibiotics are used to treat infection occurring as a complication of an existing rheumatic disease. This event is particularly common in rheumatoid arthritis as will be discussed later.
The particular advantage of extending the usual classification of drugs used in rheumatology to include not only purely anti-rheumatic agents but also adjuvant drugs serves to heighten awareness of the potential for drug interactions (see Section 4.7).

4.4 PREPARATIONS, PRESENTATIONS, AND PACKAGING OF ANTI-RHEUMATIC DRUGS

4.4.1 Preparations

In the UK there is a wide choice of anti-rheumatic preparations. Many drugs are only available as brand (proprietary) products (e.g. naproxen (Naprosyn), piroxicam (Feldene), diclofenac (Voltarol)). Some are available as both proprietary and non-proprietary preparations (e.g. aspirin, indomethacin, phenylbutazone). Colchicine is an exception in that it is not marketed as a proprietary drug in the UK where it is only available as colchicine tablets (BP, BNF). Brand versions of this drug are widely available overseas (e.g. Colgout in

Australia, and Colchineos in France and South Africa).

Details of anti-rheumatic drugs are discussed fully in the next two chapters: Chapter 5 discusses 'symptomatic drugs' and Chapter 6 'specific drugs'. Throughout these chapters and throughout the book only approved and generic names of drugs have been used in general discussion. However, introductory comments about each drug have included UK brand names and brand names of drugs available overseas.

In view of the large number of drugs available, the UK reader will find the following useful sources of reference: *British National Formulary*; *Martindale's The Extra Pharmacopoeia*, Wade (1977); the *Data Sheet Compendium* (Association of the British Pharmaceutical Industry (ABPI)), and *MIMS*. The first two list both proprietary and non-proprietary drugs. The last two contain only proprietary preparations (but not *all* proprietary preparations).

MIMS is a widely available publication, and, providing it is used in conjunction with literature including BP, BPC and BNF preparations*, is a useful source of reference containing up-to-date information about established, new and obsolete products. It also contains a directory of pharmaceutical manufacturers. Its main drawback is the lack of an index of approved names.

Appendix 4.11.3 (derived from *MIMS*) contains some currently marketed drugs appropriate to rheumatological prescribing (analgesics/antipyretics; non-steroidal anti-inflammatory drugs; local and systemic corticosteroids and corticotrophins; cytotoxic drugs; anti-gout drugs). Some of these terms are not entirely consistent with those used in the previous section in order to retain the nomenclature employed by MIMS**, the principal source of the drugs listed. Each table lists the proprietary name and manufacturer, the approved name (or ingredients), and the type of presentation available for each drug.

The very wide choice of preparations available for doctors in the UK† is more than evident from these lists. At present there are over 60 non-steroidal anti-inflammatory drugs marketed, and, indeed, this plethora of anti-rheumatic preparations will doubtless have become extended by the time this book has been published.

---

* Preparations complying with the *British Pharmacopoeia*, the *British Pharmaceutical Codex* or the *British National Formulary*, respectively.
** Note should be made of the fact that each table is not entirely 'homogeneous'. For example, among non-steroidal anti-inflammatories are included long-term rheumatoid suppressants such as gold, penicillamine, and anti-malarials – conventionally allocated to a separate group.
† The range of anti-rheumatic drugs available in the USA is more limited.

The apparent unwieldiness of such a variety of drugs is offset by the value of having a wide therapeutic choice in a group of disorders that often display individual variations in response. It is therefore of some comfort both to patient and to doctor to know that therapy can proceed within and beyond generic groups if lack of therapeutic response or toxicity should demand this.

4.4.2 Presentations

The scope for fruitful prescribing is enhanced not only by the wide availability of different chemical preparations (formulations) but also by the variety in the presentation of drugs (Appendices 4.11.3 (a)–(e)). The following examples illustrate this point:

1. Patients whose disease is satisfactorily controlled by a particular drug may have intolerable side effects which can often be circumvented by prescribing the same drug in a different presentation (e.g. patients with gastrointestinal side effects from plain aspirin may be able to tolerate the soluble, eneric-coated, or microencapsulated preparation).

2. Patients who find difficulty in swallowing tablets (particularly children and the elderly) may find the same drug given in suspension form more acceptable. Alternatively, the drug may be given as a suppository.

3. The mode of presentation may make a difference regarding the efficacy of therapeutic response. For example, suppositories may be more effective than the same drug taken as tablets.

4. Patients with severe deformity of the hands may find a suspension presented in an easy-to-handle container (e.g. the flip-off top container of benorylate) easier to take than tablets or suppositories. (Suppositories are particularly difficult to manipulate by deformed hands.)

5. Children may feel less inhibited in taking drugs if they are presented as an attractively coloured, flavoured suspension.

6. The availability of injectable forms of the drug may be invaluable in certain circumstances, particularly in patients established on oral corticosteroids who develop a gastrointestinal upset or who are undergoing surgery. For some years phenylbutazone has been available in injectable form, and this, as well as the more recently introduced injectable diclofenac preparation, may be useful in the treatment of acute gout.

4.4.3 Packaging

The packaging as well as the presentation of drugs is important, and has received the attention of many pharmaceutical companies in recent years. This has manifested itself in the following ways:

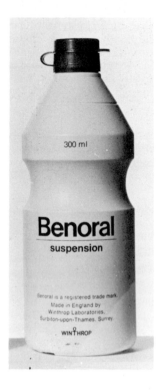
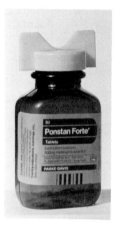
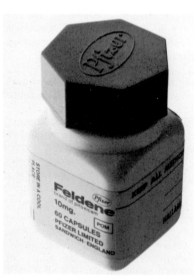
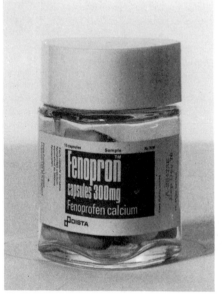

Fig. 4.1 Various anti-rheumatic drug containers featuring easily manipulable caps. The cap of the Benoral container is of the 'flip-up' type, the rest are screw caps designed in various ways to afford an easier grip for the arthritic hand.

1. Many containers (like the benorylate dispenser already mentioned) possess easily manipulable caps. Some examples of these are shown in Fig. 4.1.

2. Some drugs are now packaged in 'pop-up' form with the intention of increasing convenience and compliance (Fig. 4.2).

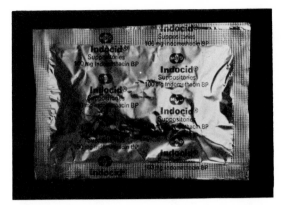

Fig. 4.3 Products covered in metal foil such as these suppositories are often found difficult to open by patients with arthritic hands.

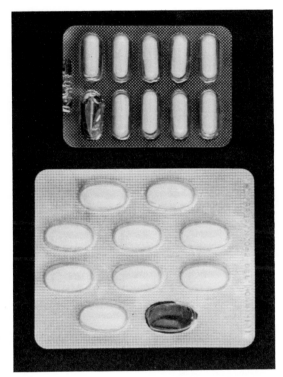

Fig. 4.2 Anti-rheumatic drugs presented in 'pop-up' form with the intention of increasing convenience and compliance.

3. Suppositories have been packaged by one pharmaceutical company to include illustrated information showing how they should be inserted (Chapter 3, Fig. 3.8). This is particularly useful as stories abound as to the alternative methods and anatomical routes patients have used to insert their suppositories. (Some patients seem to think that they are large capsules to be taken orally, whilst others have inserted them via the correct route, but still covered in their metal foil wrapper. One patient, given a finger stall for hygienic purposes, actually inserted the finger stall together with the suppository!)

4. Not all packaging is designed by the manufacturer is for easy use. Sometimes the packaging is relatively impenetrable for preservative reasons – for example, the metal foil covering certain suppositories (Fig. 4.3),

which even nursing staff have difficulty in opening. Sometimes packaging obstacles simply reflect the modern tendency to enswathe everything in a tough plastic covering.

4.5 CLINICAL APPLICATION OF DRUG THERAPY: THE CONCEPT OF 'PHASING'

Considerable variation exists in the opinions of clinicians on the stages at which to introduce individual drugs, especially in the treatment of rheumatoid arthritis (Fig. 4.4). This disagreement concerns the following particular points:

1. The division of non-steroidal anti-inflammatory drugs into 'minor' and 'major' agents.
2. The division of long-term suppressants into two categories: second-line drugs comprising gold, penicillamine, and antimalarials; and third-line drugs, the cytotoxic agents and corticosteroids.
3. The placing of corticosteroids in the scheme of therapy, or indeed, whether they should be used at all in such a scheme.

One of the most contentious points concerns the use of systemic corticosteroids. Some clinicians, including myself, believe that in *low dosage* (5–7·5 mg daily) these drugs are a valuable contribution to the scheme of management and, depending on clinical circumstances, may be prescribed at various stages of the rheumatoid disease, usually when full doses of non-steroidal inflammatory drugs have proved ineffective. Clinicians subscribing to this approach therefore tend to use corticosteroids after non-steroidal agents and before the stage of prescribing long-term suppressants (gold, penicillamine and antimalarials). Other clinicians up-

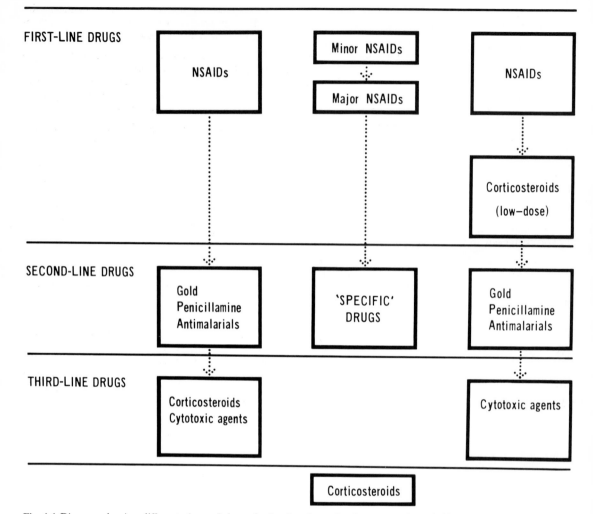

FIRST-LINE DRUGS

NSAIDs

Minor NSAIDs

Major NSAIDs

NSAIDs

Corticosteroids
(low–dose)

SECOND-LINE DRUGS

Gold
Penicillamine
Antimalarials

'SPECIFIC'
DRUGS

Gold
Penicillamine
Antimalarials

THIRD-LINE DRUGS

Corticosteroids
Cytotoxic agents

Cytotoxic agents

Corticosteroids

Fig. 4.4 Diagram showing different plans of drug phasing based on the first-, second- and third-line drug principle. Note particularly the variation in the placing of corticosteroids in the various schemes. NSAIDs = non-steroidal anti-inflammatory drugs (analgesic/anti-inflammatory drugs).

hold the opposite extreme and regard corticosteroids as applicable only for specific non-rheumatoid disorders such as polymyalgia rheumatica, giant cell arteritis, polymyositis and systemic lupus erythematosus. A further school regards the place of these drugs (in addition to the diseases just mentioned) only for specific clinical problems in rheumatoid arthritis, such as relentless progressive arthritis uncontrolled by other methods, or for threatened complete dependency.

Regarding these variations in therapeutic approach, whether to do with corticosteroids or with other drugs, much of the disparity may relate to differences between what clinicians preach and what they practise.

Apart from differences in detail, most clinicians are agreed on certain general principles to be followed in the prescribing of anti-rheumatic drugs (see Section 4.2).

4.6. FACTORS AFFECTING DRUG RESPONSE

It behoves the prescriber to remember that patients are not treated in a vacuum but in a highly complex and ever-changing environment. The multifactorial nature of this may exert subtle though important effects on the action of drugs on patients and, conversely, on the patients' reaction to drugs.

When a patient is given a drug his response is the resultant of several factors (Laurence, 1973):

1. The pharmocodynamic effect of the drug and interactions with any other drugs the patient may be taking.
2. The physiological state of the end-organ – whether, for instance, it is over- or underactive.
3. The act of medication, including the route of administration and the presence or absence of the doctor.
4. The doctor's mood, personality, attitudes and beliefs.
5. The patient's mood, personality, attitudes and beliefs.
6. What the doctor has told the patient.
7. The patient's past experience of doctors.
8. The patient's estimate of what he has received and of what ought to happen as a result.
9. The social environment, e.g. whether alone or in company.

Clearly, in any one patient, some factors may be more relevant than others, and there may also be some interplay between factors to complicate matters.

4.7 DANGERS FACING PATIENTS TAKING DRUGS

4.7.1 General

The proportion of the population taking one or more drugs continually for a large part of their lives is steadily increasing and is due to the rapidly proliferating number of prophylactic, symptomatic and suppressive medicines that have emerged from the pharmaceutical industry in recent years. Drugs for 'general medical' ailments such as hypertension, diabetes and psychiatric disorders form only a portion of this burgeoning therapeutic load, a significant proportion of which comprises drugs taken by rheumatic sufferers.

Apart from the main therapeutic benefits of short and long-term drug therapy there are also many dangers (Laurence, 1973):

1. *Dangers of the drug* – these are not markedly increased if therapy lasts years rather than months, except perhaps for addiction, renal damage (e.g. analgesic mixtures) and carcinogenesis.
2. *Dangers of stopping the drug suddenly* – dramatic illness can follow the withdrawal of anticonvulsants, corticosteroids and anti-Parkinsonian drugs.
3. *Dangers of intercurrent illness* – these are particularly prominent with hypoglycaemics, anticoagulants, corticosteroids and immunosuppressives.
4. *Dangers of interactions with other drugs or diet* – for example, monoamine oxidase inhibitor antide-

pressants interacting with sympathomimetics, including appetite suppressants; hypnotics and tranquillizers interacting with alcohol.

More specifically, it needs no emphasis that both the administration and the withdrawal of anti-rheumatic drugs can cause disease and even death. In rheumatological prescribing four particularly important additional factors need to be considered.

1. It is often necessary to prescribe more than one drug, thus introducing the additional potential for drug interactions.
2. It is often necessary to prescribe relatively toxic drugs such as gold, penicillamine and antimalarials, or even cytotoxic agents.
3. Drug therapy usually has to be maintained for long periods, and often indefinitely.
4. Rheumatic patients often have co-diseases and complications of their locomotor disturbance, manifested by disorders in other systems. This is in addition to the normal prevalence of fortuitously associated disorders such as ischaemic heart disease, chronic bronchitis, diabetes mellitus, and so forth.

For further general literature regarding iatrogenic diseases the reader is referred to the many excellent reviews on this subject (Barr, 1955; MacDonald and MacKay, 1964; Hurwitz, 1969a,b; Melmon, 1971; D'Arcy and Griffin, 1972; Girdwood, 1974; *British Medical Journal*, 1977; Weston and Weston, 1977; Davies, 1981).

4.7.2 Adverse effects associated with specific antirheumatic drugs

Disturbances due to related drug therapy may be divided into the following effects.

(a) Drug–disease effects

Throughout this book the term 'side effect' has been used although other equally apt terms include 'unwanted effects', 'toxic effects', and 'adverse effects'. Table 4.2 summarizes some of the main side effects due to anti-rheumatic drugs. In practice side effects most often affect the gut or skin, but it will be evident from the table that the spectrum of system involvement is very wide, and there are few broad categories of disease that have not been ascribed an iatrogenic cause. Further details can be found in the sections on individual drugs (Chapters 5 and 6).

(b) Drug–drug effects

Otherwise known as drug interactions, the size of the challenge encompassed by these problems in

Table 4.2 Some side effects* due to anti-rheumatic drugs[†]

System involved/ category of disease	Side effect	Examples of drugs responsible
Gastrointestinal	Dyspepsia	Many analgesic/anti-inflammatory drugs
		Corticosteroids
	Diarrhoea	Fenamates
	Gastric erosions	Salicylates
	Peptic ulceration	Indomethacin
		Phenylbutazone
		Salicylates (heavy dosage)
	Chronic blood loss	Salicylates and other analgesic/anti-inflammatory drugs
	Ileal ulceration	Indomethacin
	Hepatitis	Phenylbutazone
	Hepatic fibrosis/cirrhosis	Methotrexate
	Acute pancreatitis	Corticosteroids
	Disturbances of taste	Penicillamine
	Oral ulceration	Aspirin
	Stomatitis and glossitis	Gold
	Parotid swelling	Phenylbutazone
Integumentary	Urticaria	Salicylates
		Tetracosactrin
	Toxic erythema (e.g. morbilliform rashes)	Gold
	Vasculitis	Levamisole
		Allopurinol
		Alclofenac (withdrawn)
	Exfoliative dermatitis/toxic epidermal necrolysis	Phenylbutazone
	Life-threatening dermatosis	Gold
	Pigmentation	Corticotrophin
	Pruritus	Gold
	Erythema multiforme	Pyrazolones
		Salicylates
	Erythema nodosum	Salicylates
		Gold
	Pemphigoid reaction	PUVA (Psoralen Ultra-Violet A)
		Penicillamine
	Purpura	Allopurinol
		Indomethacin
		Antimetabolites
	Fixed drug eruptions	Oxyphenbutazone
		Dapsone
	Light-provoked drug reactions	Benoxaprofen (withdrawn)
	Nail dystrophy	Benoxaprofen (withdrawn)
	Hypopigmentation of skin and hair	Chloroquine derivatives
	Lichenoid eruptions	Gold
		Chloroquine derivatives
		Penicillamine
	Herpes simplex and other skin infections	Immunosuppressives
		Corticosteroids
	Alopecia	Cytotoxic drugs
		Allopurinol
		Colchicine
		Indomethacin
		Salicylates

Table 4.2 (*contd.*)

System involved category of disease	Side effect	Examples of drugs responsible
	Psoriasiform eruptions	Chloroquine derivatives
	Hirsutism	Corticosteroids
	Skin atrophy	Corticotrophin
	Striae	
Renal	Analgesic nephropathy	Phenacetin
	Renal failure	? Salicylates
		? Paracetamol
	Acute renal toxicity	Phenylbutazone
		Indomethacin
	Reduced renal function	Salicylates
		Indomethacin
		Ibuprofen
		Naproxen
		Fenoprofen
Pulmonary	Reactivation of tuberculosis	Corticosteroids
	Asthma	Salicylates
Cardiovascular	Precipitation/aggravation of congestive cardiac failure	Phenylbutazone
	ECG abnormality	Indomethacin
	Aggravation of hypertension	Phenylbutazone
Endocrine	Suppression of hypo-thalamic–pituitary–adrenocort-ical axis	Corticosteroids
	Cushing's syndrome	Corticosteroids
		Corticotrophin
	Dwarfism	Corticosteroids in children
	Goitre/mild hypothyroidism	Phenylbutazone
Haematological	Bone marrow depression (aplastic anaemia, agranulocytosis, thrombocytopenia)	Immunosuppressives
		Gold
		Penicillamine
		Phenylbutazone
	Haemolytic anaemia	Antimalarials
		Salicylates
	Megaloblastic anaemia	Methotrexate
		Sulphasalazine
Neoplastic disorders	Leukaemia	Phenylbutazone
	'Cancer'	Methotrexate
	Skin cancer	PUVA
Chromosome damage in certain cells (e.g. lymphocyte cultures, marrow cells)	Clastogenic changes include: poor staining, gaps, breaks, aberrations such as deletions, translocations, inversions	Cytotoxic agents (e.g. cyclo-phosphamide, methotrexate, chlorambucil)
		Certain antibiotics (e.g. mito-mycin C)
Infection	Infection encouraged or masked	Corticosteroids
		Corticotrophin
		? Indomethacin
		? Phenylbutazone
Rheumatological	Myalgia/'pseudo-rheumatism'	Corticosteroids
Neuromuscular	Proximal myopathy	Corticosteroids
		Chloroquine
	Polymyositis/dermatomyositis	Penicillamine
	Peripheral neuropathy	Chloroquine
		Dapsone
		Indomethacin
		Cytotoxic agents

Table 4.2 (*contd.*)

System involved category of disease	Side effect	Examples of drugs responsible
Neuropsychiatric	Headache, dizziness, hallucinations	Indomethacin
	Hallucinations	Pentazocine
	Hallucinations, confusional states	Salicylates
	Euphoria, depression	Corticosteroids
	Psychoses	Corticotrophin
Ophthalmological	Cataract	Corticosteroids
	Glaucoma	
	Macular lesions	Tetracosactrin
	Keratopathy	Chloroquine
	Retinopathy	
	Iritis	
Ototoxicity	Deafness, tinnitus	Salicylates
	Vertigo	Chloroquine
Disorders of the fetus and infant	Teratogenic effects (first trimester)	Cytoxic drugs (e.g. cyclophosphamide, chlorambucil, azathioprine, methotrexate). [Experimental animals.] Corticosteroids. [Experimental animals.] ? Penicillamine
	Cochleovestibular and retinal damage (second and third trimester)	Chloroquine
	Reduced birth weight	Salicylates
	Still births	? Corticosteroids
	Fetal distress	
	Congenital cataract	
	Reduction of uterine contractions in premature labour	Indomethacin Salicylates ? Other prostaglandin-synthetase inhibitors
	Premature closure of ductus arteriosus with neonatal pulmonary hypertension	? Prostaglandin-synthetase inhibitors
	Drugs in breast milk	Cyclophosphamide and other cytotoxic agents should be avoided. Analgesic/anti-inflammatory agents (e.g. aspirin, phenylbutazone, indomethacin, ibuprofen, naproxen, fenamates) enter breast milk only in low concentrations. However, caution should be exercised

* Some of these effects are the subject of only isolated reports. Others, such as some of those affecting the fetus represent observations in experimental animals.
† From Brooks *et al.* (1980); Davies (1981).

rheumatological practice is indicated in Table 4.3. It should be stressed, however, that although there is a big potential for drug interactions in rheumatology, serious interactions are unusual. Furthermore, interactions as a whole are likely to account for only a small proportion of total adverse drug effects (Volans, 1978).

The mechanisms involved in drug interaction have been summarized by Volans (1978) as follows:

Table 4.3 Some drug interactions between anti-rheumatic and other drugs*

Anti-rheumatic drug	Drug interactions	Nature of interaction
	Simple analgesics	
Paracetamol	Oral anticoagulants	Anticoagulation potentiated
	Cholestyramine	Reduced absorption of paracetamol
Pentazocine	17-Hydroxycorticosteroids, 17-ketosteroids	Urinary steroids depressed – invalidation of diagnostic tests
	Monoamine oxidase inhibitors	Enhanced effect of pentazocine (animal studies only)
	Promethazine	Maintenance requirements of pentazocine reduced
Dextropropoxyphene	17-Hydroxycorticosteroids, 17-ketosteroids	Urinary steroids depressed – invalidation of diagnostic tests
Codeine phosphate	Phenobarbitone sodium potassium iodide	Codeine–phenobarbitone and codeine–iodide complexes formed in gut
	Analgesic/anti-inflammatory drugs	
Aspirin	Alcohol	Increased gastrointestinal irritation and risk of gastric haemorrhage
	Aminosalicylic acid (PAS)	Increased risk of salicylism (particularly with large doses of aspirin)
	Ammonium chloride ascorbic acid	Increased plasma salicylate levels
	Antacids	Decreased plasma salicylate levels
	Anticoagulants	Increased risk of gastric haemorrhage (with both oral anticoagulants and heparin)
	Antidepressants	Plasma levels and side effects of nortriptyline and imipramine increased
	Corticosteroids	Accumulation of salicylate with toxicity when long-term steroid therapy withdrawn and aspirin dosage not reduced
	Hypoglycaemics	Increased hypoglycaemic effect with sulphonylureas and large doses of aspirin
	Methotrexate	Activity of methotrexate increased
	Other anti-inflammatory drugs	Plasma levels of indomethacin, fenoprofen, and naproxen lowered
	Spironolactone	Inhibition of natriuresis
	Uricosuric agents	Low-dose aspirin inhibits uricosuric action of probenecid, sulphinpyrazone, and phenylbutazone
Diflunisal	Antacids	Absorption of diflunisal decreased
Indomethacin	Buffered aspirin	Increased rate of absorption and severity of side effects of indomethacin
	Aspirin + probenecid	Total concentration of indomethacin and pain relief increased
Sulindac	Probenecid	Slightly reduced uricosuric effect of probenecid (probably not clinically significant)
Tolmetin	Aspirin	Plasma concentrations of tolmetin reduced (clinical significance uncertain)
Diclofenac	Aspirin	High salicylate levels slightly diminish protein-binding of diclofenac. Conversely, diclofenac may depress salicylate levels
Naproxen†	Aspirin	Slight reduction in naproxen plasma levels (probably not clinically significant)
	Probenecid	Increased blood concentrations of naproxen
Flufenamic acid	Oral coumarin anticoagulants, oral sulphonylurea, hypoglycaemic agents	Flufenamic acid may theoretically enhance the activity of these drugs

Table 4.3 (*contd.*)

Anti-rheumatic drug	Drug interactions	Nature of interaction
Phenylbutazone	Anticoagulants	Oral coumarin anticoagulant activity enhanced
	Cholestyramine	Absorption of phenylbutazone decreased
	Diuretics and anti-hypertensive drugs	Phenylbutazone may inhibit action of these drugs
	Hypoglycaemic drugs	Phenylbutazone enhances activity of aceto-hexamide, carbutamide, chlorpropamide, and tolbutamide
	Phenytoin	Phenylbutazone may increase phenytoin levels to toxic range
	Thyroid function tests	Phenylbutazone displaces plasma protein-bound thyroid hormone and may interfere with interpretation of thyroid function tests
	Non-analgesic/anti-inflammatory drugs	
Corticosteroids	Phenobarbitone, phenytoin, rifampicin	These drugs reduce the therapeutic effect of certain corticosteroids
	Salicylates	Salicylate concentrations may be reduced to sub-therapeutic levels
	Thiazide and related diuretics	Risk of hyperglycaemia and potassium loss increased
	Oral hypoglycaemic drugs Insulin	The effects of these anti-diabetic drugs may be diminished by corticosteroids
Corticotrophins	As above	
	Specific anti-rheumatic drugs	
Gold	Drugs that affect bone marrow (e.g. phenylbutazone, penicillamine, immunosuppressives)	It is wise to avoid giving gold with drugs tending to cause marrow aplasia, although there is no direct evidence that this is harmful
Penicillamine	See above	
Antimalarials	Hepatotoxic drugs, Drugs causing sensitization (e.g. gold)	Antimalarials may enhance the effect of these drugs
Azathioprine	Allopurinol	Allopurinol enhances the toxicity of azathioprine
	Drugs that affect bone marrow	See under gold
Cyclophosphamide	Barbiturates	The therapeutic effect and toxicity of cyclophosphamide may be increased
	Drugs that affect bone marrow	See under gold
Methotrexate	Salicylates, sulphonamides, diuretics, hypoglycaemics, diphenylhydantoins, tetracyclines, chloramphenicol, acidic anti-inflammatory agents	These and other protein-bound drugs may displace methotrexate and increase its toxicity (These potential interactions are particularly important in the management of psoriatic arthritis)
	Alcohol and other hepatotoxic agents	Risk of hepatotoxicity increased
Antibiotics	Probenecid	Side effects of nitrofurantoin and dapsone increased

Table 4.3 (*contd.*)

Anti-rheumatic drug	Drug interactions	Nature of interaction
	Antacids, dairy products, oral iron, zinc sulphate, cimetidine	Reduce absorption of tetracyclines
	Barbiturates, carbamazepine, phenytoin	Reduce blood levels of doxycycline
	Phenobarbitone	Reduces blood levels of chloramphenicol
	Ethacrynic acid, frusemide, gentamicin	Increase the nephrotoxicity of cefotamine, cephaloridine, and cephalothin

* From Hart (1981) and the *British National Formulary* (1981).
† Naproxen and certain other proprionic acid derivatives (e.g. ibuprofen, fenoprofen, and ketoprofen) can be given with oral coumarin anticoagulants.

1. Pharmaceutical incompatibility.
2. Altered absorption.
3. Altered distribution (displacement of drugs bound to plasma proteins).
4. Competition at receptor sites.
5. Competition at site of action or within same physiological system.
6. Altered metabolism (stimulation or inhibition).
7. Altered excretion.
8. Changes in fluid balance.

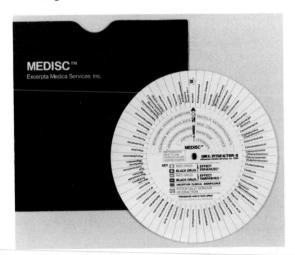

Fig. 4.5 Convenient drug interaction disc (Medisc, Excerpta Medica Services, Inc, 1976) displaying various commonly used preparations, including some anti-rheumatic drugs (aspirin, indomethacin, phenylbutazone, naproxen, corticosteroids).

A useful device to remind clinicians of main drug interactions is shown in Fig. 4.5.

(c) Disease–drug effects

This category includes those clinical circumstances where the prescribing potential or the actual effect of giving a drug is modified by a particular disease. The following serve as examples:

Diseases of the gastrointestinal tract
Patients with chronic gastrointestinal disorders (e.g. peptic ulceration, chronic inflammatory bowel disease such as ulcerative colitis and Crohn's disease) should be treated with particular caution as many anti-rheumatic agents tend to aggravate these conditions. Intestinal hurry may also complicate therapy by descreasing the absorption of drugs from the alimentary tract. Anal soreness and proctitis will contraindicate the use of suppositories.

Hepatic disease
Apart from exacerbating pre-existing disease, some anti-inflammatory agents have been implicated in certain hepatic disorders. For example, phenylbutazone and indomethacin can cause hepatitis, and methotrexate can cause hepatic fibrosis. Quite apart from these drug-induced hepatic effects, the metabolism of anti-rheumatic drugs would be expected to be disturbed if given to patients with liver disease, as most of these drugs are metabolized in the smooth endoplasmic reticulum of hepatocytes.

Renal disease

Secondary amyloidosis is an established feature of long-standing severe rheumatoses such as rheumatoid arthritis, and is seen less commonly in other chronic conditions such as ankylosing spondylitis. Other forms of renal disease may also be encountered, such as that due to systemic lupus erythematosus and analgesic nephropathy. Anti-rheumatic medication in these patients will also have to be chosen with particular care. Both phenylbutazone and indomethacin are known to cause acute renal toxicity, and even some of the relatively non-toxic proprionic acid preparations – ibuprofen, naproxen and fenoprofen – have been shown to reduce renal function (in patients with systemic lupus erythematosus). The nephrotoxic actions of gold and penicillamine have been discussed fully elsewhere.

Cardiovascular disease

This may be a complication of the rheumatic disorder (e.g. ankylosing spondylitis, systemic lupus erythematosus, rheumatoid arthritis) or it may coexist as an unrelated disease. Drugs that cause salt and water retention (e.g. phenylbutazone) should be avoided because they may precipitate congestive cardiac failure. Some drugs may also interfere with the hypotensive action of diuretics.

Respiratory disease

The risk of reactivating dormant pulmonary tuberculosis with corticosteroids should alert clinicians when treating arthritic patients with a past history of tuberculosis. Aspirin and other analgesic/anti-inflammatory drugs may provoke acute asthmatic attacks in patients with chronic asthma.

Skin disease

Patients with a hypersensitivity diathesis may develop urticaria and angioneurotic oedema in response to salicylates and related drugs. Exfoliative reactions of psoriasis may be precipitated by antimalarials in patients treated for psoriatic arthritis. Patients with Sjögren's syndrome are particularly prone to drug sensitivity reactions (e.g. penicillin, gold).

Eye disease

Patients with glaucoma should be given corticosteroids only with the utmost caution. Patients with established retinopathy should not be given antimalarials which themselves have a retinotoxic effect.

Neurological/psychiatric disease

Corticosteroids should be avoided in patients with a history of psychosis. Indomethacin may aggravate psychiatric disorders, epilepsy and Parkinsonism.

Endocrine disease

Corticosteroids may aggravate diabetes mellitus, and phenylbutazone may cause goitre and mild hypothyroidism. It would be wise, therefore, to avoid using phenylbutazone if there is evidence of thyroid disease.

Age, sex and nutritional status

Although not diseases *per se*, these biological factors may have important implications when prescribing drugs. For example, elderly patients seem more prone to the blood dyscrasia effects of phenylbutazone. Women of child-bearing age should be prescribed drugs with caution, even more so should they be pregnant. The nutritional status of patients may dictate dose levels – underweight patients in general will not need as much of a drug as more robust individuals.

4.7.3 Iatrogenic rheumatoses

Most practising rheumatologists will have encountered diagnostic problems that have ultimately been shown to be drug-induced rheumatic syndromes (iatrogenic rheumatoses). Such disorders cover a wide clinical spectrum, since there is a wide spectrum of drugs causing them (Table 4.4).

4.8 MEDICO-LEGAL IMPLICATIONS OF PRESCRIBING DRUGS

These days there is a growing awareness that medico-legal responsibilities no longer lie mainly in the domain of the orthopaedic surgeon and casualty officer. 'Today the prescription wields as much power for good or for ill as does the scalpel, and liability corresponds with power'. This comment and much of the following have been taken from Taylor (1981) – secretary of the Medical Protection Society (London). For more detailed information the reader is referred to this source, which cites many illustrative medico-legal case histories, many of them from the USA, where experience in the field is very much greater than it is in the UK. However, as the author points out, this does not mean that negligence in respect of drug administration is rare in the UK, and it is this fact that has prompted inclusion of the following, albeit brief, section.

4.8.1 Duty of care

Negligence is a civil wrong that consists of a breach of a duty of care resulting in damage. This duty is regardless of whether treatment is private, covered by a health service, or gratuitous. To prove negligence the following must be shown: (1) that there existed a duty of care; (2) that there was a dereliction of that duty; and (3) that

Table 4.4 Some iatrogenic* disorders of rheumatological significance[†]

Disorder	Examples of drugs responsible
Muscles	
Myalgia and cramps	Methysergide, oral contraceptives, guanethidine, digitalis glycosides, suxamethonium, metolazone, clofibrate, penicillamine, corticosteroids
Muscle damage	Suxamethonium, amphetamine, drug-induced myasthenia and myopathy
Joints	
Arthralgia/arthropathy/arthritis:	
Mild arthralgia and arthritis	Associated with almost any drug eruption
Severe arthropathy	Associated with certain drug eruptions, e.g. carbimazole, prazosin
Acute gout precipitated	Thiazides
Telescoping of fingers	Allopurinol
Arthritis accompanying myalgia	Steroid-withdrawal syndrome
Exacerbation of rheumatoid arthritis	Levamisole, total-dose iron dextran
Joint effusions	Practolol
Painless deforming arthropathy	Purgative abuse (? related to chronic drug-induced bowel disease)
Aches and pains associated with arteritis	Sulphonamides
Septic arthritis	Faulty intra-articular injection technique
Haemarthrosis	Anticoagulants
Shoulder-hand syndrome	Phenobarbitone, isoniazid, ? ethionamide
Bones	
Osteoporosis	Corticosteroids, heparin, alcohol
Osteomalacia	Aluminium hydroxide, anticonvulsants, barbiturates, chapattis, fluoride, glutethamide, inositol hexaphosphate. pheneturide, phenobarbitone, phenytoin, phytic acid, primidone, purgatives
Fractures and dislocations	Babiturates in the elderly increase falls and also aggravate osteomalacia
Dislocation of shoulder	Repeated i.m. injections (particularly pentazocine) may produce fibrosis around shoulder with abduction deformity leading to dislocation
Aseptic (avascular, ischaemic) necrosis	Corticosteroids, corticotrophin
Osteosclerosis	Excessive doses of fluorine, vitamin D or vitamin A. A rare feature of the milk-alkali syndrome
Ectopic calcification of muscles, tendons, ligaments, subcutaneous tissue and viscera (e.g. myocardium, aorta, kidney)	Chronic vitamin D poisoning
Ectopic calcification of tendons and periarticular tissues	Excessive intake of fluorine or vitamin A.
Local calcification	At site of intramuscular or subcutaneous injections
Bone thickening of the skull	Phenytoin
Connective tissues	
Tendons:	
Spontaneous rupture (usually Achilles' tendon, sometimes patellar tendon)	Systemic or local corticosteroids
Tendon involvement in gout	Drugs inducing gout
Adipose tissue:	
Atrophy of subcutaneous fatty tissue	Local injection of insulin or corticosteroids
Mediastinal lipomatosis	Corticosteroids
Nodular panniculitis	Withdrawal of corticosteroids
Fibrous tissue:	
Retroperitoneal fibrosis	Methysergide, ? ergotamine, ? dehydroergotamine
Pulmonary fibrosis	Busulphan, hexamethonium, mecamylamine
Fibrosing peritonitis	Practolol
Peyronie's disease (fibrous plaques in the shaft of the penis)	Propranolol, metoprolol
Dupuytren's contracture	? Propranolol

Table 4.4 (*contd.*)

Disorder	*Examples of drugs responsible*
Systemic lupus erythematosus: Whether drug-induced systemic lupus is a disease in its own right or merely spontaneous systemic lupus unmasked or aggravated by a drug has still not been resolved. For the drugs shown, there is convincing supportive evidence. Many other drugs have been implicated but the evidence is less convincing. The figures in parentheses after each drug represent the frequency of the complication.	Procainamide (5–20%). Hydrallazine (1–21%). Anticonvulsants (8% or less): ethosuximide, methoin, phenytoin, primidone, troxidone. Isoniazid (0.1%). Others: thiouracils, practolol, chlorpromazine, penicillamine
Drug-related pseudolupus: A drug-related syndrome resembling systemic lupus erythematosus but differing from it serologically	Venocuran (phenopyrazone, a horse-chestnut extract, and glycosides from several plants). This mixture is used for treatment of venous diseases
Disorders of growth	
Stunting of growth: Retarded linear growth due to inhibition of the skeletal effect of growth hormone, and consequent depression of epiphyseal growth	Corticosteroids for long periods
Reversible retardation of linear growth	Tetracyclines
Impairment of height and weight	? Stimulant drugs (e.g. methylphenidate)
Acceleration of growth: Acceleration of growth	Androgens (given before puberty)

* Not all of these disorders are 'drug' induced (e.g. chapatti-induced osteomalacia) and not all are induced by doctors (e.g. purgative-abuse-induced arthropathy, and osteomalacia).
† From Davis (1981).

there was a direct causative relationship between that dereliction and the resulting damage.

In exercising duty of care, the doctor does not *ensure* that his patient will come to no harm, but he does undertake to use *reasonable skill and care* in all that he does for his patient. The term 'reasonable skill and care' does not necessarily imply the highest standard of care in all circumstances, and a doctor will avoid a finding of negligence if he can show that: *'having regard to all the relevant circumstances, he achieved the standard of skill and care of practitioners of equal standing and experience'*.

4.8.2 Liability

A doctor found to be negligent is liable to the patient for all harm suffered as a result of that negligence. The plaintiff can enforce his claim against one or more parties. In the UK, where the involved parties may be a doctor (or doctors) and a hospital authority, an agreement between the Department of Health and the protection or defence society ensures that 'irrespective of which party may be cited, proportionate liability will reflect the degree of involvement of each party in those aspects of the care of the patient relevant to the case' (Taylor, 1981).

Interpretation of the concept of proportionate liability is not necessarily straightforward and depends on the individual facts of the case. Taking proportionate liability between a consultant and a junior hospital doctor, for example, the consultant's expectation of his junior with regard to a certain standard of knowledge and skill will depend on the junior doctor's experience and progress. It would be unreasonable, on the one hand, to expect the consultant to check a newly appointed doctor's every act, as it would, on the other hand, to delegate him responsibilities allowed a junior towards the end of his appointment.

The relationship between consultant and general practitioner may also be relevant to proportionate liability and in general depends on a two-way duty based on adequate communication regarding relevant facts about the patient, including details of drug therapy.

4.8.3 Hospital ethical committees

These committees have been set up on the recommendation of the Royal College of Physicians in all major hospitals in the UK where clinical trials and experimental procedures are carried out. Their function is to advise on the ethics of any proposed procedure, and in view of this ethical role it would seem unlikely that its members would be legally liable should a patient suffer harm from a procedure given committee approval. However, should there arise an allegation of assault based on lack of valid consent, for example, this would be directed towards the investigator (Taylor, 1981).

4.8.4 Outcome of allegations of negligence

When a solicitor confronts a doctor with an allegation of negligence, about 95% of such cases are either abandoned or settled out of court. In the special case of alleged drug-induced negligence, almost all those cases that have arisen in the UK in the past have not led to court involvement.

Errors that have resulted in settlement of one sort or another have included the following categories of negligence: (1) gross overdosage arising from misplaced or misread decimal points; (2) illegible handwriting leading to incorrect dispensing; (3) careless use of 'p.r.n.' on treatment sheets; (4) administration of the wrong drug due to failure to read the label.

4.8.5 Conclusion

With legislation as it is at present, adverse drug reactions will almost inevitably play a more prominent part in future allegations of negligence against doctors than they have previously.

New proposals arising from European Economic Community (EEC) administrative circles still lack suffi-cient precision to clarify fully the doctor's position. However, it would seem that the dispensing and, perhaps, the prescribing doctor would only avoid liability for drug-induced harm if he or she is able to (1) inform the patient of the name of the manufacturer, and (2) show that he or she passed on to the patient all relevant warnings about the use of the drug.

4.9 SUMMARY AND CONCLUSION

This chapter is intended to complement the subsequent chapters (5 and 6) devoted to individual drugs. It deals with general factors and principles involved in prescrib-ing drugs, with classification of anti-rheumatic drugs, and with the spectrum of available preparations and presentations. A section has been allocated to the question of applying drug therapy, with a note on the concept of 'phasing' drugs according to a first-, second- and third-line scheme. A further section outlines factors affecting drug response, and some detail is given to the important matter of iatrogenic disease caused by drugs (drug–disease effects, drug–drug effects, and disease–drug effects). The last section records some notes on medico-legal implications of prescribing with a cautionary reminder that 'the prescription wields as much power for good or for ill as does the scalpel...'.

It is often said that there is more to rheumatological management than writing prescriptions. To this may be added the inescapable conclusion that writing pre-scriptions is also not the only aspect of using anti-rheumatic drugs.

4.10 REFERENCES AND FURTHER READING

General factors

Baum, J. (1982) Ethical aspects of drug therapy in children. *Clin. Rheumatol.*, **1**, 45.
Bibace, R. and Walsh, M.E. (1980) Developments of children's concepts of illness. *Pediatrics*, **66**, 912.
Coleman, V. (1977) *The Medicine Men: A Shattering Analysis of the Drugs Industry*, Arrow, London.
Klass, A. (1975) *There's Gold in Them Thar Pills: An Inquiry into the Medical–Industrial Complex*, Penguin, Harmondsworth.
MIMS (April 1982) Published monthly by Haymarket Publishing, Middlesex.
Wade, A. (ed.) (1977) *Martindale. The Extra Pharmacopoeia*, 27th edn, The Pharmaceutical Press, London.

Factors affecting drug response

Laurence, D.R. (1973) *Clinical Pharmacology*, 4th edn, Churchill Livingstone, Edinburgh, pp. 1.5–1.6.

Dangers in taking drugs

Barr, D.P. (1955) Hazards of modern diagnosis and therapy. *J. Am. Med. Assoc.*, **159**, 1452.
Brooks, P.M., Kraag, G.R. and Buchanan, W.W. (1980) in *Ankylosing Spondylitis* (ed. J.M.H. Moll), Churchill Livingstone, Edinburgh, p. 203.
British Medical Journal (1977) Deaths due to drug treatment. *Br. Med. J.*, **i**, 1492.
British National Formulary (1981), Number 2, British Medical Association and The Pharmaceutical Society of Great Britain, London.
D'Arcy, P.F. and Griffin, J.P. (1972) *Iatrogenic Diseases*, Oxford University Press, London.
Davies, D.M. (ed.) (1981) *Textbook of Adverse Drug Reactions*, Oxford University Press, Oxford.
Girdwood, R.H. (1974) Deaths after taking medicaments. *Br. Med. J.*, **i**, 501.
Hart, F.D. (ed.) (1978) *Drug Treatment of the Rheumatic Diseases*, MTP Press, Lancaster.
Hurwitz, N. (1969a) Admissions to hospital due to drugs. *Br. Med. J.*, **i**, 539.
Hurwitz, N. (1969b) Predisposing factors in adverse reactions to drugs. *Br. Med. J.*, **i**, 536.

Laurence, D.R. (1973) *Clinical Pharmacology*, 4th edn, Churchill Livingstone, Edinburgh, p. 1.9.

MacDonald, M.G. and MacKay, B.R. (1964) Adverse drug reactions. *J. Am. Med. Assoc.*, **190**, 1071.

Melmon, K.L. (1971) Preventable drug reactions – causes and cures. *N. Engl. J. Med.*, **284**, 1361.

Volans, G.N. (1978) Drug interactions in rheumatoid disease – are they of any clinical importance? *Rheumatol. Rehabil.* (Supplement), p. 112.

Weston, J.K. and Weston, K. (1977) Adverse drug reactions – the scene revisited. *Clin. Toxicol.*, **10**, 129.

Medico-legal implications

Taylor, J.L. (1981) in *Textbook of Adverse Drug Reactions* (ed. D.M. Davies), Oxford University Press, Oxford, pp. 602–13.

4.11 APPENDICES

4.11.1 The persuasiveness of pharmaceutical advertising, (a) Examples from the UK. (b) Examples from the USA (see text)

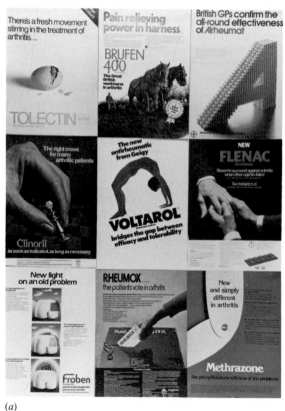

(*a*)

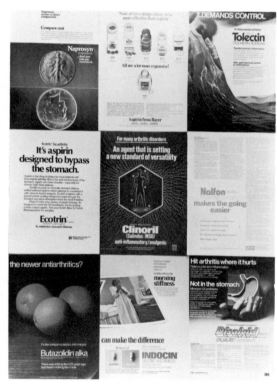

(*b*)

4.11.2 Costs of some preparations

(*a*) *Cost per tablet* of some aspirin and aspirin-containing compounds (MIMS: April, 1982)*

Preparation	mg aspirin	Manufacturer	Cost per tablet (p)[†]
	Pure aspirin		
Nu-Seals Aspirin	300	Lilly	1·18
Breoprin	648	Sterling Research Laboratories	3·88
Levius	500	Farmitalia Carlo Erba Ltd.	1·06
Solprin	300	Reckitt & Colman	0·45
Claradin	300	Nicholas	1·17
	Aspirin compounds		
Codis	500	Reckitt and Colman	2·00
Hypon	325	Calmic	2·83
Safapryn	300	Pfizer	1·63
Veganin	250	Warner	2·12
Migravess	325	Dome/Hollister-Stier	12·83
Myolgin	200	Cox	1·66
Napsalgesic	500	Dista	2·13
Antoin	400	Fox	1·54
Laboprin	300	Laboratories for Applied Biology Ltd.	2·08
Equagesic	250	Wyeth	1·81
Emprazil	300	Wellcome	4·00
Dolasan	325	Lilly	4·61
Doloxene compound	375	Lilly	4·21
Paynocil	600	Beecham	2·30
Robaxisal Forte	325	Robins	2·89
Onadox-118	300	Duncan, Flockhart	2.76
Trancoprin	300	Sterling Research Laboratories	3·03

* Retail NHS prices.
[†] Prices expressed in pence (UK) to two decimal places for comparative rather than practical purposes.

(*b*) *Cost per month of some proprionic acid preparations* (MIMS: April, 1982)*

Approved name	Proprietary name	Manufacturer	Maximal recommended dose per day	Cost per month (£)
Ibuprofen	Brufen	Boots	400 mg × 4	5·17
Naproxen	Naprosyn	Syntex	500 mg × 2	10·97
Fenoprofen	Fenopron	Dista	600 mg × 4	14·66
	Progesic	Lilly	200 mg × 12	16·73
Ketoprofen	Alrheumat	Bayer	50 mg × 4	6·52
Flurbiprofen	Froben	Boots	100 mg × 3	13·15
Fenbufen	Lederfen	Lederle	300 mg × 3	13·64
Tiaprofenic acid	Surgam	Cassenne (Roussel)	200 mg × 3	13·24

* The preparation benoxaprofen (Opren), although included in the original table, has been excluded from this table as the drug has been withdrawn from the market.

(c) *Cost per month of some analgesic/anti-inflammatory agents in different generic groups (MIMS: April, 1982)*

Generic group	Least costly preparation		Maximal recommended maintenance dosage per day	Cost per month (£)
	Approved name	Proprietary name		
Salicylic acid/ester	Aspirin	Solprin	300 mg × 24	3·02
Indole acetic acid	Indomethacin	Mobilan	50 mg × 4	7·00
Phenylacetic acid	Diclofenac	Voltarol	50 mg × 3	14·70
Proprionic acid	Ibuprofen	Brufen	400 mg × 4	5·17
Fenamic acid	Mefenamic acid	Ponstan Forte	500 mg × 3	6·64
Pyrazolone	Phenylbutazone	Butazolidin	100 mg × 3	1·12
Oxicam	Piroxicam	Feldene	10 mg × 3	12·60

4.11.3 Agents listed in MIMS

(a) *Analgesics and antipyretics listed in MIMS (April, 1982)*

Proprietary name	Manufacturer	Approved name/ ingredients	Presentation
Acupan	Carnegie	Nefopam hydrochloride	Tablet 30 mg Ampoule 1 ml (20 mg/ml) i.m. or i.v.
Cafadol	Typharm	Paracetamol 500 mg, caffeine 30 mg	Tablet
Calpol	Calmic	Paracetamol 120 mg/ 5 ml	Suspension
Cosalgesic	Cox	Dextropropoxyphene hydrochloride 32.5 mg, paracetamol 325 mg	Tablet
Cyclimorph*	Calmic	Cyclimorph – morphine tartrate	Ampoule 1 ml: Cyclimorph 10 – morphine tartrate 10 mg, cyclizine tartrate 50 mg Ampoule 1 ml: Cyclimorph 15 – morphine tartrate 15 mg, cyclizine s.c., i.m., or i.v.
Depronal	SA Warner	Dextropropoxyphene hydrochloride 150 mg	Capsule (sustained release)
DF 118	Duncan, Flockhart	Dihydrocodeine tartrate	Tablet 30 mg Elixir 10 mg/5 ml Ampoule 1 ml (50 mg/ml) s.c. or i.m.
Diconal*	Calmic	Dipanone hydrochloride 10 mg, cyclizine hydrochloride 30 mg	Tablet
Dipidolor*	Janssen	Piritramide 10 mg/ml	Ampoule 2 ml i.m.
Distalgesic	Dista	Dextropropoxyphene hydrochloride 32.5 mg, paracetamol 325 mg	Tablet

Appendix 4.11.3 (*contd.*)

Proprietary name	Manufacturer	Approved name/ ingredients	Presentation
Distalgesic Soluble	Dista	Dextropropoxyphene napsylate (equivalent to 32.5 mg hydrochloride)	Tablet
Dolasan	Lilly	Dextropropoxyphene napsylate	Tablet
Dolobid	Morson	Diflunisal	Tablet 250 mg Tablet 500 mg
Doloxene	Lilly	Dextropropoxyphene napsylate (equivalent to 65 mg hydrochloride)	Tablet
Doloxene compound	Lilly	Dextropropoxyphene napsylate (equivalent to 65 mg hydrochloride), aspirin 375 mg, caffeine 30 mg	Capsule
Dromoran*	Roche	Levorphanol tartrate	Tablet 1.5 mg Ampoule 1 ml (2mg/ml) s.c., i.m., or i.v.
Duromorph*	Laboratories for Applied Biology	Micro-crystalline morphine 64 mg/ml	Ampoule 1 ml s.c. or i.m.
Fortagesic	Winthrop	Pentazocine 15 mg (as hydrochloride), paracetamol 500 mg	Tablet
Fortral	Winthrop	Pentazocine hydrochloride	Tablet 25 mg Tablet 50 mg Suppository (as lactate) 50 mg Ampoule 1 ml (30 mg/ml) Ampoule 2 ml (30 mg/ml) s.c., i.m., or i.v.
Medocodene	Medo	Paracetamol 500 mg, codeine phosphate 8 mg, phenolphthalein 20 mg	Tablet
MST-1 Continus*	Napp	Morphine sulphate 10 mg	Tablet (sustained release)
Narphen*	Smith & Nephew Pharmaceuticals	Phenazocine hydrobromide 5 mg	Tablet
Neurodyne	Wade	Paracetamol 500 mg, codeine phosphate 8 mg	Capsule
Omnopon*	Roche	Papaveretum	Tablet 10 mg Ampoule 1 ml (20 mg/ml) s.c., i.m., or i.v.

Appendix 4.11.3 (*contd.*)

Proprietary name	Manufacturer	Approved name/ ingredients	Presentation
Palfium*	M.C.P.	Dextromoramide (as tartrate)	Tablet 5 mg Tablet 10 mg Suppository 10 mg Ampoule 1 ml (5 mg/ml) Ampoule 1 ml (10 mg/ml) s.c., i.m. or i.v.
Panadeine Co	Winthrop	Paracetamol 500 mg, codeine phosphate 8 mg	Tablet
Panadol	Winthrop	Paracetamol 500 mg	Tablet (effervescent) Elixir 120 mg/5 ml
Panasorb	Winthrop	Paracetamol 500 mg	Tablet
Paracodol	Fisons	Paracetamol 500 mg, codeine phosphate 8 mg	Tablet (effervescent)
Parahypon	Calmic	Paracetamol 500 mg caffeine 10 mg, codeine phosphate 5 mg	Tablet
Parake	Galen	Paracetamol 500 mg, codeine phosphate 8 mg	Tablet
Paralgin	Norton	Paracetamol 450 mg, caffeine 20 mg, codeine phosphate 6 mg	Tablet
Paramol-118	Duncan, Flockhart	Paracetamol 500 mg, dihydrocodeine tartrate 10 mg	Tablet
Para-Seltzer	Wander	Paracetamol 500 mg, caffeine 20 mg	Tablet (effervescent)
Pardale	Dales	Paracetamol 400 mg, codeine phosphate 9 mg, caffeine hydrate 10 mg	Tablet
Pethilorfan*	Roche	Pethidine hydrochloride 50 mg, levallorphan tartrate 0.625 mg/ml	Ampoule 1 ml Ampoule 2 ml
Pharmidone	Farmitalia	Codeine phosphate 10 mg, diphenhydramine hydrochloride 5 mg, paracetamol 400 mg, caffeine 50 mg	Tablet
Physeptone*	Wellcome	Methadone hydrochloride	Tablet 5 mg Linctus 2 mg/5 ml Ampoule 1 ml (10 mg/ml)
Propain	Farillon	Codeine phosphate 10 mg, diphenhydramine hydrochloride 5 mg, paracetamol 400 mg, caffeine 50 mg	Tablet

Appendix 4.11.3 *(contd.)*

Proprietary name	Manufacturer	Approved name/ ingredients	Presentation
Salzone	Wallace	Paracetamol 120 mg/ 5 ml	Syrup
Solpadeine	Winthrop	Paracetamol 500 mg, codeine phosphate 8 mg, caffeine 30 mg	Tablet (effervescent)
Stadol	Mead Johnson	Butorphanol tartrate 2 mg/ml	Vial 1 ml i.m. or i.v.
Syndol	Merrell	Paracetamol 450 mg, codeine phosphate 10 mg, doxylamine succinate 5 mg, caffeine 30 mg	Tablet
Temgesic	Reckitt & Colman	Buprenorphine 0.3 mg/ ml	Ampoule 1 ml Ampoule 2 ml
Unigesic	Unimed	Paracetamol 500 mg, caffeine 30 mg	Capsule
Veganin	Warner	Aspirin 250 mg, paracetamol 250 mg, codeine phosphate 9.58 mg	Tablet
Zactipar	Wyeth	Ethoheptazine citrate 75 mg, paracetamol 400 mg	Tablet
Zomax	Ortho	Zomepirac (as sodium dihydrate) 100 mg	Tablet

* Indicates products controlled under the Misuse of Drugs Act.

(b) Non-steroidal anti-inflammatory drugs* listed in MIMS (April, 1982)

Proprietary name	Manufacturer	Approved name/ ingredients	Presentation
Alrheumat	Bayer	Ketoprofen	Capsule 50 mg Suppository 100 mg
Ananase	Forte Rorer	Bromelains (proteo-lytic enzymes)	Tablet
Antoin	Cox	Aspirin 400 mg, codeine phosphate 5 mg, caffeine citrate 15 mg	Tablet
Benoral	Winthrop	Benorylate	Tablet 750 mg Suspension 4 g/10 ml Sachet 2 g
Breoprin	Sterling Research Laboratories	Aspirin (formulated for intestinal release) 648 mg	Tablet
Brufen	Boots	Ibuprofen	Tablet 200 mg Tablet 400 mg Syrup 100 mg/5 ml
Butacote	Geigy	Phenylbutazone	Tablet (enteric coated) 100 mg Tablet (enteric coated) 200 mg

Appendix 4.11.3 (*contd.*)

Proprietary name	Manufacturer	Approved name/ ingredients	Presentation
Butazolidin	Geigy	Phenylbutazone	Tablet 100 mg Tablet 200 mg Suppository 250 mg Injection 200 mg/ml i.m.
Butazolidin Alka	Geigy	Phenylbutazone 100 mg, dried aluminium hydroxide gel 100 mg, magnesium trisilicate 150 mg	Tablet
Caprin	Sinclair	Aspirin (formulated for intestinal release) 324 mg	Tablet
Chymar	Armour	Chymotrypsin 5000 units	Vial i.m.
Chymoral Forte	Armour	Tryspin and chymo-trypsin equivalent to 100 000 units proteolytic activity	Tablet (enteric coated)
Claradin	Nicholas	Aspirin 300 mg	Tablet (effer-vescent)
Clinoril	Merck Sharp & Dohme	Sulindac	Tablet 100 mg Tablet 200 mg
Codis	Reckitt & Colman	Soluble aspirin 500 mg, codeine phosphate 8 mg	Tablet
Cuprimine	Merck Sharp & Dohme	D-penicillamine 250 mg	Tablet
Delimon	Consolidated Chemicals	Morazone hydro-chloride 150 mg, salicylamide 200 mg, paracetamol 50 mg	Tablet
Disalcid	Riker	Salsalate 500 mg	Capsule
Distamine	Dista	D-penicillamine	Tablet 50 mg Tablet 125 mg Tablet 250 mg
Equagesic	Wyeth	Aspirin 250 mg, meprobamate 150 mg, ethoheptazine citrate 75 mg	Tablet
Feldene	Pfizer	Piroxicam 10 mg	Tablet
Fenopron	Dista	Fenoprofen	Tablet 300 mg Tablet 600 mg
Fenopron D	Dista	Fenoprofen	Tablet (dispers-ible) 300 mg
Flenac	Reckitt & Colman	Fenclofenac 300 mg	Tablet
Froben	Boots	Flurbiprofen	Tablet 50 mg Tablet 100 mg
Hypon	Calmic	Aspirin 325 mg, caffeine 10 mg, codeine phosphate 5 mg	Tablet
Imbrilon	Berk	Indomethacin	Capsule 25 mg Capsule 50 mg Suppository 100 mg

Appendix 4.11.3 (*contd.*)

Proprietary name	Manufacturer	Approved name/ ingredients	Presentation
Indocid	Morson	Indomethacin	Capsule 25 mg Capsule 50 mg Capsule 75 mg (sustained release) Indocid R Suspension 25 mg/ml Suppository 100 mg
Laboprin	Laboratories for Applied Biology	Aspirin 300 mg, lysine 245 mg	Tablet
Lederfen	Lederle	Fenbufen 300 mg	Capsule
Levius	Farmitalia C.E.	Aspirin 500 mg	Tablet (sustained release)
Meralen	Merrell	Flufenamic acid 100 mg	Capsule
Methrazone	WB Pharmaceuticals	Feprazone 200 mg	Capsule
Mobilan	Galen	Indomethacin	Capsule 25 mg Capsule 50 mg
Myocrisin	May & Baker	Sodium aurothiomalate	Ampoule 1 mg/0.5 ml Ampoule 5 mg/0.5 ml Ampoule 10 mg/0.5 ml Ampoule 20 mg/0.5 ml Ampoule 50 mg/0.5 ml i.m.
Myolgin	Cox	Aspirin 200 mg, paracetamol 200 mg, codeine phosphate 5 mg, caffeine citrate 15 mg	Tablet (soluble)
Naprosyn	Syntex	Naproxen	Tablet 250 mg Tablet 500 mg Suspension 250 mg/10 ml Suppository 500 mg
Napsalgesic	Dista	Dextropropoxyphene napsylate (equivalent to 32.5 mg hydrochloride), aspirin 500 mg	Tablet
Nu-Seals Aspirin	Lilly	Aspirin 300 mg	Tablet (enteric coated) 300 mg Tablet (enteric coated) 600 mg
Onadox-118	Duncan, Flockhart	Aspirin 300 mg, dihydrocodeine tartrate 10 mg	Tablet (soluble)
Opren[†]	Dista	Benoxaprofen 300 mg	Tablet
Orudis	May & Baker	Ketoprofen	Capsule 50 mg Suppository 100 mg
Palaprin Forte	Nicholas	Aloxiprin 600 mg	Tablet
Parazolidin	Geigy	Phenylbutazone 50 mg, paracetamol 500 mg	Tablet
Paynocil	Beecham	Aspirin 600 mg, amino-acetic acid 300 mg	Tablet
Plaquenil	Winthrop	Hydroxychloroquine sulphate 200 mg	Tablet

Appendix 4.11.3 (*contd.*)

Proprietary name	Manufacturer	Approved name/ ingredients	Presentation
Ponstan	Parke-Davis	Mefenamic acid	Tablet 250 mg (Ponstan) Tablet 500 mg (Ponstan Forte) Suspension 50 mg/ 5 ml (Ponstan Paediatric Suspension)
Progesic	Lilly	Fenoprofen 200 mg	Tablet
Rheumox	Robins	Azapropazone dihydrate	Capsule 300 mg Tablet 600 mg
Safapryn	Pfizer	Aspirin 300 mg (enteric-coated core), paraceta- mol 250 mg (outer layer)	Tablet
Solprin	Reckitt & Colman	Aspirin 300 mg	Tablet (soluble)
Synflex	Syntex	Naproxen (as sodium salt) 250 mg	Capsule
Tandacote	Geigy	Oxyphenbutazone 100 mg	Tablet (enteric coated)
Tanderil	Geigy	Oxyphenbutazone	Tablet 100 mg Suppository 250 mg
Tolectin	Ortho	Tolmetin	Tablet 200 mg Capsule 400 mg
Trilisate	Napp	Choline magnesium trisalicylate 500 mg	Tablet
Voltarol[†]	Geigy	Diclofenac sodium	Tablet (enteric coated) 25 mg Tablet (enteric coated) 50 mg Suppository 100 mg
Zactirin	Wyeth	Ethoheptazine citrate 75 mg, aspirin 325 mg, calcium carbonate 97 mg	Tablet

* Some of these drugs are also listed under 'analgesic and antipyretics'. Although loosely classified as 'non-steroid anti-inflammatory drugs' some of these preparations are 'specific' long-term suppressants (e.g. gold, penicillamine, antimalarials).
† Withdrawn from the market.
    Since publication of this issue of MIMS, diclofenac has also been marketed in injectable form (ampoules containing 75 mg for i.m. injection).

(*c*)   *Some* local and systemic corticosteroids and corticotrophins of rheumatological relevance listed in MIMS (April, 1982)*

Proprietary name	Manufacturer	Approved name	Presentation
Oral corticosteroid preparations			
Codelcortone	Merck Sharp & Dohme	Prednisolone 5 mg	Tablet
Decortisyl	Roussel	Prednisone	Tablet 1 mg Tablet 5 mg
Deltacortone	Merck Sharp & Dohme	Prednisone 5 mg	Tablet
Deltacortril	Pfizer	Prednisolone	Tablet (enteric coated) 2.5 mg Tablet (enteric coated) 5 mg
Deltastab	Boots	Prednisolone	Tablet 1 mg Tablet 5 mg

Appendix 4.11.3 (*contd.*)

Proprietary name	Manufacturer	Approved name/ ingredients	Presentation
Medrone	Upjohn	Methylprednisolone	Tablet 2 mg Tablet 4 mg Tablet 16 mg
Precortisyl	Roussel	Prednisolone	Tablet 1 mg Tablet 5 mg
Prednesol	Glaxo	Prednisolone (as disodium phosphate) 5 mg	Tablet (soluble)
Sintisone	Farmitalia Carlo Erba	Prednisolone steaglate 6.65 mg	Tablet
Intravenous/intramuscular corticosteroid preparations			
Efcortelan Soluble	Glaxo	Hydrocortisone (as sodium succinate) 100 mg, powder	Vial + 2 ml water for injection i.v.
Efcortesol	Glaxo	Hydrocortisone (as sodium phosphate) 100 mg/ml	Ampoule 1 ml Ampoule 5 ml i.v.
Solu-Cortef	Upjohn	Hydrocortisone (as sodium succinate) 100 mg, powder	Vial + 2 ml water for injection i.m. or i.v.
Intra-articular/peri-articular corticosteroid preparations			
Adcortyl Intra-articular/ Intradermal	Squibb	Triamcinolone acetonide 10 mg/ml	Ampoule 1 ml Vial 5 ml
Deltastab	Boots	Prednisolone acetate 25 mg/ml	Vial 5 ml
Hydrocortistab Injection	Boots	Hydrocortisone acetate 25 mg/ml	Vial 5 ml
Kenalog	Squibb	Triamcinolone acetonide 40 mg/ml	Vial 1 ml
Lederspan 20 mg	Lederle	Triamcinolone hexacetonide 20 mg/ml	Vial 1 ml Vial 5 ml
Ultracortenol	Ciba	Prednisolone pivalate 50 mg/ml	Ampoule 1 ml
Corticotrophin preparations			
Acthar Gel	Armour	Corticotrophin in hydrolysed gelatin	Vial 5 ml (20 i.u./ml) Vial 2 ml and 5 ml (40 i.u./ml) Vial 5 ml (80 i.u./ml) s.c. or i.m.
Synacthen	Ciba	Tetracosactrin 0.25 mg/ml in buffered aqueous solution	Ampoule 1 ml i.m. or i.v.
Synacthen Depot	Ciba	Tetracosactrin acetate and zinc complex	Ampoule 1 ml (1 mg/1 ml) Vial 2 ml (1 mg/ml) i.m.

* This selection of drugs to some extent reflects my preference for 'traditional' corticosteroid preparations for routine rheumatological use, and excludes the more potent systemic corticosteroids such as triamcinolone, betamethasone, dexamethasone and paramethasone.

Appendix 4.11.3 (*contd.*)

(*d*) *Some cytotoxic drugs of rheumatological relevance listed in MIMS* (April, 1982)

Proprietary name	Manufacturer	Approved name/ ingredients	Presentation
Emtexate	Nordic	Methotrexate	Ampoule 2 ml (2.5 mg/ml) Ampoule 2 ml (25 mg/ml) Vial 500 mg Vial 1 g } powder i.m., i.v.
Endoxana	WB Pharmaceuticals	Cyclophosphamide	Tablet 10 mg Tablet 50 mg Vial 107 mg Vial 214 mg Vial 535 mg Vial 1.069 g } powder i.v.
Leukeran	Wellcome	Chlorambucil	Tablet 2 mg Tablet 5 mg
Imuran	Wellcome	Azathioprine	Tablet 50 mg Vial 50 mg i.v.

(*e*) *Anti-gout drugs* listed in MIMS* (April, 1982)

Proprietary name	Manufacturer	Approved name	Presentation
Anturan	Geigy	Sulphinpyrazone 100 mg	Tablet
Benemid	Merck Sharp & Dohme	Probenecid 500 mg	Tablet
Zyloric	Calmic	Allopurinol	Tablet 100 mg Tablet 300 mg (Zyloric-300)

* Colchicine is not available as a brand product in UK. However, some pharmaceutical firms market it as the BP preparation, e.g. Colchicine **BP** (Evans) containing 500 µg colchicine.

5

Drug therapy (2): non-specific drugs

5.1 GENERAL COMMENT

There is still no general hypothesis to explain convincingly how or why anti-rheumatic drugs work. In particular there is little evidence to suggest any degree of specificity of these drugs (Rooney et al., 1975).

In considering the biological effects of anti-rheumatic agents (Famaey et al., 1975) it is important to consider effects that are observable at clinically realistic millimolar concentrations. It is also important to look for relationships between dose and therapeutic response. Dose–response curves are often bimodal and may show stimulation at low concentrations and inhibition at higher concentrations (Dick, 1978).

5.1.1 Effects on enzymes

Anti-rheumatic drugs influence a wide range of intracellular enzyme systems involved in nucleic acid, purine, pyrimidine, protein, lipid and carbohydrate metabolism. It is likely that only those effects upon oxidative phosphorylation, prostaglandin synthesis and protein biosynthesis occur at clinically realistic concentrations.

5.1.2 Effects on membranes

Thiol groups, oxygen and ion transport, water balance and the first and second messenger system are all intimately related membrane functions. These functions ultimately determine intracellular AMP:GMP ratios,

cytoplasmic and nuclear constitution, and energy availability to the cell. Specific and less specific receptors or recognition markers are present on or within the cell membrane. Anti-rheumatic drugs affect these membrane functions directly and also through the enzyme complex involved in prostaglandin synthesis (which itself exerts its effect through the cyclic AMP system). Direct effects of anti-rheumatic drugs on platelet-cell membranes have been documented and these may be a function of their capacity to bind to and acetylate membrane protein (Samter, 1969).

Membrane effects feature in the lysosomal membrane hypothesis. This is based on an assumption that these drugs act by means of their membrane labilizing or stabilizing influence, tissue destruction being modified by the ensuing change in release of lysosomal enzymes. However, it is unlikely that human disease and anti-rheumatic drug efficacy rest solely on the initiating influence of changes in lysosomal membrane permeability (Rooney et al., 1975).

5.1.3 Effects on protein-binding

It has been suggested that anti-rheumatic activity may be a function of the ability of these drugs to displace a 'natural anti-inflammatory substance' from its binding site on serum albumin (McArthur et al., 1971; Aylward, 1975). L-Tryptophan is thought to mirror the behaviour of this substance which is unduly highly bound in patients with inflammatory joint disease and therefore inactive. Release of this substance (reflected in release of L-tryptophan) allows it to exert its anti-inflammatory effect.

5.1.4 Effects on mediators

The inhibitory effect of analgesic/anti-inflammatory drugs on prostaglandin synthesis has been suggested as the mode of action of these drugs (Flower and Vane, 1974; Ferriera and Vane, 1974). However, effective anti-rheumatic regimens such as gold or corticosteroid therapy do not possess this property and do not inhibit certain other proposed chemical mediators such as kinin generation (Fauci, 1976; Sharma *et al.*, 1976). More-over, indomethacin, known to be a potent prostaglan-din and kininogen inhibitor, fails to halt the progression of the inflammatory joint disease process.

5.2 NON-SPECIFIC OR SYMPTOMATIC THERAPY

In order to provide a perspective idea of therapeutic preferences and priorities in this extensive field of non-specific anti-rheumatic drugs a series of concluding comments appear at the end of major sections. (The same policy has been adopted in the next chapter.)

5.2.1 Simple analgesic drugs

(a) General comment

This section concerns those agents that relieve pain by a central action on the central nervous system but have no peripheral anti-inflammatory action. Some have an antipyretic action (paracetamol or acetaminophen), while some do not (dextropropoxyphene). Aspirin has an anti-inflammatory effect as well as a peripheral and central analgesic action. At low dose levels, 2 g or less daily, aspirin seems to be largely analgesic.

The place of these analgesics in rheumatology is purely to relieve pain and thus make life more tolerable for the rheumatic patient, as well as enabling joint movements to be carried out more easily. Simple analgesics are often given in addition to the general programme of anti-inflammatory drugs, physical mea-sures, rest, and exercise. As a group these drugs are better tolerated, particularly by the gastrointestinal tract, than the analgesic/anti-inflammatory agents. Although modest in their effects, they represent a valuable contribution to the management of patients with both inflammatory as well as non-inflammatory rheumatic disorders.

(b) Non-addictive analgesic drugs

Much of the information comprising this section has been derived from Martindale's *The Extra Pharmacopoeia* (Wade, 1977) and *Drug Treatment of the Rheumatic Diseases* (Hart, 1978). Where necessary updating of this information has been according to more recent sources (e.g. Huskisson, 1980; Roth, 1980; *British National Formulary*, 1981; *MIMS*, April, 1982; *Data Sheet Compendium*, 1981–82). However, although every effort has been made to ensure that details are in accord with the standards accepted at the time of submission of the work for publication, pharmacology is a rapidly changing science. In view of this, some of the data contained here may need updating further by the time the book has been released.

Aspirin (Solprin, Nu-Seals Aspirin, Breoprin, Claradin, Levius)
Aspirin is analgesic in small doses and both analgesic and anti-inflammatory in large doses. For further details of its anti-inflammatory effect see Section 5.2.2(a).

Paracetamol (Calpol, Panasorb, Panadol)
Other proprietory names include: Alvedon, Panodil, Termidor (all Sweden); Anuphen, Apamide, Capital, Cen-Apap, Dolanex, Febrigesic, Febrogesic, Korum, Liquiprin, Lyteca, Nebs, Neopap, Phendex, Proval, SK-Apap, Tapar, Temlo (all USA); Atasol, Campain, Chemcetaphen, Pediaphen, Rounox (all Canada); Ben-u-ron (Germany); Ceetamol, Dolamin, Dymadon, Nevrol, Paracet, Parasin, Parmol, Placemol (all Australia); Cetamol (Eire); Doliprane (France); Napamol, Panado, Restin Elixir (all South Africa); Pacemol (New Zealand); Tempra (Australia, Canada, South Africa, USA); Tylenol (Canada, USA); Valadol (South Africa, USA).

Pharmacology and pharmacokinetics. Paracetamol (acetaminophen) is p-acetamidophenol. It has analgesic and anti-pyretic effects but little or no anti-inflam-matory action. It is the main active metabolite of phenacetin and acetanilide both of which have now been largely discarded because of their toxic side effects. Paracetamol is rapidly and almost completely absorbed from the gastrointestinal tract after oral administration. Maximal plasma concentrations are reached in 30–60 minutes. The plasma half-life is 1–3 hours. The drug is distributed relatively evenly throughout most body fluids, but binding to plasma proteins is variable. Only about 3% is excreted unchanged in the urine, some 80% being excreted by the kidney after conjugation in the liver, mainly with glucuronic acid. Hydroxylated metabolites are responsible for methaemoglobinaemia and liver toxicity.

Clinical uses, preparations and dosage. In the rheumatic disorders paracetamol is used principally to relieve pain. It is taken on demand, often in addition to regular doses of analgesic/anti-inflammatory agents. Its antipyretic effect may be useful in febrile rheumatic disorders.

Tablets contain 500 mg and the usual dose is 1 g taken as required up to 3–4 g a day. Many compound tablets are available. Most of these contain 500 mg paracetamol combined with codeine phosphate and caffeine in varying amounts.

Side effects, precautions and contraindications. Paracetamol is usually well tolerated by the gastrointestinal tract and other systems. Side effects are usually mild. Overdosage, however, may produce fatal hepatic necrosis. Thrombocytopenia and other haematological reactions have been reported; rashes and allergic reactions have also been observed.

Paracetamol should not be used in patients with liver disease. Over 7 g daily cause liver damage, and larger regular dosage may cause irreversible hepatic necrosis. In suicidal overdosage, fatal hepatic necrosis may occur several hours after apparent recovery from the suicidal attempt.

Pentazocine (Fortral)

Other proprietary names include: Fortral (Belgium, France); Fortalgesic (Sweden, Switzerland); Fortralin (Finland, Norway); Sorsegon (South Africa, Spain); Talwin (Canada, Italy, USA).

Pharmacology and pharmacokinetics. Pentazocine is a benzomorphan derivative. It has an analgesic but no anti-inflammatory action, its main action being on the central nervous system and smooth muscle.

The drug is well absorbed from the gastrointestinal tract and from subcutaneous and intramuscular injection sites. Peak plasma levels occur 1–3 hours after oral administration and 15–60 minutes after intramuscular injection. The plasma half-life is about 2 hours after intramuscular administration. The duration of action after oral administration is usually 2–6 hours. Most of the drug is metabolized in the liver. The metabolites are excreted in the urine with a small and variable amount of unchanged pentazocine. About 60% of the total dose is excreted within 24 hours.

Clinical use, preparations and dosage. Pentazocine is a mild analgesic when given orally but is more potent when given subcutaneously or intramuscularly.

The drug is available as tablets of 25 mg and capsules of 50 mg. Ampoules of 30 and 60 mg (1 and 2 ml) for subcutaneous or intramuscular injection are also available. Oral adult dosage is 25–100 mg, 3–4 hourly after meals, as required. It is also available as suppositories containing 50 mg.

Side effects, precautions and contraindications. Side effects which occasionally occur include nausea, sedation, dizziness and, rarely, hallucinations. High dosage may produce respiratory depression (reversible by naloxone but not by nalorphine), tachycardia and hypertension. In some patients, with repeated and frequent use, tolerance to the analgesic action occurs, but addiction is rare, and it is not on the Misuse of Drugs list in Great Britain (or equivalent list in the USA), whether given by mouth or injection.

There is much individual variation in its degree of hepatic metabolism and therapeutic effect. Addiction, though rare, may occur, but in these individuals there has often been previous addiction to other drugs. Addiction occurs largely with the use of parenteral preparations. Pentazocine should be used with great care in pregnancy, in patients with impaired renal, hepatic or respiratory function, with monoamine oxidase inhibitors or alcohol, or after large doses of narcotic analgesics.

Pentazocine is contraindicated in narcotic addicts, in respiratory depression, in raised intracranial pressure, head injury or pathological conditions of the brain, or after coronary occlusion where it may cause a rise in pulmonary arterial pressure.

Dextropropoxyphene (Doloxene)

Other proprietary names include: (hydrochloride) Algaphan (Australia); Antalvic (France); Darvon, Dolene, Dolocarp, Mardon, Propoxychel, Proxagesic (all USA); Develin, Erantin (both Germany); Dolotard (Sweden); Pro-65, Progesic (both Canada); (napsylate) Darvon-N (Canada, USA).

Pharmacology and pharmacokinetics. Dextropropoxyphene is (+)-a-4-dimethylamino-3-methyl-1-1, 2-diphenylbut-2yl propionate. It has a central analgesic action, but no antipyretic or anti-inflammatory action. It is readily absorbed from the gastrointestinal tract; plasma levels are apparent at 1 hour, maximal at about 2 hours, thereafter slowly declining over a further 3–4 hours. However, there is much individual variability. It has a plasma half-life of 12 hours. In man, the main route of metabolism is by N-demethylation to yield norpropoxyphene, which is excreted in the urine.

Clinical use, preparations and dosage. Dextropropoxyphene is used in the rheumatic diseases entirely for its analgesic effect. The drug is taken as required – up to 260 mg of the hydrochloride or 400 mg of the napsylate daily in divided dosage. Capsules of dextropropoxyphene napsylate contain 100 mg (equivalent to 65 mg of the hydrochloride). There are also many combinations available (e.g. with aspirin, paracetamol, caffeine), and there is a sustained-release capsule containing 150 mg dextropropoxyphene for use 8–12 hourly as required.

Side effects, precautions and contraindications. Toxicity is negligible at therapeutic dosage. However, at excessive dosage, central nervous system, cardiac and respiratory depression may occur and sometimes convulsions. Combinations with paracetamol create major treatment problems in patients with over-dosage (*Editorial*, 1977; Whittington, 1977). Continued medication with 800 mg or more daily may cause toxic psychoses or convulsions.

Dextropropoxyphene only rarely causes tolerance, euphoria or drug dependence. However, it is a narcotic analgesic and its depressant effect may be additive if given with other central nervous depressants. This may give rise to impaired mental and/or physical functions required for such tasks as driving a car or operating machinery.

Codeine phosphate

Pure codeine phosphate is only available as codeine phosphate BP. Branded preparations of codeine phosphate contain other preparations (e.g. Codis, codeine phosphate 8 mg and soluble aspirin 500 mg; Paracodol, codeine phosphate 8 mg and paracetamol 500 mg). Other proprietary names include: Codicept, Tricodein (both Germany); Codlin (Australia); Paveral (Canada).

Pharmacology and pharmacokinetics. Codeine has a mild analgesic action and causes constipation. It has a plasma half-life of 2 hours and a duration of action of 4–6 hours. The drug is metabolized by the liver and mainly excreted as inactive forms in the urine. About 10% of a given dose is demethylated to form morphine.

Clinical uses, preparations and dosage. Codeine is used in the rheumatic disorders as a mild analgesic (usually in combination with other more effective analgesics such as aspirin). In addition, through its costive effect, it may be used to control diarrhoea and it is valuable in arthropathies associated with intestinal hurry (e.g. colitic arthropathy).

Codeine is available as the phosphate in tablet form. The dosage ranges from 10–60 mg daily in divided doses. The dose in compound analgesic tablets is usually 5–10 mg per tablet.

Side effects, precautions and contraindications. Codeine constipates at ordinary dose levels, and at high levels causes respiratory depression.

The drug should be used with caution in constipated patients.

Nefopam hydrochloride (Acupan)

Other proprietary names include: Ajan (Germany).

Pharmacology and pharmacokinetics. It is an antihistamine-derived drug with moderate potency as a centrally acting analgesic agent. There is no evidence of habituation from pre-clinical research.

Clinical uses, preparations and dosage. Its usefulness has not yet been established in rheumatology, but it is indicated for musculoskeletal pain, acute traumatic pain and cancer pain. It is available in tablet form (30–90 mg three times daily) or as an injection (20 mg i.m. or i.v., repeated if necessary every 6 hours).

Side effects, precautions and contraindications. Side effects include nausea, nervousness, dry mouth and lightheadedness. Less often vomiting, blurred vision, drowsiness, sweating, insomnia, headache and tachycardia may occur.

The side effects may be additive to those of other agents having anticholinergic or sympathomimetic activity. It should be avoided in myocardial infarction. Hepatic and renal disease may interfere with the metabolism and excretion of the drug.

It is contraindicated in patients with a history of convulsive disorders.

Dihydrocodeine (DF118)

Other proprietary names include: Fortuss, Rikodeine, Tuscodin (all Australia); Paracodin (Australia, Germany, South Africa).

Pharmacology and pharmacokinetics. Dihydrocodeine tartrate is an analgesic of greater potency than codeine, but it is less potent than morphine. Sedation is also less than with morphine. It is readily absorbed from the gastrointestinal tract and after intramuscular injection, excretion being mostly via the kidneys within 24 hours of administration. The duration of therapeutic action is about 4–6 hours.

Clinical uses, preparations and dosage. Dihydrocodeine is used in the rheumatic disorders as an analgesic with mild sedative and constipating properties. It is much more effective given by intramuscular injection (when it is considered to be potentially addictive).

It is available as tablets of dihydrocodeine tartrate 30 mg: 1 or 2 as required, or as a sterile solution, 50 mg of dihydrocodeine tartrate in 1 ml with 0.9% of sodium metabisulphite for intramuscular injection. An elixir (syrup) containing 10 mg per 5 ml is also available in some countries.

Side effects, precautions and contraindications. Taken by mouth there is little risk of addiction. However, as previously stated, by intramuscular injection dihydrocodeine is potentially addictive and is controlled under the Misuse of Drugs Act in Great Britain. It is slightly constipating. The drug should be used with caution in patients with constipation, asthma or liver disease. Because of the risk of addiction, intramuscular dihydrocodeine should be avoided in individuals considered to be potential addicts.

Zomepirac (Zomax)*

Zomepirac is a benzoylpyrrole acetic acid derivative, chemically unrelated to opioids, salicylates and proprionic acid derivatives. This non-narcotic drug has been developed in the USA and has been shown to possess a high level of analgesic activity and a relatively low incidence of side effects. At the time of writing a wide-scale multicentre trial is being planned in the UK.

(c) Addictive analgesic drugs

These analgesics are never used unless the outlook is grave and pain is making reasonable life impossible. Such conditions are malignant disease of bone or joint, or advanced rheumatoid disease associated with great pain uncontrolled by other means. In such patients dipipanone, morphine or diamorphine (heroin), or levorphanol may be helpful.

Dipipanone (4, 4-diphenyl-6-piperidino-heptan-3-one hydrochloride monohydrate)

This has a strong analgesic action which begins about 15 minutes after intramuscular injection and lasts for 4–6 hours. Given alone it has relatively little hypnotic or sedative action, but 10 mg dipipanone hydrochloride mixed with 30 mg cyclizine hydrochloride (Diconal) may be given by mouth in tablet form with considerable effect 6–12 hourly. Its action may be prolonged in the presence of severe renal or hepatic disease.

Morphine (Duromorph) or diamorphine (heroin)

These may be given orally with alcohol and sometimes with cocaine (10 mg) in small doses of 5–15 mg in patients with terminal disease every 3–6 hours. The drug is used to anticipate rather than to treat severe pain as it arises, increasing the dosage if necessary. A phenothiazine, such as chlorpromazine or prochlorperazine, can be added if nausea, vomiting or agitation occurs. Such elixirs have a shelf-life of about 3 weeks and should be used within this time or discarded. Diamorphine and cocaine elixir, BPC is: diamorphine hydrochloride, 1 g; cocaine hydrochloride, 1 g; alcohol (90%), 125 ml; syrup, 250 ml; chloroform water to 1000 ml.

The use of cocaine is contentious. It is not truly euphorious or antidepressive and may cause nightmares, hallucinations, formication and occasionally excitement. It may also give rise to anorexia, nausea and tremor. Morphine can replace diamorphine, while chlorpromazine elixir, BPC can replace the simple syrup if necessary.

Dosage starts with 2.5–5 mg diamorphine and

* Temporarily withdrawn by the manufacturer in UK.

3.75–7.5 mg morphine, 3–6 hourly; the initial dosage being doubled if found insufficient. Thereafter, dose increments and spacing depend on the individual patient. Usually such a programme of oral medicine is adequate, with injections of morphine or diamorphine only being given terminally or not at all. It must be stressed that this approach is reserved for the terminal patient with an extremely poor prognosis.

Levorphanol tartrate (Dromoran Roche)

This is the dihydrate of (−)-3-hydroxy-N-methylmorphinan hydrogen tartrate. It has the therapeutic and toxic actions of morphine but is almost as effective by mouth as by injection. By mouth, the dose is 1.5–4.5 mg (1–3 tablets of 1.5 mg). The subcutaneous and intramuscular dose is 2–4 mg. It should not be give with alcohol.

(Lasagna, 1964; Beaver, 1965 and 1976; Melzack and Wall, 1965; Kantor *et al.* 1966; Stirman, 1967; Bellville *et al.*, 1968; Loan and Morrison, 1973; Marks and Sachar, 1973; Guzman *et al.*, 1974; Parkhouse, 1975; Kantor, 1976, 1980; Martin *et al.*, 1976; *Editorial*, 1977; Whittington, 1977; Sunshine *et al.*, 1978; de Andrade *et al.*, 1980; Mayer and Ruoff, 1980; Nayak *et al.*, 1980; Pruss *et al.*, 1980.)

COMMENT

Simple analgesic drugs, which reduce pain either by a local effect on the sensory nerves or by a central effect on cerebral centres associated with the appreciation of pain, have a limited place on their own in rheumatology. As most rheumatological disorders are based on inflammatory effects, adequate pain relief is more appropriately found in drugs combining an analgesic/anti-inflammatory effect. The most widely used of the analgesic drugs is paracetamol. The debate concerning its incrimination in renal disease has not yet been resolved. Dextropropoxyphene is another valuable mild analgesic, but is rarely used alone. The combination of the drug with paracetamol is more popular, and is based on claims of synergism between the two drugs. Codeine and dihydrocodeine are also widely used, but constipation often presents a problem. Pentazocine is claimed to be more potent and is non-addictive. However, its value in pain of rheumatic origin is disappointing.

The use of addictive drugs such as pethidine and the opiates has a very small place in the treatment of rheumatic disorders.

5.2.2 Analgesic/anti-inflammatory drugs

The analgesic/anti-inflammatory drugs (non-steroidal anti-inflammatory drugs) are not curative, nor are they thought to reverse permanently the disease process in any arthropathy. However, by reducing pain and swelling they improve joint function and are thus

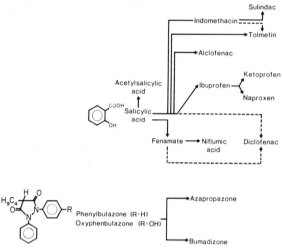

Fig. 5.1 Interrelationships between some analgesic/anti-inflammatory drugs (after Arznei-Telegramm, 1977).

valuable adjuncts in the management of inflammatory rheumatic disorders.

There is now a bewildering number of anti-inflammatory analgesics in addition to 'traditional' aspirin and the two drugs, phenylbutazone and indomethacin, that followed it in the 1950s and 1960s respectively. Many of these newer preparations belong to the proprionic acid group, of which additional members of the group appear at regular intervals.

Fig. 5.1 summarizes the interrelationships between some of these non-steroidal anti-inflammatory agents, and Fig. 5.2 provides an overall classification of these drugs based on their chemistry. This model has been used throughout this section to guide the reader through the non-steroidal 'wilderness'. It should be emphasized, however, that similarity of chemical characteristics does not necessarily imply similarity of therapeutic effect or of toxicity, and in some instances drugs in entirely different groups may be more similar in their clinical effects than drugs that are generically similar.

The choice of a particular analgesic/anti-inflamma-

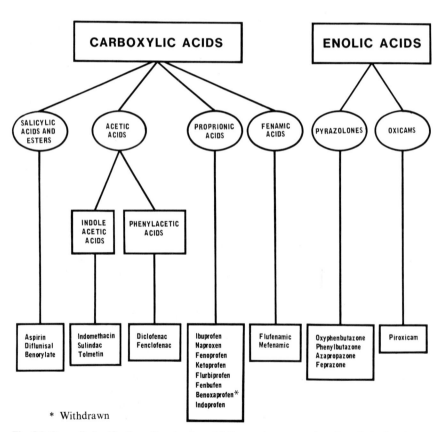

* Withdrawn

Fig. 5.2 Over all classification of analgesic anti-inflammatory agents based on their chemistry.

tory agent for a particular patient remains somewhat arbitrary, and often several drugs, either within a single generic group or in different groups will have to be tried (preferably to maximal dosage) before a response is observed. It is likely that pharmacogenetic differences between patients influence these variations in response to a considerable extent, and research is needed to provide a means by which patient-specific factors can be identified, perhaps through histocompatability typing. In this way the likely pharmacological response of individual patients to individual drugs could be anticipated and much time, frustration, effort and expense saved.

(a) Salicylic acids and esters

Aspirin (Solprin, Nu-Seals Aspirin, Breopin, Claradin, Levius)
Other proprietary names include: Acetophen, Acetyl-Sal, Ancasal, Asadrine, Cetasal, Entrophen, Monasalyl, Neopirine-25, Nova-Phase, Novasen, Sal-Adult, Sal-Infant, Supasa, Triaphen-10 (all Germany); Albyl-Selters, Apernyl, Bamyl, Dispril, Instantine, Premaspin (all Sweden); ASA, Measurin (both USA); Aquaprin, Aspasol (both South Africa); Aspégic (lysine acetylsalicylate), Aspirisucre, Claragine, Ivépirine, Juvépirine, Seclopyrine (all France); Aspisol, Bi-prin, Clariprin, Codral Junior, Elsprin, Infatabs A, Novosprin, Prodol, Provoprin-500, Solcetas, Solusal (all Australia); Babiprin (Eire); Ecotrin (Canada, USA); Rhonal (Canada, France).

Pharmacology and pharmacokinetics. Aspirin (acetylsalicylic acid, acidum acetylsalicylicum, salicylic acid acetate, polopiryna) is o-acetoxybenzoic acid. Absorption of non-ionized aspirin occurs in the stomach. Acetyl salicylates and salicylates are also readily absorbed from the intestine. Hydrolysis to salicylic acid occurs rapidly in the intestine and in the circulation. Salicylates are extensively (50–90%) bound to plasma proteins; aspirin to a lesser degree. Appreciable plasma concentrations are reached within 30 minutes and peak levels at about 2 hours. Aspirin and salicylate are rapidly distributed to all body tissues; they appear in milk and cross the placenta. The rate of excretion of aspirin varies with the pH of the urine, increasing as the pH rises and being greatest at pH 7.5 and above. A circadian excretion rhythm has been reported. Aspirin is excreted as salicylic acid, as glucuronide conjugates, and as salicyluric and gentisic acids.

Pain relief is effected by a central analgesic action and by a peripheral action. It relieves pain of low intensity, from bone and joint rather than from viscera. Salicylates inhibit the synthesis of prostaglandins in inflamed tissues and thereby prevent sensitization of pain re-

ceptors to substances such as bradykinin which appear to mediate the pain response. However, this is probably not the only mechanism of action, and it has been suggested (Morley, 1975) that aspirin not only acts at the level of prostaglandin production by the macrophage but possibly also on lymphokine action on target cells or on lymphokine production by lymphocytes. The central analgesic action probably operates at hypothalamic level. The antipyretic action is due to action on heat-regulating centres resulting in dissipation of body heat through cutaneous vasodilation.

Salicylates stimulate respiration directly and indirectly, increasing oxygen consumption and carbon dioxide production. Therapeutic doses cause an extra- and intracellular respiratory alkylosis compensated by an excretion of bicarbonate.

Aspirin at a dosage of 4 g a day decreases the plasma iron concentration and shortens erythrocyte survival time. It can cause mild haemolysis in patients with glucose-6-phosphate dehydrogenase deficiency. Aspirin also prolongs the bleeding time and inhibits many platelet functions. (A single dose of aspirin may effect these changes for several days.)

(Macpherson *et al.*, 1955; Rosenthal *et al.*, 1964; Hollister and Levy, 1965; Collier, 1969; Samter, 1969; Levy and Leonards, 1971; Martin, 1971; Levy *et al.*, 1972; Menguy *et al.*, 1972; Rowland *et al.*, 1972; Gibson *et al.*, 1975.)

Clinical uses, preparations and dosage. Aspirin is used in the treatment of acute and chronic rheumatic states. It is usually considered first choice in rheumatic fever, rheumatoid arthritis (if tolerated), juvenile rheumatoid arthritis, most seronegative arthropathies and most soft-tissue lesions. However, it is of less value in ankylosing spondylitis and of little value in acute or chronic gout. Aspirin may be of modest help in the control of osteoarthrotic pain.

If a purely analgesic effect is required aspirin is used in individual doses of 0.6–1 g. For an anti-inflammatory effect regular dosage every 3–4 hours is necessary and a total daily dosage of 4–6 g should be achieved.

The aim is to use the lowest effective dose level, which is often the highest tolerated. Only about half the patients who tolerate a lower dosage will be able to continue at the higher dosage of 4–6 g daily for many weeks because of troublesome side effects. For optimal anti-inflammatory effect in patients with rheumatoid arthritis, plasma salicylate concentrations of 15–30 g 100 ml^{-1} ($1.1–2.2 \text{ mmol l}^{-1}$) are required, but there is much variation between patients in effect and tolerance.

The accepted daily dose of aspirin for the management of juvenile chronic polyarthritis is 80 mg/kg body weight. The dosage of benorylate should be 200 mg kg^{-1} in two divided doses per day. To control the fever of the systemic phase of juvenile chronic polyarthritis it may be necessary to give 100 mg kg^{-1} of aspirin. In these patients careful watch should be made for evidence of hyperventilation. In all patients on anti-inflammatory doses of aspirin it is advisable to check the plasma salicylate level, as children rarely complain of tinnitus or nausea.

In rheumatic fever 100 mg kg^{-1} body weight should be given over 24 hours. Although having a dramatic effect on the fever and joint symptoms it has no effect on the carditis and, indeed, is contraindicated in the presence of cardiac enlargement or severe mitral valve disease, as fluid retention can occur.

(Marson, 1953; Mainland and Sutcliffe, 1965; Boardman and Hart, 1967; Halvorsen *et al.*, 1973; Multz *et al.*, 1974; Champion *et al.*, 1975.)

Prophylactic effects of aspirin. There is some evidence that aspirin may protect from either myocardial infarction or the production of atheroma (Alexander *et al.*, 1959; Boston Collaboration Drug Surveillance Group, 1974; Jick and Miettinen, 1976; Davis *et al.*, 1978). A suggestion that aspirin may protect against postoperative thrombosis has not been validated (Medical Research Council, 1972). It has also been suggested that aspirin may exert a protective effect on articular cartilage (Simmons and Chrisman, 1965; Chrisman and Snook, 1968; Ginsberg *et al.*, 1968; Farney *et al.*, 1973).

Preparations available include the following: aspirin tablets 300 g; soluble aspirin tablets (calcium aspirin) 300 g, with calcium carbonate, anhydrous citric acid and saccharin sodium; aloxiprin, a polymeric condensation compound of aluminium oxide and aspirin, as 600 g tablets (equivalent to 500 g aspirin); sustained-release aspirin (microgranular), each microgranule coated with inert methyl cellulose, 500 g tablets (various other sustained-release preparations are available); benorylate (4-acetamido-2-acetoxy benzoate) is a paracetamol ester of aspirin which is absorbed from the gastrointestinal tract as the intact molecule and then rapidly broken down into its component substances. It is available as a 750 mg tablet (1.5 g three times daily), a suspension containing 4 g (10 ml^{-1}), and a 2 g sachet (both 2–4 g twice daily). Aspirin suppositories are available in some European countries. Mixtures, powders and suspensions tend to deteriorate and are more toxic to the gastrointestinal tract. For this reason they are no longer recommended. There are also available a large number of compound tablets, as well as aspirin preparations which are enteric coated, glycinated, buffered, or coated with paracetamol. Only buffered preparations have been convincingly shown to reduce faecal blood loss, but adequate buffering causes rapid renal elimination, thereby rendering this type of formulation of little value in long-term therapy (Cooke, 1976).

Many clinical studies on the variants of aspirin preparations, particularly benorylate, were carried out in the early 1970s (Cummings *et al.*, 1963; Franke and Manz, 1964, 1972; Weill *et al.*, 1968; Alexander *et al.*, 1970; Bain and Burt, 1970; Baum, 1970; Cardoe, 1970; Hart and Nicholson, 1971; Haslock *et al.*, 1971; Beales *et al.*, 1972; Croft *et al.*, 1972; Danhof *et al.*, 1972; Robertson *et al.*, 1972; Bennett, 1973; Bitensky and Chayen, 1973; de Choisy, 1973; Hämäläinen *et al.*, 1973; Hingorani, 1973; Livingstone, 1973; Maneksha, 1973; Medrei, 1973; Pavelka *et al.*, 1973; Poore, 1973; Reizenstein and Doberl, 1973; Robertson, 1973; Rosner *et al.*, 1973; Sasisekhar *et al.*, 1973; Sperry *et al.*, 1973). (Literature details of benorylate and other aspirin derivatives are listed separate from aspirin in the reference list.)

Newer salicylate preparations. Salsalate (salicylosalicylic acid) (Disalcid), although first synthesized in 1920, has only relatively recently been introduced into clinical practice. It has been found to have significant antirheumatic activity and is claimed to cause less gastric bleeding and less gastric erosion (probably because it is virtually insoluble in gastric juice and is largely absorbed from the small intestine) (Rubin, 1964; Nordqvist *et al.*, 1965; Leonards, 1969; Deodhar *et al.*, 1977; Liyanage and Tambar, 1978).

Choline magnesium trisalicylate has also been introduced into clinical practice recently, and it has been established that it is clinically effective as an analgesic/anti-inflammatory agent and causes less blood loss than plain aspirin (Cohen and Garber, 1978; Cohen *et al.*, 1978; Zucker and Rothwell, 1978; Blechman and Lechner, 1979; Ehrlich *et al.*, 1980).

A different type of chemical modification of the salicylate molecule is represented by diflunisal (Dolobid) (5-(2, 4-difluorophenyl) salicylic acid) which will be discussed in a later section.

Side effects

Dyspepsia: This is the most frequent reason for failure of aspirin therapy. As with many of the other side effects of aspirin, it is dose related but unpredictable in individual patients. Thirty per cent of patients on high-dose aspirin therapy suffer intolerable malaise, loss of concentration and dyspepsia within the therapeutic range. A variety of methods have been proposed to reduce these side effects, and it is worth experimenting with different formulations. However, when aspirin intolerance persists it is important to change to another drug.

Gastrointestinal bleeding: There has been prolonged and intensive debate concerning aspirin and gastrointestinal bleeding from which certain facts emerge. Over 70% of those taking high-dose aspirin will have some degree of gastrointestinal bleeding. Such a loss (average 5 ml per day) may occasionally be sufficient to produce a treatable iron deficiency state, particularly in menstruating women. For the same reason it is important to identify those few patients who persistently lose more than 10–15 ml per day. Blood loss is unrelated to dyspepsia and shows a consistent pattern between patients, although there are wide variations. Bleeding occurs with acetylsalicylic acid but not with salicylic acid. A few patients taking aspirin will suffer frank haemorrhage from the gastrointestinal tract but the number of such patients must be small in proportion to the number of people taking aspirin. Furthermore, it would appear that those at greatest risk of bleeding are those patients who have other predisposing factors such as hypovitaminosis C, minor coagulation disorders or altered bile acids. Atrophic gastritis appears to protect against aspirin-induced gastrointestinal bleeding. There is no relationship between major bleeding and either minor bleeding or dyspepsia, and if aspirin is re-started after a major haemorrhage these patients do not necessarily bleed again.

Despite these comments it is important to stress that rheumatoid arthritis patients in large numbers who have been controlled on aspirin therapy show not a fall but a rise in haemoglobin concentration over a long period. However, re-exposure to aspirin after aspirin-induced bleeding is hardly justified, especially with the many alternatives now available.

(Hurst and Lintott, 1939; Kelly, 1956; Lange, 1957; Alvarez and Summerskill, 1958; Muir and Cossar, 1959; Grossman *et al.*, 1961; Pierson *et al.*, 1961; Scott *et al.*, 1961; Weiss *et al.*, 1961; Croft and Wood, 1967; Parry and Wood, 1967; Duggan, 1968; Goulston and Cooke, 1968; Gyroy and Stiel, 1968; Thune, 1968; Bouchier and Wilkins, 1969; Cooke and Goulston, 1969; Leonards, 1969; Leonards and Levy, 1969, 1970, 1972a, b; St. John and McDermott, 1970; Needham *et al.*, 1971; Croft *et al.*, 1972; Leonards *et al.*, 1973; Langman, 1974; Levy, 1974; Mills *et al.*, 1974.)

Peptic ulceration: Aspirin can produce acute mucosal erosions and is therefore 'ulcerogenic' in a sense. However, its role in the production of chronic peptic ulceration is still not established. A dose – response relationship has been shown between aspirin ingestion and peptic ulceration, particularly gastric ulceration (Cameron, 1975). The relationship between aspirin and duodenal ulceration is less certain.

(Paul, 1943; Muir and Cossar, 1955; Brown and Mitchell, 1956; Allibone and Flint, 1958; Barager and Duthie, 1960; Douglas and Johnson, 1961; Kiser, 1963; Davenport, 1964; Duggan, 1965; Menguy, 1966; Thorsen *et al.*, 1968; Chapman and Duggan, 1969; Gillies and Skyring, 1969; Edmar, 1971; Ivey *et al.*, 1972; St. John *et al.*, 1973; Spire, 1974; Cameron, 1975; Cooke, 1976.)

Liver: Some recent reports have pointed to aspirin as a cause of hepatic toxicity. In the early stages of high-dose aspirin therapy, there may be a small rise in liver enzyme activities both in adults and in children. This is sometimes associated with eosinophilia. A possible role of aspirin in causing chronic liver disease, however, is much less clear. A palpable liver without biochemical evidence of dysfunction is common in rheumatoid arthritis. Moreover, a palpable liver with raised liver enzyme activities in a patient with rheumatoid arthritis may be due to coincidental liver disease such as primary biliary cirrhosis, chronic active hepatitis or even amyloidosis.

(Russell *et al.*, 1971; Athreya *et al.*, 1973, 1975; *Editorial*, 1973; Rich and Johnson, 1973; Goldenberg, 1974; Koppes and Arnett, 1974; Seaman *et al.*, 1974; Wolfe *et al.*, 1974; Garber *et al.*, 1975; Bernstein *et al.*, 1977.)

Renal disease: After the original reports of phenacetin and analgesic nephropathy, the common practice of combining aspirin and phenacetin in certain formulations led to the incrimination of aspirin as a nephrotoxic agent. However, although it is undoubted that the acute administration of aspirin will increase exfoliation of renal cells and may alter renal blood flow, it is unlikely that aspirin alone predisposes to chronic renal disease.

(Harvald and Glausen, 1960; Scott, 1963; Scott *et al.*, 1963; Prescott, 1965, 1969; Abrahams and Levin, 1968; Campbell and MacLaurin, 1968; Manra and Kincaid-Smith, 1970; Abel, 1971; Wigley, 1971; Murray, 1972; Macklow *et al.*, 1974; Study, 1974; New Zealand Rheumatism Study, 1974.)

Gynaecological and obstetric: Although it has been suggested that aspirin might cause fetal malformation, this remains unresolved. It is thought that aspirin may contribute to various disorders in pregnancy and in the neonatal period. These include prolonged parturition, increased perinatal mortality, increased risk of postpartum haemorrhage, and carry-over of coagulation disorders into the neonatal period.

(Casteels-Van Daele *et al.*, 1972; Lewis and Schulman, 1973; McNeil, 1973; Haslam *et al.*, 1974; Collins and Turner, 1975; Faivre *et al.*, 1975; Turner and Collins, 1975; Slone *et al.*, 1976a, b.)

Haematological: Aspirin may rarely cause reversible pancytopenia. The drug (in low doses) has also been shown to produce striking changes in platelets and in coagulation and clotting factors.

(Weiss *et al.*, 1968; Kaneshiro *et al.*, 1969; Mielke *et al.*, 1969; Menon, 1970; Zucker and Peterson, 1970; Hirsch *et al.*, 1973; O'Brien, 1975; Roth and Majerus, 1975; Goldsweig *et al.*, 1976; Meade *et al.*, 1977; Moroz, 1977; Ratnoff, 1977.)

Hypersensitivity: The frequency of aspirin hypersensitivity has not been clearly established but some reports quote figures of 2–4%. Deaths have occasionally occurred from the administration of very small amounts of aspirin, often in adults with a past history of allergy, asthma or nasal polyps. Allergy to aspirin may co-exist with similar reactions to chemically dissimilar substances such as indomethacin, dextropropoxyphene or naproxen (Szczeklik *et al.*, 1977). Clinicians should therefore exercise particular caution even when prescribing non-salicylate anti-rheumatic drugs in patients with aspirin hypersensitivity.

(Friedlaender and Feinberg, 1947; Walton and Randle, 1957; Salvaggio and Crane, 1961; Giraldo *et al.*, 1969; McDonald *et al.*, 1972; Lockey *et al.*, 1973; Yunginger *et al.*, 1973; Matthews and Stage, 1974; Doeglas, 1975; Speer, 1975; Szczeklik *et al.*, 1975; Basomba *et al.*, 1976.)

Fluid retention: This effect of salicylates is sometimes important in the management of rheumatic carditis but is rarely of significance in the chronic rheumatic diseases.

(The various side effects of aspirin have been discussed in further depth by Dick (1978), to which the reader is referred for additional details.)

Precautions. Aspirin should be used with extreme caution in patients with gastric lesions on in patients taking anticoagulants. Pregnancy is not a contraindication as there is no clear evidence that therapeutic doses cause damage to the fetus, but prolonged high dosage may prolong the length of gestation and labour, probably due to inhibition of prostaglandin synthesis. Small doses of aspirin oppose the uricosuric action of both probenecid and sulphinpyrazone. Interactions between aspirin and other drugs are discussed elsewhere (Section 4.7).

Contraindications. Known aspirin hypersensitivity: active peptic ulceration.

Diflunisal (Dolobid)

Pharmacology and pharmacokinetics. The gastrointestinal absorption of diflunisal (2′, 4′-difluoro-4-hydroxy-3-biphenylcarboxylic acid) at therapeutic doses is virtually complete, peak plasma levels being reached in about 2 hours. About 95% is excreted in the urine as glucuronide conjugates and 4–5% in the faeces after 96 hours. Disappearance from the plasma is concentration dependent, with an elimination half-life of 11–12 hours, hence the rationale of a daily dosage schedule.

Its mode of action in the relief of acute and chronic pain is unknown, but activity of the drug may be related to selective blockade of prostaglandin synthetase.

(Steelman *et al.*, 1975, 1976, 1978; Tempero *et al.*, 1975, 1976, 1977; Tocco *et al.*, 1975; Majerus and

Stanford, 1977; Stone *et al.*, 1977; Dresse *et al.*, 1978; Kuehl and Egan, 1978.)

Clinical uses, praparations and dosage. The main clinical studies of diflunisal are summarized in Appendix 5.5.1. Currently, diflunisal is primarily indicated for the relief of pain. However, studies underway suggest that its anti-inflammatory activity may be sufficient to justify using the drug for inflammatory arthritides such as rheumatoid arthritis. The initial dosage is 500 mg (two tablets) given twice daily. This dosage can be reduced to 250 mg b.d. for long-term usage. Up to 1000 mg daily have been used in clinical studies.

(Hannah *et al.*, 1977; Bahous *et al.*, 1978; Huskisson *et al.*, 1978; Schulz *et al.*, 1979.)

Side effects, precautions and contraindications. Side effects are most commonly gastrointestinal (gastric pain, dyspepsia, nausea and vomiting). Less often central nervous system effects (vertigo and somnolence) occur and rarely rash and pruritus have been reported.

The drug should be used with caution in patients having a history of gastrointestinal haemorrhage or ulceration and in patients taking anticoagulant therapy. Co-administration of aluminium hydroxide suspension reduces the absorption of diflunisal by about 40%.

Diflunisal may have to be given in reduced dosage to patients with impaired renal function.

The drug should not be given to children, pregnant women or nursing mothers as its safety in those clinical areas has not yet been established.

Diflunisal is contraindicated in patients showing hypersensitivity to the drug, to aspirin or other analgesic/anti-inflammatory drugs. It is also contraindicated in patients with active gastrointestinal bleeding or active peptic ulcer.

COMMENT

Salicylates, particularly aspirin, are the most widely used of the analgesic/anti-inflammatory drugs. Despite a swing towards prescribing newer 'equivalents', they continue to be regarded as the traditional first choice. Apart from long usage, salicylates in general are the least expensive of the analgesic/anti-inflammatory group. Aspirin is usually considered as the yardstick against which the efficacy of other analgesic/anti-inflammatory drugs is assessed.

Although many clinicians prefer to start with newer non-salicylate preparations, as they may be better tolerated, tolerance to salicylates can be enhanced in some patients by using special preparations and formulations (e.g. soluble, enteric-coated micro-encapsulated, esterified forms).

Salicylates are valuable in treating a wide variety of acute and chronic rheumatic disorders. However, ankylosing spondylitis responds less well to this group of drugs than to certain other analgesic/anti-inflammatory agents (e.g. phenylbutazone, indomethacin).

(b) Acetic acids

Acetic acids may be subdivided into indole acetic acids (indomethacin, sulindac, tolmetin) and phenylacetic acids (diclofenac, fenclofenac).

Indole acetic acids

Indomethacin (Indocid, Imbrilon, Tannex, Artracin, Mobilan).
Other proprietary names include: Amuno (Germany); Confortid, Indomec (both Sweden); Inacid (Spain); Indacin, Mezolin (both Japan); Indocin (USA); Infrocin (Canada); Metindol (Poland).

Pharmacology and pharmacokinetics. Indomethacin (1-p-chlorobenzoyl)-5 methoxy-2-methylindole-3-acetic acid) is an effective anti-rheumatic drug, judicious clinical use being associated with an acceptable incidence of side effects.

Peak serum concentrations appear within 1–2 hours of ingestion. Antacids delay but do not reduce absorption. After an oral dose of 100 mg, serum concentrations will range between 2 and 5 μg (100 ml^{-1}). When given as a suppository, peak serum concentrations of about 1–3 μg (100 ml^{-1}) will be achieved. Synovial fluid concentrations are less than corresponding serum concentrations for the first 1–2 hours after an oral dose, and thereafter exceed the concentration in serum. Indomethacin is about 90% protein-bound in the circulation and is metabolized mainly in the liver by demethylation followed by deacetylation. The plasma half-life is less than 2 hours, the bulk of the ingested dose being excreted in the urine within 24 hours. There is a delay between peak serum level and the maximal reduction of pain and tenderness. In addition to circulating indomethacin, with its short half-life, there is a 'deep pool' in peripheral tissues where the active drug is re-formed from its inactive metabolites. This component turns over at a much slower rate, prolonging clinical effect beyond the period when the drug can be measured in plasma.

If probenecid is given orally with indomethacin it produces an increase in serum indomethacin concentration with an increase in clinical effect, whereas frusemide reduces the serum concentration of indomethacin. There may also be an interaction between indomethacin and aspirin and these two drugs should probably not be given together. Furthermore, in general, indomethacin should be prescribed alone if possible.

Mode of action. Indomethacin shares with all the other analgesic/anti-inflammatory drugs a wide variety of biological effects on many different systems (Famaey *et al.*, 1975). In the laboratory it is used by pharmacologists as the prototype molecule for inhibition of prostaglandin synthesis (Flower and Vane, 1974). It has also been shown that indomethacin may profoundly affect serum concentrations of kininogen, another chemical mediator of inflammation, and that it does so before, but in association with, changes in clinical indices (Sharma *et al.*, 1976).

(Sicuteri *et al.*, 1964; Holt and Hawkins, 1965; Jeremy and Towson, 1970; Champion *et al.*, 1971; Duggan *et al.*, 1972; Emori *et al.*, 1973a, b; Hridberg *et al.*, 1972; Brooks *et al.*, 1974a, b, 1975; Flower and Vane, 1974; de Gaetano *et al.*, 1974; Kunze *et al.*, 1974; Palmer *et al.*, 1974; Robinson and Levine, 1974; Barnett *et al.*, 1975; Famaey *et al.*, 1975; Fowler, 1975; Huskisson, 1976; Kwan *et al.*, 1976; Sharma *et al.*, 1976; Stanford *et al.*, 1977; Tan and Mulrow, 1977.)

Clinical uses, preparations and dosage. Indomethacin is useful in most rheumatic disorders, but is particularly helpful in ankylosing spondylitis, gout, rheumatoid arthritis and osteoarthrosis, particularly of the hip. A summary of the main clinical studies of the drug is shown in Appendix 5.5.2. About 20–30% of patients cannot tolerate it at effective dose levels, but about the same proportion do rather better with it than with most anti-inflammatory analgesics. It is effective in seronegative spondarthritides such as Reiter's disease and psoriatic arthritis. However, it may aggravate ulcerative lesions of the stomach or intestine and should be avoided in patients with peptic ulceration, ulcerative colitis or Crohn's disease.

A loading dose given at night is helpful in disorders such as ankylosing spondylitis and rheumatoid arthritis in which pain is often particularly prominent at night and in which morning stiffness is a major symptom. In such patients indomethacin suppositories are especially useful.

The usual dosage is 25 mg 2–4 times a day taken orally with or after meals. It is prudent to start with a test dose after the evening meal in case the patient proves to be an 'over-reactor'. To relieve nocturnal symptoms a dose of 50–100 mg by mouth (preferably with or after a milk drink or snack) or 100 mg in suppository form is prescribed on retiring. In acute gout, larger doses are necessary – 100 mg for night cover and 100–150 mg in the day in divided dosage. As symptoms settle the dosage is reduced. Some patients may need even larger doses initially. Indomethacin is available as capsules of 25 and 50 mg, sustained-release capsules containing 75 mg and suppositories of 100 mg. In some countries an elixir of 25 mg per 5 ml is available. Indomethacin as tablets of the sodium trihydrate (Osmosin), delivering 7 mg h^{-1} over 10 h, have recently been introduced in UK.

(Winter *et al.*, 1963; Hart and Boardman, 1965; Rothermich, 1966; Healey, 1967; Huskisson and Hart, 1972; Wright and Roberts, 1973; Calabro, 1975; Jaffe, 1976; Hobkirk *et al.*, 1977; Rhymer and Gengos, 1979.)

Side effects, precautions and contraindications. Headaches (often severe and throbbing), vertigo, mental 'muzziness', confusion and a number of other cerebral effects are dose related and diminish or disappear with reduction of dosage. Gastrointestinal symptoms, abdominal pain, vague discomfort, anorexia or peptic ulceration, sometimes with bleeding and perforation, are not dose related and may occur at any time on any dose. Diffuse gastritis with bleeding may occur, but is rare. Prepyloric gastric ulcers, also rare, may mimic carcinomatous lesions, but disappear within 4–5 weeks of stopping the drug. Haematological changes such as thrombocytopenia (sometimes with purpura) have been reported, but are rare. Severe depression, hallucinations and even psychoses have been reported. Psychiatric disorders, Parkinsonism and epilepsy may be exacerbated. Rashes are uncommon, as are hypersensitivity reactions such as urticaria, pruritus and asthma. Patients allergic to aspirin may cross-react with indomethacin. Suppositories of indomethacin may cause anal irritation in some patients, but in general are well tolerated over long periods. The use of suppositories reduces but does not necessarily abolish the tendency to gastrointestinal irritation, presumably due to a systemic effect of the drug. Patients with impaired renal function are more likely to react adversely to the drug, since elimination is probably prolonged.

Contraindications. Active peptic ulceration. A history of recurrent gastrointestinal erosions. Conditions for safe use in children have not yet been established. Safety for use during pregnancy or lactation has also not been established. Indomethacin suppositories are contraindicated in patients with a recent history of proctitis. Patients who show hypersensitivity to indomethacin or to aspirin should not be given indomethacin.

(Vecchio *et al.*, 1964; Solomon, 1966; Boardman and Hart, 1967; Burns, 1968; Taylor *et al.*, 1968; Jeremy and Towson, 1970; Carr and Siegel, 1973; Eade *et al.*, 1975; Vessel *et al.*, 1975; Rane *et al.*, 1978.)

Sulindac (Clinoril)

Pharmacology and pharmacokinetics. Sulindac ((Z)-5-fluoro-2-methyl-1-(*p*-methyl-sulphinylbenzylidene)-1 *H*-indene-3-acetic acid) is an indene derivative of indomethacin. The drug, which is a sulphoxide, is well absorbed after oral administration and has a plasma half-life of about 7 hours. Once absorbed the drug is enterohepatically recycled and converted in the gut into the sulphone and the sulphide, the latter being responsible for the pharmacological activity of sulindac. The sulphide has a half-life of 18 hours which enables sulindac to be given on a twice-daily basis. Sulindac and its sulphone metabolite are excreted in the urine and bile, either unchanged or mainly as the glucuronide conjugates. The active sulphide, on the other hand, is excreted only in the faeces.

(Shen, 1976; Van Arman *et al.*, 1976; Duggan *et al.*, 1977; Kwan and Duggan, 1977; Kwan *et al.*, 1978.)

Clinical uses, preparations and dosage. Sulindac has been found to be effective in rheumatoid arthritis, ankylosing spondylitis and osteoarthrosis, but it is doubtful if it is as potent as indomethacin. It has also been found to be effective in acute gout and soft-tissue rheumatism. A summary of the main clinical studies of sulindac is shown in Appendix 5.5.3.

Sulindac is available as a 100 mg tablet and is usually given in a dosage of 200 mg twice daily in rheumatoid arthritis. A lower dosage can be given in osteoarthrosis and in mild inflammatory disorders.

(*Editorial*, 1977; Huskisson, 1978; Huskisson and Scott, 1978; Rooney *et al.*, 1978; Sharma and Haslock, 1978; Oyemade and Onadeko, 1979; Rhymer, 1979.)

Side effects, precautions and contraindications. Side effects, precautions and contraindications are as for naproxen. Compared with indomethacin, sulindac is much less likely to cause headaches or gastric side effects than aspirin.

Sulindac can be given to patients receiving oral coumarin anticoagulants, but the prothrombin time should be checked daily for the first few days of treatment. The drug slightly reduces the uricosuric effect of probenecid but probably not to an important extent.

(Bower and Domiano, 1979a, b; Ryan *et al.*, 1977; Porro *et al.*, 1978.)

Tolmetin sodium (Tolectin)

Pharmacology and pharmacokinetics. Tolmetin (1-methyl-5-p-toluoylpyrrole-2 acetic acid) is well absorbed after ingestion and has a relatively short plasma half-life of about 1 hour. It is 99% bound to plasma proteins. It is excreted in the urine mainly as tolmetin glucuronide or as an inactive dicarboxylic acid metabolite and its glucuronide. Small amounts are excreted as the unchanged drug.

It has some chemical similarities to indomethacin but behaves more like proprionic acid derivatives.

(Wong *et al.*, 1973; Plostnieks *et al.*, 1975; Selley *et al.*, 1975; Wong, 1975; Cressman *et al.*, 1976; Brogden *et al.*, 1978.)

Clinical uses, preparations and dosage. Particularly in the USA, tolmetin has been shown to be useful in a wide range of rheumatic diseases (Appendix 5.5.4) and is well tolerated. Its clinical application is similar to that of proprionic acid derivatives.

The drug is available as a 200 mg tablet, dosages of 1200 mg or so in four divided doses being required to achieve a significant anti-inflammatory effect. The dosage range is 600–1800 mg daily.

In juvenile rheumatoid arthritis a dose of 20–25 mg kg^{-1} day^{-1} subdivided into 3 or 4 doses should be given. The dosage should not exceed 30 mg kg^{-1} day^{-1}, nor 1800 mg day^{-1} whatever the body weight. Half a tablet (100 mg) with water or milk is a suitable unit for most children's doses.

(Huskisson *et al.*, 1974; Pavelka and Susta, 1974; Cordrey, 1976; Brogden *et al.*, 1978; Ehrlich, 1979.)

Side effects, precautions and contraindications. Side effects are mainly gastrointestinal, including haemorrhage and peptic ulceration. Less common side effects are headache, dizziness, drowsiness, rashes, mild oedema and hypersensitivity reactions.

Tolmetin can be given with oral coumarin anticoagulants, but careful control initially with daily prothrombin time estimations should be carried out.

Concurrent administration of aspirin reduces plasma concentrations of tolmetin, but the clinical significance of this is unknown.

Studies indicate that the drug is poorly tolerated by peptic ulcer patients, and tolmetin should not be given to those with active ulcers and only cautiously to those with a history of peptic ulceration.

(Beirne *et al.*, 1974; Caldwell *et al.*, 1975; Ehrlich and Wortham, 1975; Mielke *et al.*, 1975; Whitsett *et al.*, 1975.)

Phenylacetic acids

Diclofenac sodium (Voltarol). Other proprietary names include: Voltaren (South Africa); Voltarène (Switzerland).

Pharmacology and pharmacokinetics. Diclofenac (the sodium salt of N-(2-6-dichlorophenyl)-O-aminophenyl acetic acid) is rapidly and completely absorbed by mouth and by rectum, and is almost completely (99%) bound to serum proteins (mostly albumin). Its metabolites are mainly excreted in the urine but also in the bile. The drug inhibits prostaglandin synthetase and also exerts an inhibiting effect on platelet aggregation.

(Krupp *et al.*, 1973; Aylward *et al.*, 1979; John, 1979; Maier *et al.*, 1979; Sallman, 1979.)

Clinical uses, preparations and dosage. Diclofenac has been found to be a useful analgesic/anti-inflammatory agent in a wide spectrum of rheumatic disorders (Appendix 5.5.5) including rheumatoid arthritis, osteoarthrosis, ankylosing spondylitis and acute gout. It has also been used in childhood polyarthritis.

The drug is available as tablets of 25 mg and 50 mg. (In some countries the drug is available as a 50 mg suppository and a 75 mg intramuscular injection.) The usual daily dosage in adults is 50–150 mg in divided doses. Dosage in children has not yet been established.

(Ciccolunghi *et al.*, 1975, 1976, 1977, 1979a; Ciccolunghi and Chaudri, 1976; Wagenhauser, 1976; Bach, 1979; Bonomo, 1979; Fowler, 1979; Haslock *et al.*, 1979; McMahon, 1979.)

Side effects, precautions and contraindications. Epigastric pain, nausea, diarrhoea, headache and slight dizziness are the commonest side effects, but these are often transient, disappearing with continued medication. Less commonly rash, peripheral oedema and abnormalities of serum transaminase have been reported.

The drug should be used with care in patients with hepatic or renal impairment, or a history of peptic ulcer. The safety of diclofenac has not yet been established in pregnancy.

(Michot *et al.*, 1975; Miura, 1975; Uthgenannt and Timm, 1975; Lehtola and Sipponen, 1977; Szezeklik *et al.*, 1977; Ciccolunghi *et al.*, 1978, 1979b; Ciucci, 1979; Fowler, 1979.)

Fenclofenac (Flenac)

Pharmacology and pharmacokinetics. Fenclofenac (2-(2, 4-dichlorophenoxy) phenylacetic acid) appears to be well absorbed from the gastrointestinal tract, giving peak plasma concentrations in 3–4 hours. The plasma half-life ranges from 20–38 hours. Fenclofenac is extensively bound to plasma proteins, mainly albumin. The major metabolite is the glucuronide. Urinary excretion is predominant in humans (93%), although a small percentage is eliminated in the faeces. The drug has been shown to be an effective prostaglandin synthetase inhibitor.

(Jordan and Rance, 1974; Atkinson and Leach, 1976, 1978; Atkinson *et al.*, 1977; Rooney *et al.*, 1977; Mowat, 1980; Phillips, 1980.)

Clinical uses, preparations and dosage. Clinical studies (Appendix 5.5.6) have established fenclofenac to be a useful analgesic/anti-inflammatory agent in rheumatoid arthritis, osteoarthrosis, ankylosing spondylitis, juvenile chronic arthritis and soft-tissue injury. There is also some preliminary evidence to suggest that the drug may exercise a more fundamental disease-modifying influence in rheumatoid arthritis.

Fenclofenac is available as 300 mg tablets and the

dose range is up to 1200 mg on a twice daily regimen, taken with or after food.

(Goldberg *et al.*, 1975; Bacon *et al.*, 1977; Glick, 1977; Goldberg and Tudor, 1977; Hingorani, 1977; Lambert and Wright, 1977; Tudor *et al.*, 1977; Glick and Loebl, 1980.)

Side effects, precautions and contraindications. Gastrointestinal discomfort and nausea have been reported. However, this has occurred infrequently and has usually been insufficient to lead to withdrawal of treatment. Mild rashes have been observed during the first month of treatment. Fenclofenac should not yet be prescribed for children or for pregnant or lactating women. Nor should the drug be co-administered with anticoagulant drugs. Patients with known renal or hepatic diseases, asthma or sensitivity to other non-steroidal anti-inflammatory drugs should also be treated cautiously. The drug is contraindicated in patients with active peptic ulceration or bleeding. Fenclofenac interferes with thyroid function tests and should be withdrawn at least 10 days before these tests are carried out.

(Atkinson *et al.*, 1974; Cardoe, 1977; Garner, 1977; Rainsford, 1977; Smith, 1977; Salmon *et al.*, 1977; Humphrey *et al.*, 1980; Ratcliffe *et al.*, 1980; Snaith, 1980; Svensen, 1980; Swain *et al.*, 1980.)

COMMENT
The principal member of this group is indomethacin, which is now a widely used analgesic/anti-inflammatory agent of potency on a par with other important anti-inflammatory drugs such as aspirin and phenylbutazone. It continues to be popular in a wide variety of inflammatory rheumatic disorders, including rheumatoid arthritis, the spondarthritides, and acute gout. Its therapeutic efficacy is marred by gastrointestinal and, more characteristically, CNS side effects such as severe throbbing headache. However, it is probably the most widely used analgesic/anti-inflammatory drug after aspirin.

(c) Proprionic acids

Ibuprofen (Brufen)
Another proprietary name is Motrin (Canada, USA).

Pharmacology and pharmacokinetics. Ibuprofen (2-(-4-isobutylphenyl) proprionic acid) is well absorbed from the gastrointestinal tract and peak concentrations in the circulation occur about $1\frac{1}{2}$ hours after ingestion. The drug is extensively bound to plasma proteins and has a half-life of about 2 hours. It is rapidly excreted in the urine and about 60% of a dose is recovered in the urine as metabolites and their conjugates. Some ibuprofen may be excreted in the faeces, possibly after excretion in the bile.

(Adams *et al.*, 1970; Davis and Avery, 1971; Brooks *et al.*, 1973; Glass and Swannell, 1978.)

Clinical uses, preparations and dosage. Ibuprofen, the first of the proprionic acid derivatives to be introduced in most countries, is an analgesic with anti-inflammatory properties. Although the potency of the drug as an anti-inflammatory agent is probably less than that of, say, aspirin or indomethacin, the drug is useful in a wide range of rheumatic disorders (Appendix 5.5.7) from the milder forms of rheumatoid arthritis to osteoarthrosis and back pain. It is less suitable for very active rheumatoid arthritis, acute Reiter's disease, acute gout, ankylosing spondylitis, and other conditions in which inflammation is prominent. Ibuprofen is available as 200 and 400 mg tablets and a 600 mg tablet has been recently introduced in UK (Brufen 600). Most reported studies have used 1200 mg daily, but more recently higher doses, up to 2400 mg daily, have been recommended for particularly active disease states. Doses smaller than 1200 mg daily are unlikely to be effective in an anti-inflammatory role. Ibuprofen can be used in children in doses up to 40 mg kg^{-1} day^{-1}.

(Nassonova *et al.*, 1973; Pipitone *et al.*, 1973, 1975; Wagenhauser, 1973; Levernieux, 1975; Miller *et al.*, 1975; Otadny, 1975.)

Side effects, precautions and contraindications. Ibuprofen is generally well tolerated, but may cause nausea, vomiting, dyspepsia, diarrhoea and, occasionally, stomatitis, or gastrointestinal haemorrhage. Other side effects include headache, dizziness, nervousness, oedema, rash, tinnitus, and blurred vision. Increased values for SGPT, bilirubin, and alkaline phosphatase have been reported, but have often returned to normal despite continued treatment. Thrombocytopenia has also been reported. Ibuprofen should be given with care to patients with peptic ulceration or a history of such ulceration. Ibuprofen can be given to patients receiving oral coumarin anticoagulants, but it is wise to check the prothrombin time daily for the first few days of combined therapy.

(Cardoe, 1970, 1975; Collum and Bowen, 1971; Goncalves, 1973; Thilo *et al.*, 1974; Buckler *et al.*, 1975; Dimitriu, 1975; Duckert, 1975; Giobanu and Zalaru, 1975; Rejholec, 1975; Sadowska-Wroblewska *et al.*, 1975; Thompson *et al.*, 1975.)

Naproxen (Naprosyn)
Other proprietary names include: Naxen (Mexico); Proxen (Austria, Germany, Switzerland).

Pharmacology and pharmacokinetics. Naproxen ((+)-2-(6-methoxy-2-naphthyl)-proprionic acid) is readily absorbed from the gastrointestinal tract. It is extensively bound to plasma proteins and has a half-life of about 14 hours. About half of a dose is excreted in the urine in 24 hours, and about 94% in 5 days, largely as glucuronide. Naproxen, like other proprionic acid derivatives has been shown to inhibit the synthesis of prostaglandins.

(Roszkowski *et al.*, 1971; Runkel *et al.*, 1972, 1973, 1976; Segre, 1975.)

Clinical uses, preparations and dosage. Naproxen is one of the more effective proprionic acid derivatives. It is useful for symptomatic treatment of a wide range of rheumatic disorders (Appendix 5.5.8) ranging from rheumatoid arthritis to soft-tissue rheumatism and backache. It is perhaps marginally less useful than aspirin in patients with particularly active rheumatoid arthritis and marginally less useful than indomethacin and phenylbutazone in ankylosing spondylitis. It has been shown to be effective in the treatment of acute gout. Naproxen is effective in only about 60% of patients with rheumatoid arthritis. Differences between patient responses to the drug are much greater than differences in response to different drugs. Naproxen is therefore a useful drug for a particular subgroup of patients. It takes effect within 24 hours of the start of treatment and a week of therapy is long enough to assess its effectiveness.

Naproxen is available as a 250 mg tablet, a 500 mg tablet, a flavoured suspension containing 25 mg ml^{-1} and as suppositories each containing 500 mg. The usual dose is 250 mg twice daily. A larger dose (500 mg) may be useful at night for the relief of morning stiffness. The recommended maximum dose is 1 g per day. In acute gout, 750 mg should be given as a starting dose, followed by 250 mg 8 hourly until the attack has passed. It has been found useful in the treatment of juvenile arthritides.

(Roszkowski *et al.*, 1971; Katona, 1973; Tiselins, 1973; Hill *et al.*, 1974; Huskisson *et al.*, 1979; Segre, 1979.)

Side effects, precautions and contraindications. On the whole, naproxen is remarkably free from side effects, and together with ibuprofen is one of the least toxic of the proprionic acid derivatives. Unwanted features which have occasionally occurred include nausea, vomiting, dyspepsia, constipation, gastrointestinal haemorrhage, insomnia or drowsiness, headache, dizziness, tinnitus, pruritus, skin changes, including angioneurotic oedema, visual disturbances, and an increase in bleeding time. Naproxen should be given with care to patients with peptic ulceration or a history of ulceration. In view of the high plasma protein binding of naproxen, patients simultaneously receiving hydantoins, coumarin anticoagulants or a highly protein-bound sulphonamide should be observed for signs of overdosage. The use of naproxen should be avoided in patients who are breast feeding.

(Halvoresen *et al.*, 1973; Beck and Hayes-Allen, 1974; Hart, 1974; Hart and Matts, 1974; Hayes-Allen, 1974; Matts, 1974; Nadell *et al.*, 1974; Roth and Boost, 1975; Fredell and Strand, 1977; Jain *et al.*, 1979; Segre, 1979; Slattery *et al.*, 1979.)

Fenoprofen (Fenopron)

Pharmacology and pharmacokinetics. Fenoprofen is the calcium salt of dl-2-(3-phenoxyphenyl) proprionic acid. The drug is readily absorbed from the gastrointestinal tract and gives rise to peak plasma concentrations 1–2 hours after a dose. The half-life is about $2\frac{1}{2}$ hours. It is extensively bound to plasma proteins. About 95% of a dose is excreted in the urine in 24 hours, chiefly as the glucuronide and as the glucuronide of hydroxylated fenoprofen. Absorption is reduced if aspirin is given concomitantly. Part of its anti-inflammatory effect is attributed to prostaglandin synthetase inhibition.

(Rubin *et al.*, 1971, 1972, 1974; Chernish *et al.*, 1972; Ho and Esterman, 1974.)

Clinical uses, preparations and dosage. Fenoprofen is useful as symptomatic therapy in a wide variety of rheumatic disorders (Appendix 5.5.9). In rheumatoid arthritis it is as effective as full doses of aspirin and it has also been shown to be effective in osteoarthrosis and in acute gout. Like naproxen, fenoprofen is effective in about 60% of patients with rheumatoid arthritis, and both of these drugs are probably more effective than ibuprofen or ketoprofen. Fenoprofen is available as a 300 mg capsule or tablet. The usual initial dosage is 2.4 mg daily in four divided doses, but in patients who respond well, 1.2–1.8 mg daily may suffice.

(Mikulaschek, 1974; Murphy *et al.*, 1978; Ridolfo *et al.*, 1979.)

Side effects, precautions and contraindications. The side effects, precautions and contraindications concerning fenoprofen are similar to those for ibuprofen, except that fenoprofen may enhance the effects of anticoagulants.

(Herrmann *et al.*, 1972; Rubin *et al.*, 1974; Lin *et al.*, 1975; Blechman and Zane, 1976; Loebl *et al.*, 1977.)

Ketoprofen (Alrheumat; Orudis)
Another proprietary name is Profénid (France).

Pharmacology and pharmacokinetics. Ketoprofen (2-(3-benzoylphenyl) proprionic acid) is readily absorbed from the gastrointestinal tract; peak plasma concentrations occur $\frac{1}{2}$–2 hours after a dose. The plasma half-life is about $1\frac{1}{2}$–2 hours. The drug is extensively bound to plasma proteins. The rate of excretion appears to be variable, 30–90% of a dose being recoverable in the urine in 24 hours, chiefly as the glucuronide. Its anti-inflammatory effect is thought at least in part to be due to inhibition of prostaglandin synthetase.

(Populaire *et al.*, 1973; Mitchell *et al.*, 1975; Kennedy, 1976; Kaller, 1979.)

Clinical uses, preparations and dosage. Ketoprofen is one of the group of analgesics with anti-inflammatory properties similar in effectiveness to ibuprofen. There is evidence for its usefulness in rheumatoid arthritis, ankylosing spondylitis, gout and osteoarthrosis (Appendix 5.5.10).

(Bocquet and Vignon, 1973; Atra and Goldenberg, 1974; Fossgrenn *et al.*, 1976; Grahame, 1976; Kirchheiner *et al.*, 1976; Renier and Boasson, 1976; Williams *et al.*, 1977; Peltola, 1978; Mason and Bolton, 1979.)

The drug is available as 50 mg capsules, and the usual dosage is 50 mg, three times daily. In some countries it is also available for injection and as a 100 mg suppository. The latter may be useful at night to allay morning stiffness in patients who are unable to tolerate the drug by mouth.

(Asch *et al.*, 1974; Asch, 1975; David-Chaussé *et al.*, 1976; Fournie and Ayrolles, 1976; Gougeon *et al.*, 1976; Le Chevallier and Valet, 1976; Griffin *et al.*, 1978.)

Side effects, precautions and contraindications. Side effects, precautions and contraindications are as for ibuprofen, except that particular care should be exercised in patients receiving coumarin anticoagulants as their effect may be enhanced by ketoprofen.

(Gomez, 1976; Lussier and Arsenault, 1976; Rahbek, 1976; Gross, 1979.)

Flurbiprofen (Froben)

Pharmacology and pharmacokinetics. Flurbiprofen (2-(2-fluoro-4-biphenylyl) proprionic acid) is well absorbed after oral medication, with peak plasma levels achieved $1\frac{1}{2}$ hours after administration. Absorption bears a linear relationship to dose. It has a relatively short plasma half-life of about 4 hours. Several metabolites have been identified but do not appear to contribute to the activity of the drug. Flurbiprofen and its metabolites are excreted in both urine and faeces. The drug is a potent inhibitor of prostaglandin synthetase and has been shown to possess significant anti-inflammatory activity in animals and humans. There is also evidence that it is an antithrombotic agent by inhibiting platelet aggregation.

(Glenn *et al.*, 1973; Nishizawa *et al.*, 1973; Davis *et al.*, 1974; Adams *et al.*, 1975a, b, 1977; Bacon *et al.*,

1975; Sim *et al.*, 1975; Yasunaga and Ryo, 1975; Cardoe *et al.*, 1977; Chalmers *et al.*, 1977; Cremoncini *et al.*, 1977; Ford-Hutchinson *et al.*, 1977; Thebault *et al.*, 1977.)

Clinical uses, preparations and dosage. Flurbiprofen has been shown to be effective in rheumatoid arthritis, osteoarthrosis and ankylosing spondylitis (Appendix 5.5.11), and its effects are comparable with those achieved by full doses of aspirin. There is some evidence that it may be a useful antithrombotic agent, but it is not yet conventionally used for this purpose. Flurbiprofen is available as a 50 mg and a 100 mg tablet. Initial dosage is 50 mg, three times daily. For pain at night or morning stiffness the evening dose can be increased to 100 mg. Doses up to 300 mg can be given.

(Doury and Pattin, 1977; Ford-Hutchinson *et al.*, 1977; Huskisson *et al.*, 1977; Innes, 1977; Joshi *et al.*, 1977; Sheldrake *et al.*, 1977.)

Side effects, precautions and contraindications. Flurbiprofen has only recently been introduced, and so far there is insufficient experience of its side effects. At the time of writing, however, side effects have included anorexia, nausea, dyspepsia, diarrhoea, constipation, gastrointestinal haemorrhage and vertigo. Rash has occasionally been reported.

The drug should not be used in pregnancy or in children. It should also be avoided in patients receiving oral anticoagulants and in patients with peptic ulceration. Care should be taken when administering the drug to asthmatics or those who have experienced bronchospasm with other anti-inflammatory or analgesic agents.

No untoward interactions with other drugs have yet been described and a recent study has shown no significant interference of flurbiprofen with oral anticoagulation.

(Brooks and Khong, 1977; Marbet *et al.*, 1977; Vakil *et al.*, 1977a, b.)

Fenbufen (Lederfen)

Pharmacology and pharmacokinetics. Fenbufen (y-oxo (1, 1'-biphenyl)-4-butanoic acid), a pro-drug, is rapidly and completely absorbed from the gastrointestinal tract with peak levels occurring at $1\frac{1}{2}$–2 hours. Its long duration of action is attributable to the prolonged half lives (10 to 17 hours) of its active metabolites. In general, the urine is the main excretory pathway (66%) although a proportion of metabolites are eliminated in the faeces (8%) and via the lungs (12%). Both fenbufen and its metabolites have been shown to inhibit prostaglandin activity and synthesis.

(Sloboda and Osterberg, 1976; Child *et al.*, 1977; van Lear, 1978; Mawdsley, 1979.)

Clinical uses, preparations and dosage. Fenbufen has been shown to be an effective and well-tolerated anti-rheumatic agent in rheumatoid arthritis and osteoarthrosis (Appendix 5.5.12). It has also been found to be effective in ankylosing spondylitis and acute gout. It is available as 300 mg capsules, the dosage being 600–900 mg daily in a single or divided dose. Many patients can be adequately controlled with a daily dosage of 600 mg taken at night.

(Coutinho *et al.*, 1976; Child *et al.*, 1977; Mawdsley, 1979.)

Side effects, precautions and contraindications. Adverse effects are uncommon, but include gastrointestinal intolerance and less often rash, dizziness, drowsiness and headache. When fenbufen and aspirin are administered together, serum concentrations of fenbufen and its metabolites are reduced by 10–20%. Fenbufen should be used with caution in patients with a history of peptic ulcer and should be used only when essential in pregnant and nursing women. The drug is contraindicated in proprionic acid or aspirin hypersensitivity.

(Panagides, 1976; Mawdsley, 1979.)

Benoxaprofen (Opren)

The product licences for this drug have recently been withdrawn on grounds of safety.

This has arisen from over 3500 reports of adverse reactions associated with this drug received by the Committee on Safety of Medicines. Included among these reports are 61 deaths, predominantly in the elderly. There have also been serious toxic effects on various organ systems, particularly the gastrointestinal tract, the liver and bone marrow, in addition to the known effects on skin, nails and eyes.

However, despite this ban, it was felt that the interest generated by this new drug justified retaining its inclusion, if only as a basis for future pharmaceutical speculation.

Pharmacology and pharmacokinetics. Benoxaprofen (dl-2-(4-chlorophenyl)-α-methyl-5-benzoxazole acetic acid), one of the most recent proprionic acid derivatives to be released in the UK (but recently withdrawn), is rapidly absorbed after oral administration, reaches a peak blood level after 2–6 hours and has an elimination half-life of about 32 hours. Benoxaprofen is excreted as the β-glucuronide in the urine, but is excreted unchanged in the faeces. The drug has pharmacological properties (and toxic effects) that differentiate it from other effective analgesic/anti-inflammatory agents: its plasma half-life allowed an optimal once-a-day dosage regimen; it is a relatively weak inhibitor of prostaglandin synthetase; it may act primarily by inhibiting mononuclear cell migration into sites of inflammation.

(Cashin *et al.*, 1977; Chatfield *et al.*, 1977; Smith *et al.*, 1977; Chatfield and Green, 1978; Meacock and Kitchen, 1979; Dawson, 1980; Jones *et al.*, 1980; Lightfoot, 1980; Nash *et al.*, 1980.)

Clinical uses, preparations and dosage. Preliminary clinical trials have demonstrated effectiveness of benoxaprofen in rheumatoid arthritis, ankylosing spondylitis and osteoarthrosis (Appendix 5.5.13). More extensive studies were underway in patients with these disorders and also in gout, soft-tissue problems, and other rheumatic disorders where analgesic/anti-inflammatory agents have been shown to be useful.

Until withdrawal benoxaprofen was available as 300 mg tablets. The usual daily dosage for rheumatoid arthritis and osteoarthrosis was 600 mg daily as a single dose 1 hour before retiring. The drug was administered twice daily.

(Chatfield *et al.*, 1977; Highton and Grahame, 1978; Huskisson *et al.*, 1978; Huskisson, 1979; Huskisson and Scott, 1979; Ridolfo *et al.*, 1979; Bacon *et al.*, 1980; Lightfoot, 1980.)

Side effects, precautions and contraindications. The side-effect profile of benoxaprofen has received considerable publicity in view of the frequency of toxic effects and their unusual nature, and has recently led to withdrawal of the drug.

In a study of 300 patients, Halsay and Cardoe (1982) found cutaneous side effects to account for almost 70% of all toxic effects. The commonest skin problem was photosensitivity*, followed by onycholysis, and then multiple subepidermal cysts (milia). Another recent report (Fenton *et al.*, 1982) has drawn attention to additional, though less common, cutaneous effects including reversal of male-pattern baldness, hypertrichosis, and accelerated hair and nail growth. These authors have also encountered the Stevens–Johnson syndrome and toxic epidermal necrolysis in patients receiving benoxaprofen. These more serious cutaneous features have also been reported by Hindson (1982). In view of these changes it was advised that particular care be taken to avoid re-challenging patients with the Stevens–Johnson syndrome as this condition is potentially lethal.

Gastrointestinal side effects, although less common than the cutaneous effects, could be troublesome, particularly in the elderly, and included dyspepsia, nausea, vomiting, constipation, abdominal pain and

---

* The side effect could be avoided by staying out of direct sunlight or by using an appropriate sunscreen. Clinicians were advised to take especial care to warn about this side effect, particularly when the drug had been prescribed in patients about to take a vacation in a sunny climate.

occult bleeding. Peptic ulceration occurred only rarely. There has been a disturbing report recently (Taggart and Alderdice, 1982) of fatal cholestatic jaundice in five elderly women who had taken the drug.

Somnolence, dizziness, weakness and headache were other side effects that had been reported, though infrequently.

Before withdrawal it was advised that benoxaprofen be given cautiously in patients with impaired liver function and a reduced dosage used in patients with impaired renal function. Although preliminary studies had not shown appreciable alteration in haemostasis in patients receiving oral anticoagulants, it was recommended that benoxaprofen should be used with caution in these patients. Administration to patients with active peptic ulceration was not recommended, although benoxaprofen probably caused less gastrointestinal bleeding than other proprionic acid derivatives.

It was stressed that the drug should not be given to patients exhibiting hypersensitivity to salicylates or other non-steroidal anti-inflammatory agents.

The safety of benoxaprofen administration in children and in pregnancy had not been established.

(Chatfield *et al.*, 1978; Jones *et al.*, 1980; Mikulaschek, 1980; Ridolfo *et al.*, 1980; Cardoe and Halsey, 1982; Fenton *et al.*, 1982; Hindson *et al.*, 1982; Taggart and Alderdice, 1982.)

Indoprofen

Indoprofen (α-[p-(1-oxoisoindolin-2-yl)-phenyl] proprionic acid) is the most recent phenylalkanoic derivative to show promise as an analgesic/anti-inflammatory agent. The drug is rapidly and completely absorbed from the gastrointestinal tract and is rapidly excreted. About 80% of the administered dose is recoverable in the urine within 24 hours (15% in unchanged form, the rest conjugated as glucuronide). Clinical trials and application were started in Italy. The drug has recently been introduced into the UK as Flosint (indoprofen 200 mg tablets 1–4 daily in divided doses). It has been found to be effective in rheumatoid arthritis, osteoarthrosis and acute gout to a degree at least comparable with conventional anti-inflammatory therapy. Most studies with rheumatoid patients have used a dose of 800 mg per day.

The drug is generally well tolerated and appears to be as troublefree as other proprionic acid preparations. The most frequent side effects are gastrointestinal (pain, heartburn, nausea, vomiting, constipation, diarrhoea).

(Buttinoni *et al.*, 1973; Fuccella *et al.*, 1973; Baldrighi and Sacchetti, 1976; Caruso *et al.*, 1977; Smith *et al.*, 1977; Berry *et al.*, 1978; Rubegni *et al.*, 1978; Chèrié Lignière *et al.*, 1979; Chiapazzo, 1979; Cooper *et al.*, 1979; Giro and Lo Presti, 1979; Huskisson and Scott, 1979; Okun *et al.*, 1979; Saba and Orlandi, 1979; Bruni *et al.*, 1980; Tirri *et al.*, 1980.)

COMMENT

This series of drugs, starting with ibuprofen, was introduced as a means of finding analgesic/anti-inflammatory agents of comparable effect to aspirin, but with fewer side effects – particularly gastrointestinal side effects. They appear to vary only slightly in anti-inflammatory effect, and the justification of dividing these drugs into those with minor and major effects would seem to be hardly justified. When used in maximal dosage, most of the drugs probably approach aspirin in efficacy, and some may equal it. In general, side effects are less than with aspirin. Naproxen is one of the most popular of this group, and has the advantage (as do several newer analgesic/anti-inflammatory drugs) of twice daily administration. This drug has also been shown to be effective in ankylosing spondylitis and acute gout, as well as in rheumatoid arthritis.

The large number of proprionic acid preparations now available, a bewildering catalogue of drugs which continues to increase, makes individual assessment difficult to measure on a comparative basis. However, considering variations in patient response, even within generic groups, it is useful to have a number of proprionic acid derivatives from which to choose.

(d) Fenamic acids

Flufenamic acid (Meralen)
Other proprietary names include: Ansatin, Flufacid, Lanceat, Nichisedan, Reumajust A, Saal-F (all Japan); Surika (Germany); Orpyrin (aluminium flufenamate) (Japan).

Pharmacology and pharmacokinetics. Flufenamic acid (n. ααα-trifluoro-m-tolyl anthranilic acid) shows peak plasma levels after oral administration at about 3–6 hours. A secondary peak in blood levels occurs after about 8 hours due to hydroxylated metabolites, probably resulting from enterohepatic circulation. Plasma protein binding is almost complete. Fifty-five per cent is eliminated via the kidneys as the unchanged drug, glucuronide conjugate and hydroxylated glucuronides, and about 36% is excreted via the faeces.

(De Salcedo *et al.*, 1966; Winder *et al.*, 1966.)

Clinical uses, preparations and dosage. Flufenamic acid has been found to be useful as an analgesic/anti-inflammatory agent (Appendix 5.5.14) and is often considered when proprionic acid derivatives have been found ineffective or poorly tolerated.

The drug is available as 100 mg and 200 mg capsules. The usual dose range is 200 mg, three times daily, reducing to 400 mg daily. Not more than $10 \, \text{mg kg}^{-1}$ daily should be given in patients weighing less than 45 kg.

(Coodley, 1963; Barnardo *et al.*, 1966; Cowan and Masheter, 1966; Fearnley and Masheter, 1966; Ferris and Pigott, 1966; Haward, 1966; Hume Kendall, 1966; Simpson *et al.*, 1966; Holmes, 1967; Rajan *et al.*, 1967.)

Side effects, precautions and contraindications. Side effects are nausea, vomiting, diarrhoea (at least 10% of patients) and epigastric discomfort. Sensitivity rash occurs infrequently.

Contraindications: inflammatory bowel disease (e.g. ulcerative colitis), peptic ulceration, renal and hepatic impairment, pregnancy, nursing mothers.

The drug should be used cautiously in patients with allergic diseases, particularly asthma. Caution should also be exercised in those on oral coumarin anticoagulants and oral sulphonylurea hypoglycaemic drugs.

(Tudhope, 1966.)

Mefenamic acid (Ponstan Forte)
Other proprietary preparations include: Coslan (Spain); Parkemed (Germany); Ponstel (USA); Ponstyl (France).

See under flufenamic acid with the following exceptions. It is probably less anti-inflammatory than flufenamic acid. Haemolytic anaemia has been reported with mefenamic acid. The drug is available as 250 capsules and 500 mg tablets and as a paediatric suspension (50 mg 5 ml^{-1}). The adult dose is 500 mg, three times daily after meals.

(Barnardo *et al.*, 1966.)

(e) Pyrazolones

Phenylbutazone (Butazolidin, Butacote)
Other proprietary names include: Algoverine, Butagesic, Chembutazone, Ecobutazone, Eributazone, Intrabutazone, Malgesic, Merizone, Nadozone, Neo-Zoline, Novophenyl, Phenbutazol, Phenylbetazone, Tazone, Wescozone (all Canada); Artrizin (Denmark); Artropen, Diossidone, Kadol, Ticinil (all Italy); Azolid (USA); Butacal, Butalan, Butalgin, Butaphen, Butarex, Butoroid, Butoz, Buzon, Phenylbute (all Australia); Butapirazol (Poland); Butina, Butozone, Butrex, Panazone (all South Africa); Elmedal, Praecirheumin (both Germany).

Pharmacology and pharmacokinetics. Phenylbutazone is 3.5 dioxo-1, 2-diphenyl-4m-butylpyrazolidine, a pyrazolone derivative. It has anti-inflammatory, analgesic and antipyretic properties in animals and man. There is little doubt that phenylbutazone possesses antirheumatic activity at least as powerful as that of either indomethacin or aspirin. It has been found to be of particular value in ankylosing spondylitis and gouty arthritis.

Plasma levels are detected within 2 hours, but peak levels occur at about 72 hours. The drug may be detected in serum as long as 15 days after the last dose and the half-life is further prolonged in patients with liver disease. There are wide variations in the serum concentration achieved after a constant dose, but equilibrium is achieved between 8 and 10 days after starting maintenance therapy. It is about 98% protein-bound, mainly to plasma albumin, the proportion falling with increasing serum concentrations. The serum concentration achieved with continuous medication is of some relevance as both efficacy and side effects are at least partially dose related. Genetic factors probably influence the metabolism of the drug.

Negligible amounts of phenylbutazone are excreted unchanged in the urine and a small proportion is recoverable in bile and faeces. Three major metabolic compounds have been identified, only one (metabolite I) being anti-inflammatory. This metabolite is identical with oxyphenbutazone and, although its rate of absorption is rather slower, the plasma binding and half-life of this compound are similar to that of phenylbutazone.

The pharmacodynamics of phenylbutazone metabolism are of some practical significance. It has been customary to administer phenylbutazone in 100 mg doses, three times daily, but in fact after the plateau has been reached in 8–10 days the drug can be given in a single daily dose of 200 or 300 mg. Higher doses on a long-term basis are neither necessary nor advisable.

(Bruck *et al.*, 1954; Bakke *et al.*, 1974; Brooks *et al.*, 1975; Fowler, 1975.)

Mode of action. Phenylbutazone inhibits the biosynthesis of prostaglandins, uncouples oxidative phosphorylation and inhibits ATP-dependent biosynthesis of mucopolysaccharide sulphates in cartilage. In addition, it has a mild uricosuric effect by diminishing tubular reabsorption of uric acid. Lower concentrations of the drug have the opposite effect, inhibiting tubular secretion of uric acid, thereby causing urate retention. Phenylbutazone causes substantial sodium chloride and water retention (probably due to a direct action on the renal tubules), and may precipitate heart failure and acute pulmonary oedema in predisposed patients. These clinical effects may be increased by a drug-induced fall in urinary output and oedema. Further, in the treatment of acute gout, although pain may be relieved dramatically, swelling in the affected area may remain unchanged because of oedema. Potassium excretion is not affected. On withdrawing the drug, a compensatory diuresis off-loads the excess of sodium and chloride and the expansion of plasma volume returns to normal. These fluid changes may be enough to cause apparent anaemia which disappears after diuresis. Water loading may be controlled by concurrent administration of diuretics. Phenylbutazone may reduce the uptake of iodine by the thyroid (apparently by a direct effect on the gland) and may thereby inhibit synthesis of organic iodine compounds. This effect may occasionally cause goitre and even frank myxoedema. Phenylbutazone inhibits enzymes of the Krebs cycle, and chromosomal damage has been reported by some workers.

(Benedek, 1962; Whittaker and Price Evans, 1970; Smyth and Percy, 1973; Bakke *et al.*, 1974; Brooks *et al.*, 1975.)

Clinical uses, preparations, dosage. Phenylbutazone is effective in almost all the rheumatic disorders (Appendix 5.5.15), particularly in acute gout, ankylosing spondylitis, osteoarthrosis, rheumatoid arthritis and in Reiter's disease and other seronegative spondarthritides. It has also been used with effect in the past in rheumatic fever. Phenylbutazone may also provide symptomatic control in prolapsed intervertebral disc disease, Paget's disease of bone and metastatic malignant disease of bone. However, though a highly effective drug, it is wise, because of its side effects and drug interactions, to use it only where a less potentially dangerous agent fails to control symptoms. It is also prudent not to continue medication indefinitely, particularly in elderly patients, without close clinical and haematological control (see under side effects). It would also seem reasonable to avoid using phenylbutazone to treat mild conditions such as trivial sports or other injuries where less toxic agents would suffice.

Phenylbutazone is prescribed as 100 and 200 mg tablets orally after food. In acute gout, a dosage of 600–800 mg is given initially on the first day, reducing the dosage as symptoms become controlled by 100–200 mg daily to a maintenance of 200–400 mg, withdrawing the drug as soon as the attack has passed. In chronic rheumatic conditions, particularly ankylosing spondylitis, after an initial dose of 200 mg 2–3 times daily, usually for 2 days, most patients can be adequately controlled on 300 mg daily, and often 100 mg is sufficient once control has been established. Every effort should be made to maintain the dose at the lowest effective level, and patients should be reviewed regularly with this in mind. Some patients manage comfortably for long periods without any medication. Phenylbutazone should always be given with or after food. Enteric-coated and antacid-incorporated tablets are available, as are suppositories of 250 mg. It is effective, though sometimes painful, given by intramuscular injection (3 ml ampoules containing 200 mg of the sodium salt per ml with xylocaine 1%).

(Graham, 1958; Strandberg, 1965; Rushford and Fowler, 1970; Lewis-Faning and Fowler, 1971; McIntosh and Fowler, 1977.)

Side effects, precautions and contraindications. The reported frequency of side effects varies widely. The most serious is marrow aplasia (Böttiger and Westerholm, 1972), which occurs at a rate of 1 per 100 to 150 000 patient/months of treatment. Aplastic anaemia tends to occur in the elderly patient, usually after prolonged treatment. Agranulocytosis, on the other hand, may be seen in younger people in the early stages of treatment. Acute sensitivity reactions and fatal blood changes from short courses of therapy are very rare. Most patients (87%) who develop agranulocytosis do so within 3 months of starting treatment, compared with only 30% of patients with aplastic anaemia. About 50% of those with aplastic anaemia develop this after at least a year of treatment (Fowler, 1967). Agranulocytosis and aplastic anaemia occur with equal frequency and are not confined to patients with rheumatoid arthritis. Phenylbutazone causes an appreciable number of deaths from blood dyscrasias. About 25 people a year die in the UK from phenylbutazone, a figure higher than that quoted for gold, although the mortality rate per prescription is higher for gold.

The pathogenesis of drug-induced aplastic anaemia remains unclear, but a direct toxic effect, an allergy produced by the production of antibodies to damaged cell membranes as a consequence of drug treatment, or true allergy have all been implicated.

Sequential blood counts do not guarantee protection, but monthly monitoring at least reminds the clinician that the patient is receiving a potentially toxic drug.

Phenylbutazone is also toxic to the gastrointestinal tract and both dyspepsia and acute and chronic blood loss have been reported (MacFarlane *et al.*, 1976), although phenylbutazone appears less likely to cause bleeding than aspirin or indomethacin. A previous history of peptic ulceration is a relative contraindication to prescribing drugs of this group.

Phenylbutazone, like radiotherapy, may induce chromosomal damage in peripheral white blood cells. However, not one instance of leukaemia or tumour of the reticuloendothelial system was detected in a survey of over 30 000 rheumatic patients treated with phenylbutazone (Leavesley *et al.*, 1969).

Other side effects that may be encountered using phenylbutazone include rashes, hepatitis, interference with anticoagulant control (Aggeler *et al.*, 1967), a febrile syndrome with lymphadenopathy, salivary gland enlargement (Murray-Bruce, 1966), hepatosplenomegaly, goitre due to blockage of intrathyroid iodide (Benedek, 1962), and abscess formation at the site of local injection.

Reference has been made to the fact that phenylbutazone also causes fluid retention, manifested as ankle oedema, weight gain and cardiac failure, particularly in elderly patients. It should therefore rarely be prescribed for the elderly.

(Bruck *et al.*, 1954; Lawrence, 1960; Benedek, 1962; Rodgers and Simpson, 1966; Aggeler *et al.*, 1967; Fowler, 1967; Fowler *et al.*, 1975; Leavesley *et al.*, 1969; Böttiger and Westerholm, 1972; Nieweg, 1973; Girdwood, 1974; MacFarlane *et al.*, 1976; Inman, 1977.)

Oxyphenbutazone (Tanderil; Tandacote)
Other proprietary names include: Butapirone, Iridil (both Italy); Oxalid (USA); Phlogase (Germany); Rheumpax (Sweden); Tandearil (Canada, USA).

Oxyphenbutazone (4-butyl-1-p-hydroxyphenyl-3, 5-dioxo-2-phenyl-pyrazolidine monohydrate) is a hydroxy analogue of phenylbutazone and one of its major metabolites. It has the same general properties and the same actions, therapeutic uses, interactions, and toxic effects as phenylbutazone, and it is more expensive than the parent drug.

Although initially it was thought that side effects might prove less common than with phenylbutazone, this has not been confirmed. Pharmacologically, therapeutically and toxicologically it may be regarded as the same substance. It is available as 100 mg tablets and 250 mg suppositories, and as enteric coated 100 mg tablets.

(Hart *et al.*, 1978.)

Azapropazone (Rheumox)
Other proprietary names include: Cinnamin (Japan); Prolix (South Africa); Prolixan (Germany).

Pharmacology and pharmacokinetics. Azapropazone (5-dimethylamino)-9-methyl-2-propyl)-(1 H-pyrazolo (1-2-α) (1, 2, 4) benzotriazine-1, 3 (2H) dione dihydrate) is well absorbed from the gastrointestinal tract. Peak plasma levels are achieved about 4–6 hours after a single dose and the plasma half-life is 12 hours. More than 95% of the drug is protein bound. About 60% of azapropazone is excreted in the urine unchanged. Most of the rest is excreted as the inactive 6-hydroxy metabolite. Dosage should therefore be reduced in patients with impaired renal function.

Although its chemical structure resembles phenylbutazone, its actions and side effects are more like those of the proprionic acid derivatives.

(Jahn and Adrian, 1969; Schatz *et al.*, 1970; Jahn, 1973; Jahn *et al.*, 1973, Klatt and Koss, 1973a, b; Jones, 1976; Leach, 1976.)

Clinical uses, preparations and dosage. Clinical trials (Appendix 5.5.16) have established azapropazone to be useful in a wide range of rheumatic disorders including rheumatoid arthritis, various seronegative spondarth-

ritides, osteoarthrosis and soft-tissue rheumatism. In general, it is probably comparable with naproxen in its clinical effects.

The drug is available as a 300 mg capsule and a 600 mg tablet has been recently introduced in UK (Rheumox 600). The normal dosage is 1200 mg, divided four times daily. Up to 1800 mg may be given, but the frequency of gastric side effects becomes appreciable at this dosage level. The drug may be given on a 12-hourly basis. Paediatric dosage has not yet been established.

(Mennet *et al.*, 1971; Grennan *et al.*, 1974; Mathies *et al.*, 1974; Brooks and Buchanan, 1976; Eberl, 1976; Eberl and Bröll, 1977; Sondervorst, 1979.)

Side effects, precautions and contraindications. Azapropazone may cause gastrointestinal disturbances. Rashes have been reported. It should be given with caution to patients with acute gastritis, impaired renal function, or with gastric or duodenal ulcers. It should also be avoided in patients receiving oral anticoagulants as azapropazone potentiates the action of these drugs. Despite its chemical similarity to phenylbutazone no blood dyscrasias have been reported. Nevertheless, for the moment regular blood tests should be performed.

Fetal abnormalities have not been reported, but safety in human pregnancy cannot yet be assumed.

(Adrian, 1973; Huntington Research Center, 1975a, b, c, d; Adrian *et al.*, 1976; Mintz and Fraga, 1976; Hradsky and Bruce, 1978.)

Feprazone (Methrazone)
Another proprietary name is Zepelin (Italy).

The introduction of the terpenyl grouping of gefarnate, an ulcer-healing drug, to the basic chemical structure of phenylbutazone has given rise to feprazone (4-prenyl-1, 2-diphenyl-3, 5-pyrazolidinedione).

Clinical studies so far have shown that this drug in a dose of 600 mg daily has analgesic/anti-inflammatory activity similar to that of major antirheumatic agents such as aspirin, indomethacin and phenylbutazone, with a reduced tendency to cause gastrointestinal symptoms. The frequency of other side effects is similar to that occurring with phenylbutazone, except that blood dyscrasias and fluid retention are probably less prevalent.

(Casadio *et al.*, 1967; Dotti *et al.*, 1972; Ghiringhelli *et al.*, 1972; Ligniere *et al.*, 1972; Pasotti *et al.*, 1972; Rooney *et al.*, 1974; Fletcher *et al.*, 1975.)

COMMENT
Phenylbutazone and oxyphenbutazone are potent analgesic/anti-inflammatory agents which have been established in rheumatological practice for over three decades. They are particularly useful in treating ankylosing spondylitis and associated spondarthritides, and in

acute gout. Their striking effect in ankylosing spondylitis is sometimes used as a therapeutic test in early cases.
The choice of using phenylbutazone or its oxy-analogue
has to be carefully measured against the risk of serious
toxic effects, particularly suppression of bone marrow.
However, with careful monitoring and meticulous attention to ensuring minimal dosage, this risk can be
reduced. These drugs should also be used with great
caution, if at all, in the elderly. Although much of the
concern regarding the usage of phenylbutazone is fully
justified, some anxiety stems from memories of therapeutic catastrophies which resulted from the much
higher dosages (up to 1 g per day) which were used when
the drug was first introduced.

The more recently introduced pyrazolone–feprazone – is probably slightly less toxic with regard to
gastrointestinal side effects, fluid retention and blood
dyscrasias.

(f) Oxicams

Piroxicam (Feldene)

Pharmacology and pharmacokinetics. Piroxicam (4-
hydroxy-2-methyl-N-(2-pyridyl)-2H-1, 2-benzothiazine
1, 1-dioxide) is absorbed smoothly after oral administration over 2 hours. Plasma concentrations rise to peak
values at 4 hours. Plasma concentrations then remain
stable over the next 24–48 hours permitting its use on a
once-a-day regimen. Piroxicam is metabolized to metabolite III which, either free or conjugated with glucuronic acid, accounts for up to 60% of a daily dose in
urine and faeces. The prostaglandin synthetase inhibition can be largely ascribed to the parent drug rather
than to any of its metabolites. Piroxicam is about 90%
bound to plasma proteins.

(Lombardino and Wiseman, 1972, 1973; Hobbs and
Twomey, 1976, 1979; Nuotio and Mäkisara, 1978;
Twomey and Hobbs, 1978; Wiseman, 1978a, b, 1980;
Ishizaki *et al.*, 1979; Bachman, 1980; Carty *et al.*, 1980a,
b; Mercier and Lesne, 1980; Milne and Twomey, 1980;
Rogers, 1980; Twomey *et al.*, 1980; Wiseman and
Lombardino, 1980.)

Clinical uses, preparations and dosage. Piroxicam has
been shown to be a useful analgesic/anti-inflammatory
drug in a variety of rheumatic disorders such as
rheumatoid arthritis, osteoarthrosis, ankylosing
spondylitis, acute gout and extra-articular rheumatic
problems (Appendix 5.5.17).

The drug is available as a 10 mg capsule in the UK
(in most countries outside the UK where the drug is
available, 20 mg capsules are also marketed) and the
recommended starting dose is 20 mg given as a single
daily dose. A relatively small group of patients with

minor inflammatory activity may be maintained on as
little as 10 mg. On the other hand, some patients, such as
those with active rheumatoid arthritis or acute gout,
may need 30–40 mg daily.

(Nussdorf, 1978; Pitts and Proctor, 1978; Günther *et
al.*, 1979; Bahr, 1980; Mathies and Wolff, 1980; Pitts,
1980.)

Side effects, precautions and contraindications. Piroxicam is generally well tolerated. Gastrointestinal symptoms are the most commonly encountered side effects,
but in most instances these do not interfere with the
course of therapy. The frequency of gastrointestinal side
effects appears to increase with increasing dosages.
Peptic ulceration and gastrointestinal bleeding have
been reported with piroxicam in a small proportion of
patients. Other side effects which have been reported
infrequently include ankle oedema and changes in liver
function tests.

The safety of the drug in children, or in pregnancy or
lactating women, has not yet been established.

Piroxicam is contraindicated in patients known to be
hypersensitive to the drug or hypersensitive to aspirin or
other analgesic/anti-inflammatory drugs.

(Di Perri *et al.*, 1979; Gaynor and Constantine, 1979;
Rau, 1980; Reubi, 1980.)

5.2.3 Pure anti-inflammatory drugs

Corticosteroids and corticotrophin prevent or diminish
all the cardinal features of inflammation (local heat,
redness, swelling and tenderness). They inhibit not only
the early microscopic features of oedema, capillary
dilatation, phagocyte activity, leucocyte migration, and
fibrin deposition, but also the later features of capillary
and fibroblast proliferation, deposition of collagen, and
scarring. This applies whatever the cause of the inflammation – mechanical, infective, allergic or immunological. These therapeutic effects are therefore non-
specific, palliative, suppressive and temporary. The
anti-inflammatory effect may be entirely beneficial but
may be hazardous if active infective agents are present.
Nevertheless, used correctly, these drugs are the most
effective anti-inflammatory agents at our disposal. Their
mode of action in rheumatic disorders is still obscure,
and the lysosomal stabilization hypothesis, previously
popular, does not satisfy all investigators.

For parts of this section I have leaned heavily on the
excellent account by Hart (1978), and the reader is
referred particularly to this source for further details.

(a) Corticosteroids

Prednisolone (Codelcortone, Cordex, Delta Phoricol,
Delta-Cortef, Deltacortril, Deltacortril Enteric,

Deltalone, Deltastab, Di-Adreson-F, Marsolone, PreCortisyl).

Other proprietary names include: Adnisolone, Deltasolone, Optocort, Panafortelone, Paracortol, Prelone, Solone (all Australia); Dacortin H, Nisolone (both Spain); Decortin-H, Hostacortin H, Keteocort H, Predni-Coelin, Predni-H (all Germany); Delcortol (Denmark); Deltacortenolo, Deltidrosol, Prednisol (all Italy); Donisolone, Predonine (both Japan); Encortolone (Poland); Hydrocortancyl, Predniretard (both France); Lenisolone, Polypred, Predeltilone (South Africa); Meticortelone (South Africa, USA); Meti-Derm (Australia, USA); Precortalon (Sweden); Prednis, Ropredlone, Sterane, Ulacort (all USA); Scherisolon (Australia, Germany); Ultracorten-H (prednisolone sodium tetrahydrophthalate) (Germany).

Prednisolone (11β, 17α, 21-trihydroxypregna-1, 4-diene-3, 20-dione) will be taken as the prototype compound.(Prednisone is converted into prednisolone in the liver.)

Pharmacology and pharmacokinetics. Prednisolone is rapidly absorbed from the gastrointestinal tract and to a lesser and more variable extent also from other sites such as synovial cavities, the conjunctival sac and skin. The corticosteroids are reversibly bound to two fractions of plasma proteins (globulin-bound and albumin-bound corticosteroid). At low or normal plasma concentrations, prednisolone is largely bound to globulin (low capacity but high affinity for corticosteroid). With increasing levels of prednisolone the globulin-bound corticosteroid changes little, but the fraction bound to albumin (high capacity but low affinity for corticosteroid) increases. Hypoalbuminaemia can therefore lead to unusually high levels of free unbound drug, particularly with high-dose therapy.

Prednisolone is rapidly metabolized in the liver, conjugated, and excreted in the urine. Although prednisolone disappears from the blood within 100–200 minutes (half-life about 1 hour), its metabolic actions, started at tissue level, last for many hours.

Adrenal steroids are chiefly used in medicine for their anti-inflammatory effects. These are only obtained when the drug is given in doses exceeding those needed for physiological effect. The normal metabolic effects, which are of the greatest importance to the normal functioning of the body, then become toxic effects. Much successful effort has gone into separating glucocorticoid from mineralocorticoid effects, and some steroids, including prednisolone, have virtually no mineralocorticoid effect. However, it has not yet proved possible to separate some of the glucocorticoid effects from each other, so that if a steroid is used for its anti-inflammatory action, the risks of osteoporosis, haematemesis, diabetes and other unwanted effects remain.

The pharmacological and physiological effects of corticosteroids are shown in Table 5.1 and Appendix 5.5.18 and, although included in the table, it should be re-stressed that mineralocorticoid effects are minimal with prednisolone.

(Long *et al.*, 1940; Copeman, 1953; Di Raimondo and Forsham, 1958; Cope, 1972; Laurence, 1973; Myles and Daly, 1974; Thompson and Lippman, 1974; Dluhy *et al.*, 1975; Fauci, 1976; Hart, 1978.)

Clinical uses. The use of corticosteroids are many (Appendix 5.5.18). Further details of clinical usage in rheumatic disorders in which corticosteroids are especially indicated are as follows.

Rheumatoid arthritis: Corticosteroids are only used in this disorder when inflammatory features have not responded to non-steroidal agents prescribed in maximal dosage and to simple physical measures such as rest and splintage. The bad reputation the corticosteroids earned during the 1950s in the treatment of rheumatoid arthritis was due to dosage levels being considerably higher than those used today.

There is much evidence that if the dosage exceeds 6–7 mg daily of prednisolone (or equivalent) in this disease some side effects will eventually follow. (In other diseases such as asthma or acute systemic lupus erythematosus, a higher dosage may be associated with fewer side effects.) A single dose of 5 mg at night may improve night pain and morning stiffness in rheumatoid arthritis. Although it has been shown that such an evening dose suppresses secretion of corticotrophin more than a morning dose, clinical improvement and the patient's opinion should be weighed against laboratory findings.

Alternate-day therapy is less likely to produce hypothalamic–pituitary–adrenal axis suppression. However, patients usually prefer daily therapy as symptoms tend to recur on the day the drug is not taken. A single morning dose of corticosteroid produces less suppression of 17-hydroxycorticosteroids than the same amount given in divided doses, but again, variations in clinical response will dictate patterns of prescribing. Myles *et al.* (1971) found that most rheumatic patients could be managed satisfactorily on a single morning dose of corticosteroids.

Injectable intramuscular prednisolone has been suggested as a means of obviating misuse by the patient. However, injections are more unpleasant for the patient and variable absorption from different injection sites may result in less certain control than that obtained by the oral route.

Further comments on the use of corticosteroids in rheumatoid arthritis are included in Section 4.5.

Systemic lupus erythematosus: Corticosteroid therapy is the main weapon in the treatment of this condition. Although the acute features of the disease are

Table 5.1 Effects of prednisolone (modified from Laurence, 1973)

General	Specific pharmacological effect		Clinical effect
	General	*Detailed*	
Glucocorticoid	Carbohydrate metabolism	Gluconeogenesis increased, peripheral glucose utilization (transport across cell membranes) decreased	Hyperglycaemia, glycosuria (sometimes), latent diabetes becomes overt
	Protein metabolism	Anabolism (conversion of amino acids to proteins) decreased, catabolism remains normal or is increased	Muscle wasting, osteoporosis, slowing of growth in children
			Skin atrophy, increased capillary fragility } Bruising, striae
			Healing of peptic ulcers and wounds delayed
	Fat deposition	Increased	Increased on shoulders, face and abdomen
	Inflammatory response	Depressed	Beneficial in reducing excessive 'useless' inflammation, harmful in limiting response to infection
	Allergic effects	Suppressed	Antigen–antibody interaction unaffected, but injurious inflammatory consequences do not follow
	Antibody production	Reduced	
	Lymphoid tissue	Reduced	
	Renal excretion of uric acid	Increased	
	Blood eosinophils	Reduced	
	CNS electrolyte changes (?)	Altered	Euphoria or psychotic states
	Vitamin D action	Reduced	Tendency to rickets and osteomalacia
	Hypercalcaemia	Reduced	Hypercalcaemic effect of sarcoidosis and vitamin D intoxication reduced
	Urinary excretion of calcium	Increased	Renal stones
	Growth in children (mechanism uncertain)	Reduced	Dwarfism
	Hypothalamic–pituitary–adrenocortical system	Suppressed	Adrenocorticoid insufficiency state
Mineralocorticoid	Retention of sodium by renal tubule	Increased	Overall effect sodium retention
	Sodium excretion	Increased	
	Potassium excretion	Increased	Potassium loss
	Glomerular filtration rate	Increased	

controlled relatively rapidly, with adequate dosage, corticosteroids may have negligible effects on severe myocarditis, renal disease and cerebral vasculitis. Even though larger amounts of prednisolone produce a more rapid clinical response, dosage levels tend to be more moderate now than they were some years ago. At high dosage, the principal concern is that therapeutic complications increase and intercurrent infections are more common. Corticosteroids would appear to do no more than suppress the inflammatory reaction of the condition, having no lasting or permanent influence on the underlying disease process.

Other rheumatic conditions: In rheumatic fever corticosteroids take second place to salicylates. Even when given early in large doses corticosteroids do not appear to prevent or minimize cardiac damage. They are effective in reversing the acute exudative phase and are probably more potent in this respect than salicylates. However, because of side effects, corticosteroids are usually confined to patients with severe renal disease or those who are intolerant of, or respond poorly to, salicylates.

Polymyalgia rheumatica: In polymyalgia rheumatica, corticosteroid therapy is the treatment of choice and probably the only medication, given soon enough in adequate dosage, that will prevent the development of blindness.

Preparations and dosage. Prednisolone is available as tablets of 1 and 5 mg, the former being used for gradual minimal dose reduction, as in steroid 'weaning' in rheumatoid arthritis and polymyalgia rheumatica. Enteric-coated tablets of 2.5 mg are useful in dyspeptic patients but may be incompletely absorbed. Soluble tablets of prednisolone disodium phosphate (5 mg) dissolved in water may be preferred. Dosage will depend entirely on the nature and severity of the clinical problem to be treated. However, as a general principle, it should be stressed that only the lowest daily dose which adequately suppresses the disorder should be prescribed. In individual patients, therapeutic effect and possible toxicity will have to be assessed and balanced against each other. For example, in more potentially dangerous conditions, such as systemic lupus erythematosus or giant cell arteritis, higher dosages may be necessary.

Alternative corticosteroids

Prednisone and prednisolone are interchangeable in therapeutics and physiologically. Prednisone is converted into prednisolone (the active form) by the liver. This biotransformation may be decreased in the presence of severe liver disease, but for practical purposes the two agents may be considered identical. Prednisone is usually prescribed as tablets of 1, 2.5 or 5 mg.

Methylprednisolone is available as 2, 4 and 16 mg tablets. The larger strength tablets are intended for alternate-day therapy.

Triamcinolone is available as tablets of 1, 2 and 4 mg. It has almost no sodium-retaining effect, and during the first few days of therapy may actually cause sodium loss in the urine and a mild diuresis. Nausea, weight loss and dizziness may also occur occasionally.

Dexamethasone is available as tablets of 0.5, 0.75 and 2 mg.

Betamethasone is available as 0.5 mg tablets and as soluble betamethasone sodium phosphate 0.5 mg tablets.

Paramethasone is available as 2 mg tablets.

Cortisone and *hydrocortisone* tablets are more suited for adrenal replacement therapy. They are less appropriate for antirheumatic (anti-inflammatory) treatment because of their greater sodium-retaining effect.

Generally there is little or no advantage in substituting any of the above for oral systemic therapy with prednisone or prednisolone. A roughly equivalent anti-inflammatory effect is obtained with 25 mg cortisone, 20 mg hydrocortisone (cortisol), 4 mg prednisone or prednisolone, 4 mg triamcinolone or methylprednisolone, 2 mg paramethasone, or 0.75 mg dexamethasone or betamethasone. Triamcinolone, paramethasone, dexamethasone and betamethasone have virtually no sodium-retaining effect at conventional dose levels.

Side effects, precautions and contraindications. Adverse effects are all too often those of overdosage. To quote Hart (1978): 'Almost all doses recommended in almost all text books for almost all disorders will in time produce some or all of the features of Cushing's disease'. The complications of systemic corticosteroid therapy have been well reviewed by David *et al.* (1970) and individual studies are summarized in Appendix 5.5.19. The three major types of adverse effects have been listed by Dujourne and Azarnoff (1975) as follows:

(1) Adrenal insufficiency after withdrawal of therapy, due to continued inhibition of hypothalamic adrenal corticotrophin releasing factor and/or adrenal atrophy from previous corticosteroid therapy.

(2) Iatrogenic hyperadrenocorticism, leading to the features of Cushing's disease – moon face, acne, hirsutism, redistribution of body fat, 'buffalo hump', atrophy of skin and subcutaneous tissues, purpura and striae (Fig. 5.3).

(3) Reactivation of the disease process that has been suppressed on stopping or reducing therapy.
    Other possible adverse effects of systemic corticosteroids are many but those of most importance include:

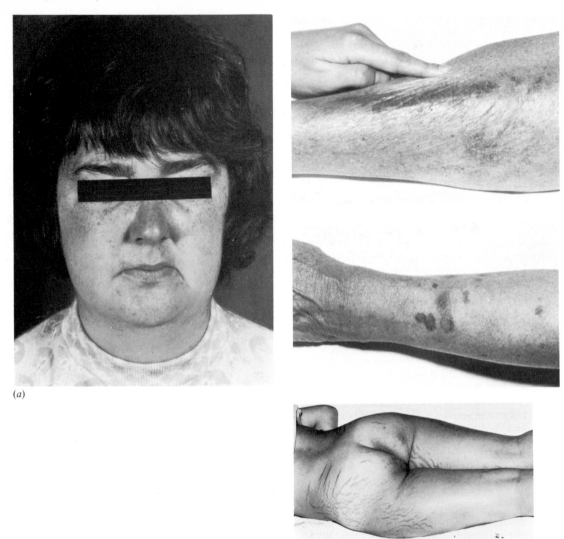

Fig. 5.3 Some features of iatrogenic hyperadrenocorticism. (*a*) Moonface. (*b*) (Above downwards): atrophic 'tissue paper' skin, purpura, striae.

(4) Impaired carbohydrate metabolism. The corticosteroids stimulate gluconeogenesis, primarily through a catabolic (or anti-anabolic) action on protein. They seem to oppose the action of insulin at cellular level and therefore may aggravate or induce diabetes mellitus. The so-called steroid diabetes is usually mild and ketosis is rare.

(5) Facilitation of growth and spread of many types of micro-organism (e.g. viruses, bacteria, fungi).

(6) Pseudotumour cerebri. The patient, usually a child, develops papilloedema during treatment which is usually reversed on stopping corticosteroids, but sometimes appears with dose reduction, particularly with triamcinolone.

(7) Psychiatric changes: insomnia, nervousness, mania, depression, and even schizophrenia and suicidal attempts. Such adverse effects may be more likely to occur in those with pre-existing personality disorders. However, they may be seen occasionally in apparently normal subjects.

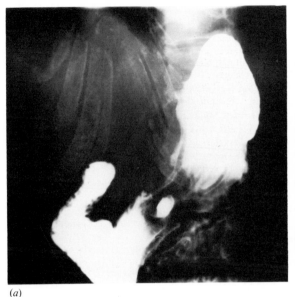
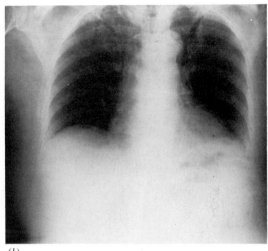

(a)   (b)

Fig. 5.4 (*a*) Barium meal showing peptic ulcer. (*b*) Plain X-ray showing air under right diaphragn after ulcer perforation in a patient on long-term corticosteroid therapy.

(8) Glaucoma and cataract formation.
(9) Peptic and intestinal ulceration and perforation (Fig. 5.4). The clinical features of perforation are often relatively masked.
(10) Pancreatitis (rare).
(11) Growth retardation in children (Fig. 5.5). Although juvenile chronic polyarthritis may suppress and delay normal growth, natural or therapeutic remission of arthritic disease induced by non-steroidal agents will lead to a return of natural growth. On the other hand, continued corticosteroid therapy leads to persistent stunting if such therapy cannot be substantially reduced or discontinued. Because of this serious effect on growth the use of corticotrophin (Zutschi *et al.*, 1971) or alternate-day corticosteroid therapy (Ansell and Bywaters, 1974) should always be considered.
(12) Osteoporosis (Fig. 5.6) and spontaneous fractures.
(13) Aseptic bone necrosis.
(14) Myopathy.
(15) Vasculitis and neuropathy. It is the experience of some workers that vasculitis and neuropathy occur more commonly in rheumatoid patients treated with corticosteroids, particularly with erratic and irregular dosage (Kemper *et al.*, 1975; Hart, 1966).

These adverse effects are summarized in Table 5.2.

Patients who have received corticosteroid therapy for more than a few weeks at a dose of 7.5 mg or more of prednisolone or equivalent must be assumed to have impaired response to stress. Such patients may develop hypotension under general anaesthesia if not given an adequate corticosteroid supplement before and during anaesthesia. Supplements should also be given in the face of other forms of major stress (e.g. coronary occlusion, intercurrent infection) and it should be emphasized that adrenocortical suppression may continue for up to 6 months after stopping treatment. All patients taking corticosteroids should carry a card specifying the details of their steroid medication; not only does this act as an *aide-mémoire* for patients, but the information may be invaluable in the event of head injury, stroke or other circumstances in which the patient is unable to communicate.

There are different views regarding the mortality and teratogenicity risk to the fetus from corticosteroid therapy taken during pregnancy. The subject has been reviewed by Hart (1978) whose conclusion represents the general policy at present – continue corticosteroids in pregnancy in patients who need it.

Prednisolone is excreted in very small amounts in breast milk and appears to be of no consequence to the nursing infant.

Corticosteroids are contraindicated in patients with peptic ulceration, osteoporosis, mental instability (psychoses or severe psychoneuroses), and they should

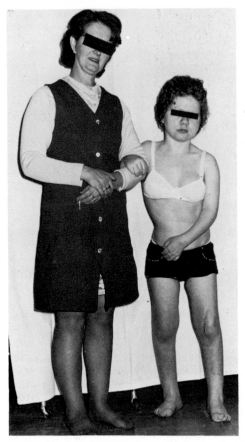

Fig. 5.5 Growth retardation in a patient treated with long-term daily corticosteroid therapy for juvenile chronic polyarthritis. (The patient was still much smaller than her mother at the age of 18, and continues at this height now aged 22.) (From Wright and Moll, 1976 with permission.)

be used only with great caution in the presence of congestive cardiac failure, diabetes mellitus, infectious diseases, chronic renal failure, and in the elderly. Patients with active or doubtfully quiescent tuberculosis should not be given corticosteroids unless as adjuncts to treatment with tuberculostatic drugs.

Corticosteroids should not be withdrawn suddenly because of the risk of causing a flare-up of the suppressed disease.

(b) Corticotrophins

Corticotrophin (Acthar, Acthar Gel, Cortico-Gel, Cortrophin ZN, Crookes acth/cmc)
Other proprietary names include: Acortan (Germany); Acton (Canada, South Africa, Sweden); Alfatrofin, Isactid, Reacthin (all Sweden); Duracton (Canada).

Table 5.2 Systemic corticosteroids: summary of adverse effects (Hart, 1978)

1. *Endocrine*: Adrenal suppression; hypotension; lack of energy; hyperglycaemia and glycosuria ('steroid diabetes mellitus'); hirsutism; amenorrhoea; growth retardation in children
2. *Electrolyte disturbances*: Hypokalaemia, sodium and fluid retention; hypertension
3. *Muscles*: Myopathy
4. *Bone and Joints*: Infection; aseptic necrosis; osteoporosis
5. *CNS*: Headaches; mental and mood changes; intracranial hypertension
6. *Eye*: Posterior subcapsular cataract; glaucoma; papilloedema
7. *Gastrointestinal*: Gastroduodenal upsets; peptic ulcer exacerbation and perforation; intussusception; perforated diverticula
8. *Skin and subcutaneous tissues*: Atrophy; 'steroid purpura'; moon face; acne; redistribution of body fat; 'buffalo hump'; increased tendency to infection

Pharmacology and pharmacokinetics

Corticotrophin (ACTH, adrenocorticotrophic hormone, adrencorticotropin, corticotropin, corticotropinum) is a polypeptide chain comprising 29 amino acids obtained from the anterior lobe of the pituitary gland of the pig and other mammals used by man for food.

It stimulates the human adrenal cortex to secrete cortisol, corticosterone, aldosterone and a number of weak androgenic substances. Prolonged medication therefore produces adrenocortical hyperplasia and increased synthesis and output of cortisol. Corticotrophin is ineffective when taken by mouth as it is destroyed by the proteolytic enzymes of the gut.

Corticotrophin activity resides largely in the first 24 amino acids of the peptide chain which are identical in pig, sheep, cow and human. It is stored in protein bound and free forms in the pituitary. The substance is readily absorbed after intramuscular and intravenous injection. It rapidly disappears from the circulation and in man the plasma half-life is about 15 minutes. Corticotrophin is inactivated in the tissues, no biological activity being present in the urine.

Clinical uses, preparations and dosage

The indications for use of corticotrophin are as under prednisolone. After courses of corticotrophin hypothalamic and pituitary activity is suppressed, but adrenal responsiveness is retained. Booster doses of corticotrophin, used in the past in patients on prolonged corticosteroid oral therapy, fail to prevent suppression of the adrenal cortex. A course of 1–3 weeks of intramus-

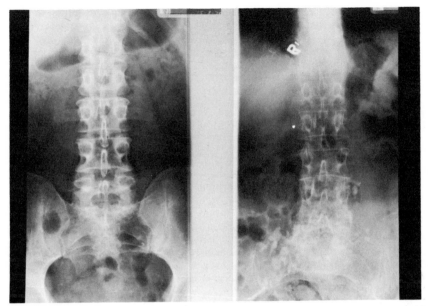

Fig. 5.6 X-rays of a patient with rheumatoid arthritis before and after long-term corticosteroid therapy showing the development of osteoporosis (right).

cular corticotrophin may be tried under hospital conditions in patients with an acute flare of inflammatory arthritis, in the hope that oral corticosteroids can be avoided. Corticotrophin is available in a number of forms: (1) hydrolysed gelatin, 20, 40 and 80 international units per ml for intramuscular or subcutaneous use; (2) adsorbed on zinc hydroxide, 40 international units per ml; (3) complexed with and dissolved in carboxylethylcellulose, 20 and 40 international units per ml. The last two are long-acting preparations. These repository forms are given once daily. Dosage depends on the disorder to be treated, averaging between 10 and 40 international units. Higher dosages are allowable in severe and intractable conditions. For intravenous use, sterile solutions of corticotrophin are available where more intense adrenocortical stimulation is required, maximal stimulation being obtained in adults with 25 units infused over 8 hours.

Side effects, precautions, contraindications
Side effects, apart from hypersensitivity reactions such as fever and anaphylaxis, are as under prednisolone – with a higher frequency of hypertension, heart failure, acne, sodium loading and hypokalaemic alkalosis. Skin pigmentation may be increased. When allergic reactions occur, therapeutic effects diminish, sometimes dramatically. Antibodies may develop to corticotrophin in patients on long-term therapy.

Cautions and contraindications are as with predni-

solone. Because of its mineralocorticoid action it should not be used in patients with hypertension and/or left ventricular failure. Acne will be aggravated. Although gastrointestinal complications may be less than with oral corticosteroids, they do occur. Allergic reactions are sometimes severe and, rarely, may be fatal.

For references, see under corticosteroids.

Tetracosactrin (Cortrosyn Depot, Synacthen, Synacthen Depot)
Tetracosactrin (Ciba 30920, cosyntrophin, tetracosactide; α^{1-24} corticotrophin; β^{1-24} corticotrophin) is a synthetic analogue of corticotrophin containing the first 24 of the 39 amino acids of that substance (Ser-Tyr-Ser-Met-Glu-His-Phe-Arg-Trp-Gly-Lys-Pro-Val-Gly-Lys-Lys-Arg-Arg-Pro-Val-Lys-Val-Tyr-Pro). It has all the therapeutic and toxic activity of corticotrophin. Although allergic reactions may be less common, local tissue reactions may occur and Glass *et al.* (1971) noted the development of antibodies in 12 of 38 patients treated over several months.

The substance is available as tetracosactrin zinc complex (long-acting form) 1 mg per ml ampoule and 2 mg per 2 ml multi-dose vial. It may be given by intramuscular injection daily or every few days. It is important to stress that small doses such as 0.1–0.15 mg daily are more effective in reducing arthritic symptoms than larger injections such as 0.25–0.50 mg given every 3–4 days. Patients receiving more than 1 mg tetracosactrin weekly, whatever the frequency of injections, are likely to develop signs of overdosage.

Tetracosactrin acetate, 0.25 mg per ml in buffered aqueous solution, is also available for intravenous or intramuscular use to test adrenocortical function. This preparation is also used to treat anaphylactic shock or drug-sensitivity reactions.

One mg of tetracosactrin given intramuscularly has roughly the clinical effect of 100–150 international units of corticotrophin intramuscularly.

COMMENT

Corticosteroids and corticotrophins are the most potent of the anti-inflammatory group, but they have no direct analgesic effect – analgesia being derived indirectly from inflammatory suppression. These valuable drugs continue to be widely used, but therapeutic circumspection lingers, and is based on important toxic effects. The choice of oral corticosteroid versus injections of corticotrophin is based largely on clinical circumstances. Generally, oral corticosteroids continue to be the most often used drugs in the 'pure anti-inflammatory' group. This is based partly on the general convenience of oral rather than parenteral administration, particularly in patients in whom self-injection would be difficult.

There continues to be a diversity of opinion regarding the use of these drugs in rheumatoid arthritis, although their indication in polymyalgia rheumatica and life-threatening circumstances (e.g. systemic lupus erythematosus) is more clear cut. In the author's view, providing dosage does not exceed 7.5 mg daily, and preferably not more than 5 mg daily, this type of therapy is a useful adjunct in some patients with rheumatoid arthritis, particularly if control is not adequate with full dosage of non-steroidal treatment.

The therapeutic antipathy towards drugs in this group, as with phenylbutazone, to some extent rests on the toxic effects due to the much larger doses used when the drugs were first introduced. However, with more cautious prescribing, particularly regarding careful attention to low/or intermittent dosage this group of drugs continues to be a useful and powerful asset to the therapeutic armoury.

5.3 SUMMARY AND CONCLUSIONS

The chapter has discussed details of analgesic, analgesic/anti-inflammatory drugs (non-steroidal anti-inflammatory drugs) and pure anti-inflammatory drugs. The analgesic drugs (e.g. paracetamol, dextropropoxyphene) relieve pain and do nothing else. The analgesic/anti-inflammatory drugs (e.g. aspirin, phenylbutazone, indomethacin, naproxen) are usually taken regularly to provide both a non-specific anti-inflammatory effect as well as an analgesic effect. Pure anti-inflammatory drugs (corticosteroids and corticotrophins) are also non-specific anti-inflammatory agents, but have no direct analgesic activity, pain relief being an indirect effect through control of inflammation. More specific anti-rheumatic agents will be discussed in the next chapter.

The drugs discussed in the chapter provide a valuable symptomatic effect in most acute and chronic rheumatoses. However, as has been stressed in Chapter 3, their usage in management is often not enough on its own, and in many patients must be combined with other therapeutic approaches in an overall management programme.

5.4 REFERENCES AND FURTHER READING

General

Aylward, M. (1975) A review of possible mechanisms of action of the antirheumatic drug-alclofenac. *Curr. Med. Res. Op.*, **3**, 249.

Dick, W.C. (1978) Drug treatment of rheumatoid arthritis. in *Copeman's Textbook of the Rheumatic Diseases* (ed. J.T. Scott), 5th edn, Churchill Livingstone, Edinburgh, p. 406.

Famaey, J.P., Brooks, P.M. and Dick, W.C. (1975) Biological effects of nonsteroidal anti-inflammatory drugs. *Sem. Arthr. Rheum.*, **5**, 63.

Fauci, A.S. (1976) Glucocorticoid therapy: mechanism of action and clinical considerations. *Ann. Int. Med.*, **84**, 304.

Ferreira, S.H. and Vane, J.R. (1974) New aspects of the mode of action of nonsteroid anti-inflammatory drugs. *Ann. Rev. Pharmacol.*, **14**, 57.

Flower, R.J. and Vane, J.R. (1974) Inhibition of prostaglandin synthesis. *Biochem. Pharmacol.*, **23**, 1439.

McArthur, J.N., Dawkins, P.D., Smith, M.J.H. and Hamilton, E.B.D. (1971) Mode of action of antirheumatic drugs. *Br. Med. J.*, **ii**, 677.

Rooney, P.J., Watkins, C., Ahola, S.J. *et al.* (1975) A short term double blind controlled trial of prenozoric (DA 2370) in rheumatoid arthritis. *Curr. Med. Res. Op.*, **2**, 43.

Samter, M. (1969) The acetyl in aspirin. *Ann. Int. Med.*, **71**, 208.

Sharma, J.N., Zeitlin, I.T., Brooks, P.M. and Dick, W.C. (1976) A novel relationship between plasma kininogen and rheumatoid. *Agents and Actions*, **6**, 148.

Simple analgesic drugs

Beaver, W.T. (1965) Mild analgesics. A review of their clinical pharmacology. *Am. J. Med. Sci.*, **250**, 577.

Beaver, W.T. (1976) Symposium on narcotics and ataractics. *Hosp. Pract. – Special Report.*

Bellville, J.W., Forrest, W.H., Elashoff, J. and Laska, E. (1968) Evaluating side effects of analgesics in a cooperative clinical study. *Clin. Pharmacol. Ther.*, **9**, 303.

British National Formulary (1981) No. 2. British Medical Association and the Pharmaceutical Society of Great Britain, London.

Cohen, A. and Hernandez, C.M. (1976) Nefopam HCL: new analgesic agent. *J. Intl. Med. Res.*, **4**, 138.

Data Sheet Compendium (1981–82) Datapharm Publications Ltd., London.

De Andrade, J.R., Honig, S., Ciccone, W.J. and Leffall, L. (1980) Clinical comparison of zomepirac with pentazocine in the treatment of post-operative pain. *J. Clin. Pharmacol.*, **20**, 292.

Editorial (1977) Dangers of dextropropoxyphene. *Br. Med. J.*, **i**, 668.

Guzman, F., Braun, C., Lim, R.K.S. *et al.* (1974) Narcotic and non-narcotic analgesics which block visceral pain evoked by intra-arterial injection of bradykinin and other analgesic agents. *Arch. Int. Pharmacodyn. Ther.*, **149**, 571.

Hart, F.D. (ed.) (1978) *Drug Treatment of the Rheumatic Diseases*. MTP Press, Lancaster.

Huskisson, E.C. (ed.) (1980) *Clinics in Rheumatic Diseases*, Vol. 6, No. 3. Antirheumatic Drugs II. Saunders, London.

Kantor, T.G. (1976), Symposium on narcotics and ataractics. *Hospital Practice – Special Report*.

Kantor, T.G. (1980) in *Clinics in Rheumatic Diseases* (ed. E.C. Huskisson), Vol. 6, No. 3, Saunders, London, p. 525.

Kantor, T.G., Sunshine, A., Laska, E. *et al.* (1966) Oral analgesic studies: pentazocine HCL; codeine; aspirin and placebo and their influence on response to placebo. *Clin. Pharmacol. Ther.*, **7**, 447.

Lasagna, L. (1964) The clinical evaluation of morphine and its substitutes as analgesics. *Pharmacol. Rev.*, **16**, 47.

Loan, W.B. and Morrison, J.D. (1973) Strong analgesics: pharmacological and therapeutic aspects. *Drugs*, **5**, 108.

Marks, R.M. and Sachar, E.J. (1973) Undertreatment of medical inpatients with narcotic analgesics. *Ann. Int. Med.*, **78**, 173.

Martin, W.R., Eades, C.G., Thompson, J.A. *et al.* (1976) The effects of morphine and nalorphine-like drugs in the non-dependent and morphine-dependent chronic spinal dog. *J. Pharmacol. Exp. Ther.*, **197**, 517.

Mayer, T.G. and Ruoff, G.E. (1980) Clinical evaluation of zomepirac in the treatment of acute orthopaedic pain. *J. Clin. Pharmacol.*, **20**, 285.

Melzack, R. and Wall, P.D. (1965) Pain mechanisms: A new theory. *Science*, **150**, 971.

MIMS (Monthly Index of Medical Specialities) (1982) April Issue. Medical Publications Ltd, London.

Nayak, R.K., Ng, K.T., Gottleib, S. and Plostnieks, J. (1980) Zomepirac kinetics in healthy males. *Clin. Pharmacol. Ther.*, **27**, 395.

Parkhouse, J. (1975) Simple analgesics. *Drugs*, **10**, 366.

Pruss, T.P., Gardocki, J.F., Taylor, R.J. and Muschek, L.D. (1980) Evaluation of the analgesic properties of zomepirac. *J. Clin. Pharmacol.*, **20**, 216.

Roth, S.H. (1980) *New Directions in Arthritis Therapy*, PSG Publishing Co. Inc., Littleton, Mass.

Stirman, J.A. (1967) A comparison of methotrimeprazine and meperidine as analgesic agents. *Anesthes. Analg.*, **46**, 176.

Sunshine, A., Slafta, J. and Gruber, C. (1978) A comparative study: propoxyphene, fenoprofen, the combination of propoxyphene and fenoprofen, aspirin and placebo. *J. Clin. Pharmacol.*, **18**, 11.

Wade, A. (ed.) (1977) *Martindale: The Extra Pharmacopoeia*, 27th edn. The Pharmaceutical Press, London.

Whittington, R.M. (1977) Dextroproxyphene (Distalgesic) overdosage in the West Midlands. *Br. Med. J.*, **ii**, 172.

Willkens, R.F. and Segre, E.J. (1976) Combination therapy with naproxen and aspirin in rheumatoid arthritis. *Arthr. Rheum.*, **19**, 677.

Non-steroidal analgesic/anti-inflammatory drugs

Salicylic acids and esters

Aspirin

Abel, J.A. (1971) Analgesic nephropathy – a review of the literature 1967–1970. *Clin. Pharmacol. Ther.*, **12**, 583.

Abrahams, C. and Levin, M.W. (1968) Analgesic nephropathy. *Lancet*, **i**, 645.

Alexander, W.D., MacDougall, A.I., Oliver, M.F. and Boyd, G.S. (1959) The effect of salicylate on the serum lipids and lipoproteins in coronary artery disease. *Clin. Sci.*, **18**, 195.

Allibone, A. and Flint, F.S. (1958) Bronchitis, aspirin, smoking and other factors in the aetiology of peptic ulcer. *Lancet*, **ii**, 179.

Alvarez, A.S. and Summerskill, W.H.J. (1958) Gastrointestinal haemorrhage and salicylates. *Lancet*, **ii**, 920.

Athreya, B.H., Gorske, A.L. and Myers, A.R. (1973) Aspirin-induced abnormalities of liver function. *Am. J. Dis. Child.*, **126**, 638.

Athreya, B.H., Moser, G., Cecil, H.S. and Myers, A.R. (1975) Aspirin-induced hepatoxicity in juvenile rheumatoid arthritis. *Arthr. Rheum.*, **18**, 347.

Austen, K.F. (1963) in *Salicylates: An International Symposium* (eds A. St. J. Dixon, B.K. Martin, M.J.H. Smith and P.H.N. Wood), Churchill, London, p. 161.

Baragar, F.D. and Duthie, J.J.R. (1960) Importance of aspirin as a cause of anaemia and peptic ulcer in rheumatoid arthritis. *Br. Med. J.*, **i**, 1106.

Basomba, A., Romar, A., Pelaez, A. *et al.* (1976) The effect of sodium cromoglycate in preventing aspirin-induced bronchospasm. *Clin. Allerg.*, **6**, 269.

Baum, J.J. (1970) Blood salicylate levels and clinical trials with a new form of enteric-coated aspirin: studies in rheumatoid arthritis and degenerative joint disease. *Clin. Pharmacol.*, **10**, 132.

Bayles, T.B. (1963) in *Salicylates* (eds A. St. J. Dixon, B.K. Martin, M.J.H. Smith and P.H.N. Wood), Churchill, London, p. 43.

Beeley, L. and Kendall, M.J. (1971) Effect of aspirin on renal clearance of ^{125}I-diatrizoate. *Br. Med. J.*, **i**, 707.

Begg, T.B. (1963) A century of salicylates. *Appl. Ther.*, **5**, 247, 257.

Bernstein, B.H., Singsen, B.H., Koster, K.K. and Hanson, V. (1977) Aspirin-induced hepatotoxicity and its effect on juvenile rheumatoid arthritis. *Am. J. Dis. Child.*, **131**, 659.

Boardman, P.L. and Hart, F.D. (1967) Clinical measurement of the anti-inflammatory effects of salicylates in rheumatoid arthritis. *Br. Med. J.*, **iv**, 264.

Boston Collaborative Drug Surveillance Group (1974) Regular aspirin intake and acute myocardial infarction. *Br. Med. J.*, i, 440.

Bouchier, I.A.D. and Williams, H.S. (1969) Determination of faecal blood-loss after combined alcohol and sodium-acetylsalicylate intake. *Lancet*, i, 178.

Brooks, P.M., Walker, J.J., Bell, M.A. *et al.* (1975) Indomethacin – aspirin interaction: a clinical appraisal. *Br. Med. J.*, iii, 69.

Brown, R.K. and Mitchell, N. (1956) The influence of some of the salicyl compounds (and alcoholic beverages) on the natural history of peptic ulcer. *Gastroenterology*, 31, 198.

Cameron, A.J. (1975) Aspirin and gastric ulcer. *Mayo Clin. Proc.*, 50, 565.

Campbell, H. (1879) *The Salicylate Treatment of Gout, Rheumatic Gout, Neuralgia and Diabetes*, 2nd edn, H. Renshaw, London.

Campbell, E.J.M. and MacLaurin, R.E. (1958) Acute renal failure in salicylate poisoning. *Br. Med. J.*, i, 503.

Casteels-Van Daele, M., Jaeken, J., Eggermont, E. *et al.* (1972) More on the effects of antenatally administered aspirin on aggregation of platelets of neonates. *J. Pediatr.*, 80, 685.

Champion, C.D., Day, R.O., Graham, G.G. and Paull, P.D. (1975) in *Clinics in the Rheumatic Diseases* (eds C.M. Pearson and W. Carson Dick), Saunders, London, p. 245.

Chapman, B.L. and Duggan, J.M. (1969) Aspirin and uncomplicated peptic ulcer. *Gut*, 10, 443.

Chrisman, O.D. and Snook, G.A. (1968) Studies on the protective effect of aspirin against degeneration of human articular cartilage. *Clin. Orth.*, 56, 77.

Collier, H.O.J. (1969) A pharmacological analysis of aspirin. *Adv. Pharmacol. Chemother.*, 7, 333.

Collins, E. and Turner, G. (1975) Maternal effects of regular salicylate ingestion in pregnancy. *Lancet*, ii, 335.

Cooke, A.R. (1976) Drugs and gastric damage. *Drugs*, 11, 36.

Cooke, A.R. and Goulston, K. (1969) Failure of intravenous aspirin to increase gastrointestinal blood loss. *Br. Med. J.*, iii, 330.

Croft, A.N., Cuddigan, J.H.P. and Sweetland, C. (1972) Gastric bleeding and benorylate, a new aspirin. *Br. Med. J.*, iii, 545.

Croft, A.N. and Wood, P.H.N. (1967) Gastric mucosa and susceptibility to occult gastrointestinal bleeding caused by aspirin. *Br. Med. J.*, i, 137.

Cummings, A.J., Martin, B.K. and Wiggins, L.F. (1963) *In vitro* and *in vivo* properties of aloxipirin; a new aluminium derivative of acetylsalicylic acid. *J. Pharm. Pharmacol.*, 15, 56.

Danhof, I.E., Kailey, J.D. and Guinn, E.C. (1972) Benorylate and gastrointestinal blood loss. *Curr. Ther.*, 14, 583.

Davenport, H.W. (1964) Gastric mucosal injury by fatty and acetylsalicylic acids. *Gastroenterology*, 46, 245.

Davis, J.W., Lewis, H.D., Phillips, P.E. *et al.* (1978) Effect of aspirin on exercise-induced angina. *Clin. Pharmacol. Ther.*, 23, 505.

Dick, W.C. (1978) in *Copemans Textbook of the Rheumatic Diseases* (ed. J.T. Scott). 5th edn, Churchill Livingstone, Edinburgh, pp. 409–11.

Doeglas, H.M. (1975) Reactions to aspirin and food additives in patients with chronic urticaria including the physical urticarias. *Br. J. Dermatol.*, 93, 135.

Douglas, R.A. and Johnson, E.D. (1961) Aspirin and chronic gastric ulcer. *Med. J. Austr.*, ii, 893.

Duggan, J.M. (1965) The relationship between perforated peptic ulcer and aspirin ingestion. *Med. J. Austr.*, ii, 259.

Duggan, J.M. (1968) Gastrointestinal haemorrhage, gastric ulcer and aspirin abuse. *Austr. Ann. Med.*, 17, 183.

Duthie, J.J.R. (1963) *Salicylates: An international symposium* (eds A. St. J. Dixon, B.K. Martin, M.J.H. Smith and P.H.N. Wood), Churchill, London, p. 288.

Edmar, D. (1971) Effects of salicylates on the gastric mucosa as revealed by roentgen examination and the gastro-camera. *Acta Radiol. (Stockholm)*, 11, 57.

Editorial (1973) Liver injury by salicylates. *Br. Med. J.*, ii, 732.

Faivre, J., Faivre, M. and Lery, N. (1975) Aspirin and pregnancy. *Lyon Med.*, 233, 725.

Forney, H.J., Bentley, G. and Matthews, R.S. (1973) Salicylates and repair in adult articular cartilage. *Orthopaedics (Oxford)*, 6, 19.

Franke, M. and Manz, G. (1972) Benorylate and indomethacin in the treatment of rheumatoid disease: a double blind clinical trial. *Curr. Ther. Res.*, 14, 113.

Friedlaender, S. and Feinberg, S.M. (1947) Aspirin allergy: its relation to chronic intractable asthma. *Ann. Intern. Med.*, 26, 734.

Garber, E., Craig, R.M. and Bahu, R.M. (1975) Aspirin hepatotoxicity. *Ann. Intern. Med.*, 82, 592.

Gibson, T., Zaphiropoulos, G., Grove, J. *et al.* (1975) Kinetics of salicylate metabolism. *Br. J. Clin. Pharmacol.*, 2, 233.

Gillies, M.A. and Skyring, A. (1969) Gastric and duodenal ulcer: the association between aspirin ingestion, smoking and family history of ulcer. *Med. J. Austr.*, ii, 280.

Ginsberg, J.M., Eyring, E.J., Lacey, S. and Tomblin, W. (1968) Inhibition of cartilage destruction by intermittent salicylate. *Arthr. Rheum.*, 11, 824.

Giraldo, B., Blumenthal, M.N. and Spink, W.H. (1969) Aspirin intolerance and asthma: a clinical and immunologic study. *Ann. Int. Med.*, 71, 479.

Goldenberg, D.L. (1974) Aspirin hepatotoxicity. *Ann. Int. Med.*, 80, 773.

Goldsweig, H.G., Kapusta, M. and Schwarty, J. (1976) Bleeding, salicylates and prolonged prothrombin time: three case reports and a review of the literature. *J. Rheumatol.*, 3, 37.

Goulston, K. and Cooke, A.R. (1968) Alcohol, aspirin and gastric bleeding. *Br. Med. J.*, iv, 664.

Graham, G.G. and Rowland, M. (1972) Application of salivary salicylate data to biopharmaceutical studies of salicylates. *J. Pharm. Sci.*, 61, 1219.

Greer, H.D., Ward, H.P. and Corbrin, K.B. (1965) Chronic salicylate intoxication in adults. *J. Am. Med. Assoc.*, 193, 555.

Gross, M. and Greenberg, L.A. (1948) *The Salicylates – A Critical Bibliographic Review*. Hillhouse Press, New Haven, CT.

Grossman, M., Matsumoto, K.K. and Lichter, R. (1961) Fecal blood loss produced by oral and intravenous administration of various salicylates. *Gastroenterology*, 40, 383.

Gyory, A.Z. and Stiel, J.N. (1968) Effect of particle size on aspirin induced gastrointestinal bleeding. *Lancet*, ii, 300.

Halvoresen, L., Dotevall, G. and Sevelius, H. (1973) Comparative effects of aspirin and naproxen on gastric mucosa. *Scand. J. Rheumatol.*, 2 (Suppl.), p. 43.

Hanzlik, P.J. (1927) *Actions and Uses of the Salicylates and Cincophen in Medicine*. William and Wilkins, Baltimore.

Harris, W.H., Salzman, E.W., Athanasoulis, C.A. *et al.* (1977), Aspirin prophylaxis of venous thromboembolism after total hip replacement. *N. Engl. J. Med.*, **23**, 1246.

Harvald, B. and Glausen, E. (1960) Nephrotoxicity of acetylsalicylic acid. *Lancet*, **ii**, 767.

Haslam, R.R., Ekert, H. and Gillam, G.L. (1974) Haemorrhage in a neonate possibly due to maternal ingestion of salicylate. *J. Pediatr.*, **84**, 556.

Hecht, A. and Goldner, M.G. (1959), Reappraisal of the hypoglycemic action of acetylsalicylate. *Metabolism*, **8**, 418.

Heggarty, H. (1974) Aspirin and anaemia in childhood. *Br. Med. J.*, **i**, 491.

Hirsh, J., Street, D., Cade, J.F. and Amy, H. (1973) Relation between bleeding time and platelet connective tissue reaction after aspirin. *Blood*, **41**, 369.

Hofmann, L.M., Krupnick, M.I. and Garcia, H.A. (1972) Interactions of spironolactone and hydrochlorothiazide with aspirin in the rat and dog. *J. Pharmacol. Exp. Ther.*, **180**, 1.

Hollister, L. and Levy, G. (1965) Some aspects of salicylate distribution and metabolism in man. *J. Pharm. Sci.*, **54**, 1126.

Hurst, A. and Lintott, G.A.M. (1939) Aspirin as a cause of haematemesis: a clinical and gastroscopic study. *Guy's Hosp. Rep.*, **89**, 173.

Iancu, T. (1972) Serum transaminases and salicylate therapy. *Br. Med. J.*, **ii**, 167.

Ivey, K.J., Morrison, S. and Gray, C. (1972) Effect of intravenous salicylates on the gastric mucosal barrier in man. *Am. J. Dig. Dis.*, **17**, 1055.

Jarvis, J.F. (1966) A case of unilateral permanent deafness following acetylsalicylic acid. *J. Laryngol. Otol.*, **80**, 318.

Jick, H. and Miettinen, O.S. (1976) Regular aspirin use and myocardial infarction. *Br. Med. J.*, **i**, 1057.

Kaneshiro, M.M., Mielke, C.H., Kasper, C.K. and Rapaport, S.I. (1969) Bleeding time after aspirin in disorders of intrinsic clotting. *N. Engl. J. Med.*, **281**, 1039.

Kelly, J.J. (1956) Salicylate ingestion: a frequent cause of gastric haemorrhage. *Am. J. Med. Sci.*, **232**, 119.

Kiser, J.R. (1963) Chronic gastric ulcer associated with aspirin ingestion. A report of 5 cases and a review of the literature. *Am. J. Dig. Dis.*, **8**, 856.

Koppes, G.M. and Arnett, F.C. (1974) Salicylate hepatotoxicity. *Postgrad. Med.*, **56**, 193.

Lange, H.F. (1957) Salicylates and gastric haemorrhage, 2. Manifest bleeding. *Gastroenterology*, **33**, 770.

Langman, M.J.S. (1974) in *Controversy in Internal Medicine* (eds F.J. Ingelfinger, R.V. Ebert, M. Finland, and A.S. Relman), Vol. 2, Saunders, Philadelphia, p. 493.

Leonard, J.R. (1969) Absence of gastrointestinal bleeding following administration of salicylic acid. *J. Lab. Clin. Med.*, **74**, 911.

Leonards, J.R. and Levy, G. (1969) Reduction and prevention of aspirin-induced occult gastrointestinal blood loss in man. *Clin. Pharmacol. Ther.*, **10**, 571.

Leonards, J.R. and Levy, G. (1970) Aspirin-induced occult gastrointestinal blood loss: local *versus* systemic effects. *J. Pharmacol. Sci.*, **59**, 1511.

Leonards, J.R. and Levy, G. (1972a) Effect of pharmaceutical formulation on gastrointestinal bleeding from aspirin tablets. *Arch. Intern. Med.*, **129**, 457.

Leonards, J.R. and Levy, G. (1972b) Gastrointestinal blood loss from aspirin and sodium salicylate tablets in man. *Clin. Pharmacol. Ther.*, **14**, 62.

Leonards, J.R., Levy, G. and Niemczura, R. (1973) Gastrointestinal blood loss during prolonged aspirin administration. *N. Engl. J. Med.*, **289**, 1020.

Levy, G. and Leonards, J.R. (1971) Urine pH and salicylate therapy. *J. Am. Med. Assoc.*, **217**, 81.

Levy, G., Tsuchiya, T. and Amsel, L.P. (1972) Limited capacity for salicyl phenolic glucuronide formation and its effect on the kinetics of salicylate elimination in man. *Clin. Pharmacol. Ther.*, **13**, 258.

Levy, M. (1974) Aspirin use in patients with upper gastrointestinal bleeding and peptic ulcer disease. *N. Engl. J. Med.*, **290**, 1158.

Lewis, R.B. and Schulman, J.D. (1973) Influence of acetylsalicylic acid, an inhibitor of prostaglandin synthesis, on the duration of human gestation and labour. *Lancet*, **ii**, 1159.

Lockey, R.F., Rucknagel, D.L. and Vanselow, N.A. (1973) Familial occurrence of asthma, nasal polyps and aspirin intolerance. *Ann. Intern. Med.*, **78**, 57.

Loh, H.S. and Wilson, C.W.M. (1975) The interactions of aspirin and ascorbic acid in normal men. *J. Clin. Pharmacol.*, **15**, 36.

Macdougall, A.I. and Alexander, W.D. (1963) in *Salicylates* (eds A. St. J. Dixon, B.K. Martin, M.J.H. Smith and P.H.N. Wood), Churchill, London, p. 92.

Macklon, A.F., Craft, A.W., Thompson, M. and Kerr, D.N.S. (1974) Aspirin and analgesic nephropathy. *Br. Med. J.*, **i**, 597.

MacLagan, T.J. (1876) The treatment of acute rheumatism by salicin. *Lancet*, **i**, 342.

Macpherson, C.R., Milne, M.D. and Evans, B.M. (1955) The excretion of salicylate. *Br. J. Pharmacol.*, **10**, 484.

Mainland, D. and Sutcliffe, M.I. (1965) Aspirin in rheumatoid arthritis: a seven day double blind trial – preliminary report. *Bull. Rheum. Dis.*, **16**, 388.

Manra, R.C. and Kincaid-Smith, P. (1970) Papillary necrosis in rats caused by aspirin and aspirin-containing mixtures. *Br. Med. J.*, **iii**, 559.

Manso, C., Taranta, A. and Nydick, I. (1956) Effect of aspirin administration on serum glutamic oxaloacetic and glutamic pyruvic transaminases in children. *Proc. Soc. Exp. Biol. Med.*, **93**, 83.

Marson, F.G.W. (1953) Studies in gout, with particular reference to the value of sodium salicylate in treatment. *Q. J. Med.*, **22**, 331.

Martin, B.K. (1971) The formulation of aspirin. *Adv. Pharm. Sci.*, **3**, 107.

Matthews, J.I. and Stage, D. (1974) Indomethacin, aspirin and urticaria. *Ann. Intern. Med.*, **80**, 771.

Mauer, I., Weinstein, D. and Solomon, H.M. (1970) Acetylsalicylic acid: no chromosome damage in human leukocytes. *Science*, **169**, 198.

McDonald, J.R., Mathison, D.A. and Stevenson, D.D. (1972) Aspirin intolerance in asthma. *J. Allergy Clin. Immunol.*, **50**, 198.

McNeil, J.R. (1973) The possible teratogenic effect of salicylates on the developing fetus. Brief summaries of eight suggestive cases. *Clin. Pediatr.*, **12**, 347.

Meade, T.W., Chakrabarti, R., Haines, A.P. *et al.* (1977) Aspirin and plasma fibrinogen. *Lancet*, **ii**, 1289.

Medical Research Council (1972) Effect of aspirin on post-operative venous thrombosis. *Lancet*, **ii**, 441.

Menguy, R. (1966) Gastric mucosal injury by aspirin. *Gastro-enterology*, **51**, 430.

Menguy, R., Desbaillets, L., Masters, Y.F. and Okabe, S. (1972) Evidence for a sex-linked difference in aspirin meta-bolism. *Nature*, **239**, 102.

Menon, I.S. (1970) Aspirin and blood fibrinolysis. *Lancet*, **i**, 364.

Mielke, C.H., Kameshiro, M.M., Mather, I.A. *et al.* (1969) The standardised ivy bleeding time and its prolongation by aspirin. *Blood*, **34**, 204.

Miller, J.J. and Weissmann, D.B. (1976) Correlation between transaminase concentrations and serum salicylate concen-trations in juvenile rheumatoid arthritis. *Arthr. Rheum.*, **19**, 115.

Mills, D.G., Barda, I.T., Philp, R.B. and Eldridge, C. (1974) Effects of *in vitro* aspirin on blood platelets of gastro-intestinal bleeders. *Clin. Pharmacol. Ther.*, **15**, 187.

Mongan, E., Kelly, P., Nies, K. *et al.* (1973) Tinnitus as an indication of therapeutic salicylate levels. *J. Am. Med. Assoc.*, **226**, 142.

Moore-Robinson, M. and Warin, R.P. (1967) Effect of sali-cylates in urticaria. *Br. Med. J.*, **iv**, 262.

Morley, J. (1975) *Proc. Aspirin Symp.*, Royal College of Surgeons, London, p. 19.

Moroz, L.A. (1977) Increased blood fibrinolytic activity after aspirin ingestion. *N. Engl. J. Med.*, **296**, 525.

Muir, A. and Cossar, I.A. (1955) Aspirin and ulcer. *Br. Med. J.*, **ii**, 7.

Muir, A. and Cossar, I.A. (1959) Aspirin and gastric haemorr-hage. *Lancet*, **i**, 539.

Multz, C.V., Bernard, G.C., Blechman, W.C. *et al.* (1974) A comparison of intermediate dose aspirin and placebo in rheumatoid arthritis. *Clin. Pharmacol. Ther.*, **15**, 310.

Murray, R.M. (1972) Analgesic nephropathy: removal of phenacetin from proprietary analgesics. *Br. Med. J.*, **iv**, 131.

Needham, C.D., Kyle, J., Jones *et al.* (1971) Aspirin and alcohol in gastrointestinal haemorrhage. *Gut*, **12**, 819.

New Zealand Rheumatism Study (1974) Aspirin and the kidney. *Br. Med. J.*, **i**, 593.

O'Brien, J.R. (1975) Annotation: aspirin, haemostasis and thrombosis. *Br. J. Haematol.*, **29**, 523.

Opelz, G., Terasaki, P.I. and Hirata, A.A. (1973) Suppression of lymphocyte transformation by aspirin. *Lancet*, **ii**, 478.

Parry, D.J. and Wood, P.H.N. (1967) Relationship between aspirin taking and gastroduodenal haemorrhage. *Gut*, **8**, 301.

Paul, W.D. (1943) The effect of acetylsalicylic acid on the gastric mucosa. *J. Iowa State Med. Soc.*, **33**, 4.

Paulus, H.E., Siegel, M., Mongan, E. *et al.* (1971) Variations of serum concentrations and half life of salicylate in patients with rheumatoid arthritis. *Arthr. Rheum.*, **14**, 527.

Pierson, R.N., Holt, P.R., Watson, R.M. and Keating, R.P. (1961) Aspirin and gastrointestinal bleeding. *Am. J. Med.*, **31**, 259.

Pinckard, R.N., Hawkins, D. and Farr, R.S. (1968a)

Permanent alteration of human albumin (HSA) by acetyl-salicylic acid (ASA). *Fed. Proc.*, **27**, 543.

Pinckard, R.N., Hawkins, D. and Farr, R.S. (1968b) *In vitro* acetylation of plasma proteins, enzymes and DNA by aspirin. *Nature*, **219**, 68.

Pinckard, R.N., Hawkins, D. and Farr, R.S. (1970) The inhibitory effect of salicylate on the acetylation of human albumin by acetylsalicylic acid. *Arthr. Rheum.*, **13**, 361.

Prescott, L.F. (1965) Effects of acetylsalicyclic acid, phen-acetin, paracetamol and caffeine on renal tubular epithe-lium. *Lancet*, **ii**, 91.

Prescott, L.F. (1969) Renal papillary necrosis and aspirin. *Scot. Med. J.*, **14**, 82.

Ratnoff, O.D. (1977) A new property of an old remedy: fibrinolysis and aspirin. *N. Engl. J. Med.*, **296**, 566.

Rich, R.R. and Johnson, J.S. (1973) Salicylate hepatotoxicity in patients with juvenile rheumatoid arthritis. *Arth. Rheum.*, **16**, 1.

Rosenthal, R.K., Bayles, T.B. and Freemont-Smith, K. (1964) Simultaneous salicylate concentrations in synovial fluid and plasma in rheumatoid arthritis. *Arthr. Rheum.*, **7**, 103.

Roth, G.J. and Majerus, O.W. (1975) The mechanism of the effect of aspirin on human platelets. I. Acetylation of a particulate fraction protein. *J. Clin. Invest.*, **56**, 624.

Rowland, M., Riegelman, S., Harris, O.A. and Sholkoff, S.D. (1972) Absorption kinetics of aspirin in man following oral administration of an aqueous solution. *J. Pharm. Sci.*, **61**, 379.

Rubin, A., Rodda, B.E., Warrich, P. *et al.* (1973) Interactions of aspirin with non-steroidal anti-inflammatory drugs in man. *Arthr. Rheum.*, **16**, 635.

Russell, A.S., Sturge, R.A. and Smith, M.A. (1971) Serum transaminase during salicylate therapy. *Br. Med. J.*, **ii**, 428.

Salvaggio, J. and Crane, E. (1961) Severe allergic reactions after ingestion of acetylsalicylic acid compounds. *J. Loui-siana State Med. Soc.*, **113**, 292.

Samter, M. (1969) The acetyl in aspirin. *Ann. Intern. Med.*, **71**, 208.

Samter, M. (1973) Intolerance to aspirin. *Hosp. Pract.*, **8**, 85.

Samter, M. and Beers, R.F. (1967) Concerning the nature of intolerance to aspirin. *J. Allergy*, **40**, 281.

Scott, J.T. (1963) In *Salicylates: An International Symposium* (eds A. St. J. Dixon, B.K. Martin, M.J.H. Smith and P.H.N. Wood), Churchill, London, p. 242.

Scott, J.T., Denman, A.M. and Dorling, J. (1963) Renal irritation caused by salicylates. *Lancet*, **i**, 344.

Scott, J.T., Porter, I.H., Lewis, S.M. and St.J. Dixon, A. (1961) Studies of gastrointestinal bleeding caused by cortico-steroids, salicylates and other analgesics. *Q. J. Med., New Series*, **30**, 167.

Seaman, W.E., Ishak, K.G. and Plotz, P.H. (1974) Aspirin-induced hepatotoxicity in patients with systematic lupus erythematosus. *Ann. Intern. Med.*, **80**, 1.

See, G. (1877) Histoire de l'acide salicylique. *Bull. Acad. Med. (Paris)*, **26**, 689.

Segre, E.J., Chaplin, M., Forchielli, E. *et al.* (1974) Nap-roxen–aspirin interactions in man. *Clin. Pharmacol. Ther.*, **15**, 374.

Simmons, D.P. and Chrisman, O.D. (1965) Salicyclate in-hibition of cartilage degeneration. *Arthr. Rheum.*, **8**, 960.

Slone, D., Heinonen, O.P., Kaufman *et al.* (1976a) Aspirin and congenital malformations. *Lancet*, **i**, 1373.

Slone, D., Siskind, V., Heinonen, O.P. *et al.* (1976b) Aspirin and congenital malformations. *Lancet*, **i**, 1373.

Smith, B.M., Skillman, J.J., Edwards, B.G. and Silen, W. (1971) Permeability of the human gastric mucosal alteration by acetylsalicylic acid and ethanol. *N. Engl. J. Med.*, **285**, 716.

Smith, M.J.H. and Smith, P.K. (1966) *The Salicylates. A Critical Bibliographic Review*, Wiley, New York.

Speer, F. (1975) Aspirin allergy: a clinical study. *S. Med. J.*, **68**, 314.

Sperryn, M.M., Hamilton, E.B.D. and Parsons, V. (1973) Double blind comparison of aspirin and 4-(acetamido) phenyl-2-acetoxyberyocite (benorylate) in rheumatoid arthritis. *Ann. Rheum. Dis.*, **32**, 157.

Spiro, H.M. (1974) in *Controversy in Internal Medicine* (eds F.J. Ingelfinger, R.V. Ebert, M. Finland and A.S.P. Relman), Vol. 2, Saunders, Philadelphia, p. 500.

St. John, D.J.B. and McDermott, F.T. (1970) Influence of achlorhydria on aspirin induced occult gastrointestinal blood loss. *Br. Med. J.*, **ii**, 450.

St. John, C.J.B., Yeomans, M.D. and de Boer, W.G.R.N. (1973) Chronic gastric ulcer induced by apsirin: an experimental model. *Gastroenterology*, **65**, 634.

Stone, E. (1763) An account of the success of the bark of the willow in the cure of agues. *Phil. Soc. Trans.*, **53**, 195.

Stricker (1876) Uber die Resultate der Behandlung der Polyarthritis rheumatica mit Salicylsaure. *Berlin Klin. Wochenschr.*, **13**, 1.

Szczeklik, A., Gryglewski, R.J., Czerniawska-Mysik, G. and Pieton, R. (1977) Asthmatic attacks induced in aspirin sensitive patients by diclofenac and naproxen. *Br. Med. J.*, **ii**, 231.

Tainter, M.L. and Ferris, A.J. (1969) *Aspirin in Modern Therapy. A Review*, Bayer Company Division of Sterling Drugs, New York, p. 1.

Thompson, H.E. and Dragstedt, C.A. (1934), Modifying action of calcium and sodium bicarbonate on salicylate intoxication. *Arch. Int. Med.*, **54**, 308.

Thorsen, W.B., Western, D., Tanaka, Y. and Morrisey, J.F. (1968) Aspirin injury to the gastric mucosa: gastrocamera observations of the effects of pH. *Arch. Int. Med.*, **121**, 499.

Thune, S. (1968) Gastrointestinal bleeding and salicylates. *Nordic Med.*, **79**, 352.

Turner, G. and Collins, E. (1975) Fetal effects of regular salicylate ingestion in pregnancy. *Lancet*, **ii**, 338.

Von Maur, K., Adkinson, N.F., Metre, T.E. *et al.* (1974) Aspirin intolerance in a family. *J. Allergy Clin. Immunol.*, **54**, 380.

Walton, C.H.A. and Randle, D.L. (1957) Aspirin allergy. *Can. Med. Assoc. J.*, **76**, 1016.

Weiss, H.J., Aledort, L.M. and Kochwa, S. (1968) The effect of salicylates on the hemostatic properties of platelets in man. *J. Clin. Invest.*, **47**, 2169.

Weiss, A., Pitman, E.R. and Graham, E.C. (1961) Aspirin and gastric bleeding. Gastroscopic observations with review of literature. *Am. J. Med.*, **31**, 266.

Wijnja, L., Snijder, J.A.M. and Nieweg, H.O. (1966) Acetylsalicylic acid as a cause of pancytopenia from bone marrow damage. *Lancet*, **ii**, 768.

Wigley, R.D. (1971) Aspirin and the kidney. *N. Z. Med. J.*, **74**, 301.

Witthauer, K. (1899) Aspirin, ein neues Salicylpreparat. *Ther. Monatschelfe*, **13**, 330.

Wohlgemut, J. (1899) Uber aspirin (acetylsalicylsaure) *Ther. Monatschelfe*, **13**, 276.

Wolfe, J.D., Metzger, A.L. and Goldstein, R.C. (1974) Aspirin hepatitis. *Ann. Int. Med.*, **80**, 74.

Wolff, J. and Austen, K.F. (1958) Salicylates and thyroid function II. The effect on the thyroid-pituitary inter-relation. *J. Clin. Invest.*, **37**, 1144.

Yu, T.F. and Gutman, A.B. (1959) A study of the paradoxical effects of salicylate in low, intermediate and high dosage on the renal mechanisms for excretion of urate in man. *J. Clin. Invest.*, **38**, 1298.

Yunginger, J.W., O'Connell, E.J. and Logan, G.B. (1973) Aspirin-induced asthma in children. *J. Pediatr.*, **82**, 218.

Zucker, M.B. and Peterson, J. (1970) Effect of acetylsalicylic acid, other nonsteroidal anti-inflammatory agents, and dipyridamole on human blood platelets. *J. Lab. Clin. Med*, **76**, 66.

Choline magnesium trisalicylate

Blechman, W.J. and Lechner, B.L. (1979) Clinical comparative evaluation of choline magnesium trisalicylate and acetylsalicylic acid in rheumatoid arthritis. *Rheumatol. Rehabil.*, **18**, 119.

Cohen, A. and Garber, H.E. (1978) Comparison of choline magnesium trisalicylate and acetylsalicylic acid in relation to fecal blood loss. *Curr. Ther. Res.*, **23**, 187.

Cohen, A., Thomas, G.B. and Cohen, E.B. (1978) Serum concentration, safety and tolerance of oral doses of choline magnesium trisalicylate. *Curr. Ther. Res.*, **23**, 358.

Ehrlich, G.E., Miller, S.B. and Zeiders, R.S. (1980) Choline magnesium trisalicylate versus ibuprofen in rheumatoid arthritis. *Rheumatol. Rehabil.*, **19**, 30.

Zucker, M.B. and Rothwell, K.G. (1978) Differential influences of salicylate compounds on platelet aggregation and serotonin release. *Curr. Ther. Res.*, **23**, 194.

Salicylsalicylic acid

Fraser, T.N. (1945) Gold therapy in rheumatoid arthritis. *Ann. Rheum. Dis.*, **4**, 771.

Deodhar, S.D., McLeod, M.M., Dick, W.C. and Buchanan, W.W. (1977) A short-term comparative trial of salsalate and indomethacin in rheumatoid arthritis. *Curr. Med. Res. Op.*, **5**, 185.

Leonards, J.R. (1969) Absence of gastro-intestinal bleeding following administration of salicylsalicylic acid. *J. Lab. Clin. Med.*, **74**, 911.

Liyanage, S.P. and Tambar, P.K. (1978) Comparative study of salsalate and aspirin in osteoarthrosis of the hip or knee. *Curr. Med. Res. Op.*, **5**, 450.

Nordqvist, P., Harthan, J.G.L. and Karlsson, R. (1965) Metabolic kinetics of salicylsalicylic acid, aspirin and sodium salicylate in man. *Nor. Med.*, **79**, 352.

Ré, O.N. (1979) Salicylsalicylic acid revisited: a multicentre study. *J. Int. Med. Res.*, **7**, 90.

Rubin, H.S. (1964) Serum salicylate levels in osteoarthritis following oral administration of a preparation containing salicyl salicylic acid. *Am. J. Med. Sci.*, **248**, 31.

Benorylate

Alexander, F., Flahaut, J., Reveschot, H. and Drykoningen, G. (1970), Étude de l'activité antipyrétique d'une nouvelle substance, le benorylate dan la clinique pédiatrique. *Bruxelles-Médical*, **6**, 439.

Bain, L.S. and Burt, R.A.P. (1970) The treatment of rheumatoid disease. A double-blind trial comparing buffered aspirin with benorylate. *Clin. Trials J.*, **7**, 307.

Beales, D.L., Burry, H.C. and Grahame, R. (1972) Comparison of aspirin and benorylate in the treatment of rheumatoid arthritis. *Br. Med. J.*, **ii**, 483.

Bennett, A. (1973) Inhibition of prostaglandin synthesis by benorylate. *Rheumatol. Rehabil.* (Suppl.: A Symposium on Benorylate), p. 101.

Bitensky, L. and Chayen, J. (1973) Quantitative assay of action on the synovium in human rheumatoid arthritis *Rheumatol. Rehabil.* (Suppl.: A Symposium on Benorylate), p. 92.

Cardoe, N. (1970) Preliminary assessment of a new drug: benorylate. *Clin. Trials J.*, **7**, 313.

Croft, D.N., Cuddigan, J.H.P. and Sweetland, C. (1972) Gastric bleeding and benorylate, a new aspirin. *Br. Med. J.*, **3**, 545.

Danhof, I.E., Kailey, J.D. and Gunn, E.C. (1972) Benorylate gastrointestinal blood loss. *Curr. Ther. Res.*, **14**, 583.

De Choisy, J. (1973) A new method of assessing grip strength and wrist and arm movement in the arthritic patient. *Rheumatol. Rehabil.* (Suppl.: A Symposium on Benorylate), p. 81.

Franke, M. and Menz, B.K. (1964) Benorylate and indomethacin in the treatment of rheumatoid disease: a double-blind clinical trial. *Curr. Ther. Res.–Clin. Exp.*, **14**, 112.

Hämäläinen, M., Laine, V.A., Penn, R.G. and Vainio, K. (1973) The passage of benorylate into the synovial fluid and tissue of rheumatoid patients. *Rheumatol. Rehabil.* (Suppl.: A Symposium on Benorylate), p. 85.

Hart, G. and Nicholson, P.A. (1971) The analgesic activity of benorylate, aspirin and placebo. *Clin. Trials J.*, **8**, 51.

Haslock, D.I., Nicholson, P.A. and Wright, V. (1971) The treatment of rheumatoid arthritis: a comparison of phenylbutazone and benorylate. *Clin. Trials J.*, **8**, 43.

Hingorani, K. (1973) A double-blind study of benorylate and ibuprofen in rheumatoid arthritis. *Rheumatol. Rehabil.* (Suppl: A Symposium on Benorylate), p. 39.

Livingstone, J.L. (1973) Benorylate pharmaceutics. *Rheumatol Rehabil.* (Suppl: A Symposium on Benorylate), p. 16.

Maneksha, S. (1973) Safapryn and benorylate – a comparative trial of two new preparations of aspirin and paracetamol in the treatment of rheumatoid arthritis and osteoarthritis. *Curr. Med. Res. Op.*, **1**, 563.

Medvei, V.C. (ed.) (1973) A Symposium on Benorylate. *Rheumatol. Rehabil.* (Suppl.).

Parelkon, K., Geirregat, R., Vojtisek, O. and Bremova, A. (1973) A study of the long term treatment of rheumatoid arthritis with benorylate suspension. *Rheumatol. Rehabil.* (Suppl: A Symposium on Benorylate), p. 48.

Poore, A.C.G. (1973) The development of a special packing concept for benorylate suspension. *Rheumatol. Rehabil.* (Suppl: A Symposium on Benorylate), p. 20.

Reizenstein, P.G. and Döberl, A. (1973) Relevance of gastrointestinal symptoms and blood loss after long term treatment with a salicylate-paracetamol ester, a new anti-inflammatory

agent (benorylate). *Rheumatol. Rehabil.* (Suppl: A Symposium on Benorylate), p. 66.

Robertson, A. (1973) Benorylate – the rationale. *Rheumatol. Rehabil.* (Suppl: A Symposium on Benorylate), p. 7.

Robertson, A., Glynn, J.P. and Watson, A.K. (1972) The absorption and metabolism in man of 4-acetamidophenyl-2-acetoxybenzoate (benorylate), *Xenobiotica*, **2**, 339.

Rosner, I., Mottot, G., Khalihi-Varasteh, H. and Legros, J. (1973) Experimental data on benorylate and their clinical relevance. *Rheumatol. Rehabil.* (Suppl: A Symposium on Benorylate), p. 59.

Sasisekhar, P.R., Penn, R.G., Haslock, I, and Wright, V. (1973) A comparison of benorylate and aspirin in the treatment of rheumatoid arthritis. *Rheumatol. Rehabil.* (Suppl: A Symposium on Benorylate), p. 31.

Spooner, J.B. (1973) Side effects encountered with benorylate. *Rheumatol. Rehabil.* (Suppl: A Symposium on Benorylate), p. 75.

Weill, J., Gaillon, R., Rendu, C., Lejeune, C. (1968) Un nouvel antipyrétique d'usage pédiatrique: l'acétoxybenzoate 2-(acetamido) phényl 4. *Thérapie*, **23**, 541.

Diflunisal

*Ackermann, K. and Braun, H.D. (1978) in *Diflunisal in Clinical Practice* (ed. K. Miehlke), Futura Publishing, New York, pp. 143–8.

*Adams, I.D. (1978) Diflunisal in the management of sprains. *Curr. Med. Res. Op.*, **5**, 544.

*Andrew, A., Rodda, B., Verhaest, L. and van Winzum, C. (1977) Diflunisal: six-month experience in osteoarthritis. *Br. J. Clin. Pharmacol.*, **4**, 455.

*Axler, A. (1978) in *Symposium on Diflunisal: New Perspectives in Analgesia*, Abstract 9.

Bahous, I., Lutterbeck, P.M. and Tempero, K.F. (1978) Diflunisal: a novel long-acting analgesic. *Clin. Ther.*, **1** (Suppl. A), 10.

*Barrau, J. (1978) Double-blind comparison of efficacy and tolerance of diflunisal and oxyphenbutazone in the treatment of strains and sprains. *Clin. Ther.*, **1** (Suppl. A), 43.

*Bernett, P., Primbs, P. and Braun, H.D. (1978) in *Symposium on Diflunisal: New Perspectives in Analgesia*, Abstract 7.

*Bresnihan, B., Hughes, G. and Essigman, W.K. (1978) Diflunisal in the treatment of osteoarthritis: a double-blind study comparing diflunisal with ibuprofen. *Curr. Med. Res. Op.*, **5**, 556.

*Brom, H.L.F. (1978) in *Symposium on Diflunisal: New Perspectives in Analgesia*, Abstract 11.

*Christodoulopoulos, J., Houssianakou, E. and Seitnides, B. (1978) in *Symposium on Diflunisal: New Perspectives in Analgesia*, Abstract 15.

*Cirillo, V.J., Bahous, I., Franchimont, P. *et al.* (1978) Diflunisal in the treatment of osteoarthritis of the hip: a double-blind comparison with placebo. *Clin. Trials J.*, **15**, 40.

DeSchepper, P.J., Tjandramaga, T.B., Kramp, R. and Getson, A. (1978a) in *Symposium on Diflunisal: New Perspectives in Analgesia*, Abstract 18.

DeSchepper, P.J., Tjandramaga, T.B., Verhaest, L. *et al.* (1978b) Diflunisal (MK-647) versus acetylsalicylic acid: a comparative study of their effect upon faecal blood loss, in the presence and absence of alcohol. *Clin. Ther.*, **1**, 49.

*Devroey, P. (1978) The treatment of postoperative pain with a single dose of diflunisal. *Clin. Ther.*, **1** (Suppl. A), 30.

*Devroey, P., Steelman, S.L., Caudron, J. *et al.* (1977) A double-blind, placebo-controlled, single-dose study comparing three dose levels of diflunisal with aspirin and placebo in patients with pain due to episiotomy. *Acta Therapeutica*, **3**, 205.

Dieppe, P.A. and Huskisson, E.C. (1978) in *Diflunisal in Clinical Practice* (ed. K. Miehlke), Futura Publishing, New York, pp. 57–62.

Dresse, A., Delapierre, D., Baudinet, G. and Kramp, R. (1978) in *Symposium on Diflunisal: New Perspectives in Analgesia*, Abstract 1.

*Essigman, W.K., Chamberlain, M.A. and Wright, V. (1978) Diflunisal in osteoarthrosis of the hip and the knee. *Curr. Med. Res. Op.*, **5**, 551.

*Goutallier, D., Debeyre, J. and Block, F. (1978a) in *Diflunisal in Clinical Practice* (ed. K. Miehlke), Futura Publishing, New York, pp. 119–132.

*Goutallier, D., Debeyre, J. and Bock, F. (1978b) in *Symposium on Diflunisal: New Perspectives in Analgesia*, Abstract 14.

*Grayson, M.F. (1978) Two trials of diflunisal in osteoarthritis. *Curr. Med. Res. Op.*, **5**, 567.

Hannah, J., Ruyle, W.F., Jones, H. *et al.* (1977) Discovery of diflunisal. *Br. J. Clin. Pharmacol.*, **4**, 7.

*Hayat, M.M., Delgado, M. and Bock, F. (1978) in *Symposium on Diflunisal: New Perspectives in Analgesia*, Abstract 16.

*Hazleman, B.L. (1978) in *Symposium on Diflunisal: New Perspectives in Analgesia*, Abstract 4.

*Honig, W.J. (1978) in *Diflunisal in Clinical Practice* (ed. K. Miehlke), Futura Publishing, New York, pp. 105–18.

Huskisson, E.C., Williams, T.N., Shaw, L.D. and Kerry, J. (1978) Diflunisal in general practice. *Curr. Med. Res. Op.*, **5**, 589.

*Jaegemann, V. (1978) in *Symposium on Diflunisal: New Perspectives in Analgesia*, Abstract 5.

*Jaffe, G.V., Roylance, P.J. and Grimshaw, J.J. (1978) A controlled study of diflunisal in sprains and strains. *Clin. Med. Res. Op.*, **5**, 584.

*Keet, J.G.M. (1979) A comparative clinical trial of diflunisal and ibuprofen in the control of pain in osteoarthritis. *J. Intl. Med. Res.*, **7**, 272.

*Kolsen Petersen, J. (1978a) in *Diflunisal in Clinical Practice* (ed. K. Miehlke), Futura Publishing, New York, pp. 133–42.

*Kolsen Peterson, J.K. (1978b) The analgesic and anti-inflammatory efficacy of diflunisal and codeine after removal of impacted third molars. *Curr. Med. Res. Op.*, **5**, 525.

Kuehl, F.A. and Egan, R.W. (1978) in *Diflunisal in Clinical Practice* (ed. K. Miehlke), Futura Publishing, New York, pp. 13–20.

Majerus, P.W. and Stanford, N. (1977) Comparative effects of aspirin and diflunisal on prostaglandin synthetase from human platelets and sheep seminal vesicles. *Br. J. Clin. Pharmacol.*, **4**, 15.

*Paalzow, L., Edman, P., Ekman, A. and Lindstrom, B. (1978) in *Symposium on Diflunisal: New Perspectives in Analgesia*, Abstract 3.

Schulz, P., Perrier, C.V., Ferber, F. *et al.* (1979) Diflunisal, a new-acting analgesic and prostaglandin inhibitor: effect of concomitant acetylsalicylic acid therapy on ototoxicity and on disposition of both drugs. *J. Intl. Med. Res.*, **7**, 61.

*Semb, H. and Persson, B.M. (1978) in *Diflunisal in Clinical Practice* (ed. K. Miehlke), Futura Publishing, New York, pp. 133–42.

Smit Sibinga, C.T., Tempero, K.F. and Breault, G.O. (1976) in *Microcirculation* (eds J. Grayson and W. Zingg), Plenum Press, New York, pp. 211–12.

Smit Sibinga, C.T. (1977) Effect of diflunisal on platelet function and blood coagulation. *Br. J. Clin. Pharmacol.*, **4**, 375.

Steelman, S.L., Breault, G.O., Tocco, D. *et al.* (1975) Pharmacokinetics of MK-647, a novel salicylate. *Clin. Pharmacol. Ther.*, **17**, 245.

Steelman, S.L., Smit Sibinga, C.T., Schulz, P. *et al.* (1976) The effect of diflunisal on urinary prostaglandin excretion, bleeding time and platelet aggregation in normal human subjects. *Thirteenth International Congress of Internal Medicine*, Abstract 215.

Steelman, S.L., Tempero, K.F. and Cirillo, V.J. (1978) The chemistry, pharmacology, toxicology and clinical pharmacology of diflunisal. *Clin. Ther.*, **1**, 6.

Stone, C.A., Van Arman, C.G., Lotti, V.J. *et al.* (1977) Pharmacology and toxicology of diflunisal. *Br. J. Clin. Pharmacol.*, **4**, 19S.

*Tait, G.B.W., Lim, C.M., Highton, T.C. *et al.* (1978) in *Diflunisal in Clinical Practice* (ed. K. Miehlke), Futura Publishing, New York, pp. 43–56.

Tempero, K.F., Cirillo, V.J. and Steelman, S.L. (1977) Diflunisal: A review of pharmacokinetic and pharmacodynamic properties, drug interactions, and special tolerability studies in humans. *Br. J. Clin. Pharmacol.*, **4**, 31.

Tempero, K.F., Franklin, J., Reger, B. and Kappas, A. (1976) The influence of diflunisal, a novel anlagesic on serum uric acid and uric acid clearance. *Clin. Res.*, **24**, 258.

Tempero, K.F., Steelman, S.L., Besselaar, G.H. *et al.* (1975) Special studies on diflunisal, a novel salicylate. *Clin. Res.*, **23**, 224.

Tocco, D.J., Breault, G.O., Zacchei, A.G. *et al.* (1975) Physiological disposition and metabolism of 5-(2′, 4′-difluorophenyl) salicylic acid, a new salicylate. *Drug Metab. Disp.*, **3**, 453.

*Van Winzum, C. and Rodda, B. (1977) Diflunisal: efficacy in postoperative pain. *Br. J. Clin. Pharmacol.*, **4**, 39.

*Van Winzum, C., Cook, T., Verhaest, L. and Andrew, A. (1978) in *Diflunisal in Clinical Practice* (ed. K. Miehlke), Futura Publishing, New York, pp. 83–104.

Warren, J.S. (1978) Cholestatic jaundice due to diflunisal. *Br. Med. J.*, **ii**, 736.

*Wes, B.J. (1978) Diflunisal in oral surgery. *Clin. Ther.*, **1** (Suppl. A), 34.

*Wojtulewski, J.A., Walter, J. and Gray, J. (1978) Diflunisal compared with naproxen in the treatment of osteoarthritis of hip or knee: a double-blind trial. *Curr. Med. Res. Op.*, **5**, 562.

Acetic acids

Indole acetic acids

Indomethacin

*Aylward, M., Parker, R.J., Holly, F. *et al.* (1975) Long term study of indomethacin and alclofenac in the treatment of rheumatoid arthritis. *Br. Med. J.*, **ii**, 79.

Barnett, D.B., Edwards, I.R. and Smith, A.J. (1975) Antagonism by indomethacin of diuretic response to calcitonin in man. *Br. Med. J.*, iii, 686.

Boardman, P.L. and Hart, F.D. (1967) Side effects of indomethacin. *Ann. Rheum. Dis.*, **26**, 127.

*Brewer, E.J. (1968), A comparative evaluation of indomethacin acetominophen and placebo as antipyretic agents in children. *Arthr. Rheum.*, **11**, 645.

*Brodie, G.N. (1974) Indomethacin and bone pain. *Lancet*, i, 1160.

† Broll, H., Tausch, G. and Eberl, R. (1976) in *Inflammatory Arthropathies* (eds E.C. Huskisson and G.P. Velo), Excerpta Medica, Amsterdam, pp. 175–8.

Brooks, P.M., Bell, M.A., Lee, P. *et al.* (1974a) The effect of frusemide on indomethacin plasma levels. *Br. J. Clin. Pharmacol.*, **1**, 485.

Brooks, P.M., Bell, M.A., Sturrock, R.D. *et al.* (1974b) The clinical significance of indomethacin-probenicid interaction. *Br. J. Clin. Pharmacol.*, **1**, 287.

Brooks, P.M., Walker, J.J., Bell, M.A. *et al.* (1975) Indomethacin aspirin interaction: a clinical appraisal. *Br. Med. J.*, ii, 69.

Burns, C.A. (1968) Indomethacin: reduced retinal sensitivity and corneal deposits. *Am. J. Ophthalmol.*, **66**, 825.

Calabro, J.J. (1975) Long-term reappraisal of indomethacin. *Drug Ther.*, **5** (2), 46.

Carr, R.E. and Siegel, I.M. (1973) Retinal function in patients treated with indomethacin. *Am. J. Ophthalmol.*, **75**, 302.

Champion, D., Mongan, E., Paulus, H. *et al.* (1971) Effect of concurrent aspirin administration on serum concentration of indomethacin. *Arthr. Rheum.*, **14**, 375.

Cooperating Clinics Committee of the American Rheumatism Association (1967) A three month trial of indomethacin in rheumatoid arthritis with special reference to analysis and inference. *Clin. Pharmacol. Ther.*, **8**, 11.

De Gaetano, G., Vermylen, J., Donati, M.B. *et al.* (1974) Indomethacin and platelet aggregation in chronic glomerulonephritis: existence of non-responders. *Br. Med. J.*, i, 301.

Duggan, D.E., Hogans, A.F., Kwan, K.C. and MacMahon, F.G. (1972) The metabolism of indomethacin in man. *J. Pharmacol. Exp. Ther.*, **181**, 563.

Duggan, D.E., Hooke, K.F., Noll, R.M. and Kwan, K.C. (1975) Enterophepatic circulation of indomethacin and its role in intestinal irritation. *Biochem. Pharmacol.*, **25**, 1749.

Eade, O.E., Acheson, E.D., Curthbert, M.F. and Hawkes, C.H. (1975) Peripheral neuropathy and indomethacin. *Br. Med. J.*, ii, 66.

Emmerson, B.T. (1967) Regimen of indomethacin therapy in acute gouty arthritis. *Br. Med. J.*, ii, 272.

Emori, H.W., Champion, G.D., Bluestone, R. and Paulus, H.E. (1973a) Simultaneous pharmacokinetics of indomethacin in serum and synovial fluid. *Ann. Rheum. Dis.*, **32**, 433.

Emori, H.W., Paulus, H.E., Bluestone, R. and Pearson, C.M. (1973b) The pharmacokinetics of indomethacin in serum. *Clin. Pharmacol. Ther.*, **14**, 134.

Famaey, J.P., Brooks, P.M. and Dick, W. (1975) Biological effects of non-steroidal anti-inflammatory drugs. *Sem. Arthr. Rheum.*, **5**, 63.

*Fitch, K.D. and Gray, S.D. (1974) Indomethacin in soft tissue sports injuries. *Med. J. Austr.*, i, 260.

† Focan-Henrard, D. and Franchimont, P. (1976) in *Inflammatory Arthropathies* (eds E.C. Huskisson and G.P. Velo), Excerpta Medica, Amsterdam, pp. 185–90.

Flower, R.J. and Vane, J.R. (1974) Inhibiting prostaglandin synthesis. *Biochem. Pharmacol.*, **23**, 1439.

Fowler, P.D. (1975) in *Clinics in the Rheumatic Diseases*, Vol. 1, No. 2, *Current Management of Rheumatoid Arthritis* (eds C.M. Pearson and W.C. Dick), Saunders, London.

Hart, F.D. and Boardman, P.L. (1963) Indomethacin: a new non-steroidal anti-inflammatory agent. *Br. Med. J.*, ii, 965.

Hart, F.D. and Boardman, P.L. (1965) Indomethacin and phenylbutazone: a comparison. *Br. Med. J.*, ii, 1281.

† Haslock, I. (1976) in *Inflammatory Arthropathies*. (eds E.C. Huskisson and G.P. Velo), Excerpta Medica, Amsterdam, pp. 197–205.

Healey, L.A. (1967) An appraisal of indomethacin. *Bull. Rheum. Dis.*, **18**, 483.

Hobkirk, D., Rhodes, M. and Haslock, I. (1977) Night medication in rheumatoid arthritis. II. Combined therapy with indomethacin and diazepam. *Rheumatol. Rehabil.*, **16**, 125.

*Hodgkinson, R. and Woolf, D. (1973) A five year clinical trial of indomethacin in osteoarthritis of the hip. *Practitioner*, **210**, 392.

Holt, L.P.J. and Hawkins, C.F. (1965) Indomethacin: studies of absorption and the use of indomethacin suppositories. *Br. Med. J.*, i, 1354.

Huskisson, E.C. (1976) in *Inflammatory Arthropathies* (eds E.C. Huskisson and G.P. Velo), Exerpta Medica, Amsterdam, pp. 99–105.

*Huskisson, E.C. and Grayson, M.F. (1974) Indomethacin or amylobarbitone sodium for sleep in rheumatoid arthritis with some observations on the use of sequential analysis. *Br. J. Clin. Pharmacol.*, **1**, 151.

Huskisson, E.C. and Hart, F.D. (1972) The use of indomethacin and aloxiprin at night. *Practitioner*, **208**, 248.

*Huskisson, E.C., Berry, H., Street, F.G. and Medhurst, H.E. (1973) Indomethacin for soft-tissue injuries: a double-blind study in football players. *Rheumatol. Rehabil.*, **12**, 159.

*Huskisson, E.C., Taylor, R.T., Burston, D. *et al.* (1970) Evening indomethacin in the treatment of rheumatoid arthritis. *Ann. Rheum. Dis.*, **29**, 393.

Hvidberg, E., Lausen, H.H. and Jansen, J.A. (1972) Indomethacin: plasma concentrations and protein binding in man. *Eur. J. Clin. Pharmacol.*, **4**, 119.

Jacobs, J.C. (1967) Sudden death in arthritic children receiving large doses of indomethacin. *J. Am. Med. Assoc.*, **199**, 932.

*Jacobs, J.H. (1965) in *Recenti Acquisizione nella Terapia Antirheumatica Non Steroidea*, Minerva Medica, Milan, pp. 73–81.

Jaffe, G. (1976) A double-blind, multi-centre comparison of naproxen and indomethacin in acute musculo-skeletal disorders. *Curr. Med. Res. Op.*, **4**, 373.

Jeremy R. and Towson, J. (1970) Interaction between aspirin and indomethacin in the treatment of rheumatoid arthritis. *Med. J. Austr.*, ii, 127.

*Kinsella, T.D., MacKenzie, K.R., Kim, S.O. and Johnson, L.G. (1967) Evaluation of indomethacin by a controlled, crossover technique in 30 patients with ankylosing spondylitis. *Can. Med. Assoc. J.*, **96**, 1454.

Kunze, M., Stein, G., Kunze, E. and Traeger, A. (1974) The

pharmacokinetics of indomethacin in relation to age in patients with occlusion of bile ducts, with reduced renal function and with signs of intolerance. *Dtsche Gesundkeitswesen*, **29**, 351.

Kwan, K.C., Breault, G.C., Umbenhauer, E.R. *et al.* (1976) Kinetics of indomethacin absorption, elimination, and enterohepatic circulation in man. *J. Pharmacokinetics Biopharmaceutics*, **4**, 255.

*Marcolongo, R. (1976) in *Inflammatory Arthropathies* (eds E.C. Huskisson and G.P. Velo), pp. 207–23. Excerpta Medica, Amsterdam.

*Marion, W.F. van (1973) Indomethacin in the treatment of soft tissue lesions: a double-blind study against placebo. *J. Intl. Med. Res.*, **1**, 151.

Murthy, M.H.V., Rhymer, A.R. and Wright, V. (1978) Indomethacin or prednisolone at night in rheumatoid arthritis? *Rheumatol. Rehabil.*, **17**, 8.

Palmer, L., Bertilsson, L., Alvan, G. *et al.* (1974) in *Prostaglandin Synthetase Inhibitors* (eds H. Robinson and J.R. Vane), Raven Press, New York, pp. 91–7.

*Patterson, J.H., Tyston, W.R. and Gey, B.B. (1971) in *Eighth International Congress of Pediatrics*, Feilhaur, Neunkirechen, Austria, pp. 175–82.

*Perkins, E.S. and MacFaul, P.A. (1965) Indomethacin in the treatment of uveitis. A double-blind trial. *Trans. Ophthalmol. Soc. UK*, **85**, 53.

Rane, A., Oelz, O., Frolich, J.C. *et al.* (1978) Relation between plasma concentration of indomethacin and its effect on prostaglandin synthesis and platelet aggregation in man. *Clin. Pharmacol. Ther.*, **23**, 658.

Rhymer, A.R. and Gengos, D.C. (1979) in *Clin. Rheum. Dis.* Vol. 5, No. 2, (ed. E.C. Huskisson). Saunders, London, p. 541.

Robinson, D.R. and Levine, L. (1974) in *Prostaglandin Synthetase Inhibitors* (eds H.J. Robinson and J.R. Vane), Raven Press, New York, pp. 223–8.

*Roth, S.H. and Englund, D.W. (1967) Indomethacin in the treatment of juvenile rheumatoid arthritis. *Arthr. Rheum.*, **10**, 307.

Rothermich, N.O. (1966) An extended study of indomethacin: 1. Clinical Pharmacology. *J. Am. Med. Assoc.*, **195**, 531.

*Sänger, L., Stoeber, E. and Kölle, G. (1967) Long term therapy with indomethacin in juvenile rheumatoid arthritis and Still's disease. *Arzneimittelforschschrift*, **17**, 1414.

Sharma, J.N., Zeitlin, I.T., Brooks, P.M. and Dick, W.C. (1976) A novel relationship between plasma kininogen and rheumatoid arthritis. *Agents and Actions*, **6**, 148.

Sicuteri, F., Michelacci, S. and Anselmi, B. (1964) Characterisation of vasoconstrictor and antimigraine properties of indomethacin, a new anti-inflammatory drug derived from indole. *Settimeina Med.*, **52**, 335.

Smyth, C.J. and Percy, J.S. (1973) Comparison of phenylbutazone and indomethacin in acute gout. *Ann. Rheum. Dis.*, **32**, 351.

Solomon, L. (1966) Activation of latent infection by indomethacin: a report of three cases. *Br. Med. J.*, **iv**, 961.

Stanford, N., Roth, G.J., Shen, T.Y. and Majerus, P.W. (1977) Lack of covalent modification of prostaglandin synthetase (cyclooxygenase) by indomethacin. *Prostaglandins*, **13**, 669.

Tan, S.Y. and Mulrow, P.J. (1977) Inhibition of the renin-aldosterone response to furosemide by indomethacin. *J. Clin. Endocrinol. Metab.*, **45**, 174.

Taylor, R.T., Huskisson, E.L., Whitehouse, G.H., *et al.* (1968) Gastric ulceration occurring during indomethacin. *Br. Med. J.*, **iv**, 734.

Vecchio, C., Fontana, A. and Tavazzi, L. (1964) Effects of prolonged indomethacin administration on the gastric musoca of the rat. *Reumatismo*, **16**, 404.

Vessel, E.S., Passananti, G.T. and Johnson, A.O. (1975) Failure of indomethacin and warfarin to interact in normal human volunteers. *J. Clin. Pharmacol.*, **15**, 486.

Wanka, J. and Dixon, A. St. J. (1964) Treatment of osteoarthritis of the hip with indomethacin. *Ann. Rheum. Dis.*, **23**, 288.

Winter, C.A., Risley, E.A. and Nuss, G.W. (1963) Anti-inflammatory and antipyretic activities of indomethacin, 1-(p-chlorobenzoyl)-5-methoxy-2-methylindole-3-acetic acid. *J. Pharmacol. Exp. Ther.*, **141**, 369.

Wright, V. and Roberts, M. (1973) Indomethacin in the treatment of rheumatoid diseases. *Clin. Med.*, **1**, 12.

*Wright, V., Walker, W.C. and McGuire, R.J. (1969) Indomethacin in the treatment of rheumatoid arthritis. *Ann. Rheum. Dis.*, **28**, 157.

Sulindac

*Andelman, S.Y. (1977) A long-term double-blind multicenter study of Clinoril (sulindac) in the treatment of osteoarthritis. *Abstracts of the XIV International Congress of Rheumatology*, San Francisco, 1977, p. 233.

†Andrade, L. and Fernandez, A. (1976) in *Clinoril in the Treatment of Rheumatic Disorders* (eds E.C. Huskisson and P. Franchimont), Raven Press, New York, pp. 49–58.

*Ballabio, C.B., Gigante, D., Pipitone, V. *et al.* (1976) in *Clinoril in the Treatment of Rheumatic Disorders* (eds E.C. Huskisson and P. Franchimont,), Raven Press, New York, pp. 87–98.

*Bernett, P., Prokscha, G.W. and Braun, H.D. (1976) in *Clinoril in the Treatment of Rheumatic Disorders* (eds E.C. Huskisson and P. Franchimont), Raven Press. New York pp. 141–50.

*Bordier, Ph. and Kuntz, D. (1978) Sulindac: Clinical results of treatment of osteoarthritis. *Eur. J. Rheumatol. Infl.*, **1**, 27.

*Borrachero del Campo, J. (1978) Comparative double-blind and open studies of sulindac and acetylsalicylic acid in the treatment of rheumatoid arthritis. *Eur. J. Rheumatol. Infl.*, **1**, 16.

Bower, R.J. and Damiano, R.E. (1977a) Human tolerability of sulindac. *Abstracts of the XIV International Congress of Rheumatology*, San Francisco, 1977, p. 254.

Bower, R.J. and Damiano, R.E. (1977b) Human tolerability of sulindac. *A paper presented at XIV International Congress of Rheumatology*, San Francisco, 1977, p. 254.

*Britton, M., Calin, J. and Calin, A. (1977) Objective criteria in the assessment of ankylosing spondylitis, exemplified by a six-month double-blind parallel trial of sulindac and indomethacin. *Abstracts of the XIV International Congress of Rheumatology*, San Francisco, 1977, p. 254.

*Calabro, J.J. (1978) Sulindac in the treatment of gout: multicenter studies. *Eur. J. Rheumatol. Inf.*, **1**, 21.

*Calabro, J.J., Khoury, M.I. and Smyth, C.J. (1976) Clinoril in acute gout. *Acta Rheumatol. Port*, **11**, 163.

*Chahade, W.H. and Federico, W.A. (1976) in *Clinoril in the Treatment of Rheumatic Disorders* (eds E.C. Huskisson and P. Franchimont), Raven Press, New York, pp. 69–76.

*Ciocci, A. (1978) Sulindac in the treatment of rheumatic arthritis. *Eur. J. Rheumatol. Infl.*, **1**, 55.

*Cohen, A. (1976) Intestinal blood loss after a new anti-inflammatory drug, sulindac. *Clin. Pharmacol. Ther.*, **20**, 238.

*Demetriades, P., Seitanides, B., Vezyroglou, G. *et al.* (1976) in *Clinoril in the Treatment of Rheumatic Disorders* (eds E.C. Huskisson and P. Franchimont), Raven Press, New York, pp. 37–48.

*Diamond, H.S., Bankhurst, A.D., Wilkens, R.F. *et al.* (1977) Sulindac in the treatment of acute gout. *Abstracts of XIV International Congress of Rheumatology*, San Francisco, 1977, p. 255.

*Dieppe, P.A., Burry, H.C., Grahame, R. and Perera, T. (1976), Sulindac in osteoarthrosis of the hip. *Rheumatol. Rehabil.*, **15**, 112.

Duggan, D.E., Hare, L.E., Ditzler, C.A. *et al.* (1977) The disposition of sulindac. *Clin. Pharmacol. Ther.*, **21**, 326.

Editorial (1977) Sulindac. *Lancet*, **i**, 462.

*Fasching, M. and Eberl, R. (1976) Sulindac: clinical test of a new anti-inflammatory agent in rheumatoid arthritis. *Wiener Klin. Wochenschr.*, **88** (Suppl. 3), 59.

*Gadomski, M., Singer-Bakker, H. and Braun, H.D. (1976) in *Clinoril in the Treatment of Rheumatic Disorders* (eds E.C. Huskisson and P. Franchimont), Raven Press, New York, pp. 133–9.

*Gibson, T. and Laurent, R. (1980) Sulindac and indomethacin in the treatment of ankylosing spondylitis: a double-blind cross-over study. *Rheumatol. Rehabil.*, **19**, 189.

*Gigante, D., Zorzin, L. and Carratelli, L. (1976) in *Clinoril in the Treatment of Rheumatic Disorders* (eds E.C. Huskisson and P. Franchimont), Raven Press, New York, pp. 151–9.

*Highton, T.C. and Jeremy, R. (1976) in *Clinoril in the Treatment of Rheumatic Disorders* (eds E.C. Huskisson and P. Franchimont), Raven Press, New York, pp. 99–112.

†Huskisson, E.C. (1976) Experience with sulindac in rheumatoid and osteoarthritis. *Eur. J. Rheumatol. Infl.*, **1**, 12.

Huskisson, E.C. (1978) Sulindac. *Eur. J. Rheumatol. Infl.*, **1**, 3.

Huskisson, E.C. and Scott, J. (1978) Sulindac. Trials of a new anti-inflammatory drug. *Ann. Rheum. Dis.*, **37**, 89.

*Ingberg, L. and Holopainen, O. (1976) in *Clinoril in the Treatment of Rheumatic Disorders* (eds E.C. Huskisson and P. Franchimont), Raven Press, New York, pp. 59–68.

Kwan, K.C. and Duggan, D.E. (1977) Pharmacokinetics of sulindac. *Acta Rheumatol. Belg.*, **1**, 168.

Kwan, K.C., Duggan, D.E., Van Arman, E.G. and Shen, T.Y. (1978) Sulindac: chemistry, pharmacology and pharmacokinetics. *Eur. J. Rheumatol. Infl.*, **1**, 9.

Liebling, M.R., Altman, R.D., Benedek, T.G. *et al.* (1975) A double-blind, multiclinic trial of sulindac (MK-231) in the treatment of ankylosing spondylitis. *Arthr. Rheum.*, **18**, 411 (Abstract).

*Mavrikakis, M.E., Madkour, M.M., Spencer, D.M. and Balint, G.P. (1977) Double-blind study comparing the therapeutic effect of a new non-steroidal, anti-inflammatory drug, sulindac, with benorylate in tablet form in rheumatoid arthritis. *Pharmatherapeutica*, **1**, 681.

*Mowat, A.M., Mowat, A.G., Wojtulewski, J.A. *et al.* (1977) Sulindac in ankylosing spondylitis. *Abstracts of the XIV International Congress of Rheumatology*, San Francisco, 1977, p. 253.

*Nahir, A.M. and Scharf, Y. (1980) A comparative study of diclofenac and sulindac in ankylosing spondylitis. *Rheumatol. Rehabil.*, **19**, 193.

*Nissila, M. and Koota, K. (1976) in *Clinoril in the Treatment of Rheumatic Disorders* (eds E.C. Huskisson and P. Franchimont), Raven Press, New York, pp. 113–22.

Oyemade, G.A.A. and Onadeko, B.O. (1979) A controlled clinical study comparing sulindac with ibuprofen and aspirin in the treatment of musculo-skeletal diseases. *J. Intl. Med. Res.*, **7**, 556.

*Pingeon, R.A., Harman, R.E., Walford, L.G. and Daurio, C.P. (1977) Sulindac in rheumatoid arthritis. *Abstracts of the XIV International Congress of Rheumatology*, San Francisco, 1977, p. 256.

Porro, G.B., Petrillo, M., Fumagalli, M. and Carratelli, L. (1978) Endoscopic evaluation of the effects of a new anti-inflammatory drug, sulindac, on the gastric mucosa. *Eur. J. Rheumatol. Infl.*, **1**, 34.

*Reynolds, P.M.G., Rhymer, A.R., MacLeod, M.M. and Buchanan, W.W. (1977) Comparison of sulindac and aspirin in rheumatoid arthritis. *Curr. Med. Res. Op.*, **4**, 485.

Rhymer, A.R. (1979) in *Clinics in Rheumatic Diseases: Anti-Rheumatic Drugs* (ed. E.C. Huskisson), Vol. 5, No. 2, Saunders, London, p. 553.

Rooney, P., Buchanan, W.W., Haigh, B.S., Roylance, P.J. and Rhymer, A.R. (1978) A clinical assessment in general practice of sulindac. *Eur. J. Rheumatol. Infl.*, **1**, 66.

Ryan, J.R., Jain, A.K., McMahon, F.G. and Vargas, R. (1977) On the question of an interaction between sulindac and tolbutamide in the control of diabetes. *Clin. Pharmacol. Ther.*, **21**, 231.

Shams-Eldeen, M.A., Vallner, J.J. and Needham, T.E. (1978) Interaction of sulindac and metabolite with human serum albumin. *J. Pharm. Sci.*, **67**, 1077.

Sharma, B.K. and Haslock, I. (1978) Night medication in rheumatoid arthritis. III. The use of sulindac. *Curr. Med. Res. Op.*, **5**, 472.

Shen, T.Y. (1976) in *Clinoril in the Treatment of Rheumatic Disorders* (eds E.C. Huskisson and P. Franchimont), Raven Press, New York, pp. 1–8.

*Simon, F., de Gery, A., Mankes, C.J. and Delbarre, F. (1976) in *Clinoril in the Treatment of Rheumatic Disorders* (eds E.C. Huskisson and P. Franchimont), Raven Press, New York, pp. 77–86.

Van Arman, C.G., Risley, E.A., Nuss, G.W. *et al.* (1976) in *Clinoril in the Treatment of Rheumatic Disorders* (eds E.C. Huskisson and P. Franchimont), Raven Press, New York, pp. 9–36.

*Villiaumey, J. and Di Menza, C. (1976) in *Clinoril in the Treatment of Rheumatic Disorders* (eds E.C. Huskisson and P. Franchimont), Raven Press, New York, pp. 161–5.

*Worthington, W.W. (1976) in *Clinoril in the Treatment of Rheumatic Disorders* (eds E.C. Huskisson and P. Franchimont), Raven Press, New York, pp. 167–73.

*Zollner, N., Adam, O. and Wolfram, G. (1976) in *Clinoril in the Treatment of Rheumatic Disorders* (eds E.C. Huskisson and P. Franchimont), Raven Press, New York, pp. 175–81.

Tolmetin

†April, P., Albert, M., Deighton, M.N. and Termulo, C. (1975) in *Tolmetin, a New Non-Steroidal Anti-inflammatory Agent* (ed. J.R. Ward), Excerpta Medica, Princeton, pp. 47–56.

*Aylward, M., Holly, F., Maddock, J. and Wheeldon, R. (1977) Treatment of rheumatoid arthritis with tolmetin: a comparison with alclofenac. *Curr. Med. Res. Op.*, **4**, 695.

*Aylward, M., Maddock, J., Parker, R.J. *et al.* (1976) Evaluation of tolmetin in the treatment of active chronic rheumatoid arthritis: open and controlled double-blind studies. *Curr. Med. Res. Op.*, **4**, 158.

*Bachmann, F., Stroescu, D. and Hartl, W. (1975) Double-blind and dose range studies with Tolectin in rheumatoid arthritis. *Zeitschr. für Allgemeinmedizin*, **30**, 1382.

*Bain, L.S., El-Ghobarey, A.R., Collins, R.M. and Sargent, N.W. (1975) Tolmetin: an evaluation of a new preparation in the treatment of rheumatoid arthritis. *Br. J. Clin. Pract.*, **29**, 208.

Beirne, J.A., Bianchine, J.R., Johnson, P.C. and Wartham, G.P. (1974) Gastrointestinal blood loss caused by tolmetin aspirin and indomethacin. *Clin. Pharmacol. Ther.*, **16**, 821.

*Berkowitz, S., Bernhard, G., Bilka, P.J. *et al.* (1974) Tolmetin versus placebo for the treatment of rheumatoid arthritis: a sequential double-blind clinical trial. *Curr. Ther. Res. – Clin. Exp.*, **16**, 442.

*Bernhard, G.C., Poiley, J. and Tarpley, E.L. (1975) in *Tolmetin, a New Non-Steroidal Anti-inflammatory Agent* (ed. J.R. Ward), Excerpta Medica, Princeton, pp. 108–18.

*Brewer, E.J., Baum, J., Fink, C. *et al.* (1975) A multi-clinic open study of tolmetin in the treatment of juvenile rheumatoid arthritis. *Scand. J. Rheumatol.*, **4**, 11.

Brogden, R.N., Heel, T.M., Speight, T.M. and Avery, G.S. (1978) Tolmetin: a review of its pharmacological properties and therapeutic efficacy in rheumatic disease. *Drugs*, **15**, 429.

*Brown, J.H., Hull, J. and Biundo, J.J. (1975) Results of a one-year trial of tolmetin in patients with rheumatoid arthritis. *J. Clin. Pharmacol.*, **15**, 455.

Caldwell, J., Brandon, M.L., Franz, K.H. *et al.* (1975) in *Tolmetin, a New Non-Steroidal Anti-Inflammatory Agent* (ed. J.R. Ward), Excerpta Medica, Princeton, pp. 57–70.

*Cardoe, N. and Steele, C.E. (1977) A double-blind crossover comparison of tolmetin sodium and phenylbutazone in the treatment of rheumatoid arthritis. *Curr. Med. Res. Op.*, **4**, 688.

Cordrey, L.J. (1976) Tolmetin sodium, a new anti-arthritis drug: double-blind and long-term studies. *J. Am. Ger. Soc.*, **24**, 440.

Cressman, W.A., Wortham, G.F. and Plostnieks, J. (1976) Absorption and excretion of tolmetin in man. *Clin. Pharmacol. Ther.*, **19**, 224.

Ehrlich, G.E. (1979) in *Clinics in Rheumatic Diseases. Anti-Rheumatic Drugs* (ed. E.C. Huskisson), Vol. 5, No. 2, Saunders, London, p. 481.

*Ehrlich, G.E., Hobbs, T.R., Cordrey, L.J. and Hamaty, D. (1975) in *Tolmetin a New Non-Steroidal Anti-Inflammatory Agent* (ed. J.R. Ward), Excerpta Medica, Princeton, pp. 71–87.

*Ehrlich, G.E. and Roth, S. (1976) Rheumatoid arthritis: long-term therapy with tolmetin sodium. *Orth. Dig.*, **4**, 16.

Ehrlich, G.E. and Wortham, G.F. (1975) Pseudoproteinuria in tolmetin-treated patients. *Clin. Pharmacol. Ther.*, **17**, 467.

Huskisson, E.C., Berry, H., Scott, J. and Balme, H.W. (1974) Tolectin for rheumatoid arthritis. *Rheumatol. Rehabil.*, **13**, 132.

*Jentsch, D.D. (1973) Tolectin treatment of rheumatoid arthritis and gout. *Excerpta Medica Intl. Congress Ser.*, **299**, 114.

*Klemp, P. and Meyers, D.L. (1970) Clinical trial of tolmetin and aspirin in the treatment of rheumatoid arthritis. *S. Afr. Med. J.*, **52**, 167.

Mielke, C.H., Heiden, D. and Amadio, P. (1975) in *Tolmetin, a New Non-Steroidal Anti-Inflammatory Agent* (ed. J.R. Ward), Excerpta Medica, Princeton, pp. 174–82.

*Muller, F.O., Goslin, J.A. and Erdmann, G.H. (1977) A comparison of tolmetin with aspirin in the treatment of osteo-arthritis of the knee. *S. Afr. Med. J.*, **51**, 794.

Pavelka, K. and Susta, A. (1974) Tolmetin, a new non-steroidal antirheumatic. *Arzneimittelforschung*, **24**, 1353.

Plostnieks, J., Cressman, W.A., Lemanowicz, E.F. *et al.* (1975) in *Tolmetin, a New Non-Steroidal Anti-Inflammatory Agent* (ed. J.R. Ward), Excerpta Medica, Princeton, pp. 23–33.

*Rau, R., Lobsiger, M. and Gross, D. (1975) Tolmetin treatment in patients with osteoarthritis of the hip and the knee. *Scand. J. Rheumatol.*, **4**, 510.

*Rau, R., Lobsiger, M. and Gross, D. (1977) Treatment of severe osteoarthrosis of the knee and the hip with tolmetin. (A double-blind comparison with indomethacin). *Praxis*, **66**, 147.

*Robinson, H., Abruzzo, J.L., Miyara, A. and Ward, J.R. (1975) in *Tolmetin, a New Non-Steroidal Anti-Inflammatory Agent* (ed. J.R. Ward), Excerpta Medica, Princeton, pp. 88–97.

*Roth, S.H. and Simson, J. (1975) in *Tolmetin, a New Non-Steroidal Anti-Inflammatory Agent* (ed. J.R. Ward), Excerpta Medica, Princeton, pp. 119–33.

*Schattenkirchner, M., Schattenkirchner, U. and Muller-Fassbender, H. (1977) Clinical experience with Tolectin in the long-term treatment of ankylosing spondylitis. *Therapiewoche*, **27**, 2298.

*Schneyer, J. (1974) Tolmetin *versus* aspirin in the treatment of rheumatoid arthritis, a controlled double-blind study. *J. Rheumatol.*, **1** (Suppl. 1), 60.

Selley, M.L., Glass, J., Triggs, E.J. and Thomas, J. (1975) Pharmacokinetics studies of tolmetin in man. *Clin. Pharmacol. Ther.*, **17**, 599.

*Setoyama, M., Nagase, A., Nishijima, Y. *et al.* (1979) Analgesic effect of tolmetin in surgical patients. *Basic Pharmacol. Ther.*, **4**, 193.

Whitsett, T.L., Barry, J.P., Czerwinski, A.W., Hall, W.H. and Hampton, J.W. (1975) in *Tolmetin, a New Non-Steroidal Anti-Inflammatory Agent* (ed. J.R. Ward), Excerpta Medica, Princeton, pp. 134–41.

Wong, S. (1975) in *Tolmetin, a New Non-Steroidal Anti-Inflammatory Agent* (ed. J.R. Ward), Excerpta Medica, Princeton, pp. 1–22.

Wong, S., Gardocki, J.F. and Priss, T.P. (1973) Pharmacologic evaluation of Tolectin (tolmetin, McN 2559) and McN2981, two anti-inflammatory agents. *J. Pharmacol. Exp. Ther.*, **185**, 127.

Phenylacetic acids

Diclofenac

*Abrams, G.J., Solomon, L. and Meyers, O.L. (1978) A long-term study of diclofenac sodium (Voltaren) in the treatment of patients with rheumatoid arthritis or osteoarthritis. *S. Afr. Med. J.*, **53**, 442.

Aylward, M., Fowler, P.D., John, V., Maddock, J. and Seldrup, J. (1979) The influence of diclofenac sodium

(Voltarol) on free, protein-bound and total plasma L-tryptophan in adult healthy male subjects. *Rheumatol. Rehabil.* (Suppl. 2), 47.

Bach, G.L. (1979) Comparative clinical trials with diclofenac sodium (Voltarol) and naproxen in rheumatic conditions: investigation of possible changes in diclofenac dose and dose interval. *Rheumatol. Rehabil.* (Suppl. 2), 69.

†Barnes, C.G., Berry, H., Carter, M.E. *et al.* (1979) Diclofenac sodium (Voltarol) and indomethacin: a multicentre comparative study in rheumatoid arthritis and osteoarthritis. *Rheumatol. Rehabil.* (Suppl. 2), 144.

*Bijlsma, A. (1977) Voltaren bij reumatoide artritis. *Reuma Wereldwijd*, **1**, 4.

*Bijlsma, A. (1978) The long-term efficacy and tolerability of Voltaren (diclofenac sodium) and indomethacin in rheumatoid arthritis. *Scand. J. Rheumatol.*, **22** (Suppl.), 74.

Bonomo, I. (1979) Critical analysis of the Brazilian literature on diclofenac sodium (Voltarol). *Rheumatol. Rehabil.* (Suppl. 2), 72.

*Cardoe, N. (1979) Diclofenac sodium (Voltarol): a double-blind comparative study with ibuprofen in patients with rheumatoid arthritis. *Rheumatol. Rehabil.* (Suppl. 2), 89.

Ciccolunghi, S.N. and Chaudri, H.A. (1976) in *Chronic Forms of Polyarthritis*. International Symposium, Torremolinos, March 1975 (ed. F.J. Wagenhäuser), Huber, Bern, p. 345.

Ciccolunghi, S.N., Chaudri, H.A. and Schubiger, B.I. (1977) Long-term trials in rheumatic conditions – a series of compromises. *EULAR Bull. Monogr.*, **1**, 135.

Ciccolunghi, S.N., Chaudri, H.A. and Schubiger, B.I. (1979a) The value and results of long-term studies with diclofenac sodium (Voltarol). *Rheumatol. Rehabil.* (Suppl. 2), 100.

Ciccolunghi, S.N., Chaudri, H.A., Schubiger, B.I. and Reddrop, R. (1978) Report on a long-term tolerability study of up to two years with diclofenac sodium (Voltaren). *Scand. J. Rheumatol.* (Suppl. 22), 86.

Ciccolunghi, S.N., Levi, B. and Chaudri, H.A. (1975) Klinische Erfahrungen mit Voltaren, einem neuen micht-steroiden Antirheumatikum. *Wienen Med. Wochenschr.*, **125**, 66.

Ciccolunghi, S.N., Schubiger, B.I. and Reddrop, R. (1979b) Comparison of tolerability findings in international clinical trials. *Rheumatol. Rehabil.* (Suppl. 2), 122.

Ciccolunghi, S.N., Schubiger, B.I. and Walker, A.N. (1976) Summary of international experience in Voltaren in clinical trials. *Proceedings III Congress, South East Asia and Pacific Area*, Singapore, 1976 (ed. R. Robinson), Hans Huber, Bern, p. 17–31.

Ciucci, A.G. (1979) A review of spontaneously reported adverse drug reactions with diclofenac sodium (Voltarol). *Rheumatol. Rehabil.* (Suppl. 2), 116.

*Doreen, M.S., Boardman, P.L., Fowler, P.D. and Poole, P.H. (1979) Diclofenac sodium (Voltarol) in rheumatoid arthritis. A report of a double-blind trial. *Rheumatol. Rehabil.* (Suppl. 2), 78.

Fowler, P.D. (1979a) Diclofenac sodium (Voltarol): drug interactions and special studies. *Rheumatol. Rehabil.* (Suppl. 2), 60.

*Fowler, P.D. (1979b) A double-blind comparison of diclofenac sodium (Voltarol) and placebo in inpatients with rheumatoid arthritis. *Rheumatol. Rehabil.* (Suppl. 2), 75.

Fowler, P.D. (1979) in *Clinics in Rheumatic Diseases: Anti-Rheumatic Drugs* (ed. E.C. Huskisson), Vol. 5, No. 2,

Saunders, London, p. 427.

*Ghazi, S.A. and Fowler, P.D. (1973) A clinical trial of a new anti-inflammatory/analgesic compound in rheumatoid arthritis – GP45, 840. *J. Intl. Med. Res.*, **1**, 591.

Haslock, I., Eade, A. and Woolf, D. (eds) (1979), Diclofenac (Voltarol) in the treatment of rheumatic diseases: a conspectus of international experience. *Rheumatol. Rehabil.* (Suppl. 2).

John, V.A. (1979), The pharmacokinetics and metabolism of diclofenac sodium (Voltarol) in animals and man. *Rheumatol. Rehabil.* (Suppl. 2), 22.

Kendall, M.J., Thornhill, D.P. and Willis, J.V. (1979) Factors affecting the pharmacokinetics of diclofenac sodium (Voltarol). *Rheumatol. Rehabil.* (Suppl. 2), 38.

*Kirchheiner, B. Trang, L. and Wollheim, F.A. (1976) Diclofenac sodium (Voltaren) in rheumatoid arthritis. A double-blind comparison with indomethacin and placebo. *Intl. J. Clin. Pharmacol.*, **13**, 292.

Krupp, P.J., Nenasse-Gdynia, R., Sallmann, A. *et al.* (1973) Sodium [0-[(2, 6-dichlorophenyl)-amino]-phenyl]-acetate (GP45,840), a new non-steroidal anti-inflammatory agent. *Experientia* (Basle), **29**, 450.

Lehtola, J. and Sipponen, P. (1977) A gastroscopic and histological double-blind study of the effects of diclofenac sodium and naproxen on the human gastric mucosa. *Scand. J. Rheumatol.*, **6**, 97.

Maier, R., Menassé, R., Riesterer, L. *et al.* (1979) The pharmacology of diclofenac sodium (Voltarol). *Rheumatol. Rehabil.* (Suppl. 2), 11.

McMahon, M.F. (1979) An open assessment of the efficacy and tolerability of diclofenac sodium (Voltarol) in patients with rheumatic disease and a comparative study of diclofenac sodium (Voltarol) with indomethacin in patients with osteoarthritis and rheumatoid arthritis. *Rheumatol. Rehabil.* (Suppl. 2), 81.

Michot, F., Ajdacic, K. and Glaus, L. (1975) A double-blind clinical trial to determine if an interaction exists between diclofenac sodium and the oral anticoagulant acenoconmarol (Nico-amolone). *J. Intl. Med. Res.*, **3**, 153.

†Mohing, W. (1976) in *Voltaren, a New Non-Steroidal Antirheumatic Agent (Diclofenac)*. Proceedings of the VIIIth Symposium of the European Rheumatology Congress, Helsinki, 1975 (ed. F.J. Wagenhäuser), Huber, Bern, p. 40.

Miura, T. (1975) Long-term tolerability study of Voltaren. *J. Intl. Med. Res.*, **3**, 145.

*Pinheiro, G.C., Gouveia, O.S., Moreira Filho, J.M.L. *et al.* (1975) Clinical trial in osteoarthritis comparing Voltaren (GP45,840) with indomethacin. *Folha Médica*, **71**, 341.

*Rossi, F.A. and Baroni, L. (1975) A double-blind comparison between diclofenac sodium and ibuprofen in osteoarthritis. *J. Intl. Med. Res.*, **3**, 267.

*Sacks, S. (1974) Diclofenac sodium in rheumatoid arthritis and osteoarthritis. *S. Afr. Med. J.*, **48**, 213.

Sallmann, A. (1979) The chemistry of diclofenac sodium (Voltarol). *Rheumatol. Rehabil.* (Suppl. 2), 4.

*Schubiger, B.I., Ciccolunghi, S.N. and Tanner, K. (1980) Once daily dose treatment with a non-steroidal anti-rheumatic drug (diclofenac) in osteoarthritis. *J. Intl. Med. Res.*, **8**, 167.

*Seda, H. and Cardoza, P.C. (1976) Eficácia e tolerabilidade do diclofenac sódico versus ibuprofen en portadores de osteoartrose. *Folha médica*, **72**, 633.

†Shiokawa, Y., Takatori, M., Sakuma, A. (1972) Multicentre trial of Voltaren (GP45,840) on rheumatoid arthritis by double-blind technique. *J. Jap. Rheumatol. Assoc.*, **12**, 271.

*Siegmeth, W. and Placheta, P. (1978) Langzeit vergleichsstudie: Diclofenac (Voltaren) und Naproxen (Proxen) bei Arltrosen. *Schweizerische Med. Wochenschr.*, **108**, 349.

Szezeklik, A., Gryglewski, R.J., Czerniawska-Mysik, G. and Pieton, R. (1977) Asthmatic attacks induced in aspirin sensitive patients by diclofenac and naproxen. *Br. Med. J.*, **2**, 231.

Uthgenannt, H. and Timm, H. (1975) The effect of Voltarol(R) on the gastro-intestinal excretion of blood. *Munchener Med. Wozhenschr.*, **117**, 1987.

Von Manz, G. and Franke M. (1977), Diclofenac-Na bei ankylosierender Spondylitis. *Fortschritt der Medizin*, **95**, 1706.

Wagenhäuser, F.J. (ed.) (1976) Voltaren – a new, non-steroid antirheumatic agent (diclofenac). *Proceedings of a Symposium held during the VIIIth European Rheumatology Congress*, Helsinki, 1975. Huber, Bern.

*Wagenhäuser, F.J. and Narozna, H. (1975) Behandlung der Arthrose mit einem neuem micht-steroiden Antirheumatikum (Voltaren). *Schweizerische Med. Wochenschr.*, **105**, 652.

Fenclofenac

*Akyol, M.S., Anderson, M. and Thompson, M. (1977) Fenclofenac in the treatment of rheumatoid arthritis and ankylosing spondylitis. *Proc. R. Soc. Med.*, **70** (Suppl. 6), 37.

*Ansell, B.M., Peskett, S., Hazleman, B. *et al.* (1930) Fenclofenac in juvenile chronic arthritis. *R. Soc. Med. Intl. Congr. Symp. Ser.*, No. 28, 53.

Atkinson, D.C. and Leach, E.C. (1976) Anti-inflammatory and related properties of 2-(2, 4-dichlorophenoxy) phenylacetic acid (fenclofenac). *Agents and Actions*, **6**, 657.

Atkinson, D.C. and Leach, E.C. (1978) Effects of fenclofenac on prostaglandin production in carragenin air bleb exudates in rats. *Agents and Actions*, **8**, 263.

Atkinson, D.C., Godfrey, K.E., Jordan, B.J. *et al.* (1974) 2-(2, 4-dichlorophenoxy) phenylacetic acid (fenclofenac): one of a novel series of anti-inflammatory compounds with low ulcerogenic potential. *J. Pharm. Pharmacol.*, **26**, 357.

Atkinson, D.C. Green, D. and Leach, E.C. (1977) Pharmacology and toxicology of fenclofenac. *Proc. R. Soc. Med.*, **70**, (Suppl. 6), 1.

*Aylward, M., Bater, P.A., Davies, D.E. *et al.* (1980) Interim report on the results from a double-blind, controlled therapeutic evaluation of fenclofenac and indomethacin in the extended treatment of patients with active rheumatoid disease. *R. Soc. Med. Intl. Congr. Symp. Ser.*, No. 28, 101.

*Bachmann, P. (1980) Fenclofenac and indomethacin in rheumatoid arthritis: a double-blind cross-over comparison. *R. Soc. Med. Intl. Congr. Symp. Ser.*, No. 28, 31.

Bacon, P.A., Davies, J. and Ring, E.F.J. (1977) The use of quantitative thermography to assess the anti-inflammatory dose range for fenclofenac. *Proc. R. Soc. Med.*, **70** (Suppl. 6), 18.

*Bird, H.A., Rhind, V.M., Leatham, P.A. and Wright, V. (1980) A comparative study of fenclofenac and fenoprofen in osteoarthrosis. *R. Soc. Med. Intl. Congr. Symp. Ser.*, No. 28, 23.

*Camp, A.V., Berry, H., Heywood, D. *et al.* (1980) A trial of fenclofenac, D-penicillamine and placebo in rheumatoid arthritis. *R. Soc. Med. Intl. Congress Symp. Ser.*, No. 28, 95.

Cardoe, N. (1977) Side-effects of fenclofenac with special reference to the gastrointestinal tract. *Proc. R. Soc. Med.*, **70** (Suppl. 6), 51.

*Crean, D.M. (1980) The add-on value of fenclofenac and ibuprofen in the treatment of actively-managed soft-tissue injury. *R. Soc. Med. Intl. Congr. Symp. Ser.*, No. 28, 41.

*Davies, J.E., Billings, R.A., Burry, H.C. *et al.* (1977) Fenclofenac in osteoarthrosis. *Proc. R. Soc. Med.*, **70** (Suppl. 6), 34.

*Essigman, W.K. (1980) Fenclofenac in osteoarthrosis. *R. Soc. Med. Intl. Congr. Symp. Ser.*, No. 28, 1.

Garner, A. (1977) Assessment of gastric mucosal damage: comparative effects of aspirin and fenclofenac on the gastric mucosa of the guinea-pig. *Toxicol. Appl. Pharmacol.*, **42**, 477.

Glick, E.N. (1977) Preliminary clinical evaluation of fenclofenac (32 patients). *Proc. R. Soc. Med.*, **70** (Suppl. 6), 43.

Glick, E.N. and Loebl, W.Y. (1980) Fenclofenac – a trial of single versus divided dosage. *R. Soc. Med. Intl. Congr. Symp. Ser.*, No. 28, 49.

Goldberg, A.A.J., Smith, R.B., Tudor, R. and Clarke, D.R. (1975) Fenclofenac: methodological considerations in the design and implementation of phase II studies. *Scand. J. Rheumatol.*, **6** (Suppl. 8), 71.

Goldberg, A.A.J. and Tudor, R. (eds) (1977) A seminar on fenclofenac. *Proc. R. Soc. Med.*, **70** (Suppl. 6), 1.

*Goode, J.D. (1980) Long-term use of fenclofenac in rheumatoid arthritis. *R. Soc. Med. Intl. Congr. Symp. Ser.*, No. 28, 57.

*Haslock, I. and Laycock, T. (1980) A comparison of fenclofenac and aspirin in the treatment of rheumatoid arthritis: preliminary results. *R. Soc. Med. Intl. Congr. Symp. Ser.*, No. 28, 13.

†Hill, H.F.H. and Hill, A.G.S. (1977) Fenclofenac and soluble aspirin in rheumatoid arthritis: a comparative trial. *Proc. R. Soc. Med.*, **70** (Suppl. 6), 27.

Hingorani, K. (1977) Fenclofenac therapy in rheumatic disease. *Proc. R. Soc. Med.*, **70** (Suppl. 6), 40.

Humphrey, M.J., Capper, S.J. and Kurtz, A.B. (1980) Fenclofenac and thyroid hormone concentrations. *Lancet*, **i**, 487.

Jordan, B.J. and Rance, M.J. (1974) Taurine conjugation of fenclofenac in the dog. *J. Pharm. Pharmacol.*, **26**, 359.

*Kadir, N. and Grayson, M.F. (1980) Fenclofenac compared with Distalgesic in cervical spondylosis: a short-term trial using a new neck goniometer. *R. Soc. Med. Intl. Congr. Symp. Ser.*, No. 28, 35.

Lambert, J.R. and Wright, V. (1977) Therapeutic dose range of fenclofenac. *Proc. R. Soc. Med.*, **70** (Suppl. 6), 16.

*Lipani, J.A. (1980) The efficacy and safety of fenclofenac in the treatment of rheumatoid arthritis. *R. Soc. Med. Intl. Congr. Symp. Ser.*, No. 28, 67.

*Loebl, W.H. (1977) Fenclofenac in rheumatoid arthritis – comparative studies. *Proc. R. Soc. Med.*, **70** (Suppl. 6), 31.

*McGill, P.E., Ferguson, H. and Stillings, J. (1980) Fenclofenac in the treatment of rheumatoid arthritis. *R. Soc. Med. Intl. Congr. Symp. Ser.*, No. 28, 109.

Mowat, A.G. (1980) The effect of fenclofenac on neutrophil movement. *R. Soc. Med. Intl. Congr. Symp. Ser.*, No. 28, 89.

*Nicholls, A. (1980) A comparison of fenclofenac and ketoprofen in rheumatoid arthritis. *R. Soc. Med. Intl. Congr. Symp. Ser.*, No. 28, 17.

Phillips, N.C. (1980) Immuno-inflammatory pharmacology of fenclofenac: a preliminary report. *R. Soc. Med. Intl. Congr. Symp. Ser.*, No. 28, 83.

*Pritchard, M.H., Evans, P.H. and Nuki, G. (1977) Fenclofenac in rheumatoid arthritis: sequential double-blind cross-over comparisons with placebo and naproxen. *Proc. R. Soc. Med.*, **70** (Suppl. 6), 23.

Rainsford, K.D. (1977) Comparative studies of gastric ulcerogenesis by non-steroid anti-inflammatory drugs: effects of fenclofenac. *Proc. R. Soc. Med.*, **70** (Suppl. 6), 4.

Ratcliffe, W., Hazelton, R.A. and Thomson, J.A. (1980) Effect of fenclofenac on thyroid-function tests. *Lancet*, **i**, 432.

Rooney, P.J., McLeod, M., Madkour, M. and Mavrikakis, M. (1977) Studies on the anti-inflammatory effects of fenclofenac using 99-technetium joint scanning. *Proc. R. Soc. Med.*, **70** (Suppl. 6), 20.

Salmon, P.R., O'Drisoll, S.L., Fedail, S. and Jayson, M.I.V. (1977) Fenclofenac tolerance in the dyspeptic patients. *Proc. R. Soc. Med.*, **70** (Suppl. 6), 49.

Smith, R.B. (1977) Analysis of the side-effect patterns presenting during the course of a continuing long-term open study of fenclofenac. *Proc. R. Soc. Med.*, **70** (Suppl. 6), 46.

Snaith, M.L. (1980) Fenclofenac in patients with dyspepsia. *R. Soc. Med. Intl. Congr. Symp. Ser.*, No. 28, 79.

Svensen, S. (1980) An assessment of the efficacy and tolerance of fenclofenac in patients intolerant of naproxen. *R. Soc. Med. Intl. Congr. Symp. Ser.*, No. 28, 61.

Swain, M.C., Goldberg, A.A.J. and Smith, D.W. (1980) Fenclofenac: a review of drug-associated effects and their relationship to diagnosis and age. *R. Soc. Med. Intl. Congr. Symp. Ser.*, No. 28, 73.

Tudor, R., Goldberg, A.A.J. and Clarke, D.R. (1977) The methodology of the fenclofenac clinical research programme and results obtained with particular reference to the therapeutic dose range. *Proc. R. Soc. Med.*, **70** (Suppl. 6), 11.

Proprionic acids

Ibuprofen

Adams, S.S., Bough, R.G., Cliffe, E.E. *et al.* (1970) Some aspects of the pharmacology, metabolism and toxicology of ibuprofen. *Rheumatol. Rehabil.* (Suppl.), 9.

Adams, S.S., Bresloff, P. and Mason, C.G. (1975) The optical isomers of ibuprofen. *Curr. Med. Res. Op.*, **3** (Special Issue), 552.

Adams, S.S. and Buckler, J.W. (1959) in *Clinics in Rheumatic Diseases: Anti-Rheumatic Drugs* (ed. E.C. Huskisson), Vol. 5, No. 2, Saunders, London, pp. 359–80.

*Alfieri, G., Signorelli, I. and Cremoncini, C. (1975) Use of ibuprofen in obstetric and gynaecological pathology. *Curr. Med. Res. Op.*, **3** (Special Issue), 502.

*Ballabio, C.B. and Colombo, B. (1973) Controlled clinical evaluation of Brufen and indomethacin in rheumatoid arthritis with endoscopic control. *Abstracts of XIII International Congress of Rheumatology*, Kyoto, 19.

*Brackertz, B. and Busson, M. (1978) Comparative study of sulindac (Clinoril) and ibuprofen (Brufen) in osteoarthrosis. *Br. J. Clin. Pract.*, **32**, 78.

Brooks, C.D., Schlagel, C.A., Sekhar, N.C. and Sobota, J.T. (1973) Tolerance and pharmacology of ibuprofen. *Curr. Ther. Res.*, **15**, 180.

Brooks, C.D. and Ulrich, J.E. (1980) Effect of ibuprofen or aspirin on probenecid-induced uricosuria. *J. Intl. Med. Res.*, **8**, 283.

Buckler, J.W., Hall, J.E., Rees, J.A. *et al.* (1975) The tolerance and acceptability of ibuprofen ('Brufen') in the elderly patient. *Curr. Med. Res. Op.*, **3** (Special Issue), 558.

Cardoe, N. (1970) A review of long term experience with ibuprofen with special reference to gastric tolerance. *Rheumatol. Phys. Med.* (Suppl. 10), 28.

Cardoe, N. (1975) 'Brufen' in the treatment of rheumatoid disease in patients with gastric intolerance. *Curr. Med. Res. Op.*, **3** (Special Issue), 518.

*Chalmers, T.M. (1969) Clinical experience with ibuprofen in the treatment of rheumatoid arthritis. *Ann. Rheum. Dis.*, **28**, 513.

Ciobanu, V. and Zalaru, M. (1975) The activity and tolerance of ibuprofen in patients with rheumatism and associated conditions. *Curr. Med. Res. Op.*, **3** (Special Issue), 566.

Collum, L.M.T. and Bowen, D.I. (1971) Ocular side-effects of ibuprofen. *Br. J. Ophthalmol.*, **55**, 472.

*Cosh, J.A. and Ring, F.J. (1973) Thermographic evaluation of the anti-inflammatory activity of ibuprofen in rheumatoid arthritis. *Abstracts of XIII International Congress of Rheumatology*, Kyoto, p. 53.

*Cremoncini, C., Mola, V. and Alfieri, G. (1975) Use of ibuprofen as an anti-inflammatory drug in the treatment of phlebitis. *Curr. Med. Res. Op.*, **3** (Special Issue), 547.

Davies, E.F. and Avery, G.S. (1971) Ibuprofen: a review of its pharmacological properties and therapeutic efficiency in rheumatic disorders. *Drugs*, **2**, 416.

*De Blecourt, J.J. (1975) A comparative study of ibuprofen ('Brufen') and indomethacin in uncomplicated arthrosis. *Curr. Med. Res. Op.*, **3** (Special Issue), 477.

*De Carvalho, P.M. (1975) An evaluation of the anti-inflammatory effects of ibuprofen ('brufen') in osteoarthrosis of the knee using radioactive technetium (^{99m}Tc). *Curr. Med. Res. Op.*, **3**, 580.

*Dick-Smith, J.B. (1969) Ibuprofen, aspirin and placebo in the treatment of rheumatoid arthritis. *Med. J. Austr.*, **ii**, 853.

Dimitriu, C. (1975) Nephropathine in rheumatic diseases: therapeutic problems. *Curr. Med. Res. Op.*, **3** (Special Issue), 551.

*Dragomir-Naghiu, M. (1975) Algodystrophies in the upper and lower limbs treated with ibuprofen. *Curr. Med. Res. Op.*, **3** (Special Issue), 582.

*Dragomir-Naghiu, M. and Stoia, I. (1975) Ibuprofen ('Brufen') in the treatment of catarrhal and respiratory viral diseases with rheumatismal manifestations. *Curr. Med. Res. Op.*, **3** (Special Issue), 584.

Duckert, F. (1975) The absence of effect of the antirheumatic drug ibuprofen on oral anticoagulation with phenoprocoumon. *Curr. Med. Res. Op.*, **3** (Special Issue), 556.

*Giansiracuso, J.E., Donaldson, M.S., Koonce, M.L. *et al.* (1975) Ibuprofen in osteoarthritis. *Curr. Med. Res. Op.*, **3** (Special Issue), 481.

Glass, R.C. and Swannell, A.J. (1978) Concentrations of ibuprofen in serum and synovial fluid from patients with arthritis. *Br. J. Clin. Pharmacol.*, **6**, 453.

*Godfrey, R.G. and De la Cruz, S. (1975) Effect of ibuprofen dosage on patient response in rheumatoid arthritis. *Arthr. Rheum.*, **18**, 135.

Goncalves, L. (1973) Influence of ibuprofen on haemostasis in patients on anticoagulant therapy. *J. Intl. Med. Res.*, **1**, 180.

*Guagliano, G., Cironni, S., Bagliani, A. *et al.* (1975) Thrombophlebitis of the lower limbs: therapy with 2-(4-isobutyl phenyl) proprionic acid. *Curr. Med. Res. Op.*, **3** (Special Issue), 542.

*Hadidi, T.S., Asar, D.K. and Esmat, A. (1973) A double-blind cross-over study of ibuprofen, metiazinic acid, aspirin and a placebo in rheumatoid arthritis. *Abstracts of XIII International Congress of Rheumatology*, Kyoto, p. 5.

*Jasani, M.K., Downie, W.W., Samuels, B.M. and Buchanan, W.W. (1968) Ibuprofen in rheumatoid arthritis. Clinical study of analgesic and anti-inflammatory activity. *Ann. Rheum. Dis.*, **27**, 457.

*Joshipura, J.C.N. and Dongaonkar, D.G. (1976) Comparative evaluation of ibuprofen and oxyphenbutazone in soft-tissue rheumatism. *Proceedings of 3rd S.E.A.P.A.L. Congress*, Singapore.

*Lequesne, M. (1975) Clinical evaluation of ibuprofen, given orally and rectally, in degenerative arthroses. *Curr. Med. Res. Op.*, **3** (Special Issue), 570.

Lessel, B. and Shaw, J.W. (1973) The respiratory stimulant action of ibuprofen and salicylates. *Abstracts of XIII International Congress of Rheumatology*, Kyoto, p. 63.

Levernieux, J. (1975) Ibuprofen at high dosage. *Curr. Med. Res. Op.*, **3** (Special Issue), 485.

*Løkken, P., Norman-Pedersen, K., Bruaset, I. and Olsen, I. (1975) Ibuprofen ('Brufen') tested with bilateral oral surgery as a model for evaluation of anti-inflammatory effects. *Curr. Med. Res. Op.*, **3** (Special Issue), 493.

Lukačević, D., Djilas, D. and Nikolic, J. (1975) Clinical experience with ibuprofen in the treatment of rheumatic diseases. *Curr. Med. Res. Op.*, **3** (Special Issue), 576.

*Marsili, M.T. and Conte, C. (1975) The use of ibuprofen in ophthalmology. *Curr. Med. Res. Op.*, **3** (Special Issue), 509.

Melluish, J.W., Brooks, C.D., Ruoff, G. *et al.* (1975) Ibuprofen and visual function. *Arch. Ophthalmol.*, **93**, 781.

*Mena, H.R., Ehrlich, G.E., Giansiracusa, J. *et al.* (1976) Response of osteoarthritis to ibuprofen or flurbiprofen. *J. Intl. Med. Res.*, **4**, 152.

*Menon, N.D., Whetton, J.J., Ansell, B.M. and Goldberg, A.A.J. (1973) A comparative study of ibuprofen and aspirin in Still's disease (juvenile chronic polyarthritis). *Abstracts of XIII International Congress of Rheumatology*, Kyoto, p. 17.

Miller, A.C., Buckler, J.W. and Sheldrake, F.E. (1975) Clinical studies of ibuprofen. *Curr. Med. Res. Op.*, **3** (Special Issue), 589.

*Mitchell, D.M. and MacDonald, G. (1974) Controlled trial of ibuprofen in rheumatoid arthritis. *J. Rheumatol.*, **1** (Suppl. 1), 59.

*Montezuma de Carvalho, P. (1975) An evaluation of the anti-inflammatory effects of ibuprofen ('Brufen') in osteoarthrosis of the knee using radioactive technetium (^{99m}Tc). *Curr. Med. Res. Op.*, **3** (Special Issue), 580.

*Muckle, D.S. (1975) Ibuprofen ('Brufen') in soft-tissue injuries. *Curr. Med. Res. Op.*, **3** (Special Issue), 488.

Nassonova, V.A., Denissov, L.N., Sidelnikova, S.M. *et al.* (1973) Results of clinical studies of Brufen in antirheumatic therapy. *Abstracts of XIII International Congress of Rheumatology*, Kyoto, p. 16.

*Nikolić, J. and Lukačević, D. (1975) Ibuprofen ('Brufen') in the treatment of ankylosing spondylitis. *Curr. Med. Res. Op.*, **3** (Special Issue), 573.

Otadny, A.U. (1975) Comparative clinical trial of three proprionic acid derivatives (ibuprofen, ketoprofen and naproxen) in rheumatic diseases. *Curr. Med. Res. Op.*, **3** (Special Issue), 536.

Panayi, G.S. (1975) The effect of ibuprofen on lymphocyte stimulation by phytohaemagglutinin *in vitro*. *Curr. Med. Res. Op.*, **3** (Special Issue), 513.

*Pavelka, K., Susta, A., Vojtisek, O., *et al.* (1973) Double-blind comparison of ibuprofen and phenylbutazone in a short-term treatment of progressive polyarthritis. *Arz. Forsch.*, **23**, 842.

*Pavelka, K., Vojtišek, O., Šusta, A. *et al.* (1978) Experience with high doses of ibuprofen in the long-term treatment of rheumatoid arthritis. *J. Intl. Med. Res.*, **6**, 355.

*Pavelka, K., Vojtišek, O., Šusta, A. and Salavcova, V. (1975) Ibuprofen in the long-term treatment of coxarthrosis. *Curr. Med. Res. Op.*, **3** (Special Issue), 528.

Pipitone, V., Carrozzo, M. and Loizzi, P. (1973) A clinical study of Brufen in comparison with phenylbutazone and indomethacin. *Abstracts of XIII International Congress of Rheumatology*, Kyoto, p. 134.

Pipitone, V., Loizzi, P. and Bonomo, G.M. (1975) A multi-centre clinical evaluation, with proctoscopic control, of the use of ibuprofen suppositories in rheumatic conditions. *Curr. Med. Res. Op.*, **3** (Special Issue), 568.

Rejholec, V. (1975) Long-term ibuprofen therapy of rheumatic disease in patients with a past history of peptic ulceration. *Curr. Med. Res. Op.*, **3** (Special Issue), 522.

Sadowska-Wroblewska, M., Kawenoki-Minc, E., Graff-Wroblewska, T. and Maldyk, H. (1975) The effect of ibuprofen on the liver function tests in chronic rheumatic diseases. *Curr. Med. Res. Op.*, **3** (Special Issue), 563.

*Sheldrake, F.E. and Ansell, B.M. (1975) The use of 'Brufen' (ibuprofen) in the treatment of juvenile chronic polyarthritis. *Curr. Med. Res. Op.*, **3** (Special Issue), 604.

*Siegmeth, W. and Sieberer, W. (1978) A comparison of the short-term effects of ibuprofen and diclofenac in spondylosis. *J. Intl. Med. Res.*, **6**, 369.

Šusta, A., Pavelka, K. and Vojtišek, O. (1975) The comparison of four non-steroidal antirheumatic agents in the treatment of rheumatic disease. *Curr. Med. Res. Op.*, **3** (Special Issue), 525.

Thilo, D., Nyman, D. and Duckert, F. (1974) A study of the effects of the anti-rheumatic drug, ibuprofen (Brufen) on patients being treated with the oral anti-coagulant phenprocoumon (Marcoumar). *J. Intl. Med. Res.*, **2**, 276.

Thompson, M., Craft, A.W., Akyol, M.S. and Porter, R. (1975) Ibuprofen in the treatment of rheumatic diseases: long-term experience with observations on lack of adverse effects. *Curr. Med. Res. Op.*, **3** (Special Issue), 594.

*Van Wering, R.F. and Bleker, O.P. (1972) Oral analgesia in post-partum pain: a comparison of ibuprofen ('Brufen') and dextropropoxyphene. *Curr. Med. Res. Op.*, **1**, 49.

*Vojtišek, O., Pavelka, K. and Susta, A. (1975) 'Brufen' in the short-term treatment of rheumatoid arthritis. *Curr. Med. Res. Op.*, 3 (Special Issue), 532.

Wagenhauser, F.J. (1973) Long-term study with Brufen. *Abstracts of XIII International Congress of Rheumatology*, Kyoto, p. 106.

Naproxen

*Ansell, B.M., Hanna, B., Moran, H. *et al.* (1979a) Naproxen in juvenile chronic polyarthritis. *Eur. J. Rheumatol. Infl.*, 2, 79.

Ansell, B.M., Major, G., Liyanage, S.D. *et al.* (1978) A comparative study of Butacote and Naprosyn in ankylosing spondylitis. *Ann. Rheum. Dis.*, 37, 436.

*Ansell, B.M., Major, G., Liyanage, S.P. *et al.* (1979b) A comparative study of Butacote and Naprosyn in ankylosing spondylitis, *Eur. J. Rheumatol. Infl.*, 2, 45.

*Aromaa, U. and Asp, K. (1978) A comparison of naproxen, indomethacin and acetylsalicylic acid in pain after varicose vein surgery. *J. Intl. Med. Res.*, 6, 152.

*Backhouse, C.I., Engler, C. and English, J.R. (1980) Naproxen sodium and indomethacin in acute musculoskeletal disorders. *Rheumatol. Rehabil.*, 19, 113.

Beck, E.R. and Hayes-Allen, M.C. (1974) Naproxen (Naprosyn) and gastrointestinal haemorrhage. *Br. Med. J.*, 2, 51.

*Berry, H., Fernandez, L., Clarke, A.K. *et al.* (1978) Indoprofen and naproxen in the treatment of rheumatoid arthritis: a clinical trial. *Br. Med. J.*, i, 274.

*Berry, H., Swinson, D., Jones, J. and Hamilton, E.B.D. (1979) Indomethacin and naproxen suppositories in the treatment of rheumatoid arthritis. *Eur. J. Rheumatol. Infl.*, 2, 65.

*Binzus, G. and Josenhans, G. (1973) Ergebnisse eines offenen Therapieversuches mit Naproxen bei Patienten mit degenerativen Gelenkerkrankungen. *Scand. J. Rheumatol.* (Suppl. 2), 80.

*Blechman, W.J., Willkens, R., Boncaldo, G.L. *et al.* (1978) Naproxen in osteoarthritis: double-blind crossover trial. *Ann. Rheum. Dis.*, 37, 80.

*Borrachero, J. and Alcalde, A. (1973) Estudio sobre la efectividad de naproxen en la artritis reumatoidea. *Scand. J. Rheumatol.* (Suppl. 2), 140.

*Bowers, D.E., Dyer, H.R., Forsdick, W.M. *et al.* (1975) Naproxen in rheumatoid arthritis – a controlled trial. *Ann. Int. Med.*, 83, 470.

Capell, H.A., McLeod, M.M., Hernandez, L.A. *et al.* (1976) Comparison of azapropazone and naproxen in rheumatoid arthritis. *Curr. Med. Res. Op.*, 4, 285.

*Castles, J.J., Moore, T.L., Vaughan, J.H. *et al.* (1978) Multicenter comparison of naproxen and indomethacin in rheumatoid arthritis. *Arch. Intl. Med.*, 138, 362.

*Clark, A.K., Barnes, C.G., Goodman, H.V. *et al.* (1975) A double-blind comparison of naproxen against indomethacin in osteoarthrosis. *Drug Res.*, 25, 302.

*Cochrane, G.M. (1973) A double-blind comparison of naproxen with indomethacin in osteoarthritis. *Scand. J. Rheumatol.* (Suppl. 2), 89.

*Cuq, P. (1973) Experience française du du traitement de la crise de goutte aiguë par le naproxen-C1674. *Scand. J. Rheumatol.* (Suppl. 2), 64.

†Diamond, H., Alexander, S., Kuzell, W. *et al.* (1973) A multicenter double-blind crossover comparison study of naproxen and aspirin in patients with rheumatoid arthritis. *Scand. J. Rheumatol.* (Suppl. 2), 171.

*D'Omézon, Y. (1973) Etude des cliniciens français sur l'action du Naproxène dans la P.C.E. *Scand. J. Rheumatol.* (Suppl. 2), 164.

Dumas, K. (ed.) (1973) Naproxen: Proceedings from an International Medical Symposium presented by Syntex Corporation. *Scand. J. Rheumatol.* (Suppl. 2).

*Eberl, R., Tausch, G., Sochor, H. and Binzus, G. (1973) Ergebrusse eines offenen Versuches mit Naproxen bei Polyarthritis Chronica und anderen Erkrankungen des rheumatischen Formenkreises. *Scand. J. Rheumatol.* (Suppl. 2), 150.

*Fernandez del Vallado, P., Gijón Baños, J. and Prostigo Alvarez, J.L. (1973) Enzayo clinico albierto con naproxen en las artropatiás degenerativas (osteoarthritis). *Scand. J. Rheumatol.* (Suppl. 2), 72.

*Flores, J.B. (1973) Naproxen: efecto aharrador de corticosteroides en artritis reumatoid. *Scand. J. Rheumatol.* (Suppl. 2), 127.

Fredell, E.W. and Strand, L.J. (1977) Naproxen overdose. *J. Am. Med. Assoc.*, 238, 938.

Frenger, W. and Marbach, H.J. (1973) Klinische Untersuchung von Naproxen, von allem mit Bezug auf seine Verträghchkeit. *Scand. J. Rheumatol.* (Suppl. 2), 137.

Halvorsen, L., Dotevall, G. and Sevelins, H. (1973) Comparative effects of aspirin and naproxen on gastric mucosa. *Scand. J. Rheumatol.* (Suppl. 2), 43.

Harrison, I.T., Lewis, B., Nelson, P. *et al.* (1970) Nonsteroidal anti-inflammatory agents. I. 6-substituted 2-naphthyl-acetic acids. *J. Med. Chem.*, 13, 203.

Hart, F.D. (1974) Naproxen (Naprosyn) and gastrointestinal haemorrhage. *Br. Med. J.*, ii, 51.

Hart, F.D. and Matts, S.G.F. (1974) Naproxen and gastro-intestinal haemorrhage. *Br. Med. J.*, ii, 51.

Hayes-Allen, M.C. (1974) Naproxen and gastro-intestinal haemorrhage. *Br. Med. J.*, i, 572.

*Hazleman, B.L., Mowat, A.G., Sturge, N.A. *et al.* (1979) A long-term trial of a higher dose of naproxen in the treatment of rheumatoid arthritis, ankylosing spondylitis and osteoarthritis. *Eur. J. Rheumatol. Infl.*, 2, 56.

*Helby-Petersen, P., Ibfelt, H. and Rossel, I. (1973) A double-blind crossover comparison of naproxen and placebo in rheumatoid arthritis. *Scand. J. Rheumatol.* (Suppl. 2), 145.

Hernandez, L.A., MacLeod, M., Grennan, D.M. *et al.* (1975) Clinical evaluation of two daily doses of naproxen and indomethacin: result of a double-blind crossover trial. *Curr. Med. Res. Op.*, 3, 359.

*Hill, H.F.H. and Hill, A.G.S. (1973) Naproxen in ankylosing spondylitis. *Scand. J. Rheumatol.* (Suppl. 2), 121.

*Hill, H.F.H. and Hill, A.G.S. (1976) Naproxen in treatment of ankylosing spondylitis. *Ann. Rheum. Dis.*, 35, 287.

Hill, H.F.H., Hill, A.G.S. and Mowat, A.G. (1974) Naproxen: a new nonhormonal anti-inflammatory agent. *Ann. Rheum. Dis.*, 33, 12.

†Hill, H.F.H, Hill, A.G.S., Mowat, A.G. *et al.* (1973) Multicentre double-blind crossover trial comparing naproxen and aspirin in rheumatoid arthritis. *Scand. J. Rheumatol.* (Suppl. 2), 176.

*Hill, H.F.H., Hill, A.G.S., Mowat, A.G. *et al.* (1974) Naproxen. A new non-hormonal anti-inflammatory agent. Studies in rheumatoid arthritis. *Ann. Rheum. Dis.*, 33, 12.

Huskisson, E.C., Woolf, D.L., Balme, H.W. *et al.* (1979a) Four new anti-inflammatory drugs: responses and variations. *Eur. J. Rheumatol. Infl.*, **2**, 29.

Huskisson, E.C., Woolf, D.L., Doyle, D.V. and Scott, J. (1979b) A trial of naproxen, flurbiprofen, indomethacin and placebo in the treatment of osteoarthritis. *Eur. J. Rheumatol. Infl.*, **2**, 69.

Huskisson, E.C., Woolf, D.L. and Scott, J. (1979c) One year follow-up of patients treated with naproxen. Time, cause and factors affecting response. *Eur. J. Rheumatol. Infl.*, **2**, 33.

Jaffe, G. (1976) A double-blind, multi-centre comparison of naproxen and indomethacin in acute musculoskeletal disorders. *Curr. Med. Res. Op.*, **4**, 373.

Jain, A., McMahon, F.G., Slattery, J.T. and Levy, G. (1979) Effect of naproxen on the steady-state serum concentration and anti-coagulant activity of warfarin. *Clin. Pharmacol. Ther.*, **25**, 61.

*Kageyama, T. (1973) Clinical evaluation of naproxen in the treatment of osteoarthritis – a double-blind, cross-over trial. *Scand. J. Rheumatol.* (Suppl. 2), 94.

Katona, G. (1973) Four years of clinical experience with naproxen – and objective methods of evaluation. *Scand. J. Rheumatol.* (Suppl. 2), 101.

*Katona, G., Ortega, E. and Robles-Gil, J. (1971) The treatment of rheumatoid arthritis – a new non-steroidal anti-inflammatory drug, naproxen. *Clin. Trials J.*, **8**, 3.

*Kogstad, O. (1973) A double-blind cross-over study of naproxen and indomethacin in patients with rheumatoid arthritis. *Scand. J. Rheumatol.* (Suppl. 2), 159.

*Luftschein, S., Bienen Stock, H., Varady, J.C. and Stiff, F.W. (1979) Increasing dose of naproxen in rheumatoid arthritis: use with and without corticosteroids. *J. Rheumatol.*, **6**, 397.

*Lussier, A., Myhal, D., Boost, G. *et al.* (1973a) Long-term study of naproxen challenged by a short-term double-blind cross-over study with placebo in rheumatoid patients. *Scand. J. Rheumatol.* (Suppl. 2), 113.

*Lussier, A., Regoli, D., Gysling, E. *et al.* (1973b) Methoxypropiocin (RS-3540-Naproxen); clinical study on 40 patients suffering from rheumatoid arthritis. *Intl. J. Clin. Pharmacol. Ther. Toxicol.*, **7**, 6.

*Lussier, A., Segre, E.J., Multz, C.V. *et al.* (1973c) Naproxen – a novel approach to dose-finding efficacy trials in rheumatoid arthritis. *Clin. Pharmacol. Ther.*, **14**, 434.

*Makela, A.L. (1977) Naproxen in the treatment of juvenile rheumatoid arthritis. *Scand. J. Rheumatol.*, **6**, 193.

*Martinez-Lavin, M., Holman, K.I., Smyth, C.J. and Vaughan, J.H. (1980) A comparison of naproxen, indomethacin and aspirin in osteoarthritis. *J. Rheumatol.*, **7**, 711.

Matts, S.G.F. (1974) Naproxen (Naprosyn) and gastrointestinal haemorrhage. *Br. Med. J.*, **ii**, 52.

*Mayhew, S.R. (1978) A comparison of benorylate and naproxen in degenerative arthritis. *Rheumatol. Rehabil.*, **17**, 29.

*Melton, J.W., Lussier, A., Ward, J.R. *et al.* (1978) Naproxen vs. aspirin in osteoarthritis of the hip and knee. *J. Rheumatol.*, **5**, 338.

Mowat, A.G., Ansell, B.M., Gumpel, J.M. *et al.* (1976) Naproxen in rheumatoid arthritis. Extended trial. *Ann. Rheum. Dis.*, **35**, 498.

*Mowat, A.G., Ansell, B.M., Gumpel, J.M. *et al.* (1979) Naproxen in rheumatoid arthritis extended trial; further report. *Eur. J. Rheumatol. Infl.*, **2**, 19.

*Mowat, A.M. and Mowat, A.G. (1979) A comparative trial of naproxen and benorylate suspensions in the treatment of rheumatoid arthritis. *Eur. J. Rheumatol. Infl.*, **2**, 74.

Nadell, J., Bruno, J., Varady, J. and Segre, E.J. (1974) Effect of naproxen and of aspirin on bleeding time and platelet aggregation. *J. Clin. Pharmacol.*, **14**, 176.

*Poal, J., de Anta, J. and Reyes, J. (1973) Estudio de naproxen en osteoarthritis. *Scand. J. Rheumatol.* (Suppl. 2), 77.

*Reynolds, P.M.G. and Wharwell, P.J. (1974) A single-blind crossover comparison of fenoprofen, ibuprofen and naproxen in rheumatoid arthritis. *Curr. Med. Res. Op.*, **2**, 461.

Roszkowski, A.P., Rooks, W.H., II, Tomolonis, A.J. and Miller, L.M. (1971) Anti-inflammatory and analgesic properties of d-2-(6′-methoxy-2′-naphthyl)-proprionic acid (naproxen). *J. Pharmacol. Exp. Ther.*, **179**, 114.

Roth, S.H. and Boost, G. (1975) An open trial of naproxen in rheumatoid arthritis patients with significant oesophageal, gastric and duodenal lesions. *J. Clin. Pharmacol.*, **15**, 378.

*Ruedy, J. and McCullough, W. (1973) A comparison of the analgesic efficacy of naproxen and propoxyphene in patients with pain after orthopaedic surgery. *Scand. J. Rheumatol.* (Suppl. 2), 56.

Runkel, R., Chaplin, M. and Boost, G. (1972) Absorption distribution metabolism and excretion of naproxen in various laboratory animals and human subjects. *J. Pharm. Sci.*, **61**, 703.

Runkel, R.A., Chaplin, M.D., Sevelius, H. *et al.* (1976) Pharmacokinetics of naproxen overdoses. *Clin. Pharmacol. Ther.*, **20**, 269.

Runkel, R., Forchielli, E., Boost, G. *et al.* (1973) Naproxen – metabolism, excretion and comparative pharmacokinetics. *Scand. J. Rheumatol.* (Suppl. 2), 29.

Segre, E.J. (1975) Naproxen metabolism in man. *J. Clin. Pharmacol.*, **15**, 316.

Segre, E.J. (1979) Drug interactions with naproxen. *Eur. J. Rheumatol. Infl.*, **2**, 12.

Segre, E.J. (1979) in *Clinics in Rheumatic Diseases: Anti-Rheumatic Drugs* (ed. E.C. Huskisson), Vol. 5, No. 2, Saunders, London, p. 411.

Slattery, J.T., Levy, G., Jain, A. and McMahon, F.G. (1979) Effect of naproxen on the kinetics of elimination and anticoagulant activity of a single dose of warfarin. *Clin. Pharmacol. Ther.*, **25**, 51.

*Stetson, J.B., Robrusan, K., Wardell, W. and Lasagna, L. (1973) Analgesic activity of oral naproxen in patients with postoperative pain. *Scand. J. Rheumatol.* (Suppl. 2), 50.

†Sturge, R.A., Scott, J.T., Hamilton, E.B.D. *et al.* (1977) Multicentre trial of naproxen and phenylbutazone in acute gout. *Ann. Rheum. Dis.*, **36**, 80.

*Sturge, R.A., Scott, J.T., Hamilton, E.B.D. *et al.* (1979) Multicentre trial of naproxen and phenylbutazone in acute gout. *Eur. J. Rheumatol. Infl.*, **2**, 40.

*Szanto, E. (1974) A double-blind cross-over study of naproxen and indomethacin in rheumatoid arthritis. *Scand. J. Rheumatol.*, **3**, 118.

*Thompson, M., Akyol, M.S., Cosh, J. *et al.* (1979) Naproxen in patients with osteoarthritis and intolerance to other non-steroidal anti-inflammatory drugs. *Eur. J. Rheumatol. Infl.*, **2**, 25.

Tiseluis, P. (1973) Hydroxyproline excretion in the urine as a measure of anti-inflammatory effect in rheumatic patients using naproxen. *Scand. J. Rheumatol.* (Suppl. 2), 109.

*Van Gerwen, F., Van Der Korst, J.K. and Gribnau, F.W.J. (1978) Double-blind trial of naproxen and phenylbutazone in ankylosing spondylitis. *Ann. Rheum. Dis.*, **37**, 85.

*Vetter, G. (1975) Double-blind crossover study of clopirac and naproxen in rheumatoid arthritis. *J. Belge de Rheumatol.*, **30**, 107.

*Williams, J.G.P. and Engler, C. (1977) A double-blind comparative trial of naproxen and indomethacin in sports injuries. *Rheumatol. Rehabil.*, **16**, 265.

*Willkens, R.F. (1973) Double-blind crossover trial and naproxen and placebo in patients with rheumatoid arthritis. *Scand. J. Rheumatol.* (Suppl. 2), 132.

*Willkens, R.F. and Case, J.B. (1973) Treatment of acute gout with naproxen. *Scand. J. Rheumatol.* (Suppl. 2), 69.

Willkens, R.F., Case, J.B. and Hiux, F.J. (1975) The treatment of acute gout with naproxen. *J. Clin. Pharmacol.*, **15**, 363.

*Willkens, R.F. and Segre, E.J. (1976) Combination therapy with naproxen and aspirin in rheumatoid arthritis. *Arthr. Rheum.*, **19**, 677.

*Winer, J., Wagenhäuser, F. and Nárožná, H. (1973) Klinischer Vergleich von Naproxen und Indomethacin in der Behandlung der prozredient chronischen Polyarthritis (ein Zwischenbericht). *Scand. J. Rheumatol.* (Suppl. 2), 155.

Fenoprofen

Blechman, W.J. and Zane, S. (1976) Fenoprofen calcium in steroid treatment of rheumatoid arthritis: efficacy, safety, and steroid-sparing effect. *J. Rheumatol.*, **3** (Suppl. 2), 34.

*Brooke, J.W. (1976) Fenoprofen therapy in large-joint osteoarthritis: double-blind comparison with aspirin and long-term experience. *J. Rheumatol.*, **3** (Suppl. 2), 71.

*Chakravorty, N.K. and Annan, G. (1980) Fenoprofen in the treatment of osteoarthrosis of hips and knee joints in the elderly. *J. Intl. Med. Res.*, **8**, 270.

Chernish, S.M., Rubin, A., Rodda, B.E. *et al.* (1972) The physiological disposition of fenoprofen in man: IV. The effects of position of subject, food ingestion and antacid ingestion on the plasma levels of orally administered fenoprofen. *J. Med. Clin. Exp. Theoret.*, **3**, 249.

*Davis, J., Turner, R., Collins, R. and Kaufmann, J. (1976) Comparison of fenoprofen calcium and aspirin therapy during gold induction in rheumatoid arthritis. *Clin. Pharmacol. Ther.*, **19**, 105.

*Diamond, H.S. (1976) Double-blind crossover study of fenoprofen and aspirin in osteoarthritis. *J. Rheumatol.*, **3** (Suppl. 2), 67.

*Duff, I.F., Neukom, J.E. and Himes, J.E. (1976) Fenoprofen in patients with rheumatoid arthritis receiving maintenance gold therapy. *J. Rheumatol.*, **3** (Suppl. 2), 32.

*Franke, M. and Manz, G. (1977) Comparison of fenoprofen and oxyphenbutazone in patients with rheumatoid arthritis. *Curr. Ther. Res. Clin. Exp.*, **21**, 43.

*Fries, J.F. and Britton, M.C. (1973) Fenoprofen calcium in rheumatoid arthritis. *Arth. Rheum.*, **16**, 629.

*Godfrey, R., Gum, O.B. and Maltz, B.A. (1977) Evaluation of fenoprofen calcium (Nalfon) in ankylosing spondylitis. *Abstract of the XIV International Congress of Rheumatology*, San Francisco, 1977, p. 168.

†Gum, O.B. (1976) Fenoprofen in rheumatoid arthritis: a controlled crossover multi-centre study. *J. Rheumatol.*, **3**

(Suppl. 2), 26.

Herrmann, R.G., Marshall, W.S., Crowe, V.G. *et al.* (1972) Effect of a new anti-inflammatory drug, fenoprofen, on platelet aggregation and thrombus formation. *Proc. Soc. Exp. Bio. Med.*, **139**, 548.

Ho, P.P.K. and Esterman, A. (1974) Fenoprofen: inhibitor of prostaglandin synthesis. *Prostaglandins*, **6**, 107.

*Huskisson, E.C. (1974) Long-term use of fenoprofen in rheumatoid arthritis: the therapeutic ratio. *Curr. Med. Res. Op.*, **2**, 545.

*Huskisson, E.C., Wojtulewski, J.A., Berry, H. *et al.* (1974) Treatment of rheumatoid arthritis with fenoprofen: comparison with aspirin. *Br. Med. J.*, **i**, 176.

Lin T.M., Warrick, M.W., Evans, D.C. and Nash, J.F. (1975) Action of the anti-inflammatory agents, acetylsalicylic acid, indomethacin and fenoprofen on the gastric mucosa of dogs. *Res. Commun. Chem. Pathol. Pharmacol.*, **2**, 1.

Loebl, D.H., Craig, R.M., Culic, D.D. *et al.* (1977) Gastrointestinal blood loss: effect of aspirin, fenoprofen, and acetaminophen in rheumatoid arthritis as determined by sequential gastroscopy and radioactive fecal markers. *J. Am. Med. Assoc.*, **237**, 976.

McMahon, F.G., Jain, A. and Onel, A. (1976) Controlled evaluation of fenoprofen in geriatric patients with osteoarthritis. *J. Rheumatol.*, **3** (Suppl. 2), 76.

Mikulaschek, W.M. (1974) Clinical experience with fenoprofen, a new antirheumatic agent. *Curr. Med. Res. Op.*, **2**, 556.

Murphy, J.E., Donald, J.F. and Layes Molla, A. (1978) Analgesic efficacy and acceptability of fenoprofen combined with paracetamol and coupled with dihydrocodeine tartrate in general practice. *J. Intl. Med. Res.*, **6**, 375.

Nickander, R., Marshall, W., Emmerson, J.L. et al. (1977) in *Pharmacological and Biochemical Properties of Drug Substances* (ed. M.E. Goldberg), Vol. 1, American Pharmaceutical Association. Academy of Pharmaceutical Sciences, Washington, D.C., pp. 183–213.

Panusch, R.S. (1978) Effects of fenoprofen and benoxaprofen on human lymphocytes: inhibition of tritiated thymidine uptake. *Agents and Actions*, **8**, 238.

*Reynolds, P.M.G. and Whorwell, P.J. (1974) A single-blind crossover comparison of fenoprofen, ibuprofen and naproxen in rheumatoid arthritis. *Curr. Med. Res. Op.*, **2**, 461.

Ridolfo, A.S., Nickander, R. and Mikulaschek, W.M. (1979) in *Clinics in Rheumatic Diseases: Anti-Rheumatic Drugs* (ed. E.C. Huskisson), Vol. 5, No. 2, Saunders, London, p. 393.

Rubin, A., Chernish, S.M., Crabtree, R. *et al.* (1974) A profile of the physiological disposition and gastrointestinal effects of fenoprofen in man. *Curr. Med. Res. Op.*, **2**, 529.

Rubin, A., Rodda, B.E., Warrick, P. *et al.* (1971) Physiological disposition of fenoprofen in man: I. Pharmacokinetic comparison of calcium and sodium salts administered orally. *J. Pharm. Sci.*, **60**, 1797.

Rubin, A., Rodda, B.E., Warrick, P. *et al.* (1972) Physiological disposition of fenoprofen in man: II. Plasma and urine pharmacokinetics after oral and intravenous administration. *J. Pharm. Sci.*, **61**, 739.

*Sigler, J.W., Ridolfo, A.S. and Bluhm, G.B. (1976) Comparison of benefit-to-risk ratios of aspirin and fenoprofen: controlled multicentre study in rheumatoid arthritis. *J. Rheumatol.*, **3** (Suppl. 2), 49.

*Steele, D.N. (1977) Evaluation of fenoprofen in acute inflammatory conditions in soft tissue. *Abstracts of the XIV International Congress of Rheumatology*, San Francisco, 1977, p. 168.

*Wanasukapunt, S., Lertratanakul, Y. and Rubinstein, H.M. (1977) Effect of fenoprofen calcium on acute gouty arthritis. *Abstracts of the XIV International Congress of Rheumatology*, San Francisco, 1977, p. 167.

*Wojtulewski, J.A. (1974) Fenoprofen in the treatment of osteoarthrosis. *Curr. Med. Res. Op.*, **2**, 551.

*Wojtulewski, J.A., Hart, F.D. and Huskisson, E.C. (1974) Fenoprofen in treatment of osteoarthrosis of hip and knee. *Br. Med. J.*, **ii**, 475.

Ketoprofen

Amor, B., de G.A. and Delbarre, F. (1973) Etude du Kétoprofène en rhumatologie. *Revue du Rhumatisme et des Maladies Ostéo-articulaires*, **40**, 451.

*Anderson, J.A., Lee, P., Webb, J. and Buchanan, W.W. (1974) Evaluation of the therapeutic potential of ketoprofen in rheumatoid arthritis. *Curr. Med. Res. Op.*, **2**, 189.

*Aritomi, H., Kashiwazaki, S., Tadenuma, T. and Taba, H. (1977) Long-term administration of ketoprofen in patients with rheumatoid arthritis. *XIV International Congress of Rheumatology*, San Francisco, 1977, p. 41.

Asch, L., Kuntz, J.L., Richard, D. and Menneson, H. (1974) Utilisation en rhumatologie du kétoprofène injectable. *Med. Intl.*, **9**, 547.

Asch, L. (1975) Expérimentation clinique des suppositories de kétoprofène. *Gazette Med. France*, **82**, 2241.

Atra, E. and Goldenberg, J. (1974) Clinical trial with an anti-inflammatory agent ketoprofen in rheumatic diseases. *Revista Brasileira de Clinica e Terapeutica*, **3**, 237.

Bocquet, B. and Vignon, E. (1973) Etudes cliniques en rhumatologie d'un anti-inflammatoire nouveau: le kétoprofène. *Cahiers Medicaux Lyonnais*, **49**, 3365.

*Bresnihan, F.P., Grahame, R. and Burry, H.C. (1974) Ketoprofen in the management of osteoarthrosis of the hip: comparison with phenylbutazone. *Rheumatol. Rehabil.*, **13**, 125.

*Cardoe, N. (1979) Double-blind cross-over study of ketoprofen and phenylbutazone in patients with chronic osteoarthrosis of the hip. *Rheumatol. Rehabil.* (Suppl: A Symposium on Ketoprofen), p. 27.

*Caroit, M., Forette, B., Hubault, A. and Pasquier, P. (1976) Double-blind study of ketoprofen against placebo in osteoarthritis of the hip. *Scand. J. Rheumatol.*, **14**, (Suppl.), 123.

Cathcart, B.J. (1973) Studies on 2-(3-benzoylphenyl) proprionic acid (Orudis). *Ann. Rheum. Dis.*, **32**, 62.

Cathcart, B.J., Vince, J.D., Gordon, A.J. *et al.* (1973) Studies on 2-(3-benzoylphenyl) proprionic acid (Orudis). *Ann. Rheum. Dis.*, **32**, 62.

*Chlud, K. and Paugerl, S. (1979) Ketoprofen in the treatment of soft tissue injury. *Rheumatol. Rehabil.* (Suppl: New Aspects in Diagnosis and Therapy of Rheumatoid Arthritis), p. 114.

David-Chaussé, J., Dehais, J. and Bulhier, R. (1976) Results of the rectal administration of ketoprofen in fifty-two patients. *Rheumatol. Rehabil.* (Suppl: A Symposium on Ketoprofen), p. 57.

*Doury, P. and Pattin, S. (1973) Traitement de la spondylarthrite ankylosante par le kétoprofène. *Rhumatologie*, **15**, 381.

*Eberl, R., Tausch, G., Siegmeth, W. and Broll, H. (1973) Essai comparatif kétoprofène contre phénylbutazone dans la goutte. *XIII International Congress of Rheumatology*, Kyoto, 1973, published in *Rhumatologie*, Special Issue, p. 199.

*Famaey, J.P. and Colinet, E. (1976) A double-blind trial of ketoprofen in the treatment of osteoarthritis of the hip. *Rheumatol. Rehabil.* (Suppl: A Symposium on Ketoprofen), p. 45.

Fossgrenn, J., Kirchheiner, B., Petersen, F.O. *et al.* (1976) Clinical evaluation of ketoprofen (19, 583 RP). Double-blind crossover trial against indomethacin. *Scand. J. Rheumatol.*, **14**, (Suppl.), 93.

Fournie, A. and Ayrolles, C. (1976) A clinical study of ketoprofen suppositories. *Rheumatol. Rehabil.* (Suppl: A Symposium on Ketoprofen), p. 59.

*Goldman, A.L. (1977) Cross-over trial of ketoprofen and indomethacin in rheumatoid arthritis. *XIV International Congress of Rheumatology*, 1977, p. 35.

Gomez, G. (1976) Long-term safety study of ketoprofen. *Rheumatol. Rehabil.* (Suppl: A Symposium on Ketoprofen), p. 87.

Gougeon, J., Moreau-Hottin, J. and Gaillard, F. (1976) Clinical trial of the injectable form of ketoprofen. *Rheumatol. Rehabil.* (Suppl: A Symposium on Ketoprofen), p. 75.

Grahame, R. (1976) Ketoprofen-clinical efficacy. *Rheumatol. Rehabil.* (Suppl: A Symposium on Ketoprofen), p. 22.

*Grahame, R., Bresnihan, F.B., Bloch, M. and Burry, H.C. (1973) Ketoprofen ('Orudis') in the management of osteoarthrosis of the hip: comparison with phenylbutazone. *XIII International Congress of Rheumatology*, Kyoto, 1973, published in *Rhumatogie*, Special Issue, p. 203.

Grahame, R. and Huskisson, E.C. (eds) (1976) A Symposium on Ketoprofen. *Rheumatol. Rehabil.* (Suppl.).

Griffin, A.J., Grahame, R., Bloch, M. and Gibson, T. (1978) Ketoprofen: double-blind cross-over study with indomethacin administered as a combined suppository/capsule regime in patients with rheumatoid arthritis: a preliminary report. *Rheumatol. Rehabil.* (Suppl: Trends in the Drug Treatment of Rheumatic Diseases), 84.

Gross, W. (1979) Long-term studies on therapy and tolerance of ketoprofen. *Rheumatol. Rehabil.* (Suppl: New Aspects in Diagnosis and Therapy of Rheumatoid Arthritis), 112.

*Gyory, A.N., Bloch, M., Burry, H.C. and Grahame, R. (1972) Orudis in management of rheumatoid arthritis and osteoarthritis of the hip: compared with indomethacin. *Br. Med. J.*, **iv**, 398.

*Hubault, A., Caroit, M., Forette, B. and Pasquier, P. (1976) Double-blind trial of ketoprofen compared with placebo in osteoarthrosis of the hip. *Rheumatol. Rehabil.* (Suppl: A Symposium on Ketoprofen), 52.

*Jessop, J.D. (1976) Double-blind study of ketoprofen and phenylbutazone in ankylosing spondylitis. *Rheumatol. Rehabil.* (Suppl: A Symposium on Ketoprofen), 37.

Kaller, H. (1979) The pharmacological properties of ketoprofen and its place in antirheumatic therapy. *Rheumatol. Rehabil.* (Suppl: New Aspects in Diagnosis and Therapy of Rheumatoid Arthritis), 99.

*Kennedy, A.C. (1976a) Ketoprofen in the treatment of rheumatoid arthritis. *Rheumatol. Rehabil.* (Suppl: A Symposium on Ketoprofen), 34.

Kennedy, A.C. (1976b) Synovial fluid pharmacokinetics of

ketoprofen. *Rheumatol. Rehabil.* (Suppl: A Symposium on Ketoprofen), 34.

Kirchheiner, B., Fossgreen, J., Tophøj, E. and Zachariae, E. (1976) Clinical evaluation of ketoprofen (Orudis in rheumatoid arthritis: a double-blind cross-over comparison with indomethacin). *Rheumatol. Rehabil.* (Suppl: A Symposium on Ketoprofen), 50.

Le Chevallier, P.L. and Valat, J.P. (1976) Clinical therapeutic study of intramuscular ketoprofen in rheumatic diseases. *Rheumatol. Rehabil.* (Suppl: A Symposium on Ketoprofen), 79.

Lussier, A. and Arsenault, A. (1976) Gastrointestinal blood loss induced by ketoprofen, aspirin and placebo. *Scand. J. Rheumatol.*, **14** (Suppl.), 73.

Mason, J. and Bolton, M.S. (1979) A general practice assessment of Alrheumat (ketoprofen). *Rheumatol. Rehabil.* (Suppl: New Aspects in Diagnosis and Therapy of Rheumatoid Arthritis), 111.

*Mathies, H. (1979) Clinical studies with ketoprofen in rheumatoid arthritis. *Rheumatol. Rehabil.* (Suppl: New Aspects in Diagnosis and Therapy of Rheumatoid Arthritis), 114.

*Meyer, H. (1979) Clinical studies with ketoprofen in rheumatoid arthritis. *Rheumatol. Rehabil.* (Suppl: New Aspects in Diagnosis and Therapy of Rheumatoid Arthritis), 116.

*Mills, S.B., Bloch, M. and Bruckner, F.E. (1973) Double-blind crossover study of ketoprofen and ibuprofen in management of rheumatoid arthritis. *Br. Med. J.*, iv, 82.

Mitchell, W.S., Scott, P., Kennedy, *et al.* (1975) Clinicopharmacological studies on ketoprofen (Orudis). *Curr. Med. Res. Op.*, **3**, 423.

*O'Brien, W.M. and Grunwaldt, E. (1976) Ketoprofen in the treatment of rheumatoid arthritis double-blind cross-over placebo comparison. *Scand. J. Rheumatol.*, **14** (Suppl.), 105.

*Peltola, P. (1976) Double-blind cross-over study of ketoprofen and phenylbutazone in rheumatoid arthritis. *Rheumatol. Rehabil.* (Suppl: A Symposium on Ketoprofen), 56.

Peltola, P. (1978) Ketoprofen experiences. *Rheumatol. Rehabil.* (Suppl: Trends in the Drug Treatment of Rheumatic Diseases), 109.

Populaire, P., Terlain, B., Pascal, S. *et al.* (1973) The biological behaviour, serum levels, excretion and biotransformation of ketoprofen in animals and men. *Annales Pharmaceutiques Françaises*, **31**, 735.

Queneau, P., Amourdedieu, J. and Daumont, A. (1976) Clinical study of ketoprofen administered rectally in rheumatology. *Rheumatol. Rehabil.* (Suppl: A Symposium on Ketoprofen), 61.

Rahbek, I. (1976) Gastroscopic evaluation of the effect of a new anti-rheumatic compound, ketoprofen (19, 583 RP) on the human gastric mucosa. A double-blind cross-over trial against acetylsalicylic acid. *Scand. J. Rheumatol.*, **14** (Suppl.), 63.

Renier, J.C. and Boasson, M. (1976) Clinical use of ketoprofen: a retrospective study. *Rheumatol. Rehabil.* (Suppl: A Symposium on Ketoprofen), 81.

Roudier, J., Cayla, J. and Menkes, C.J. (1976) A controlled trial of ketoprofen (administered rectally) in arthritis of the hip and knee. *Rheumatol. Rehabil.* (Suppl: A Symposium on Ketoprofen), 71.

*Sany, J. and Serre, H. (1976) A study of ketoprofen in rheumatoid arthritis. *Rheumatol. Rehabil.* (Suppl: A Symposium on Ketoprofen), 67.

*Serry, M.M. (1980) A low-dosage ketoprofen preparation in the management of osteoarthrosis of the knee joint. *J. Intl. Med. Res.*, **8**, 388.

*Shiokawa, Y. (1973) Clinical evaluation of ketoprofen in rheumatoid arthritis. *Rheumatism*, **13**, 255.

Simon, L. and Blotman, F. (1976) Ketoprofen suppositories in rheumatological practice. *Rheumatol. Rehabil.* (Suppl: A Symposium on Ketoprofen), 65.

†Sydnes, O.A., Bratt, H.K., Haerum, L.B. and Straume, S. (1976) Clinical evaluation of ketoprofen (Orudis) in rheumatoid arthritis: results of a multi-centre double-blind trial against phenylbutazone. *Rheumatol. Rehabil.* (Suppl: A Symposium on Ketoprofen), 43.

*Treadwell, B.L.J. and Tweed, J.M. (1975) Ketoprofen (Orudis) in ankylosing spondylitis. *N. Z. Med. J.*, **81**, 411.

*Viara, M., Franchi, R., Liverta, C. *et al.* (1975) Ketoprofen and indomethacin in the treatment of rheumatoid arthritis. A double-blind cross-over trial. *Eur. J. Clin. Pharmacol.*, **8**, 205.

Vignon, G. (1976) Comparative study of intravenous ketoprofen *versus* aspirin. *Rheumatol. Rehabil.* (Suppl: A Symposium on Ketoprofen), 83.

Williams, M.J., Digby, J.W. and Topp, J.R. (1977) A multicenter long-term evaluation of Orudis (ketoprofen) in the treatment of arthritic disease. *XIV International Congress of Rheumatology*, 1977, p. 71.

*Wollheim, F.A., Lindroth, Y. and Sjöblom, K.G. (1978) A comparison of ketoprofen and naproxen in rheumatoid arthritis. *Rheumatol. Rehabil.* (Suppl: Trends in the Drug Treatment of Rheumatic Diseases), 78.

*Zutschi, D.W., Stern, D., Bloch, M. and Mason, R.M. (1974) Ketoprofen: a double-blind crossover study with indomethacin in patients with rheumatoid arthritis. *Rheumatol. Rehabil*, **13**, 10.

Flurbiprofen

Adams, S.S., Bresloff, P. and Risdall, P.C. (1975a) The contributions of metabolites to the anti-inflammatory activity of flurbiprofen. *Curr. Med. Res. Op.*, **3**, 27.

Adams, S.S., Burrows, C.A., Skeldon, N. and Yates, D.B. (1977) Inhibition of prostaglandin synthesis and leucocyte migration by flurbiprofen. *Curr. Med. Res. Op.*, **5** (Special Issue), 11.

Adams, S.S., McCullough, K.F. and Nicholson, J.S. (1975b) Some biological properties of flurbiprofen, an anti-inflammatory, analgesic and antipyretic agent. *Arzne.-Forsch.*, **25**, 1786.

*Bacon, P.A., Collins, A.J. and Cosh, J.A. (1975) Thermographic assessment of the anti-inflammatory effect of flurbiprofen in rheumatoid arthritis. *Curr. Med. Res. Op.*, **3**, 20.

*Brewis, I.D.L. (1977) A comparative study of flurbiprofen and indomethacin in rheumatoid arthritis. *Curr. Med. Res. Op.*, **5** (Special Issue), 48.

Brooks, P.M. and Khong, T.K. (1977) Flurbiprofen – aspirin interaction: a double-blind cross-over study. *Curr. Med. Res. Op.*, **5** (Special Issue), 53.

*Cardoe, N. (1977) A double-blind crossover study to compare the efficacy of three dosage levels of flurbiprofen in the treatment of rheumatoid disease and osteoarthrosis. *Curr. Med. Res. Op.*, **5** (Special Issue), 99.

Cardoe, N., de-Silva, M., Glass, R.C. and Risdall, P.N. (1977) Serum concentrations of flurbiprofen in rheumatoid patients receiving flurbiprofin over long periods of time. *Curr. Med. Res. Op.*, **5** (Special Issue), 21.

Chalmers, T.M., Glass, R.C. and Risdall, P.C. (1977) Concentrations of flurbiprofen in serum and synovial fluid from patients with active rheumatoid disease: some preliminary observations. *Curr. Med. Res. Op.*, **5** (Special Issue), 17.

Cremoncini, C., Vignati, E., Valente, C. and Dossena, M.G. (1977) Platelet adhesiveness, thromboclastogram, prothrombin activity and partial thromboplastin time during treatment with flurbiprofen. *Curr. Med. Res. Op.*, **5** (Special Issue), 135.

Davis, T., Lederer, D.A., Spencer, A.A. and McNicol, G.P. (1974) The effect of flurbiprofen [2-(2-fluoro-4-biphenyl) proprionic acid] on platelet function and blood coagulation. *Thromb. Res.*, **5**, 667.

Doury, P. and Pattin, S. (1977) Comparative study of effectiveness of flurbiprofen given twice or 3-times daily. *Curr. Med. Res. Op.*, **5** (Special Issue), 127.

Ford-Hutchinson, A.W., Walker, J.R., Connor, N.S. *et al.* (1977) Separate anti-inflammatory effects of indomethacin, flurbiprofen and benoxaprofen. *J. Pharm. Pharmacol.*, **29**, 372.

*Franco, P.A., Ferri, S. and Di Mummo, O. (1977) Controlled clinical trial comparing flurbiprofen and phenylbutazone in patients with rheumatoid arthritis. *Curr. Med. Res. Op.*, **5** (Special Issue), 74.

*Frank, O. (1977) A double-blind comparative study of 150 mg flurbiprofen daily and 75 mg indomethacin daily in the treatment of osteoarthrosis of the hip joint. *Curr. Med. Res. Op.*, **5** (Special Issue), 91.

Glenn, E.M., Rohloff, N., Bowman, B.J. and Lyster, S.C. (1973) The pharmacology of 2-(2-fluoro-4-biphenyl) proprionic acid (flurbiprofen). A potent non-steroidal anti-inflammatory drug. *Agents and Actions*, **3**, 210.

*Good, A. and Mena, H. (1977) Treatment of ankylosing spondylitis with flurbiprofen and indomethacin. *Curr. Med. Res. Op.*, **5** (Special Issue), 117.

*Grahame, R. and Calin, A. (1975) A controlled trial of 'Froben' (flurbiprofen) in ankylosing spondylitis – a comparison with phenylbutazone. *Curr. Med. Res. Op.*, **3**, 42.

*Hazeleman, B.L. and Bulgen, D.Y. (1977) A comparative study of the long-term efficacy of flurbiprofen and indomethacin in the treatment of rheumatoid arthritis, with special reference to iron metabolism. *Curr. Med. Res. Op.*, **5** (Special Issue), 58.

Huskisson, E.C., Scott, P.J., Boyle, S. and Patrick, M. (1977) Flurbiprofen at night. *Curr. Med. Res. Op.*, **5** (Special Issue), 85.

Innes, E.H. (1977) Efficacy and tolerance of flurbiprofen in the elderly using liquid and tablet formulations. *Curr. Med. Res. Op.*, **5** (Special Issue), 122.

Joshi, V.R., Lele, R.D., Virani, A.R. *et al.* (1977) Steroid-sparing action of flurbiprofen: use of an additional parameter of joints scans with ^{99}m technetium. *Curr. Med. Res. Op.*, **5** (Special Issue), 120.

*Kay, B. (1975) Oral flurbiprofen for post-operative pain. *Curr. Med. Res. Op.*, **3**, 49.

*Kogstad, O.A. (1973) Flurbiprofen in patients with osteoarthrosis. *Abstracts of XIII International Congress of Rheumatology, Kyoto*, p. 156.

*Kruger, H.H. (1977) Flurbiprofen and indomethacin in the treatment of rheumatoid arthritis: a double-blind cross-over study. *Curr. Med. Res. Op.*, **5** (Special Issue), 77.

Marbet, G.A., Duckert, F., Walter, M. *et al.* (1977) Interaction study between phenprocoumon and flurbiprofen. *Curr. Med. Res. Op.*, **5** (Special Issue), 26.

*Mena, H.R. and Willkens, R.F. (1977) Treatment of ankylosing spondylitis with flurbiprofen or phenylbutazone. *Eur. J. Clin. Pharmacol.*, **11**, 263.

*Muckle, D.S. (1977) A double-blind trial of flurbiprofen and aspirin in soft tissue trauma. *Rheumatol. Rehabil.*, **16**, 58.

Nishizawa, E.E., Wynalda, D.J., Fuydam, D.E. and Molony, B.A. (1973) Flurbiprofen, a new potent inhibitor of platelet aggregation. *Thromb. Res.*, **3**, 577.

*Pipitone, V., Numo, R. and Loizzi, P. (1977) Flurbiprofen in rheumatoid arthritis therapy. *Curr. Med. Res. Op.*, **5** (Special Issue), 88.

Sheldrake, F.E., Webber, J.M. and Marsh, B.D. (1977) A long-term assessment of flurbiprofen. *Curr. Med. Res. Op.*, **5** (Special Issue), 106.

*Siegmeth, W. (1977) A comparative study of flurbiprofen and indomethacin in rheumatoid arthritis. *Curr. Med. Res. Op.*, **5** (Special Issue), 64.

Sim, A.K., McCraw, A.P. and Sim, M.F. (1975) An evaluation of the effect of flurbiprofen [2-(2-fluoro-4-biphenyl) proprionic acid] on platelet behaviour. *Thomb. Res.*, **7**, 655.

Thebault, J.J., Lagrue, G. *et al.* (1977) Clinical pharmacology of flurbiprofen: a novel inhibitor of platelet aggregation. *Curr. Med. Res. Op.*, **5** (Special Issue), 130.

*Tiselius, P. (1973) Flurbiprofen in the treatment of osteoarthrosis. *Abstracts of XIII International Congress of Rheumatology, Kyoto*, p. 172.

Vakil, B.J., Kulkarni, R.D., Kulkarni, V.N. *et al.* (1977a) Estimation of gastro-intestinal blood loss in volunteers treated with non-steroidal anti-inflammatory agents. *Curr. Med. Res. Op.*, **5** (Special Issue), 32.

Vakil, B.J., Shah, P.N., Dalal, N.J. *et al.* (1977b) Endoscopic study of gastro-intestinal injury with non-steroidal anti-inflammatory drugs. *Curr. Med. Res. Op.*, **5** (Special Issue), 38.

Woodland, J., Currey, H.L.F. and Vernon-Roberts, B. (1977) The effect of anti-inflammatory and antirheumatic drugs on inflammation in the rat. *Curr. Med. Res. Op.*, **5** (Special Issue), 3.

Yasunaga, K. and Ryo, R. (1975) Evaluation of flurbiprofen as an anti-thrombotic agent. *Jap. Arch. Int. Med.*, **22**, 43.

Fenbufen

*Ammitzboll, F. (1979) Fenbufen and indomethacin in the treatment of rheumatoid arthritis. *Scand. J. Rheumatol.*, (Suppl. 23), 5.

*Bianchi, W. (1977) Long-term therapeutic efficacy and tolerance with two oral dosage regimens of fenbufen in 21 patients suffering from classical and definite rheumatoid arthritis – comparative trial with indomethacin. *A Folha Medica*, **74**, 479.

*Bonomo, I. (1977) Clinical trial with fenbufen in a double-blind cross-over study with oxyphenbutazone in degenerative joint disease. *A Folha Medica*, **74**, 225.

*Brenol, J.C. (1977) The treatment of osteoarthritis with a new therapeutic agent – fenbufen. *A Folha Medica*, **74**, 335.

*Buxton, R. (1978) Fenbufen compared with indomethacin in osteoarthritis. *Curr. Med. Res. Op.*, **5**, 682.

*Chalem, F., Pena, M., Lizarazo, H. and Farias, P. (1977) Comparison of fenbufen and aspirin in the treatment of rheumatoid arthritis. *Curr. Ther. Res.*, **22**, 679.

Child, R.G., Osterberg, A.C., Sloboda, A.E. and Tomcufcik, A.S. (1977) A new anti-inflammatory analgesic arylalkanoic acid 3-(4-biphenyl carbonyl) propionic acid, fenbufen. Synthesis and structure – activity relationships of analogs. *J. Pharm. Sci.*, **66**, 466.

Coutinho, A., Bonelli, J. and de Carvalho, P.C.N. (1976) A double-blind comparative study of the analgesic effects of fenbufen, codeine, aspirin, propoxyphene and placebo. *Curr. Ther. Res.*, **19**, 58.

*Da Gama, G.G. (1976) Fenbufen in comparison to ibuprofen in patients with rheumatoid arthritis. *A Folha Medica*, **73**, 625.

*De Freitas, G.G. (1977) Clinical and laboratory evaluation of fenbufen versus naproxen in rheumatoid arthritis. *A Folha Medica*, **74**, 217.

*De Salcedo, I., Arias, L.F. and Greenberg, B.P. (1975) Fenbufen – a new nonsteroidal anti-inflammatory agent: comparison with phenylbutazone in rheumatoid arthritis. *Curr. Ther. Res.*, **18**, 295.

*Dunky, A. and Eberl, R. (1977) Anti-inflammatory efficacy of a new anti-rheumatic drug – fenbufen – in rheumatoid arthritis. *XIV International Congress of Rheumatology*, 203 (Abstract).

*Guedes, M.S. and Coutinho, A. (1975) Atividade analgesica do Fenbufen en odontalgia: comparacao com aspirina, codeina, propoxifeno e placebo. *A Folha Medica*, **71**, 593.

*Henrikson, P.A., Tjernberg, A., Ashlstrom, U. and Peterson, L.-E. (1979) Analgesic efficacy and safety of fenbufen following surgical removal of a lower wisdom tooth. *J. Intl. Med. Res.*, **7**, 107.

*Katona, G. (1975) Double-blind cross-over study with fenbufen and indomethacin in 30 rheumatoid arthritis patients. *Scand. J. Rheumatol.*, **4** (Suppl. 8), 119 (Abstract).

*Mathias-Filho, A.P. and Bianchi, W. (1975) A double-blind crossover study with fenbufen and indomethacin in patients with rheumatoid arthritis. *A Folha Medica*, **71**, 459.

Mawdsley, P. (1979) in *Clinics in Rheumatic Diseases* (ed. E.C. Huskisson), Vol. 6, No. 3, Anti-Rheumatic Drugs II, Saunders, London, p. 615.

*Nunes, C.V. (1975) Rheumatoid arthritis: a double-blind comparative trial of fenbufen and phenylbutazone. *A Folha Medica*, **71**, 335.

Panagides, J. (1976) Effects of fenbufen and other anti-inflammatory drugs on rat liver lysosomes. *Biochem. Pharmacol.*, **25**, 2303.

*Roden, D.F. (1979) Double-blind comparison of fenbufen and aspirin in the treatment of osteoarthritis. *J. Irish Med. Assoc.*, **72**, 250.

Sloboda, A.E. and Osterberg, A.C. (1976) The pharmacology of fenbufen. 3-(4-biphenylactic acid, interesting anti-inflammatory-analgesic agents. *Inflammation*, **1**, 415.

*Sunshine, A. (1975) Analgesic value of fenbufen in postoperative patients. *Clin. Pharmacol. Ther.*, **15**, 476.

*Valtonen, E.J. (1979) Clinical comparison of fenbufen and aspirin in osteoarthritis. *Scand. J. Rheumatol.* (Suppl. 27), 1.

Van Lear, G.E. (1978) Quantitation of the anti-inflammatory agent fenbufen and its metabolites in human serum and urine using high pressure liquid chromatography. *J. Pharm. Sci.*, **67**, 1662.

*Vergara-Castro, J.M., Arias, L.F. and Greenberg, B.P. (1976) A comparative clinical trial of fenbufen and indomethacin in patients with rheumatoid arthritis. *J. Intl. Clin. Res.*, **4**, 418.

*Villela-Nunes, C. (1975) A double-blind crossover comparison of fenbufen and phenylbutazone in rheumatoid arthritis. *A Folha Medica*, **71**, 335.

Benoxaprofen

*Alarcon-Segovia, D. (1980) Long-term treatment of symptomatic OA with benoxaprofen. Double-blind comparison with aspirin and ibuprofen. *J. Rheumatol.*, **7** (Suppl. 6), 89.

*Atkinson, M.H., Brown, T.A., Robinson, H.S. and Willkens, R.F. (1980) Crossover comparison of benoxaprofen and naproxen in RA. *J. Rheumatol.*, **7** (Suppl. 6), 109.

Bacon, P.A., Davies, J. and Ring, F.J. (1980) Benoxaprofen – dose-range studies using quantitative thermography. *J. Rheumatol.*, **7** (Suppl. 6), 46.

Bang, N.U., Dwyer, A.M., Marks, C.A. *et al.* (1980) The effects of benoxaprofen and indomethacin on platelet function and biochemistry. *J. Rheumatol.*, **7** (Suppl. 6), 27.

Berry, H., Bloom, B., Hamilton, E.B.D. *et al.* (1980) Dose–range studies of benoxaprofen compared with placebo in patients with active RA. *J. Rheumatol.*, **7** (Suppl. 6), 54.

*Bird, H.A., Rhind, V.M., Pickup, M.E. and Wright, V. (1980) A comparative study of benoxaprofen and indomethacin in AS. *J. Rheumatol.*, **7** (Suppl. 6), 139.

*Blechman, W.J. (1980) Crossover comparison of benoxaprofen and naproxen in OA. *J. Rheumatol.*, **7** (Suppl. 6), 116.

Cardoe, N. and Halsey, J.P. (1982) Benoxaprofen: side-effect profile in 300 patients. *Br. Med. J.*, **284**, 1365.

Cashin, C.H., Dawson, W. and Kitchen, E.A. (1977) The pharmacology of benoxaprofen (2-[4-chlorophenyl]-α-methyl-5-benzoxazole acetic acid), LRCL 3794, a new compound with anti-inflammatory activity apparently unrelated to inhibition of prostaglandin synthesis. *J. Pharm. Pharmacol.*, **29**, 330.

Chatfield, D.H. and Green, J.N. (1978) Disposition and metabolism of benoxaprofen in laboratory animals and man. *Xenobiotica*, **8**, 133.

Chatfield, D.H., Cashin, C.H., Kitchen, E.A. and Green, J.N. (1977) Relation between plasma concentration and therapeutic efficacy of a new anti-inflammatory compound, benoxaprofen (LRCL 3794) in rats with adjuvant-induced arthritis. *J. Pharm. Pharmacol.*, **29**, 371.

Chatfield, D.H., Tarrant, M.E., Smith, G.L. and Speirs, C.F. (1977) Pharmacokinetics studies with benoxaprofen in man: prediction of steady-state levels from single-dose data. *Br. J. Clin. Pharmacol.*, **4**, 579.

Chatfield, D.H., Green, J.N., Kao, J.C. *et al.* (1978) Plasma protein binding and interaction studies with benoxaprofen. *Biochem. Pharmacol.*, **27**, 887.

Dawson, W. (1980) The comparative pharmacology of benoxaprofen. *J. Rheumatol.*, **7** (Suppl. 6), 5.

Fenton, D.A., English, J.S. and Wilkinson, J.D. (1982) Reversal of male-pattern baldness, hypertrichosis, and accelerated hair and nail growth in patients receiving benoxaprofen. *Br. Med. J.*, **284**, 1228.

*Gum, O.B. (1980) Long-term efficacy and safety of benoxaprofen: comparisons with aspirin and ibuprofen in patients with active RA. *J. Rheumatol.*, **7** (Suppl. 6), 89.

*Highton, J. and Grahame, R. (1978) A comparative trial of benoxaprofen and naproxen. *Rheumatol. Rehabil.*, **17**, 259.

Highton, J. and Grahame, R. (1980) Benoxaprofen in the treatment of OA – a comparison with ibuprofen. *J. Rheumatol.*, **7** (Suppl. 6), 125.

Hindson, C., Daymond, T., Diffey, B. and Lawlor, F. (1982) Side effects of benoxaprofen. *Br. Med. J.*, **284**, 1368.

Huskisson, E.C. (1979) Clinical studies with benoxaprofen. The story so far. *Eur. J. Rheumatol. Infl.*, **3**, 29.

Huskisson, E.C. and Scott, J. (1979) Treatment of rheumatoid arthritis with a single daily dose of benoxaprofen. *Rheumatol. Rehabil.*, **18**, 110.

Huskisson, E.C., Scott, J. and Dieppe, P. (1978) Benoxaprofen: a clinical trial with an unusual design. *Rheumatol. Rehabil.*, **17**, 254.

Jones, R.W., Waugh, A.E., Woodage, T.J., Wild, R.N. and Glynne, A. (1980) The pharmacokinetics and acceptability of benoxaprofen following rectal administration. *J. Rheumatol.*, **7** (Suppl. 6), 20.

*Lambert, J.R. and Wright, V. (1977) A double-blind comparison of benoxaprofen and placebo in rheumatoid arthritis. *Curr. Med. Res. Op.*, **5**, 269.

Lightfoot, R.W. (1980) Benoxaprofen administered once a day: determination of optimum dosage schedule. *J. Rheumatol.*, **7** (Suppl. 6), 61.

Meacock, S.C.R. and Kitchen, A.E. (1979) Effects of the non-steroidal anti-inflammatory drug benoxaprofen on leucocyte migration. *J. Pharm. Pharmacol.*, **31**, 366.

Mikulaschek, W.M. (1980) Long-term safety of benoxaprofen. *J. Rheumatol.*, **7** (Suppl. 6), 100.

Nash, J.F., Carmichael, R.H., Ridolfo, A.S. and Spradlin, C.T. (1980) Pharmacokinetic studies of benoxaprofen after therapeutic doses with a review of related pharmacokinetic and metabolic studies. *J. Rheumatol.*, **7** (Suppl. 6), 12.

Ridolfo, A.S., Crabtree, R.E., Johnson, D.W. and Rockhold, F.W. (1980) Gastrointestinal micro bleeding: comparisons between benoxaprofen and the non-steroidal anti-inflammatory agents. *J. Rheumatol.*, **7** (Suppl. 6), 36.

Ridolfo, A.S., Nicklander, R. and Mikulaschek, W.M. (1979) in *Clinics in Rheumatic Diseases*. (ed. E.C. Huskisson), Vol. 5, No. 2. Saunders, London, p. 393.

*Ridolfo, A.S., Simpson, P.J. and Ceremele, B.J. (1978) A comparison of once daily with twice daily dosage of benoxaprofen in patients with rheumatoid arthritis. *Clin. Pharmacol. Ther.*, **23**, 127.

*Roth, S.H. (1980) Benoxaprofen: once a day vs twice a day in patients with RA or OA. *J. Rheumatol.*, **7** (Suppl. 6), 68.

Smith, G.L., Goulbourn, R.A., Burt, R.A.P. and Chatfield, D.H. (1977) Preliminary studies of absorption and excretion in benoxaprofen in man. *Br. J. Clin. Pharmacol.*, **4**, 585.

Taggart, H. McA. and Alderdice, J.M. (1982) Fatal cholestatic jaundice in elderly patients taking benoxaprofen. *Br. Med. J.*, **284**, 1372.

*Tyson, V.C.H. and Glynne, A. (1980) A comparative study of benoxaprofen and ibuprofen in OA in general practice. *J. Rheumatol.*, **7** (Suppl. 6), 132.

Indoprofen

Baldrighi, G. and Sacchetti, G. (1976) Studio preliminare di emodinamica in pazienti cardiopatici trattati con dose unica endovenosa di indoprofene. *Clin. Ther.*, **79**, 339.

Berry, H., Fernandes, L., Clarke, A.K. *et al.* (1978) Indoprofen and naproxen in the treatment of rheumatoid arthritis: a clinical trial. *Br. Med. J.*, **i**, 274.

Bruni, G., Croppi, W., Fanfani, A. and Sacchetti, G. (1980) in *Clinics in Rheumatic Diseases. Anti-Rheumatic Drugs II*, (ed. E.C. Huskisson), Vol. 6, No. 3, Saunders, London, p. 499.

Buttinoni, A., Cuttica, A., Franceschini, J. *et al.* (1973) Pharmacological study on a new analgesic anti-inflammatory drug: 4-(1-oxo-2-iso-indolinyl)-phenyl-proprionic acid or K4277. *Arzneimittelforschrift*, **23**, 1100.

Caruso, I., Fumagalli, M., Marcolongo, R. and Sacchetti, G. (1977) Indoprofen for acute gouty arthritis. *Arthr. Rheum.*, **20**, 1438.

Chériè Lignière, G., Molteni, M. and Colombo, B. (1979) L'indoprofene per via endovenosa. *Reumatismo*, **31**, 291.

Chiapuzzo, A. (1979) A comparison of indoprofen and indomethacin in the supportive treatment of soft-tissue injuries in football players: a pilot study. *J. Intl. Med. Res.*, **7**, 57.

Cooper, S.A., Breen, J.F. and Giuliani, R.I. (1979) Replicate studies comparing the relative efficacies of aspirin and indoprofen in oral surgery out-patients. *J. Clin. Pharmacol.*, **19**, 151.

Fuccella, L.M., Goldaniga, G.C., Moro, E. *et al.* (1973) Fate of the analgesic and anti-inflammatory drug K4277 after oral administration to man. *Eur. J. Clin. Pharmacol.*, **6**, 256.

Giro, C. and Lo Presti, R. (1979) Confronto in doppio cieco tra indoprofene ed ibuprofen in pazienti affetti da osteoartrosi. *Giornale di Clinica Medica*, **60**, 65.

Huskisson, E.C. and Scott, J. (1979) Analgesic and anti-inflammatory properties of indoprofen. *Rheumatol. Rehabil.*, **18**, 49.

Okun, R., Green, J.W. and Shackleford, R.W. (1979) An analgesic comparison study of indoprofen *versus* aspirin and placebo in surgical pain. *J. Clin. Pharmacol.*, **19**, 487.

Rubegni, M., Bellini, P.G. and Ferrati, G. (1978) Ricerca terapeutica nell' osteoartrosi del vecchio; prova controllata con indoprofene e ibuprofene. *Clin. Ter.*, **86**, 119.

Saba, G.C. and Orlandi, G. (1979) A short-term therapeutic trial with indoprofen *versus* indomethacin in osteoarthrosis. *Curr. Ther. Res.*, **25**, 260.

Smith, R.V., Humphrey, D.W. and Escalona-Castillo, H. (1977) GLC determination of indoprofen in plasma. *J. Pharm. Sci.*, **66**, 132.

Tirri, G., Gallo, M. and La Montagna, G. (1980) Ricerca controllata sul trattamento dell'artrite zeumatoide con indorpfene. *Reumatismo*, **32**, 51.

Fenamic acids

*Bain, L.S. and Masheter, H.C. (1966) Flufenamic acid and indomethacin in rheumatoid arthritis. *Ann. Phys. Med.* (Suppl: Fenamates in Medicine), 104.

*Barnardo, D.E., Currey, H.L.F., Mason, R.M. *et al.* (1966) Mefenamic acid and flufenamic acid compound with aspirin and phenylbutazone in rheumatoid arthritis. *Br. Med. J.*, **ii**, 342.

*Brocks, B.E. (1966) A comparison of flufenamic acid and

phenylbutazone in osteoarthritis of the hip. *Ann. Phys. Med.* (Suppl: Fenamates in Medicine), 114.

*Cardoe, N. (1966) A clinical trial of flufenamic acid in rheumatoid arthritis. *Ann. Phys. Med.* (Suppl: Fenamates in Medicine), 99.

*Coodley, E.L. (1963) Evaluation of drug therapy in rheumatoid arthritis – study of flufenamic acid. *W. Med.*, 4, 228.

*Cowan, I.C. and Masheter, H.C. (1966) Flufenamic acid in rheumatoid arthritis. A placebo controlled study. *Clin. Trials J.*, 3, 503.

De Salcedo, I., Fouseca Ferreira, F.M., Silva, J.L. and Carrington, M.D. (1966) Some metabolic and hormonal effects of flufenamic acid. *Ann. Phys. Med.* (Suppl: Fenamates in Medicine), 62.

*Fearnley, M.E. and Masheter, H.C. (1966) Controlled trial of flufenamic acid therapy in rheumatoid arthritis. *Ann. Phys. Med.*, 6, 206.

Ferris, J.E. and Pigott, P.V. (1966) Evaluation of mefenamic acid and flufenamic acid in clinical pain. *Ann. Phys. Med.* (Suppl: Fenamates in Medicine), 84.

Haward, L.R.C. (1966) Effects of the fenamates on the threshold of pain. *Ann. Phys. Med.* (Suppl: Fenamates in Medicine), 55.

†Hill, A.G.S. (1966) Review of flufenamic acid in rheumatoid arthritis. *Ann. Phys. Med.* (Suppl: Fenamates in Medicine), 87.

Holmes E.L. (1967) Fenamates in medicine. *Ann. Phys. Med.* (Suppl.), 36.

Hume Kendall, P. (ed.) (1966) Fenamates in Medicine: A Symposium. *Ann. Phys. Med.* (Suppl.).

*Rajan, K.T., Hill, A.G.S., Barr, A. and Whitehall, E. (1967) Flufenamic acid in rheumatoid arthritis. *Ann. Rheum. Dis.*, 26, 43.

*Simpson, M.R., Simpson, N.R.W. and Masheter, H.C. (1966a) Flufenamic acid in rheumatoid arthritis. Comparison with aspirin and the results of extended treatment. *Ann. Phys. Med.*, 8, 208.

*Simpson, M.R., Simpson, N.R.W., Masheter, H.C. and Hardy, S.M. (1966b) Flufenamic acid in rheumatoid arthritis – the second six months of treatment. *Ann. Phys. Med.* (Suppl: Fenamates in Medicine), 111.

*Simpson, M.R., Simpson, N.R.W., Scott, B.O. and Beathy, D.C. (1966c) A controlled study of flufenamic acid in ankylosing spondylitis. *Ann. Phys. Med.* (Suppl: Fenamates in Medicine), 126.

*Sydnes, O.A. (1966) A controlled clinical trial of flufenamic acid in rheumatoid arthritis. *Ann. Phys. Med.* (Suppl: Fenamates in Medicine), 93.

Tudhope, G.R. (1966) Comparison of flufenamic acid with aspirin and paracetamol in terms of gastrointestinal blood loss. *Ann. Phys. Med.* (Suppl: Fenamates in Medicine), 58.

Winder, C.V., Kaump, D.H., Glazko, A.J. and Holmes, E.L. (1966) Experimental observations on flufenamic, mefenamic, and meclofenamic acids. *Ann. Phys. Med.* (Suppl: Fenamates in Medicine), 7.

Pyrazolones

Phenylbutazone and oxyphenbutazone

Aggeler, P.M., O'Reilly, R.A., Leong, L. and Kowitz, P.E. (1967) Potentiation of anticoagulant effect of warfarin by phenylbutazone. *N. Engl. J. Med.*, 276, 496.

Bakke, O., Draffen, G.H. and Davies, D.S. (1974) The metabolism of phenylbutazone in the rat. *Xenobiotica*, 4, 237.

Benedek, T.G. (1962) Blockage of intrathyroidal organification by phenylbutazone. *J. Clin. Endocrinol. Metab.*, 22, 959.

*Boersma, J.W. (1976) Retardation of ossification of the lumbar vertebral column in ankylosing spondylitis by means of phenylbutazone. *Scand. J. Rheumatol.*, 5, 60.

Böttiger, L.E. and Westerholm, B. (1972) Aplastic anaemia II: drug-induced aplastic anaemia. *Acta Med. Scand.*, 192, 319.

†Brooks, P.M., Walker, J.J., Dick, W.C. *et al.* (1975) Phenylbutazone: a clinico-pharmacological study in rheumatoid arthritis. *Br. J. Clin. Pharmacol.*, 2, 437.

Bruck, E., Fearnley, M.E., Meanock, I. and Patley, H. (1954) Phenylbutazone therapy: relation between the toxic and therapeutic effects and the blood level. *Lancet*, i, 225.

Calabro, J.J. (1967) Cancer and arthritis. *Arthr. Rheum.*, 10, 553.

*Calabro, J.J. (1968) An appraisal of the medical and surgical management of ankylosing spondylitis. *Clin. Orth. Rel. Res.*, 60, 1068.

Chen, W., Vrindtien, P.A., Dayton, P.G. and Banns, J.A. (1962) Accelerated aminopyrine metabolism in human subjects pretreated with phenylbutazone. *Life Sci.*, 1, 35.

Fowler, P.D. (1967) Marrow toxicity of the pyrazoles. *Ann. Rheum. Dis.*, 26, 344.

†Fowler, P.D. (1975) in *Clinics in the Rheumatic Diseases* (eds C.M. Pearson and W.C. Dick) Vol. 1, No. 2, Saunders, London, p. 267.

Fowler, P.D., Woolf, D. and Alexander, S. (1975) Phenylbutazone and hepatitis. *Rheumatol. Rehabil.*, 14, 71.

Girdwood, R.H. (1974) Death after taking medicaments. *Br. Med. J.*, i, 501.

*Godfrey, R., Calabro, T.J. and Mills, D. (1972) A double blind crossover trial of aspirin, indomethacin and phenylbutazone in ankylosing spondylitis. *Arthr. Rheum.*, 15, 110.

Graham, W. (1958) The status of phenylbutazone (Butazolidin) in the treatment of rheumatic disorders. *Can. Med. Assoc. J.*, 79, 634.

*Hart, F.D. (1954) Ankylosing spondylitis: a survey. *Ann. Rheum. Dis.*, 13, 186.

*Hart, F.D. (1955) The treatment of ankylosing spondylitis. *Proc. R. Soc. Med.*, 48, 207.

Hart, F.D. (ed.) (1978) *Drug Treatment of the Rheumatic Diseases*, MTP Press, Lancaster, p. 21.

Inman, W.H.W. (1977) Study of fatal bone marrow depression with reference to phenylbutazone and oxyphenbutazone. *Br. Med. J.*, i, 1500.

*Kinsella, T.D., MacDonald, F.R. and Johnson, L.G. (1966) Ankylosing spondylitis: a late re-evaluation of 92 cases. *Can. Med. Assoc. J.*, 95, 1.

Lawrence, A. (1960) Generalised lymphadenopathy with phenylbutazone. *Br. Med. J.*, ii, 1736.

Leavesley, G.M., Stenhouse, H.S., Dougan, L. and Woodliff, H.J. (1969) Phenylbutazone and leukaemia: is there a relationship? *Med. J. Austr.* (November), 963.

*Levernieux, J. (1965) L'évolution de la pelvispondylite rheumatismale traitée par la phenylbutazone pendant 10 ans. *Semaine Thérapeutique*, 41, 357.

Lewis-Faning, E. and Fowler, P.D. (1971) Drug treatment of rheumatic disorders in general practice: a comparative study of aspirin and an alkali-phenylbutazone preparation. *Br. J. Clin. Pract.*, **25**, 123.

MacFarlane, J.D., Masey, M.N., Grahame, R. and Burry, H.C. (1976) Gastrointestinal blood loss and phenylbutazone and feprazone. *Rheumatol. Rehabil.*, **15**, 108.

*Mason, R.M. and Hawes, R.G. (1963) The treatment of ankylosing spondylitis. *Proc. Austr. Rheum. Cong.*, Sept. 1963, 51.

McIntosh, I.B. and Fowler, P.D. (1977) Phenylbutazone suppositories: a multi-centre general practitioner study. *Practitioner*, **219**, 391.

Murray-Bruce, D.J. (1966) Letter. *Br. Med. J.*, **i**, 1599.

Nieweg, H.O. (1973) Aplastic anemia (panmyelopathy). in *Blood Disorders Due to Drugs and Other Agents* (ed. R.H. Goodwood), Excerpta Medica, Amsterdam, p. 83.

*Pearson, C.M. (1964) Management of ankylosing spondylitis. *Mod. Treat.*, **1**, 1221.

Rodgers, R.D. and Simpson, R.W. (1966) Salivary gland enlargement and phenylbutazone. *Br. Med. J.*, **ii**, 113.

Rushford, W.A.I. and Fowler, P.D. (1970) Assessment of enteric coated phenylbutazone in general practice. *Practitioner*, **205**, 671.

†Smyth, C.J. and Percy, J.S. (1973) Comparison of phenylbutazone and indomethacin in acute gout. *Ann. Rheum. Dis.*, **32**, 351.

*Sturge, R.A., Scott, J.T., Hamilton, E.B.D. *et al.* (1977) Multicentre trial of naproxen and phenylbutazone in acute gout. *Ann. Rheum. Dis.*, **36**, 80.

Strandberg, B. (1965) Phenylbutazone in the treatment of rheumatic diseases. A survey and clinical report. *Acta Rheumatol. Scand.* (Suppl.), **10**, 1.

*Van Gerwen, F., Van der Kost, J.K. and Gribnan, F.W. (1978) Double blind trial of naproxen and phenylbutazone in ankylosing spondylitis. *Ann. Rheum. Dis.*, **37**, 85.

Whittaker, J.A. and Price Evans, D.A. (1970) Genetic control of phenylbutazone metabolism in man. *Br. Med. J.*, **iv**, 323.

Azapropazone

Adrian, R.W. (1973) Reproduktionstoxikologische Untersuchungen mit Azapropazon. *Arz. Forsch.*, **23**, 658.

Adrian, R.W., Walker, F.S. and Noel, P.R.B. (1976) Toxicological studies on azapropazone. *Curr. Med. Res. Op.*, **4** (Special Issue), 17.

Brooks, P.M. and Buchanan, W.W. (1976) Azapropazone: its place in the management of rheumatoid conditions. *Curr. Med. Res. Op.*, **4**, 94.

*Brooks, P.M., Mason, D.I.R., McNeil, R. *et al.* (1976) An assessment of the therapeutic potential of azapropazone in rheumatoid arthritis. *Curr. Med. Res. Op.*, **4**, 50.

Eberl, R. (1976) Prolonged treatment with azapropazone. *Curr. Med. Res. Op.*, **4** (Special Issue), 76.

Eberl, R. and Bröll, R.H. (1977) in *Azapropazon bei Erkrankungen des Rheumatischen Formenkreises* (eds H. Fenner and R. Eberl), G. Braun GmbH, Karlsruhe, pp. 7–10.

Frank, O. (1971) Untersuchungen zur urikosurischen Wirkung von Azapropazon. *Zeitsch. Rheumaforsch.*, **30**, 368.

Grennan, D.M., Watkins, C. and Kennedy, A.C. (1974) Preliminary clinical evaluation of azapropazone in rheumatoid arthritis. *Curr. Med. Res. Op.*, **2** (Special Issue), 67.

*Grennan, D.M., McLeod, M., Watkins, C. and Dick, W.C. (1976) Clinical assessment of azapropazone in rheumatoid

arthritis. *Curr. Med. Res. Op.*, **4**, 44.

*Hingorani, K. (1976) A comparative study of azapropazone and ibuprofen in the treatment of osteoarthrosis of the knee. *Curr. Med. Res. Op.*, **4**, 57.

Hradsky, M. and Bruce, L. (1978) Endoscopic evaluation of the effect of azapropazone on the gastric mucosa. *Scand. J. Rheumatol.*, **7**, 31.

Huntington Research Center (HRC) (1975a) *Teratology Study in Rabbits.* February 5 (T-11-037-75).

Huntington Research Center (HRC) (1975b) AHR-3018: *Perinatal and Postnatal Study in Rats.* February 20 (T-11-038-75).

Huntington Research Center (HRC) (1975c) AHR-3018: *Fertility and General Reproductive Performance Study in Rats.* March 14 (T-11-078-75).

Huntington Research Center (HRC) (1975d) AHR-3018: *Teratology Study in Rats.* March 14 (T-11-079-75).

Jahn, U. (1973) Pharmakologische Prüfung von 6-Hydroxy-Azapropazon. *Arz. Forsch.*, **23**, 666.

Jahn, U. and Adrian, R.W. (1969) Pharmakologische und toxikologische Prüfung des neuen Antiphlogistikums Azapropazon = 3-Dimethyl-amino-7methyl-1, 2-(n-propyl-malonyl)-1, 2-dihydro-1, 2, 4-benzotriazin. *Arz. Forsch.*, **19**, 36.

Jahn, U., Reller, J. and Schatz, F. (1973) Pharmakokinetische Untersuchungen mit Azapropazon bei Tieren. *Arz. Forsch.*, **23**, 660.

Jones, C.J. (1976) The pharmacology and pharmacokinetics of azapropazone – a review. *Curr. Med. Res. Op.*, **4** (Special Issue), 3.

*Kageyama, T. (1969) Clinical results of azapropazone for periarthritis humeroscapularis (painful shoulder). *Shinryo to Shinyaka*, **22**, 1161.

Klatt, L. and Koss, F.W. (1973a) Pharmacokinetic studies with azapropazone dihydrate labelled with Carbon-14 in the rat. *Arz. Forsch.* (Drug Research), **23**, 913.

Klatt, L. and Koss, F.W. (1973b) Human pharmacokinetic studies with ^{14}C-tagged azapropazone dihydrate. *Arz. Forsch.* (Drug Research), **23**, 920.

*Lassus, A. (1976) A comparative pilot study of azapropazone and indomethacin in the treatment of psoriatic arthritis and Reiter's disease. *Curr. Med. Res. Op.*, **4** (Special Issue), 65.

Leach, H. (1976) The determination of azapropazone in blood plasma. *Curr. Med. Res. Op.*, **4**, 35.

*Mathies, H. and Kilani, S. (1970) Untersuchungen zur Glukokortikoid-Einsparung durch Azapropazon bei chronischer Polyarthritis. *Fortschritte der Medizin*, **88**, 942.

Mathies, H., Olbrich, E., Kilani, S. and Sausgruber, H. (1974) Glukokortikoideinsparung durch Azapropazone und Phenylbutazon im Doppelblind-cross-over-Vergleich. *Therapiewoche*, **24**, 3646.

Mennet, P., Olbrich, E., Ulrych, I. *et al.* (1971) Perorale Azapropazon-Behandlung beim Weichteilrheumatismus. *Schw. Med. Wochenschr.*, **101**, 647.

Mintz, G. and Fraga, A. (1976) Gastro-intestinal bleeding in patients with rheumatoid arthritis: the effects of azapropazone treatment. *Curr. Med. Res. Op.*, **4**, 89.

*Pavelka, K., Vojtisek, O. and Kankova, D. (1975) in *Azapropazon bei Erkrankungen des Rheumatischen Formenkreises* (eds H. fenner and R. Eberl), G. Braun GmbH, Karlsruhe, pp. 31–5.

Schatz, F., Adrian, R.W., Mixich, G. *et al.* (1970) Pharmacokinetic studies of the anti-inflammatory agent, azapropazone (Prolixan ® 300) in man. *Therapiewoche*, **20**, 39.

Sondervorst, M. (1979) in *Clinics in Rheumatic Diseases* (ed. E.C. Huskisson), Vol. 5, No. 2. Saunders, London, p. 465.

*Sugiyama, T., Okazaki, T. and Onoda, T. (1969) Examination of medicinal effect of azapropazone in chronic articular rheumatism. *Off. J. Jap. Rheum. Assoc.*, **9**, 16.

Thune, S. (1976a) A comparative study of azapropazone and indomethacin in the treatment of rheumatoid arthritis. *Curr. Med. Res. Op.*, **4**, 70.

*Thune, S. (1976b) Long-term use of azapropazone in rheumatoid arthritis. *Curr. Med. Res. Op.*, **4**, 80.

Feprazone

Casadio, S., Mantegani, A., Coppi, G. and Pala, G. (1967) On the healing properties of esters with D-panthenol with terpene acids, with particular reference to D-pantothenyl trifarnesylacetate. *Arz. Forsch.*, **17**, 1122.

Dotti, F., Ongari, R., Carazzi, R. and Chierichetti, S. (1972) Clinical study of a new anti-inflammatory drug: 4-prenyl-1, 2-diphenyl-3, 5-pyrazolidinedione (DA 2370). *Arz. Forsch.*, **22**, 265.

Fletcher, M.R., Loebl, W. and Scott, T.J. (1975) Feprazone, a new anti-inflammatory agent. Studies of potency and gastrointestinal tolerance. *Ann. Rheum. Dis.*, **34**, 190.

Ghiringelli, F., Mazzi, C. and Chierichetti, S. (1972) Metabolic and clinical effects of 4-prenyl-1, 2-diphenyl-3, 5-pyrazolidinedione (Da 2370). *Arz. Forsch.*, **22**, 268.

Harris, P.G. (1980) A monitored-release study of methrazone in general practice. *J. Intl. Med. Res.*, **8**, 276.

Ligniere, G.C., Colombo, B., Carrabba, M. *et al.* (1972) Clinical and laboratory evaluation of 4-prenyl-1, 2-diphenyl-3, 5-pyrazolidinedione (Da 2370) in rheumatoid arthritis and ankylosing spondylitis). *Arz. Forschschr.*, **22**, 253.

Macfarlane, J.D., Maisey, M.N., Grahame, R. and Burry, H.C. (1976) Gastrointestinal blood loss on phenylbutazone and feprazone. *Rheumatol. Rehabil.*, **15**, 108.

Pasotti, C., Barbieri, C., Buniva, G. and Chierichetti, S. (1972) Clinical trial of 4-prenyl-1, 2-diphenyl-3, 5-pyrazolidinedione (DA 2370) in painful osteoarticular conditions. *Arz. Forschschr.*, **22**, 262.

Rooney, P.J., McLeod, M., Grennan, D.M. and Dick, W.C. (1976) Feprazone (DA 2370) long-term experience in the management of rheumatoid arthritis complicated by severe dyspepsia. *Curr. Med. Res. Op.*, **3**, 642.

Rooney, P.J., Watkins, C., Ahola, S.J. *et al.* (1974) A short term double-blind controlled trial of prenazone (DA 2370) in rheumatoid arthritis. *Curr. Med. Res. Op.*, **2**, 43.

Oxicams

Piroxicam

Bachmann, F. (1979) Piroxicam ein neues nichtsteroidales antirheumatikum in der rheumatoiden arthritis. *Therapiewoche*, **29**, 5666.

Bachman, F. (1980) in *Rheumatology in the Eighties: An Advance in Therapy – Piroxicam* (ed. J.A. Boyle), Excerpta Medica, Princeton.

Bahr, R. (1980) Piroxicam, ein neues nichsteroides antirheumatikum. Ergebenisse einer multizentrischen prufung.

Zeitschr. Allgemeine Med., **56**, 199.

*Balogh, Z., Papazoglou, S.N., MacLeod, M. and Buchanan, W.W. (1979) A cross-over clinical trial of piroxicam, indomethacin and ibuprofen in rheumatoid arthritis. *Curr. Med. Res. Op.*, **6**, 148.

*Blum, W. and Wagenhauser, F. (1980) in *Rheumatology in the Eighties: An Advance in Therapy – Piroxicam* (ed. J.A. Boyle), Excerpta Medica, Princeton, New Jersey.

Box, J., Box, P., Turner, R. and Pisko, E. (1978) Piroxicam and rheumatoid arthritis: a double-blind 16-week study comparing piroxicam and phenylbutazone. *R. Soc. Med. Intl. Congr. Symp. Ser.*, **1**, 41.

Carty, T.J., Eskra, J.D., Lombardino, J.G. and Hoffman, W.W. (1980b) Piroxicam, a potent inhibitor of prostaglandin production in cell culture. Structure-activity study. *Prostaglandins*, **19**, 51.

Carty, T.J., Stevens, J.S., Lombardino, J.G. *et al.* (1980b) Piroxicam, a structurally novel anti-inflammatory compound. Mode of prostaglandin synthesis inhibition. *Prostaglandins*, **19**, 51.

*Commandré, F. (1980) in *Rheumatology in the Eighties: An Advance in Therapy – Piroxicam* (ed. J.A. Boyle), Excerpta Medica, Princeton, New Jersey.

†Dessain, P., Estabrooks, T.F. and Gordon, A.J. (1979) Piroxicam in the treatment of osteoarthrosis: a multicentre study in general practice involving 1218 patients. *J. Intl. Med. Res.*, **7**, 335.

DiPerri, T., Pasini, L.F., Auteri, A. *et al.* (1979) Effect of a single dose of piroxicam on human platelet aggregation *in vivo*. *Intl. J. Tiss. React.*, **1**, 161.

*Dixon, A.S. and Davies, J. (1980) in *Piroxicam, a new nonsteroidal anti-inflammatory agent. Proceedings of the Ninth European Congress of Rheumatology*, Academy Professional Information Services, New York, pp. 14–21.

Gaynor, B.J. and Constantine, J.W. (1979) The effects of piroxicam on platelet aggregation. *Experientia*, **35**, 797.

†Gordon, G.V., Abruzzo, J.L., Meyers, A.R. and Boyle, J.A. (1980) in *Rheumatology in the Eighties: An Advance in Therapy – Piroxicam* (ed. J.A. Boyle) Excerpta Medica, Princeton, New Jersey.

*Grewin, B. (1979) Piroxicam in rheumatoid arthritis. *Intl. J. Tiss. React.*, **1**, 163.

Günther, R., Egg, D. and Herold, M. (1979) Efficacy and safety of piroxicam and indomethacin in the treatment of musculoskeletal disorders. A double blind comparative study. *Zeitschr. Rheumatol.*, **38**, 330.

Hobbs, D.C. and Twomey, T.M. (1976) Biotransformation of piroxicam by the rat, dog and monkey. *Pharmacologist*, **18**, 152.

Hobbs, D.C. and Twomey, T.M. (1979) Piroxicam pharmacokinetics in man: aspirin and antacid interaction studies. *J. Clin. Pharmacol.*, **19**, 270.

Ishizaki, T., Nomura, T. and Abe, T. (1979) Pharmacokinetics of piroxicam, a new nonsteroidal anti-inflammatory agent, under fasting and postprandial states in man. *J. Pharmacokin. Biopharm.*, **7**, 369.

Jain, A.K., McMahon, F.G., Ryan, J.R. *et al.* (1978) Piroxicam, a novel analgesic in post partum pain. *Eur. J. Rheumatol. Infl.*, **1**, 356.

*Lee, H.K., Hong, J.Y., Lee, S.H. and Song, H.S. (1979) Clinical effects of piroxicam in orthopedic field. *Korean Central J. Med.*, **36**, 425.

Lombardino, J.G. and Wiseman, E.H. (1972) Sudoxicam and related N-heterocylic carboxamides of 4-hydroxy-2H-1, 2-benzothiazine 1, 1-dioxide. Potent nonsteroidal anti-inflammatory agents. *J. Med. Chem.*, **15**, 848.

Lombardino, J.G. and Wiseman, E.H. (1973) Potent anti-inflammatory N-heterocylic 3-carboxamides of 4-hydroxy-2-methyl-2H-1, 2-benzothiazine 1, 1-dioxide. *J. Med. Chem.*, **16**, 493.

Mäkisara, P. and Nuotio, P. (1978) Piroxicam and rheumatoid arthritis: comparative study of piroxicam and ibuprofen. *R. Soc. Med. Intl. Congr. Symp. Ser.*, **1**, 65.

Mathies, H. and Wolff, E. (1980) Klinische wirkung des antirheumatikums: piroxicam. *München Med. Wochenschr.*, **122**, 99.

Mercier, M. and Lesne, M. (1980) in *Rheumatology in the Eighties: An Advance in Therapy* – Piroxicam (ed. J.A. Boyle), Excerpta Medica, Princeton, New Jersey.

Milne, G.M. and Twomey, T.M. (1980) The analgesic properties of piroxicam in animals and correlation with experimentally determined plasma levels. *Agents and Actions*, **10**, 31.

Murphy, J.E. (1979) Piroxicam in the treatment of acute gout: a multicentre open study in general practice. *J. Intl. Med. Res.*, **7**, 507.

Nuotio, P. and Mäkisara, P. (1978) Pharmacokinetic and clinical study of piroxicam. *R. Soc. Med. Intl. Congr. Symp. Ser.*, **1**, 25.

Nussdorf, R.T. (1978) Piroxicam and acute musculoskeletal disease: a double blind 14-day study comparing piroxicam and phenylbutazone. *R. Soc. Med. Intl. Congr. Symp. Ser.*, **1**, 93.

*Ostermann, K. (1980) in *Rheumatology in the Eighties: An Advance in Therapy* – Piroxicam (ed. J.A. Boyle), Excerpta Medica, Princeton.

*Otte, J. (1980) in *Rheumatology in the Eighties: An Advance in Therapy* – Piroxicam (ed. J.A. Boyle), Excerpta Medica, Princeton.

Pitts, N.E. (1980) in *Piroxicam, a new Non-steroidal Anti-inflammatory Agent. Proceedings of the Ninth European Congress of Rheumatology*, Academy Professional Information Services, New York, pp. 48–66.

Pitts, N.E. and Proctor, R.R. (1978) Summary: efficacy and safety of piroxicam. *Proc. R. Soc. Med. Intl. Congr. Symp. Ser.*, **1**, 97.

Radi, I., Matoso, L., Posmantir, A. and Papalexiou, P. (1978) Safety and efficacy of piroxicam in the treatment of ankylosing spondylitis. *Eur. J. Rheumatol. Infl.*, **1**, 349.

*Rahman, M., Turner, R., Pisko, E. and Agudelo, C. (1979) Long term efficacy and safety of piroxicam in the treatment of rheumatoid arthritis. *Clin. Pharmacol. Ther.*, **25**, 243.

Rau, R. (1980) in *Piroxicam, a New Non-steroidal Anti-inflammatory Agent. Proceedings of the Ninth European Congress of Rheumatology*, Academy Professional Information Services, New York, pp. 41–5.

Reubi, F. (1980) in *Piroxicam, a New Non-steroidal Anti-inflammatory Agent. Proceedings of the Ninth European Congress on Rheumatology*, Academy Professional Information Services, New York, pp. 37–40.

Rogers, H.J. (1980) in *Rheumatology in the Eighties: An Advance in Therapy* – Piroxicam (ed. J.A. Boyle), Excerpta Medica, Princeton, New Jersey.

*Santilli, G., Tuccimei, U. and Cannistrà, F.M. (1980) Comparative study with piroxicam and ibuprofen versus placebo in the supportive treatment of minor sports injuries. *J. Intl. Med. Res.*, **8**, 265.

*Schattenkirchner, M., Müller-Fassbender, H. and Melzer, H. (1980) in *Piroxicam: a New Non-steroidal Anti-inflammatory Agent. Proceedings of the Ninth European Congress of Rheumatology*, Academy Professional Information Services, New York, pp. 28–31.

Steigerwald, J.C. (1978) Piroxicam and rheumatoid arthritis: a double-blind 16 week study comparing piroxicam and indomethacin. *Eur. J. Rheumatol. Infl.*, **1**, 360.

†Sydnes, O.A. (1980) in *Rheumatology in the Eighties: An Advance in Therapy* – Piroxicam (ed. J.A. Boyle), Excerpta Medica, Princeton.

*Tausch, G. (1980) in *Piroxicam, a New Non-steroidal Anti-inflammatory Agent. Proceedings of the Ninth European Congress of Rheumatology*, Academy Professional Information Services, New York, pp. 22–70.

Tausch, G. and Eberl, R. (1978) Efficacy, tolerance and safety of piroxicam in the treatment of acute gout. *Eur. J. Rheumatol. Infl.*, **1**, 365.

Tausch, G., Eberl, R. and Bröll, H. (1978) Piroxicam and rheumatoid arthritis: long-term open treatment. *R. Soc. Med. Intl. Congr. Symp. Ser.*, **1**, 59.

Telhag, H. (1978) Safety and efficacy of piroxicam in the treatment of osteoarthrosis. *Eur. J. Rheumatol. Infl.*, **1**, 352.

Twomey, T.M. and Hobbs, D.C. (1978) Biotransformation of piroxicam by man. *Fed. Proc.*, **37**, 271.

Twomey, T.M., Bartolucci, R.N. and Hobbs, D.C. (1980) The analysis of piroxicam by high performance liquid chromatography. *J. Chromatogr. Biomed. Appl.*, **183**, 104.

*Tyndall, A. de V., Piper, S., Lyanage, S. and Ansell, B.M. (1980) in *Rheumatology in the Eighties: An Advance in Therapy* – Piroxicam (ed. J.A. Boyle), Excerpta Medica, Princeton.

Weintraub, M., Jacox, R.F., Angevine, C.D. and Atwater, E.C. (1977) Piroxicam (CP-16, 171) in rheumatoid arthritis: a controlled clinical trial with novel assessment techniques. *J. Rheumatol.*, **4**, 393.

Weintraub, M., Jacox, R.F., Angevine, C.D. and Atwater, E.C. (1978) Piroxicam and rheumatoid arthritis. An 18-month open-label continuation of a double-blind study. *R. Soc. Med. Intl. Congr. Symp. Ser.*, **1**, 53.

Widmark, P. (1978) Safety and efficacy of piroxicam in the treatment of acute gout. *Eur. J. Rheumatol. Infl.*, **1**, 346.

Wiseman, E.H. (1978a) Piroxicam (Feldene) pharmacokinetics and the clinical management of inflammation. *Eur. J. Rheumatol. Infl.*, **1**, 338.

Wiseman, E.H. (1978b) Review of preclinical studies with piroxicam: pharmacology, pharmacokinetics and toxicology. *R. Soc. Med. Intl. Congr. Symp. Ser.*, **1**, 11.

Wiseman, E.H. (1980) in *Piroxicam, a New Non-steroidal Anti-inflammatory Agent. Proceedings of the Ninth European Congress of Rheumatology*, Academy Professional Information Services, New York, pp. 2–9.

Wiseman, E.H., Chang, Y.H. and Lombardino, J.G. (1976a) Piroxicam, an anti-inflammatory agent in the 4-hydroxy-2H-1, 2-benxothiazine 1, 1-dioxide series. *Pharmacologist*, **18**, 219.

Wiseman, E.H., Chang, Y.H. and Lombardino, J.G. (1976b) Piroxicam, a novel anti-inflammatory agent. *Arz. Forsch.*, **26**, 1300.

Wiseman, E.H. and Lombardino, J.G. (1980) in *Chronicles of*

Drug Discovery (eds J.S. Bindra and D. Lednicer), Wiley-Interscience, New York.

Zizic, T.M., Sutton, J.D. and Stevens, M.B. (1978) Piroxicam and osteoarthritis: a controlled study. *R. Soc. Med. Intl. Congr. Symp. Ser.*, **1**, 71.

Pure anti-inflammatory drugs

Corticosteroids

*Ainger, L.E., Ely, R.S., Done, A.K. and Kelly, V.C. (1955) Sydenham's chorea. II. Effects of hormone therapy. *Am. J. Dis. Child.*, **89**, 580.

*Albright, F. (1947) The effect of hormones on osteogenesis in man. *Rec. Progr. Horm. Res.*, **1**, 293.

*Ansell, B.M. and Bywaters, E.G.L. (1974) Alternate-day corticosteroid therapy in juvenile chronic polyarthritis. *J. Rheumatol.*, **1**, 176.

*Ansell, B.M., Bywaters, E.G.L. and Isdale, I.C. (1956) Comparison of cortisone and aspirin in treatment of juvenile rheumatoid arthritis. *Br. Med. J.*, **i**, 1075.

*Bennett, G. (1956) Cortisone therapy of visual loss in temporal arteritis. *Br. J. Ophthalmol.*, **40**, 430.

†Bernstein, C.A. and Freyberg, R.H. (1961) Rheumatoid patients after five or more years of corticosteroid treatment: a comparative analysis of 183 cases. *Ann. Int. Med.*, **54**, 938.

*Bernstein, B., Stobie, D., Singsen, B.H. *et al.* (1977) Growth retardation in juvenile rheumatoid arthritis (JRA). *Arthr. Rheum.*, **29** (Suppl.), 212.

*Black, R.L., Oglesby, R.B., Sallman, L.V. and Bunim, J.J. (1960) Posterior subcapsular cataracts induced by corticosteroids in patients with rheumatoid arthritis. *J. Am. Med. Assoc.*, **174**, 166.

Bohus, B. and Strashimorov, D. (1970) Localisation and specificity of corticosteroid 'feed back receptors' at the hypothalamo-hypophyseal level: comparative effects of various steroids implanted in the median eminence of the anterior pituitary of the rat. *Neuroendocrinol. Intl. J. Basic Clin. Stud. Neuroendocr. Rel.*, **6**, 197.

*Bongiovanni, A.M. and McPadden, A.J. (1960) Steroids during pregnancy and possible fetal consequences. *Fertil. Steril.*, **11**, 181.

*British and U.S. Rheumatological Associations (1955) The treatment of acute rheumatic fever in children. A cooperative clinical trial of ACTH, cortisone and aspirin. *Br. Med. J.*, **i**, 555 and *Circulation*, **11**, 343.

*Bywaters, E.G.L. and Thomas, G.T. (1961) Bed rest, salicylates and steroid in rheumatic fever. *Br. Med. J.*, **i**, 1628.

*Carpenter, J.R., Bunch, T.W., Engel, A.G. and O'Brien, P.C. (1977) Survival in polymyositis: corticosteroids and risk factors. *J. Rheumatol.*, **4**, 207.

*Christianson, H.B., Brunsting, L.A. and Perry, H.O. (1956) Dermatomyositis. Unusual features, complications and treatment. *Arch. Dermatol.*, **74**, 581.

*Combined Rheumatic Fever Study Group (1960) A comparison of the effect of prednisone and acetyl acid on the incidence of residual rheumatic heart disease. *N. Engl. J. Med.*, **262**, 895.

Cope, G.L. (1972) *Adrenal Steroids and Disease*, Pitman Medical, London.

Copeman, W.S.C. (ed.) (1953) *Cortisone and ACTH in Clinical Practice*, Butterworth, London.

*Curtiss, P.H., Clark, W.S. and Herndon, C.H. (1954) Vertebral fractures resulting from prolonged cortisone and corticotrophin therapy. *J. Am. Med. Assoc.*, **156**, 467.

David, D.S., Grieco, M.H. and Cushman, P.J.R. (1970) Adrenal glucocorticoids after twenty years: a review of their clinically relevant consequences. *J. Chron. Dis.*, **22**, 637.

*De Costa, E.J. and Abelman, M.A. (1952) Cortisone and pregnancy. An experimental and clinical study of the effects of cortisone on gestation. *Am. J. Obstet. Gynaecol.*, **64**, 746.

Di Raimondo, V.L. and Forsham, P.H. (1958) Pharmacophysiologic principles in the use of corticoids and adrenocorticotrophin. *Metab. Clin. Exp.*, **7**, 5.

Dluhy, R.G., Newmark, S.R., Lauler, D.P. and Thorn, G.W. (1975) *Pharmacology and Chemistry of Adrenal Glucosteroids in Steroid Therapy* (ed. D.L. Azarnoff), Saunders, Philadelphia, p. 8.

*Done, A.K., Ely, R.S., Ainger, L.E. *et al.* (1955) Therapy of acute rheumatic fever. *Pediatrics*, **15**, 22.

*Dorfman, A., Gross, J.I. and Lorincz, A.E. (1961) The treatment of acute rheumatic fever. *Pediatrics*, **27**, 692.

Downie, W.W. (1976) Steroid therapy. *Scot. Med. J.*, **21**, 188.

*Dubois, E.L. (1956) Systemic lupus erythematosus: recent advances in its diagnosis and treatment. *Ann. Int. Med.*, **45**, 163.

Editorial* (1957) Hormone therapy in rheumatoid arthritis. *Br. Med. J.*, **ii, 1291.

†Empire Rheumatism Council (1957) Multicentre controlled trial comparing cortisone acetate and acetylsalicylic acid in the long term treatment of rheumatoid arthritis. *Ann. Rheum. Dis.*, **16**, 277.

*Esselinckx, W., Doherty, S.M. and Dixon, A.S. (1977) Polymyalgia rheumatica. Abrupt and gradual withdrawal of prednisolone treatment, clinical and laboratory observations. *Ann. Rheum. Dis.*, **36**, 219.

*Fainstat, T. (1954) Cortisone-induced congenital cleft palate in rabbits. *Endocrinology*, **55**, 502.

Fauci, A.S. (1976) Glucocorticoid therapy: mechanism of action and clinical considerations. *Ann. Int. Med.*, **84**, 304.

Folb, T.I. and Troune, J.J. (1970) Immunological aspects of candida infection complicating steroid and immuno suppressive drug therapy, *Lancet*, **ii**, 1112.

Forsham, P.H., Thorn, G.W., Frawley, T.F. and Wilson, D.L. (1950) Studies on carbohydrate metabolism in adrenal cortical hypersecretion. *J. Clin. Endocrinol.*, **10**, 825.

Francois, J. (1954) Cortisone et tension oculaire. *Annals des Oculistes*, **187**, 805.

Franke, M. (1977) What has proved its worth in the therapy of rheumatism? Steroids. *Therapiewoche*, **27**, 274.

*Fraser, F.C. (1962) Pregnancy and adrenocortical hormones. *Br. Med. J.*, **ii**, 479 (letter).

*Fraser, F.C. and Fainstat, T.D. (1951) Production of congenital defects in the offspring of pregnant mice treated with cortisone. *Pediatrics*, **8**, 527.

*Fürst, C., Smiley, W.K. and Ansell, B.M. (1966) Steroid cataract. *Ann. Rheum. Dis.*, **25**, 364.

*Giles, C.L., Mason, G.L., Duff, I.F. and McLean, J.A. (1962) The association of cataract formation and systemic corticosteroid therapy. *J. Am. Med. Assoc.*, **182**, 719.

Glass, D. and Daly, J.R. (1971) Development of antibodies

during long term therapy with corticotrophin in rheumatoid arthritis. *Ann. Rheum. Dis.*, **30**, 589.

*Goldgraber, M.B., Kirsner, J.B. and Palmer, W.L. (1957) The role of ACTH and adrenal steroids in perforation of the colon in ulcerative colitis. A clinical-pathologic study. *Gastroenterology*, **33**, 434.

*Golding, D.N. and Begg, T.B. (1960) Dexamethasone myopathy. *Br. Med. J.*, ii, 1129.

*Gordon, I. (1960) Polymyalgia rheumatica. *Q. J. Med.*, **29**, 473.

Good, R.A., Vernier, R.L. and Smith, R.T. (1957) Serious untoward reactions to therapy with cortisone and adrenocorticotropin in pediatric practice (Part 1). *Pediatrics*, **19**, 95.

Grant, J.K. (1968) The biosynthesis of adrenocortical steroids. *J. Endocrinol.*, **41**, 111.

*Harman, J.B. (1959) Muscle wasting and corticosteroid therapy. *Lancet*, i, 887.

Harris, T.N., Friedman, S., Needleman, H.L. and Saltzman, H.A. (1956) Therapeutic effects of ACTH and cortisone in rheumatic fever: cardiologic observations in controlled series of 100 cases. *Pediatrics*, **17**, 11.

Hart, F.D. (1966) Complicated rheumatoid arthritis. *Br. Med. J.*, ii, 131.

Hart, F.D. (ed.) (1978) *Drug Treatment of the Rheumatic Diseases*, MTP Press, Lancaster.

Hench, P.S. (1950) The reversibility of certain rheumatic and non-rheumatic conditions by the use of cortisone or of the pituitary adrenocorticotropic hormone. *Ann. Int. Med.*, **36**, 1.

†Hench, P.S., Kendall, E.C., Slocumb, C.H. and Polley, H.F. (1949a) The effect of a hormone of the adrenal cortex (17-hydroxy-11-dehydrocorticosterone: Compound E) and of pituitary adrenocorticotropic hormone on rheumatoid arthritis: preliminary report. *Proc. Staff Meetings Mayo Clin.*, **24**, 181.

*Hench, P.S., Slocumb, C.H., Barnes, A.R. *et al.* (1949b) The effects of the adrenal cortical hormone 17-hydroxy-11-dehydro-corticosterone (Compound E) on the acute phase of rheumatic fever: Preliminary report. *Rep. Staff Meetings Mayo Clin.*, **24**, 277.

Henneman, D.H. and Bunker, J.P. (1957) The pattern of intermediary carbohydrate metabolism in Cushing's syndrome. *Am. J. Med.*, **23**, 34.

*Howard, J.E. (1958) Osteoposisis in hyperadrenocorticism. *J. Clin. Endocrinol.*, **18**, 1131.

Huber, W. and Menander-Huber, K.B. (1980) in *Clinics in Rheumatic Diseases* (ed. E.C. Huskisson), Vol. 6, No. 3, Saunders, London, p. 467.

*Iannaccone, A., Gabrilove, J.L., Brahms, S.A. and Soffer, L.J. (1960) Osteoporosis in Cushing's syndrome. *Ann. Int. Med.*, **52**, 570.

Jasani, M.K. (1972) Possible modes of action of ACTH and glucocorticoids in allergic diseases. *Clin. Allergy*, **2**, 1.

Jasani M.K., Boyle, J.A., Dick, W.C. *et al.* (1968) Corticosteroid induced hypothalamo-pituitary adrenal axis suppression. Prospective study using two regimens of corticosteroid therapy. *Ann. Rheum. Dis.*, **27**, 352.

*Johnsson, S. and Leonhardt, T. (1957) Polyarteritis nodosa and its treatment with ACTH or cortisone. *Acta Med. Scand.*, **157**, 479.

*Kammerer, W.H., Freiberger, R.H. and Rivelis, A.L. (1958) Peptic ulcer in rheumatoid patients on corticosteroid therapy. A clinical, experimental and radiologic study. *Arthr. Rheum.*, **1**, 112.

Kemper, J.W., Baggenstoss, A.H. and Slocumb, C.H. (1957) The relationship of therapy with cortisone to the incidence of vascular lesions in rheumatoid arthritis. *Ann. Int. Med.*, **46**, 831.

*Kern, F., Clark, G.M. and Lukens, J.G. (1957) Peptic ulceration occurring during therapy for rheumatoid arthritis. *Gastroenterology*, **33**, 25.

Klinenberg, J.R. and Miller, R. (1965) Effect of corticosteroids on blood salicylate concentrations. *J. Am. Med. Assoc.*, **194**, 601.

*Latham, B.A. and Mason, R.M. (1962) Prednisolone phosphate in rheumatoid arthritis. A new approach to steroid-induced dyspepsia. *Lancet*, ii, 1190.

Laurence, D.R. (1973) *Clinical Pharmacology*, Churchill Livingstone, Edinburgh.

Long, C.N.H., Katzin, B. and Fry, E.G. (1940) The adrenal cortex and carbohydrate metabolism. *Endocrinology*, **26**, 309.

MacGregor, R.R., Sheagren, J.N., Lipsett, M.B. and Wolff, S.M. (1969) Alternate-day prednisone therapy. *N. Engl. J. Med.*, **280**, 1427.

MacGregor, R.R., Spagnuolo, P.J. and Lentnek, A.L. (1974) Inhibition of granulocyte adherence by ethanol prednisolone and aspirin. *N. Engl. J. Med.*, **291**, 642.

*MacLean, K. and Schurr, P.H. (1959) Reversible amyotrophy complicating treatment with fludrocortisone. *Lancet*, i, 701.

†Medical Research Council (1955) A comparison of cortisone and aspirin in the treatment of early cases of rheumatoid arthritis. *Br. Med. J.*, ii, 695.

†Medical Research Council (1957a) Long-term results in early cases of rheumatoid arthritis treated with either cortisone or aspirin. *Br. Med. J.*, i, 847.

*Medical Research Council (1957b) Treatment of polyarteritis nodosa with cortisone: results after one year. *Br. Med. J.*, i, 608.

*Medical Research Council (1960) Treatment of polyarteritis nodosa with cortisone: results after three years. *Br. Med. J.*, i, 1399.

*Medical Research Council (1961) Treatment of systemic lupus erythematosus with steroids. *Br. Med. J.*, ii, 915.

*Meltzer, L.E., Bockman, A.A., Kanenson, W. and Cohen, A. (1958) Incidence of peptic ulcer among patients on long-term prednisone therapy. *Gastroenterology*, **35**, 351.

*Mulder, D.W., Winkelmann, R.K., Lambert, E.H. *et al.* (1963) Steroid therapy in patients with polymyositis and dermatomyositis. *Ann. Int. Med.*, **58**, 969.

Myles, A.B. and Daly, J.R. (1974) *Corticosteroid and A.C.T.H. Treatment, Principles and Problems*. Arnold, London.

Myles, A.B., Bacon, P.A. and Daly, J.R. (1971) Single daily dose corticosteroid treatment, Effect on adrenal function and therapeutic efficacy in various diseases. *Ann. Rheum. Dis.*, **30**, 149.

Nuki, G. and Downie, W.W. (1973) in *Modern Trends in Rheumatology* (ed. A.G.S. Hill), Vol. 2, Butterworths, London, pp. 199–239.

*Oglesby, R.B., Black, R.L., Sallman, L.V. and Bunim, J.J. (1961a) Cataracts in rheumatoid arthritis patients treated with corticosteroids. Description and differential diagnosis. *Arch. Ophthalmol.*, **66**, 519.

*Oglesby, R.B., Black, R.L., Sallman, L.V. and Bunim, J.J. (1961b) Cataracts in patients with rheumatic diseases treated with corticosteroids. Further observations. *Arch. Ophthalmol.*, **66**, 625.

*Palmer, W.L. and Kirsner, J.B. (1959) Therapeutic and side effects of the anti-inflammatory steroids on the gastro-intestinal tract. *Ann. N. Y. Acad. Sci.*, **82**, 947.

*Pearson, C.M. (1962) in *Clinical Uses of Adrenal Steroids* (eds J. Brown and C.M. Pearson), McGraw-Hill, London.

*Perkoff, G.T., Silber, R., Tyler, F.H. *et al.* (1959) Studies in disorders of muscle: XII. Myopathy due to administration of therapeutic amounts of 17-hydroxycorticosteroids. *Am. J. Med.*, **26**, 891.

Persellin, R.H. and Ku, L.C. (1974) Effects of steroid hormones on human polymorphonuclear leukocyte lysosomes. *J. Clin. Invest.*, **54**, 919.

Peterson, R. (1959) The miscible pool and turnover rate of adrenocortical steroids in man. *Rec. Progr. Horm. Res.*, **15**, 231.

*Pollack, V.E., Pirani, C.L., Muehrcke, R.C. and Kark, R.M. (1959) Lupus glomerulonephritis: the effect of two therapeutic regimens on renal function and renal histology. *J. Lab. Clin. Med.*, **54**, 924 (Abstract).

*Reifenstein, E.C. (1956) The rationale for the use of anabolic steroids in controlling the adverse effects of corticoid hormones upon protein and osseous tissue. *S. Med. J.*, **49**, 934.

*Richards, R.L. (1960) Steroid therapy in collagen diseases. *Br. J. Dermatol.*, **72**, 22.

*Rosenberg, E.F. (1958) Rheumatoid arthritis. Osteoporosis and fractures related to steroid therapy. *Acta Med. Scand.*, **162** (Suppl.), 341.

*Ross, L. and Goldsmith, E.D. (1955) Histochemical studies of effects of cortisone on fetal and newborn rats. *Proc. Soc. Exp. Biol. N. Y.*, **90**, 50.

*Russek, H.I., Zohman, B.L. and Russek, A.S. (1954) Risk of thrombo-embolic complications from cortisone therapy. *Am. Heart J.*, **47**, 653.

Sarrett, L.H., Patchett, A.A. and Steelman, S. (1963) The effects of structural alteration on the anti-inflammatory properties of hydrocortisone. *Progr. Drug Res.*, **5**, 111.

*Savage, O., Chapman, L., Robertson, J.D. *et al.* (1957) The clinical course and corticosteroid excretion of patients with rheumatoid arthritis during long-term treatment with corticotropin. *Br. Med. J.*, **ii**, 1257.

*Savage, O., Copeman, W.S.C., Chapman, L. *et al.* (1962) Pituitary and adrenal hormones in rheumatoid arthritis. *Lancet*, **i**, 232.

*Schaller, J.G., (1977) Corticosteroids in juvenile rheumatoid arthritis. *Arthr. Rheum.*, **20** (Suppl.), 537.

Scott, J.T. (1972) The use of steroids in the treatment of rheumatic diseases. *Practitioner*, **208**, 18.

*Scott, J.T., Porter, J.H., Lewis, S.M. and Dixon, A. St. J. (1961) Studies of gastrointestinal bleeding caused by corticosteroids, salicylates and other analgesics. *Q. J. Med. New Series*, **30**, 167.

*Shick, R.M. (1958) Periarteritis nodosa and temporal arteritis: Treatment with adrenal corticosteroids. *Med. Clin. N. Am.*, **42**, 959.

*Skeels, R.F. (1958) Reversibility of osteoporosis in Cushing's disease. *J. Clin. Endocrinol.*, **18**, 61.

Skrabal, F., Arnot, R.N., Joplin, G.F. and Fraser, T.R. (1972) The effect of glucocorticoid withdrawal on body water and electrolytes in hypopituitary patients with adrenocortical insufficiency as investigated with ^{77}Br ^{43}K ^{24}Na and ^{3}H$_2$O. *Clin. Sci.*, **43**, 79.

*Smith, L.R. and Rosenberg, E.F. (1955) Rheumatoid arthritis: spontaneous and traumatic fractures during hormone therapy. *Bull. Inst. Med. Chicago*, **20**, 248.

*Soffer, L.J., Ludeman, H.H. and Brill, G. (1955) The effect of corticotropin and adrenal steroids on the management of acute disseminated lupus erythematosus. *Ann. N. Y. Acad. Sci.*, **61**, 418.

Soyka, L.F. (1972) Alternate-day corticosteroid therapy. *Adv. Paediatr.*, **19**, 47.

*Spiro, H.M. and Milles, S.S. (1960) Clinical and physiologic implications of the steroid-induced peptic ulcer. *N. Engl. J. Med.*, **263**, 286.

Stenlake, J.B., Williams, W.D., Davidson, A.G. *et al.* (1969) The effect of anti-inflammatory drugs on the protein binding of 11-hydroxysteroids in human plasma *in vitro*. *J. Pharm. Pharmacol.*, **21**, 451.

*Stolzer, B.L., Barr, J.H., Eisenbeis, C.H. *et al.* (1957) Prednisone and prednisolone therapy in rheumatoid arthritis: clinical evaluation with emphasis on gastro-intestinal manifestations in 156 patients observed for periods of 4 to 14 months. *J. Am. Med. Assoc.*, **165**, 13.

Thompson, E.B. and Lippman, M.E. (1974) Mechanism of action of glucocorticoids. *Metabolism*, **23**, 159.

*Toogood, J.H., Dyson, C., Thompson, C.A. and Mularchyk, E.J. (1962) Posterior subcapsular cataracts as complication of adrenocortical steroid therapy. *Can. Med. Assoc. J.*, **86**, 52.

*Van Metre, T.E., Niermann, W.A. and Rosen, L.J. (1960) A comparison of the growth suppressive effect of cortisone, prednisone and other adrenal cortical hormones. *J. Allergy*, **31**, 531.

Werk, E.E., Choi, Y., Sholiton, L. *et al.* (1969) Interference in the effect of dexamethasone by diphenylhydantoin. *N. Engl. J. Med.*, **281**, 32.

Werk, E.E., Macgee, J. and Sholiton, L.J. (1964) Effect of diphenylhydantoin on cortisol metabolism in man. *J. Clin. Invest.*, **43**, 1824.

West, H.F. (1956) Acquired resistance to corticotropins. *Ann. Rheum. Dis.*, **15**, 124.

*West, H.F. (1957) Effects of prolonged adrenocortical stimulation on patients with rheumatoid arthritis. *Ann. Rheum. Dis.*, **16**, 322.

*West, H.F. (1958a) Protein metabolism during corticosteroid therapy. *Lancet*, **ii**, 877.

*West, K.M. (1958b) Relative eosinopenic and hyperglycemic potencies of glucocorticoids in man. *Metabolism*, **7**, 441.

*Williams, R.S. (1959) Triamcinolone myopathy. *Lancet*, **i**, 698.

Wright, V. and Moll, J.M.H. (1976) *Seronegative Polyarthritis*, North-Holland, Amsterdam.

*Zutshi, D.W., Friedman, M. and Ansell, B.M. (1971) Corticotrophin therapy in juvenile chronic polyarthritis (Still's disease) and the effect on growth. *Arch. Dis. Childh.*, **46**, 584.

Corticotrophins

Carter, M.E. and James, V.H.T. (1970) An attempt at combining corticotrophin with long-term corticosteroid therapy. *Ann. Rheum. Dis.*, **30**, 589.

Copeman, W.S.C. (1953) *Cortisone and ACTH in Clinical Practice*, Butterworths, London.

Fahey, J.L. (1951) Effect of ACTH on whole blood coagulability. *Proc. Soc. Exp. Biol. N. Y.*, **77**, 491.

Glass, D, Nuki, G. and Daly, J.R. (1971) Development of antibodies during long-term therapy with corticotrophin in rheumatoid arthritis, II. Zinc tetrocosactrin (depot synacthen). *Ann. Rheum. Dis.*, **30**, 593.

Glass, D., Roffe, L., Maini, R.N. *et al.* (1975) Adverse reactions to Zn^{1-24}ACTH therapy associated with specific cellular immunity. *Clin. Exp. Immunol.*, **20**, 55.

Nuki, G., Jasani, M.K., Downie, W.W. *et al.* (1970) Clinico-pharmacological studies on depot tetrocosactrin in patients with rheumatoid arthritis. *Pharmacol. Clin.*, **2**, 99.

Thorn, G.W., Forsham, P.H., Frawley, T.F. *et al.* (1950) The clinical usefulness of ACTH and cortisone. *N. Engl. J. Med.*, **242**, 783, 824 and 865 (Review).

Travis, R.H. and Sayers, G. (1975) in *The Pharmacological Basic of Therapeutics* (eds L.S. Goodman and A. Gilman), Macmillan, New York, p. 1611.

5.5 APPENDICES: CLINICAL STUDIES OF VARIOUS AGENTS

5.5.1 Diflunisal

Author(s)	Date	Disorder	Author(s)	Date	Disorder
Andrew *et al.*	1977	Osteoarthrosis	Grayson	1978	Osteoarthrosis
Devroey *et al.*	1977	Post-episiotomy pain	Hayat *et al.*	1978	Cancer pain
Van Winzum and Rodda	1977	Postoperative pain	Hazleman	1978	Low back pain
Ackermann and Braun	1978	Post-dental surgery pain	Honig	1978	Post menisectomy pain
Adams	1978	Sprains	Jaegemann	1978	Acute low back pain
Axter	1978	Osteoarthrosis	Jaffe *et al.*	1978	Sprains and strains
Barran	1978	Strains and sprains	Kolsen Petersen	1978a,b	Post-dental surgery pain
Bernett *et al.*	1978	Strains and sprains	Paalzow *et al.*	1978	Experimental pain in man
Bresnihan *et al.*	1978	Osteoarthrosis	Semb and Persson	1978	Osteoarthrosis
Brown	1978	Minor surgery	Tait *et al.*	1978	Osteoarthrosis
Christodonlopoulos			Van Winzum *et al.*	1978	Osteoarthrosis
et al.	1978	Cancer pain	Wes	1978	Oral surgery
Cirillo *et al.*	1978	Osteoarthrosis of hip	Wojtulewski *et al.*	1978	Osteoarthrosis of hip or knee
Devroey	1978	Postoperative pain			
Essigman *et al.*	1978	Osteoarthrosis of hip and knee	Keet	1979	Osteoarthrosis
Goutallier *et al.*	1978a, b	Postoperative pain			

5.5.2 Indomethacin

Author(s)	Date	Disorder	Author(s)	Date	Disorder
Wanka and Dixon	1964	Osteoarthrosis of hip	Hodgkinson and Woolf	1973	Osteoarthrosis of hip
Jacobs	1965	Painful stiff shoulder	Huskisson *et al.*	1973	Soft-tissue sports injuries
Perkins and MacFail	1965	Uveitis	Smyth and Percy	1973	Acute gout
Cooperating Clinics			Van Marion	1973	Soft-tissue lesions
Committee of ARA	1967	Rheumatoid arthritis	Brodie	1974	Bone pain
Emmerson	1967	Acute gout	Fitch and Gray	1974	Soft-tissue sports injuries
Kinsella *et al.*	1967	Ankylosing spondylitis	Huskisson and Grayson	1974	Rheumatoid arthritis
Roth and England	1967	Juvenile rheumatoid arthritis	Aylward *et al.*	1975	Rheumatoid arthritis
Sänger *et al.*	1967	Juvenile rheumatoid arthritis	Broll *et al.*	1976	Rheumatoid arthritis
			Focan-Henrard and Franchimont	1976	Ankylosing spondylitis
Brewer	1968	Fever in children	Haslock	1976	Rheumatoid arthritis
Wright *et al.*	1969	Rheumatoid arthritis	Marcolongo	1976	Febrile states
Huskisson *et al.*	1970	Rheumatoid arthritis			
Patterson *et al.*	1971	Juvenile rheumatoid arthritis			

5.5.3 Sulindac

Author(s)	Date	Disorder	Author(s)	Date	Disorder
Jimenea *et al.*	1975	Ankylosing spondylitis	Villaumey and Di Menza	1976	Acute gout
Liebling *et al.*	1975	Ankylosing spondylitis	Worthington	1976	Acute gout
Andrade and Fernandez	1976	Osteoarthrosis	Zollner *et al.*	1976	Acute gout
Ballabio *et al.*	1976	Osteoarthrosis of hip and knee	Andalman	1977	Osteoarthrosis
			Britton *et al.*	1977	Ankylosing spondylitis
Bernett *et al.*	1976	Acute painful shoulder	Diamond	1977	Acute gout
Calabro *et al.*	1976	Acute gout	Mavrikakis *et al.*	1977	Rheumatoid arthritis
Chaliade and Federico	1976	Osteoarthrosis	Mowat *et al.*	1977	Ankylosing spondylitis
Demetriades *et al.*	1976	Osteoarthrosis of hip and knee	Pingeon *et al.*	1977	Rheumatoid arthritis
			Reynolds *et al.*	1977	Rheumatoid arthritis
Dieppe *et al.*	1976	Osteoarthrosis of hip	Bordier and Kuntz	1978	Osteoarthrosis
Fasching and Eberl	1976	Rheumatoid arthritis	Borrachero del Campo	1978	Rheumatoid arthritis
Gadomski *et al.*	1976	Ankylosing spondylitis	Calabro	1978	Gout
Gigante *et al.*	1976	Acute painful shoulder	Ciocci	1978	Rheumatoid arthritis
Highton and Jeremy	1976	Rheumatoid arthritis	Huskisson	1978	Rheumatoid arthritis
Ingberg and Holopainen	1976	Osteoarthrosis			Osteoarthrosis
Nissila and Koota	1976	Rheumatoid arthritis	Gibson and Laurent	1980	Ankylosing spondylitis
Simon *et al.*	1976	Osteoarthrosis of hip and knee	Mahir and Scharf	1980	Ankylosing spondylitis

5.5.4 Tolmetin

Author(s)	Date	Disorder	Author(s)	Date	Disorder
Jentsch	1973	Gout	Robinson *et al.*	1975	Rheumatoid arthritis
Berkowitz	1974	Rheumatoid arthritis	Roth and Simson	1975	Rheumatoid arthritis
Schneyer	1974	Rheumatoid arthritis	Aylward *et al.*	1976	Rheumatoid arthritis
April *et al.*	1975	Rheumatoid arthritis	Ehrlich and Roth	1976	Rheumatoid arthritis
Bachmann *et al.*	1975	Rheumatoid arthritis	Aylward *et al.*	1977	Rheumatoid arthritis
Bain *et al.*	1975	Rheumatoid arthritis	Cardoe and Steele	1977	Rheumatoid arthritis
Bernhard *et al.*	1975	Rheumatoid arthritis	Klemp and Meyers	1977	Rheumatoid arthritis
Brewer *et al.*	1975	Juvenile rheumatoid arthritis	Muller *et al.*	1977	Osteoarthrosis of knee
			Ran *et al.*	1977	Osteoarthrosis of hip and knee
Brown *et al.*	1975	Rheumatoid arthritis			
Ehrlich *et al.*	1975	Rheumatoid arthritis	Schattenkirchner *et al.*	1977	Ankylosing spondylitis
Ran *et al.*	1975	Osteoarthrosis of hip and knee	Setoyama *et al.*	1979	Surgical patients

5.5.5 Diclofenac

Author(s)	Date	Disorder	Author(s)	Date	Disorder
Shiokawa *et al.*	1972	Rheumatoid arthritis	Von Manz and Franke	1977	Ankylosing spondylitis
Ghazi and Fowler	1973	Rheumatoid arthritis	Abrams *et al.*	1978	Rheumatoid arthritis
Sacks	1974	Rheumatoid arthritis Osteoarthrosis			Osteoarthrosis
Pinheiro *et al.*	1975	Osteoarthrosis	Siegmeth and Placheta	1978	Osteoarthrosis
Rossi and Baroni	1975	Osteoarthrosis	Barnes *et al.*	1979	Rheumatoid arthritis
Wagenhauser and Narozna	1975	Osteoarthrosis			Osteoarthrosis
			Cardoe	1979	Rheumatoid arthritis
Kirchheiner *et al.*	1976	Rheumatoid arthritis	Doreen *et al.*	1979	Rheumatoid arthritis
Mohing	1976	Osteoarthrosis	Fowler	1979	Rheumatoid arthritis
Seda and Cardoza	1976	Osteoarthrosis	Schubiger *et al.*	1980	Osteoarthrosis
Bijlsma	1977, 1978	Rheumatoid arthritis			

5.5.6 Fenclofenac

Author(s)	Date	Disorder	Author(s)	Date	Disorder
Akyol *et al.*	1977	Rheumatoid arthritis Ankylosing spondylitis	Bird	1980	Osteoarthrosis
			Camp *et al.*	1980	Rheumatoid arthritis
			Crean	1980	Soft-tissue injury
Davies *et al.*	1977	Osteoarthrosis	Essigman	1980	Osteoarthrosis
Hill and Hill	1977	Rheumatoid arthritis	Coode	1980	Rheumatoid arthritis
Loebl	1977	Rheumatoid arthritis	Haslock and Laycock	1980	Rheumatoid arthritis
Pritchard *et al.*	1977	Rheumatoid arthritis	Kadir and Grayson	1980	Cervical spondylosis
Ansell *et al.*	1980	Juvenile chronic arthritis	Lipani	1980	Rheumatoid arthritis
			McGill *et al.*	1980	Rheumatoid arthritis
Aylward *et al.*	1980	Rheumatoid arthritis	Nicholls	1980	Rheumatoid arthritis
Bachmann	1980	Rheumatoid arthritis			

5.5.7 Ibuprofen

Author(s)	Date	Disorder	Author(s)	Date	Disorder
Jasani *et al.*	1968	Rheumatoid arthritis	Giansiracuso *et al.*	1975	Osteoarthrosis
Chalmers	1969	Rheumatoid arthritis	Godfrey and Dela Cruz	1975	Rheumatoid arthritis
Dick-Smith	1969	Rheumatoid arthritis	Guaghano *et al.*	1975	Lower limb thrombophlebitis
van Wering and Bleker	1972	Post-partum pain			
Ballabio and Colombo	1973	Rheumatoid arthritis	Lequesne	1975	Degenerative arthroses
Cosh and Ring	1973	Rheumatoid arthritis	Lokken *et al.*	1975	Oral surgery
Hadidi *et al.*	1973	Rheumatoid arthritis	Marsili and Coute	1975	Ophthalmic disorders
Menon *et al.*	1973	Still's disease	Montezuma de Carvalho	1975	Osteoarthrosis of knee
Pavelka *et al.*	1973,		Muckle	1975	Soft-tissue injuries
	1978	Rheumatoid arthritis	Nikolić and Lukačević	1975	Ankylosing spondylitis
Mitchell and			Pavelka *et al.*	1975	Osteoarthrosis of hips
MacDonald	1974	Rheumatoid arthritis	Sheldrake and Ansell	1975	Juvenile chronic polyarthritis
Alfieri *et al.*	1975	Obstetric and gynaecological disorders	Voftišek *et al.*	1975	Rheumatoid arthritis
de Blécourt	1975	Osteoarthrosis	Joshipura and		
de Carvalho	1975	Osteoarthrosis of knee	Dongaonkar	1976	Soft-tissue rheumatism
Cremoncini *et al.*	1975	Phlebitis	Mena *et al.*	1976	Osteoarthrosis
Dragomir-Naghiu	1975	Algodystrophy of upper and lower limb	Brackertz and Busson	1978	Osteoarthrosis
			Siegmeth and Sieberer	1978	Spondylosis
Dragomir-Naghiu and Stoia	1975	Catarrhal and respiratory nasal diseases with rheumatic manifestations			

5.5.8 Naproxen

Author(s)	Date	Disorder	Author(s)	Date	Disorder
Katona *et al.*	1971	Rheumatoid arthritis	Fernandez de Vallado *et al.*	1973	Osteoarthrosis
Binzus and Josenhaus	1973	Osteoarthrosis	Flores	1973	Rheumatoid arthritis
Borrachero and Alcalde	1973	Rheumatoid arthritis	Helby-Petersen *et al.*	1973	Rheumatoid arthritis
Cochrane	1973	Osteoarthrosis	Hill and Hill	1973	Ankylosing spondylitis
Cuq	1973	Acute gout	Hill *et al.*	1973	Rheumatoid arthritis
Diamond	1973	Rheumatoid arthritis	Kageyama	1973	Osteoarthrosis
D'Omézon	1973	Rheumatoid arthritis	Kogstad	1973	Rheumatoid arthritis
Eberl *et al.*	1973	Rheumatoid arthritis	Lussier *et al.*	1973a	Rheumatoid arthritis

Appendix 5.5.8 (*Contd.*)

Author(s)	Date	Disorder	Author(s)	Date	Disorder
Lussier *et al.*	1973b	Rheumatoid arthritis	Aromaa and Asp	1978	Pain after varicose vein surgery
Lussier *et al.*	1973c	Rheumatoid arthritis			
Poal *et al.*	1973	Osteoarthrosis	Berry *et al.*	1978	Rheumatoid arthritis
Ruedy and McCullough	1973	Pain after orthopaedic surgery	Blechman *et al.*	1978	Osteoarthrosis
			Castles *et al.*	1978	Rheumatoid arthritis
Stetson *et al.*	1973	Postoperative pain	Mayhew	1978	Osteoarthrosis
Willkens	1973	Rheumatoid arthritis	Melton *et al.*	1978	Osteoarthrosis of hip and knee
Willkens and Case	1973	Acute gout			
Winer *et al.*	1973	Rheumatoid arthritis	Van Gerwen *et al.*	1978	Ankylosing spondylitis
Hill *et al.*	1974	Rheumatoid arthritis	Ansell *et al.*	1979a	Juvenile chronic poly-arthritis
Reynolds and Whorwell	1974	Rheumatoid arthritis	Ansell *et al.*	1979b	Ankylosing spondylitis
Szanto	1974	Rheumatoid arthritis	Barry *et al.*	1979	Rheumatoid arthritis
Bowers *et al.*	1975	Rheumatoid arthritis	Hazleman *et al.*	1979	Rhematoid arthritis Ankylosing spondylitis Osteoarthrosis
Clark *et al.*	1975	Osteoarthrosis			
Vetter	1975	Rheumatoid arthritis			
Wilkens *et al.*	1975	Acute gout	Huskisson *et al.*	1979	Osteoarthritis
Capell *et al.*	1976	Rheumatoid arthritis	Luftschein *et al.*	1979	Rheumatoid arthritis
Hill and Hill	1976	Ankylosing spondylitis	Mowat *et al.*	1979	Rheumatoid arthritis
Jaffe	1976	Acute musculoskeletal disorders	Mowat and Mowat	1979	Rheumatoid arthritis
			Sturge *et al.*	1979	Acute gout
Mowat *et al.*	1976	Rheumatoid arthritis	Thompson *et al.*	1979	Osteoarthrosis
Willkens and Segre	1976	Rheumatoid arthritis	Backhouse *et al.*	1980	Acute musculoskeletal disorders
Makela	1977	Juvenile rheumatoid arthritis	Martinez-Lavin *et al.*	1980	Osteoarthrosis
Sturge *et al.*	1977	Acute gout			
Williams and Eyler	1977	Sports injuries			

5.5.9 Fenoprofen

Author(s)	Date	Disorder	Author(s)	Date	Disorder
Fries and Britton	1973	Rheumatoid arthritis	Duff *et al.*	1976	Rheumatoid arthritis
Huskisson	1974	Rheumatoid arthritis	Gum	1976	Rheumatoid arthritis
Huskisson *et al.*	1974	Rheumatoid arthritis	McMahon *et al.*	1976	Osteoarthrosis
Reynolds and Whorwell	1974	Rheumatoid arthritis	Sigler *et al.*	1976	Rheumatoid arthritis
			Franke and Manz	1977	Rheumatoid arthritis
Wojtulewski	1974	Osteoarthrosis	Godfrey *et al.*	1977	Ankylosing spondylitis
Wojtulewski *et al.*	1974	Osteoarthrosis of hip and knee	Steele	1977	Inflammatory disorders of soft tissue
Brooke	1976	Large-joint osteo-arthrosis	Wanasukapunt *et al.*	1977	Acute gout
			Chakravorty and Annan	1980	Osteoarthrosis of hips
Davis *et al.*	1976	Rheumatoid arthritis			
Diamond	1976	Osteoarthrosis			

5.5.10 Ketoprofen

Author(s)	Date	Disorder	Author(s)	Date	Disorder
Gyory *et al.*	1972	Osteoarthrosis of hip	Anderson *et al.*	1974	Rheumatoid arthritis
Doury and Pattin	1973	Ankylosing spondylitis	Bresnihan *et al.*	1974	Osteoarthrosis of hip
Eberl *et al.*	1973	Gout	Zutshi *et al.*	1974	Rheumatoid arthritis
Grahame *et al.*	1973	Osteoarthrosis of hip	Treadwell and Tweed	1975	Ankylosing spondylitis
Mills *et al.*	1973	Rheumatoid arthritis			
Shiokawa	1973	Rheumatoid arthritis	Viara *et al.*	1975	Rheumatoid arthritis

Appendix 5.5.10 (*Contd.*)

Author(s)	Date	Disorder	Author(s)	Date	Disorder
Caroit *et al.*	1976	Osteoarthrosis of hip	Sydnes *et al.*	1976	Rheumatoid arthritis
Famaey and Colinet	1976	Osteoarthrosis of hip	Aritomi *et al.*	1977	Rheumatoid arthritis
Hubault *et al.*	1976	Osteoarthrosis of hip	Goldman	1977	Rheumatoid arthritis
Jessop	1976	Ankylosing spondylitis	Wollheim *et al.*	1978	Rheumatoid arthritis
Kennedy	1976	Rheumatoid arthritis	Cardoe	1979	Osteoarthrosis of hip
O'Brien and			Chlud and Paugerl	1979	Soft-tissue injury
Grunwaldt	1976	Rheumatoid arthritis	Mathies	1979	Rheumatoid arthritis
Peltola	1976	Rheumatoid arthritis	Meyer	1979	Rheumatoid arthritis
Sany and Serre	1976	Rheumatoid arthritis	Serry	1980	Osteoarthrosis of knee

5.5.11 Flurbiprofen

Author(s)	Date	Disorder	Author(s)	Date	Disorder
Kogstad	1973	Osteoarthrosis	Good and Mena	1977	Ankylosing spondylitis
Tiselius	1973	Osteoarthrosis	Hazleman and		
Bacon *et al.*	1975	Rheumatoid arthritis	Bulgen	1977	Rheumatoid arthritis
Grahame and Calin	1975	Ankylosing spondylitis	Kruger	1977	Rheumatoid arthritis
Kay	1975	Postoperative pain	Menon and Willkens	1977	Ankylosing spondylitis
Brewis	1977	Rheumatoid arthritis	Muckle	1977	Soft tissue trauma
Cardoe	1977	Rheumatoid arthritis	Pipitone *et al.*	1977	Rheumatoid arthritis
Franco *et al.*	1977	Rheumatoid arthritis	Siegmeth	1977	Rheumatoid arthritis
Frank	1977	Osteoarthrosis of hip			

5.5.12 Fenbufen

Author(s)	Date	Disorder	Author(s)	Date	Disorder
Cuedes and			Biauchi	1977	Rheumatoid arthritis
Continho	1975	Toothache	Bonomo	1977	Osteoarthrosis
De Salcedo *et al.*	1975	Rheumatoid arthritis	Brenol	1977	Osteoarthrosis
Katona	1975	Rheumatoid arthritis	Chalem *et al.*	1977	Rheumatoid arthritis
Mathias-Filko			De Freitas	1977	Rheumatoid arthritis
and Bianchi	1975	Rheumatoid arthritis	Dunky and Eberl	1977	Rheumatoid arthritis
Nunes	1975	Rheumatoid arthritis	Buxton	1978	Osteoarthrosis
Sunshine	1975	Post-operative pain	Ammitzboll	1979	Rheumatoid arthritis
Villela-Nunes	1975	Rheumatoid arthritis	Henrikson *et al.*	1979	After dental surgery
Da Gama	1976	Rheumatoid arthritis	Roden	1979	Osteoarthrosis
Vergara-Castro			Valtonen	1979	Osteoarthrosis
et al.	1976	Rheumatoid arthritis			

5.5.13 Benoxaprofen

Author(s)	Date	Disorder	Author(s)	Date	Disorder
Lambert and			Berry *et al.*	1980	Rheumatoid arthritis
Wright	1977	Rheumatoid arthritis	Gunn	1980	Rheumatoid arthritis
Ridolfo *et al.*	1978	Rheumatoid arthritis	Highton and		
Alarcon-Segovia	1980	Osteoarthrosis	Grahame	1980	Osteoarthrosis
Atkinson *et al.*	1980	Rheumatoid arthritis	Roth	1980	Rheumatoid arthritis
Bird *et al.*	1980	Ankylosing spondylitis			Osteoarthrosis
Blechman	1980	Osteoarthrosis	Tyson and Glynne	1980	Osteoarthrosis

5.5.14 Fenamic acids

Author(s)	Date	Disorder	Author(s)	Date	Disorder
Coodley	1963	Rheumatoid arthritis	Fearnley and		
Bain and			Masheter	1966	Rheumatoid arthritis
Masheter	1966	Rheumatoid arthritis	Hill	1966	Rheumatoid arthritis
Barnardo *et al.*	1966	Rheumatoid arthritis	Simpson *et al.*	1966a, b	Rheumatoid arthritis
Brocks	1966	Osteoarthrosis of hip			
*Buchmann	1966	Osteoarthrosis	Simpson *et al.*	1966c	Ankylosing spondylitis
Cardoe	1966	Rheumatoid arthritis	Sydnes	1966	Rheumatoid arthritis
Cowan and			Rajan *et al.*	1967	Rheumatoid arthritis
Masheter	1966	Rheumatoid arthritis			

* Mefenamic acid, unmarked flufenamic acid

5.5.15 Phenylbutazone

Author(s)	Date	Disorder	Author(s)	Date	Disorder
Hart	1954	Ankylosing spondylitis	Godfrey *et al.*	1972	Ankylosing spondylitis
Hart	1955	Ankylosing spondylitis	Smyth and Percy	1973	Acute gout
Mason and Howes	1963	Ankylosing spondylitis	Brooks *et al.*	1975	Rheumatoid arthritis
Pearson	1964	Ankylosing spondylitis	Fowler	1975	Rheumatoid arthritis
Levernieux	1965	Ankylosing spondylitis	Boersma	1976	Ankylosing spondylitis
Kinsella *et al.*	1966	Ankylosing spondylitis	Sturge *et al.*	1977	Acute gout
Calabro	1968	Ankylosing spondylitis	Van Gerwen *et al.*	1978	Ankylosing spondylitis

5.5.16 Azapropazone

Author(s)	Date	Disorder	Author(s)	Date	Disorder
Kageyama	1969	Painful shoulder	Grennan *et al.*	1976	Rheumatoid arthritis
Sugiyama *et al.*	1969	Chronic articular	Hingorani	1976	Osteoarthrosis of knee
		rheumatism	Lassus	1976	Psoriatic arthritis
Matthies and					Reiter's disease
Kilani	1970	Rheumatoid arthritis	Thune	1976a, b	Rheumatoid arthritis
Pavelka *et al.*	1975	Rheumatoid arthritis			
Brooks *et al.*	1976	Rheumatoid arthritis			

5.5.17 Piroxicam

Author(s)	Date	Disorder	Author(s)	Date	Disorder
Wientraub *et al.*	1977,		Zizic *et al.*	1978	Osteoarthrosis
	1978,	Rheumatoid arthritis	Bachmann	1979	Rheumatoid arthritis
Box *et al.*	1978	Rheumatoid arthritis	Balogh *et al.*	1979	Rheumatoid arthritis
Jain *et al.*	1978	Post-partum pain	Dessain *et al.*	1979	Osteoarthrosis
Mäkisara and			Grewin	1979	Rheumatoid arthritis
Nuotio	1978	Rheumatoid arthritis	Lee *et al.*	1979	Orthopaedic disorders
Radi *et al.*	1978	Ankylosing spondylitis	Murphy	1979	Acute gout
Steigerwald	1978	Rheumatoid arthritis	Rahman *et al.*	1979	Rheumatoid arthritis
Tausch and			Blum and		
Eberl	1978	Acute gout	Wagenhauser	1980	Osteoarthrosis
Tausch *et al.*	1978	Rheumatoid arthritis	Commandré	1980	Extra-articular rheumatism
Telhag	1978	Osteoarthrosis	Dixon and		
Widmark	1978	Acute gout	Davies	1980	Rheumatoid arthritis

Appendix 5.5.17 (*Contd.*)

Author(s)	Date	Disorder	Author(s)	Date	Disorder
Gordon *et al.*	1980	Osteoarthrosis	Sydnes	1980	Rheumatoid arthritis
Ostermann	1980	Osteoarthrosis	Tausch	1980	Rheumatoid arthritis
Otte	1980	Osteoarthrosis	Tyndall *et al.*	1980	Juvenile chronic arthritis
Santilli *et al.*	1980	Minor sports injuries			
Schattenkirchner *et al.*	1980	Ankylosing spondylitis			

5.5.18 Systemic corticosteroids (clinical studies)

Author(s)	Date	Disorder	Author(s)	Date	Disorder
Hench *et al.*	1949	Rheumatoid arthritis	Schick	1958	Periarteritis nodosa
Hench *et al.*	1949	Acute rheumatic fever			Temporal arteritis
Ainger *et al.*	1955	Sydenham's chorea	Pollack *et al.*	1959	Lupus glomerulo-nephritis
British and US Rheumatological Association	1955	Acute rheumatic fever	Combined Rheumatic Fever Study		
Done *et al.*	1955	Acute rheumatic fever	Group	1960	Rheumatic heart disease
Medical Research Council	1955	Rheumatoid arthritis	Medical Research Council	1960	Polyarteritis nodosa
Soffer *et al.*	1955	Acute disseminated lupus erythematosus	Richards	1960	Collagen diseases
			Gordon	1960	Polymyalgia rheumatica
Ansell *et al.*	1956	Juvenile rheumatoid arthritis	Bernstein and Freyberg	1961	Rheumatoid arthritis
Bennett	1956	Temporal arteritis	Bywaters and Thomas	1961	Rheumatic fever
Christianson *et al.*	1956	Dermatomyositis	Dorfman *et al.*	1961	Acute rheumatic fever
Dubois	1956	Systemic lupus erythematosus	Medical Research Council	1961	Systemic lupus erythematosus
Harris *et al.*	1956	Rheumatic fever	Latham and Mason	1962	Rheumatoid arthritis
Editorial	1957	Rheumatoid arthritis	Pearson	1962	Systemic lupus erythematosus
Empire Rheumatism Council	1957	Rheumatoid arthritis	Savage *et al.*	1962	Rheumatoid arthritis
Johnsson and Leonhardt	1957	Polyarteritis nodosa	Mulder *et al.*	1963	Polymyositis and dermatomyositis
Medical Research Council	1957	Rheumatoid arthritis	Ansell and Bywaters	1974	Juvenile chronic polyarthritis
Medical Research Council	1957	Polyarteritis nodosa	Carpenter *et al.*	1977	Polymyositis
Savage *et al.*	1957	Rheumatoid arthritis	Schaller	1977	Juvenile rheumatoid arthritis
West	1957	Rheumatoid arthritis	Esselincky *et al.*	1977	Polymyalgia rheumatica

5.5.19 Systemic corticosteroids (adverse effects)

Author(s)	Date	Effect	Author(s)	Date	Effect
Albright	1947	Osteogenetic abnormality	Russek *et al.*	1954	Thromboembolism
Fraser and Famstat	1951	Congenital defects in mice	Ross and Goldsmith	1955	Fetal abnormalities in rats
De Costa and Abelman	1952	Gestational abnormality	Smith and Rosenberg	1955	Spontaneous and traumatic fractures
Curtiss *et al.*	1954	Vertebral fractures	Reifenstein	1956	Wasting of protein and osseous tissue
Famstat	1954	Cleft palate in rabbits	Goldgraber *et al.*	1957	Perforation of colon in ulcerative colitis
Francois	1954	Glaucoma-like reaction			

Appendix 5.5.19 (*Contd.*)

Author(s)	Date	Effect	Author(s)	Date	Effect
Kern *et al.*	1957	Peptic ulcer	Bongiovanni and		
Stolzer *et al.*	1957	Gastrointestinal effects	McPadden	1960	Fetal abnormality
Howard	1958	Osteoporosis	Golding and Begg	1960	Myopathy
Kammerer *et al.*	1958	Peptic ulcer	Iannaccone *et al.*	1960	Osteoporosis
Meltzer *et al.*	1958	Peptic ulcer	Spiro and Milles	1960	Peptic ulcer
Rosenberg	1958	Osteoporosis and fractures	Van Metre *et al.*	1960	Growth retardation
Skeels	1958	Osteoporosis	Oglesby *et al.*	1961a	Cataract
West	1958	Effects on protein meta-bolism	Oglesby	1961b	Cataract
			Scott *et al.*	1961	Gastrointestinal bleeding
West	1958	Hyperglycaemia	Fraser	1962	Pregnancy
Harman	1959	Muscle wasting	Giles *et al.*	1962	Cataract
Maclean and			Toogood *et al.*	1962	Posterior subcapsular cataracts
Schurr	1959	Amyotrophy			
Palmer and		Gastro-intestinal	Fürst *et al.*	1966	Cataract
Kirsner	1959	symptoms	Zutshi *et al.*	1971	Growth retardation
Perkoff *et al.*	1959	Myopathy	Bernstein *et al.*	1977	Growth retardation
Williams	1959	Myopathy			
Black *et al.*	1960	Posterior subcapsular cataract			

6
Drug therapy (3): 'specific' drugs

6.1 INTRODUCTORY COMMENT

The previous chapter has discussed non-specific (symptomatic) anti-rheumatic drugs. These act independently of the nature of the disease process to relieve symptoms. This chapter will deal with 'specific' agents which act on some aspect of the disease process itself, whether this be, for example, rheumatoid arthritis or gout. Their action can be distinguished from that of symptomatic remedies by their slow onset, effects on aspects of the disease other than inflammation and, in some disorders, alteration of the natural history of the disease.

This chapter also includes short notes on some commonly used adjuvant drugs (e.g. hypnotic and psychotropic drugs, haematinics, antibiotics).

6.2 RHEUMATOID ARTHRITIS

There is still much disagreement as to what this group of anti-rheumatoid drugs should be named. Though the term 'specific' has some truth, it can be criticized as some drugs are effective in more than one disease (e.g. the antimalarials in rheumatoid arthritis as well as in systemic lupus erythematosus). Other suggested terms for this group of drugs have included 'slow-acting', 'long-acting', 'remission-inducing' and 'basic'. Perhaps

the term 'long-term rheumatoid suppressants', though long, is as good as any.

Only the fully established drugs such as gold salts, antimalarials and penicillamine, and to a lesser extent, immunosuppressives, will be discussed here. Less well-established, though currently used drugs in this category (e.g. levamisole, dapsone), will be discussed in Chapter 12.

Most of the drugs described in the section are also used, in varying degree, in disorders other than rheumatoid arthritis. Only brief reference to these non-rheumatoid applications will be mentioned here, more detailed accounts being presented elsewhere (e.g. Section 6.3.1 and Chapter 12).

6.2.1 Gold salts (Myocrisin)

Other proprietary names include: Myochrysine (Canada, USA), Tauredon (Germany).

Gold salts (sodium aurothiomalate; sodium aurothiosulphate) are the oldest members of the group of 'specific' drugs for long-term use in rheumatoid arthritis. Perhaps a testimony to their effectiveness is the fact that they have survived in clinical usage since their introduction in the 1920s. However, only in the last 10 years has the 'correct' way of using gold become established.

(a) *Pharmacology and pharmacokinetics*

Sodium aurothiomalate consists mainly of the disodium salt of aurothiosuccinic acid ($C_4H_3AuNa_2O_4S$). It is rapidly absorbed from the site of intramuscular injection, and peak plasma levels of 400–700 μg (100 ml^{-1}) are achieved within 2–6 hours of injection. It has a long half-life of 5–6 days, plasma levels declining to about half of peak level after a week, when the next dose is given. After a few weeks of regular injections, equilibrium between input and output is achieved. Gold is found in both urine and faeces, but the precise mode of excretion has not been established. It is taken up by macrophages and is identifiable in the reticuloendothelial system and in the synovium, where it remains for a long time.

There is a wide individual variation in plasma levels achieved during gold therapy, and there is no convincing evidence that this is related to clinical response which is probably the best guide to therapy response. Gold plasma levels are not related to its toxic effects and are not of value in predicting them. The mode of action of the drug is unknown.

(Freberg, 1942; Lorber *et al.*, 1973; Gerber and Paulus, 1975.)

(b) *Clinical uses, preparations and dosage*

Gold is useful in rheumatoid arthritis and produces a response in about 80% of patients. Appendix 6.10.1 summarizes the main clinical studies using gold since its introduction. It acts both in seronegative (including psoriatic arthritis) and in seropositive patients, and exerts its main effect on the synovitis, reflected by reduction in joint pain, stiffness and swelling. This effect occurs slowly, most patients showing a response after 4–16 weeks of treatment. The maximal effect of the drug is achieved after 3–6 months. As with penicillamine, the number and size of nodules are reduced, and there may be improvement in some other extra-articular features of the disease. There is a reduction in the requirements for other drugs, including corticosteroids. The titre of rheumatoid factor and the ESR fall, but these changes do not reliably parallel clinical response in individual patients.

Gold is prescribed in patients with persistently active or progressive disease, despite the use of non-specific anti-inflammatory drugs, and should be considered early in the course of the disease before destructive changes have developed. There is a reasonably close relationship between response to gold and response to penicillamine, so that patients who respond to one are likely to respond to the other and *vice versa*. Gold has been shown to have a small effect on delaying the progression of X-ray changes in one study (Sigler *et al.*, 1974).

Gold is also effective in palindromic rheumatism and in juvenile chronic polyarthritis, especially juvenile rheumatoid arthritis.

The drug is given by intramuscular injection. The conventional dosage schedules to be described have been derived empirically over many years. Using sodium aurothiomalate, a test dose of 10 mg is followed in 1 week by a dose of 25 mg. Thereafter, 50 mg is given at weekly intervals. Once a response is obtained, the interval between injections is increased at first to 2, then to 4 or 6 weeks. Most clinicians would consider discontinuing the drug if no response has occurred after the administration of 500–700 mg. Others would increase the dose to 75–100 mg weekly for a few weeks in an attempt to stimulate a response. Maintenance doses are required to prevent relapse, and this is particularly important since second courses are usually ineffective and are more likely to produce toxic effects. (However, some prefer to give the drug to a total of 1 g in the first instance, repeating the course later if necessary.) At the first sign of relapse in a patient on maintenance doses, the interval between injections should be reduced until the disease is again controlled.

Another preparation, the thioglucose, is available in some countries. It is equally effective and may have a lower tendency to cause side effects (Rothermich *et al.*, 1976).

(Freyberg, 1942; *Editorial*, 1974, 1975; Gerber and Paulus, 1975; Gottlieb, 1977.)

(c) *Side effects, precautions and contraindications*

Side effects

The three major side effects of gold are blood dyscrasias, proteinuria and rashes. These are important because they may threaten life and because they may prevent the continuation of therapy. Reports relating to these and other side effects are summarized in Appendix 6.10.2.

Rashes represent the most common side-effect. They occur most often after a few months of treatment and develop in about 30% of patients. Gold dermatitis may mimic almost any skin eruption. It is often an itchy, scaly rash (Fig. 6.1), is sometimes mild and rapidly resolving, and sometimes severe (even exfoliative), and may continue for as long as a year. Pruritus sometimes precedes the rash, or may occur alone. Although some clinicians advocate using small doses of gold after the rash has resolved, it often recurs.

Proteinuria and nephrotic syndrome probably occur with about the same frequency as with penicillamine, the condition resolving slowly on withdrawing treatment.

Agranulocytosis and aplastic anaemia may develop at any time during the course of gold therapy. The precise frequency of these complications is not estab-

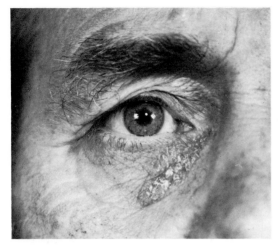

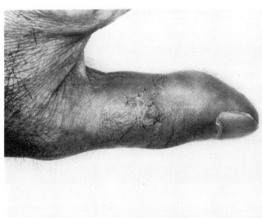

Fig. 6.1 Examples of typical gold-induced dermatitis; both patients had persistent, itchy, scaly lesions.

lished but they are rare. Thrombocytopenia, however, is not uncommon. Because of this risk, full blood and platelet counts must be carried out at least monthly in these patients.

Mouth ulcers may occur with or without skin changes in patients receiving gold. Hypersensitivity reactions may occur and it is mandatory to give a small test dose of 10 mg before proceeding with long-term therapy.

Precautions
It is prudent to avoid giving gold with other drugs that are known to suppress bone-marrow function (e.g. phenylbutazone, penicillamine, immunosuppressives). Monthly blood counts and weekly urinalysis are required during treatment. Care should be taken to ensure that once requested, the results of these tests are actually checked, preferably by the clinician responsible for introducing therapy. Patients should be warned to report any possible adverse reactions. The results of the previous blood and urine tests must always be known before the next injection is given. Gold therapy should be avoided in pregnancy.

Contraindications
Gold salts are contraindicated for the treatment of systemic lupus erythematosus.

(Campion *et al.*, 1974; Westwick *et al.*, 1974; Gordon *et al.*, 1975; Jalava *et al.*, 1977; Kean and Anastassiades, 1979.)

6.2.2 Antimalarials: Chloroquine phosphate (Arabis; Avloclor; Elestol; Malarivon; Resochin); Hydroxy-chloroquine sulphate (Plaquenil)

Other proprietary names for chloroquine phosphate include, Aralen (Australia, Canada, USA); Arechin (Poland); Chloroquin (Australia); Malaquin (Australia); Malarex (Denmark); Siragan (Australia); Tresochin (Sweden), and for hydroxychloroquine sulphate Ercoquin (Norway, Sweden); Plaquinol (Portugal); Quensyl (Germany).

Chloroquine and hydroxychloroquine, 4-aminoquinoline compounds, are antimalarials that are also used for the long-term treatment of rheumatoid arthritis and systemic lupus erythematosus. In rheumatoid arthritis they have a slow, delayed therapeutic action resembling that of gold.

(a) Pharmacology and pharmacokinetics

Chloroquine (7-chloro-[4-(4-diethylamino-1-methyl-butylamino) quinoline) and hydroxychloroquine (7-chloro-4-4-(N-ethyl-N-Z-hydroxyethylamino)-1-methyl-butylamino] quinoline sulphate) have similar actions. They are well absorbed from the gastrointestinal tract, steady-state plasma levels of chloroquine being reached after about 10 days of regular treatment. The drug has a long plasma half-life of about 6 days. Chloroquine is mainly excreted unchanged in the urine (70%), but a small amount is metabolized. In renal failure, excretion occurs to some extent via non-renal routes, but dosage should be adjusted for prolonged treatment in those with severely impaired renal function. Chloroquine is concentrated in the liver, spleen, kidney, lung, central nervous system and white blood cells. When the drug is stopped, it may take months or years for the retained drug to be excreted.

(Prouty and Kuroda, 1958; McChesney *et al.*, 1962, 1964, 1967a, b; Gabourel, 1963; Rubin *et al.*, 1963; Cohen and Yielding, 1964; Gerber, 1964; Zvaifler, 1964; Benecze and Johnson, 1965; Hurvitz and

Hirschhorn, 1965; Whitehouse and Boström, 1965; Fabre *et al.*, 1966; Rubin and Slonicki, 1966; Fedorko, 1967; Sams, 1967; Yielding, 1967; Abraham *et al.*, 1968; Kohno *et al.*, 1968; Read and Bay, 1971; Wibo and Poole, 1974.)

(b) *Clinical uses, preparations and dosage*

Although antimalarials are included under the general heading of rheumatoid arthritis, their application in the treatment of systemic lupus erythematosus and other disorders will also be discussed here. Therapeutic studies of antimalarials are summarized in Appendix 6.10.3.

In rheumatoid arthritis, chloroquine has an effect resembling that of gold, and clinical trials have shown that these two drugs are about equally effective. There is a slow amelioration of symptoms and signs which develops over a few months. There is improvement in extra-articular features of the disease, and there is reduction in ESR and in the titre of rheumatoid factor. However, there is little evidence of any influence on radiological progression of the disease. Chloroquine is generally considered to be an alternative to gold, penicillamine and immunosuppressives. Many clinicians avoid using antimalarials because of ocular toxicity, but the significance of this hazard may have been over-stressed and the use of these drugs still has some supporters who, indeed, would use it before other long-term suppressant drugs.

Indications for using antimalarials in rheumatoid arthritis are the same as for gold and penicillamine, namely, persistently active disease despite optimal anti-inflammatory therapy in patients with progressive disease.

In view of the ocular risks with long-term therapy many clinicians prefer to discontinue the drug after 12 or 18 months. It appears that retinal damage is more likely to occur if therapy is continued daily for longer than a year or if total dosage has exceeded 1.6 g/kg body weight. Chloroquine is sometimes useful in milder forms of systemic lupus erythematosus, and especially in those with troublesome chronic skin lesions. It is occasionally used in juvenile chronic arthritis as an alternative to gold salts (Laaksonen *et al.*, 1974). Antimalarials should not be used in psoriatic arthritis as the rash may be exacerbated, with the risk of an exfoliative reaction.

The following preparations may be used: chloroquine phosphate (250 mg tablet; 155 mg base), chloroquine sulphate (200 mg tablet; 150 mg base), or hydroxychloroquine sulphate (200 mg tablet: 156 mg base). Usual daily dosages for adults with rheumatoid arthritis are 200 or 250 mg of chloroquine sulphate or phosphate, respectively or 400–600 mg of hydroxychloroquine sul-

phate. It is safer to start with a low dose, increasing after 3 months in the absence of an adequate response. The paediatric dosage of chloroquine is $3\,\mathrm{mg\,kg^{-1}\,day^{-1}}$ and of hydroxychloroquine $5\,\mathrm{mg\,kg^{-1}\,day^{-1}}$.

(c) *Side effects, precautions and contraindications*

Side effects

Therapy with chloroquine and allied drugs may be associated with oculotoxicity. This may consist of a reversible keratopathy due to corneal deposition of the drug (Fig. 6.2(a)) and/or a retinopathy (Fig. 6.2(b)). The latter is by far the more serious in that it is usually irreversible and may be associated with significant visual impairment and even blindness. Retinal changes are due to selective accumulation of the drug in the pigment cells of the retina, an effect caused by both chloroquine and hydroxychloroquine (Bernstein *et al.*, 1969). This toxic effect, which leads to destruction both of rods and of cones (Wetterholm and Winter, 1964), is related to the total dose of the drug administered, the average threshold dose being about 500 g chloroquine. However, ocular lesions can occur with lower total doses (Scherbel *et al.*, 1965). The pigment-binding propensity of chloroquine may be reflected in blanching of the hair and eyebrows, changes which may be associated with retinal toxicity. The precise frequency of chloroquine toxicity has never been satisfactorily established, but is probably about 10% of patients treated with 250 mg or more per day of the drug for at least a year. However, reports vary widely from under 1% to as much as 15%. Various tests are available which have been claimed to detect early retinopathy (Carr *et al.*, 1966). These include the electrooculogram, tests of colour vision, and tests of retinal sensitivity. Despite the value of these tests, none guarantees identifying the very earliest ocular changes. It is imperative that all patients taking long-term antimalarials have regular, expert ophthalmological monitoring, and the earliest evidence of visual impairment should lead to immediate cessation of therapy. Most rheumatologists who use antimalarial drugs have a close liaison with an ophthalmology unit which enables efficient 'feedback' should the results of ocular testing be adverse. Oculotoxicity can be minimized by such a watchful approach, as well as by using low-dose or intermittent therapy. In addition to these precautions, especial care should be taken to provide patients with sufficient information about toxic effects. For example, they should be told to report immediately 'haloes around lights' (an early indication of keratopathy) as this change, although not serious in itself, will alert the clinician to the possible development of more serious ocular effects.

There is no effective treatment for the drug-induced retinopathy, which only rarely recovers after stopping

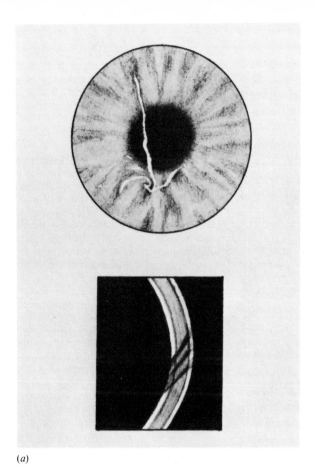

(a)

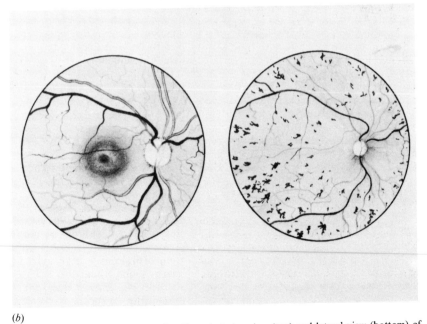

(b)

Fig. 6.2 (a) Chloroquine keratopathy. Top: Anterior view (top) and lateral view (bottom) of typical corneal changes revealed by slit-lamp examination. (b) Patterns of chloroquine retinopathy. Left: 'perimacular halo' or 'bull's eye lesion'. Right: changes resembling retinitis pigmentosa, including optic atrophy.

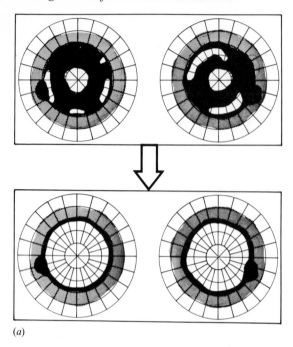

(a)

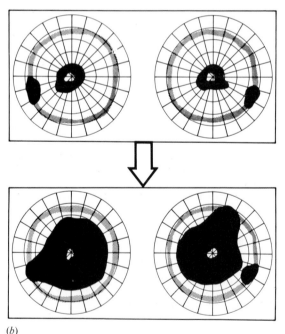

(b)

Fig. 6.3 (a) Chloroquine retinopathy: pattern of regression of bilateral visual field defects after drug withdrawal. (b) Pattern of progression of bilateral visual field defects after drug withdrawal.

therapy (Fig. 6.3(a)). Indeed, as Burns (1966) has indicated, retinal changes may actually progress for several years after drug withdrawal (Fig. 6.3(b)).

Apart from ocular changes, chloroquine is usually well tolerated. Indeed, it is probably the best tolerated of the drugs in this 'specific' group. Nausea, vomiting, pruritus and rashes occur occasionally and, in addition to the depigmentation mentioned previously, there may be loss of hair. Various forms of fetal damage (loss of eighth-nerve function, posterior column defects, mental retardation and neonatal convulsions) have been reported (Hart and Naunton, 1964). Other infrequent side effects that have been documented include myopathy, neuromyopathy and behavioural changes.

Appendix 6.10.4 summarizes the main studies concerning antimalarial-induced side effects since the introduction of these drugs in rheumatological practice.

Precautions
Ophthalmic examination including examination of visual fields with red and white light should be carried out before the start of treatment, carefully documented and repeated every 3 months (see under 'side effects'). Some clinicians prefer to stop treatment temporarily after 1 or 2 years. Reference has already been made to the fact that patients should be warned of the possibility of visual changes and advised to report at once if this occurs. It should be further stressed that evidence of oculotoxicity, either from the patient or from ophthalmic examination, should lead to discontinuation of therapy even when there is doubt.

Contraindications
Chloroquine should not be co-administered with phenylbutazone, gold salts, penicillamine or immunosuppressive drugs. A full blood count should be carried out every 6 months, although blood dyscrasias are unusual.

Chloroquine should never be given in pregnancy, to patients with visual abnormalities or to patients with psoriasis. (See under 'side effects'.)

6.2.3 D-Penicillamine (Cuprimine, Depamine, Distamine)

Other proprietary names include: Cuprenil (Poland); D-Penamine (Australia); Metalcaptase, Trolovol (both Germany).

D-penicillamine is β, β-dimethylcysteine, a degradation product of penicillin. D-penicillamine is used in preference to the L or DL forms as these inhibit pyridoxine and have caused optic neuritis. It is one of a group of drugs that can be said to have a 'specific' long-term action in rheumatoid arthritis. Its action is slow, and selective, since it does not benefit all types of inflammatory arthritis. It exerts its effects on extra-articular features of the disease as well as on joints, and there is reduction in rheumatoid factor and in ESR. In patients able to tolerate treatment, there is improvement in the outcome of the disease, although it is still debatable whether there is a delay in radiological progression.

(Jaffe, 1970 and 1978; Mackenzie, 1970; Huskisson, 1976a; Ansell and Hall, 1977; Lyle and Kleinman, 1977; Annotation, *British Medical Journal*, 1973.)

(a) Pharmacology and pharmacokinetics

Penicillamine is readily absorbed from the gastrointestinal tract and reaches peak concentrations in the blood in 1 hour. It is rapidly excreted in the urine, but traces remain in the plasma after 48 hours due to protein binding. About 80% of an intravenous dose is excreted in 24 hours, mainly as the disulphide, but small amounts of free penicillamine and of the mixed sulphide of penicillamine and cysteine also appear in the urine. Penicillamine has an established place in the treatment of three unrelated disorders – Wilson's disease, cystinuria and rheumatoid arthritis. In the first two, its mode of action is fairly well understood, but in rheumatoid arthritis it remains speculative, although it could be immunomodulatory (Roath and Wills, 1974; Huskisson and Berry, 1974). Other possibly relevant biological effects of the drug in rheumatoid arthritis include: interference with cross-linking of collagen (Francis and Mowat, 1974); interference with RNA and protein synthesis and structural alteration of protein (Roath and Wills, 1974); dissociation of macromolecular complexes (Bluestone and Goldberg, 1973); and interference with free radical metabolism (Lorber *et al.*, 1964).

(Jaffe, 1963, 1965, 1968a; Jaffe and Merryman, 1968; Assem, 1974; Chwalinska-Sadowska and Baum, 1976; Mohammed *et al.*, 1976; Arrigoni-Martelli *et al.*, 1977; Czekalowski *et al.*, 1977; Friedman, 1977; Huskisson, 1977; Jullunn *et al.*, 1977; Stanworth *et al.*, 1977.)

(b) Clinical uses, preparations and dosage

Penicillamine is effective in rheumatoid arthritis, producing a reasonable response in about 80% of patients. The present use of the drug is based on controlled multicentre clinical trials conducted in the UK (Multicentre Trial Group, 1973), confirmed by subsequent studies (Hill, 1974; Huskisson and Berry, 1974; Huskisson *et al.*, 1974). Seronegative patients respond as well as those who are seropositive; patients with juvenile chronic polyarthritis are thought to respond less well than adults. Active inflammation and proliferation of synovial tissues is suppressed in patients who respond to treatment. This action is achieved slowly, the greatest effect of the drug being seen in the second month of treatment, with the maximal effect occurring at 4–6

months. There is a reduction in the number and size of rheumatoid nodules, improvement in tenosynovitis, extensor sheath swellings and lymphadenopathy, and sometimes in peripheral neuropathy, splenomegaly and leg ulcers. There is also some evidence that rheumatoid lung disease may be improved (Lorber, 1966). Penicillamine is probably the most useful drug for patients with vasculitis. However, although initial results were encouraging and dramatic results reported in some patients with peripheral gangrene, more recent experience has been disappointing (Huskisson and Hart, 1972). Penicillamine therapy leads to a reduction in the requirements for other drugs, including corticosteroids.

The proper use of penicillamine is for patients with persistently active or progressive disease. In general, it should not be used in the first 6 months of the disease in view of the frequency of spontaneous improvement during this stage. Nor should the start of treatment be delayed much after 6 months because complete recovery is impossible once permanent anatomical changes have developed.

Penicillamine is probably as effective as gold or azathioprine. Although it causes more side effects than gold, it is less likely to be withdrawn. For these reasons, some clinicians regard penicillamine as the first choice of drugs of this group.

Penicillamine is effective in about 50% of patients with juvenile chronic polyarthritis, particularly those with juvenile rheumatoid arthritis. It is also useful in palindromic rheumatism, and it appears to have a useful role in modifying the proliferative changes of scleroderma. Less well established rheumatological indications for penicillamine include the seronegative spondarthritides and polymyositis. The drug has been used to treat gold dermatitis, and has been shown to have an antiviral effect in polio but not in vaccinia or herpes. It has no effect on the adjuvant arthritis of rats. Principal rheumatological studies relating to the therapeutic effect of penicillamine are summarized in Appendix 6.10.5.

Penicillamine is an established drug in Wilson's disease (hepatolenticular degeneration) and in cystinuria. It has also been shown to be effective in arsenical polyneuropathy and poisoning due to lead and mercury.

Penicillamine is available as 50, 125 or 250 mg tablets. (1.25 g of penicillamine hydrochloride is about equal to 1 g penicillamine). Clinical experience has shown that side effects may be reduced and compliance increased by introducing the drug at lower initial doses and with longer intervals between each increment. In adults with rheumatoid arthritis, it should be started at a dose of 125–250 mg daily. This is increased by 125–250 mg daily at intervals of 2–8 weeks, depending on clinical demand. If side effects such as nausea develop, no further increase in dosage is made until the problem has been resolved.

Similarly, once patients start to improve, no further increase in dosage is made. The usual maintenance dose is 0·5–1 g daily. A few patients need less and a few require more. In palindromic rheumatism, a dose of 250 mg daily is often enough to control the disorder. In juvenile chronic polyarthritis, the initial daily dose is 50 mg increasing to between 250 and 600 mg, depending on the patient's size.

Penicillamine has recently been approved for use in the USA.

(c) Side effects, precautions and contraindications

Side effects tend to occur at particular times during the course of treatment. The overall frequency of side effects is maximal in the first few months, problems being infrequent after 18 months of treatment.

Studies relating to the side effects of penicillamine are summarized in Appendix 6.10.6. In the main, toxic effects are dermatological, haematological, renal and gastrointestinal.

Rashes are of two main types: an 'allergic' type rash developing within the first few months of treatment and disappearing within a few days of stopping treatment; and an itchy, scaly rash consisting of raised irregular plaques appearing after 6 or more months of treatment. This rash (Fig. 6.4) disappears slowly after drug withdrawal, and, unlike the 'allergic' rash often recurs when therapy is re-introduced. It is unresponsible to treatment with topical corticosteroids. Less frequently the rash may be elastosis perforans serpiginosa, epidermolysis bullosa, pemphigus, urticaria, or rashes characteristic of systemic lupus erythematosus.

The most threatening complication is acute neutropenia or thrombocytopenia, or both. Should such a haematological crisis occur, medication must be stopped immediately and supportive medical measures, including corticosteroids, given.

Nephropathy, including the nephrotic syndrome and, rarely, a Goodpasture-like syndrome, may complicate penicillamine therapy. Proteinuria usually develops after 4 or more months of treatment and is of variable severity. Up to one third of patients developing proteinuria become nephrotic, usually within a few weeks of its appearance. Progression of proteinuria or the appearance of microscopic haematuria are indications to stop treatment. There is still no general agreement as to what constitutes an 'acceptable' degree of proteinuria, but levels below 300 mg per 24 hours in the face of major disease response may allow continuation of a moderate dosage with close monitoring (Roth, 1980).

Secondary immune complex diseases, including the lupus diathesis, can evolve into systemic lupus erythematosus. Systemic lupus is a rare and late complication, developing after 1–2 years of treatment. The patient

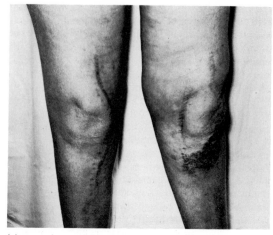

(a)

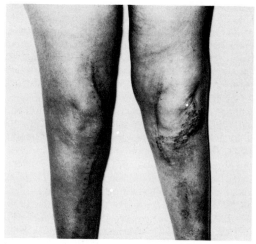

(b)

Fig. 6.4 (a) Penicillamine rash during drug therapy. (b) 3 weeks after stopping drug, showing some fading of the skin lesions.

may note a distinct change in the nature of his joint pain, and the antinuclear factor becomes strongly positive. The disease disappears on withdrawing penicillamine. A myasthenia-like syndrome has also been reported in patients with a lupus diathesis.

Anorexia and nausea are among the earliest side effects, usually developing within the first few weeks of treatment. These side effects, and others involving the gastrointestinal tract (epigastric pain, vomiting, diarrhoea), have been reported in up to one fifth of patients. However, because of concomitant anti-rheumatic therapy, it is often difficult to pin the blame on penicillamine, and it may be reasonable when there is doubt to suspect non-steroidal agents or corticosteroids in the first instance. Impairment or loss of taste may develop after about 6 weeks of treatment. Patients should be warned about this side effect which resolves after about 6 weeks whether or not the drug is withdrawn. Mouth ulcers are an occasional problem in patients on penicillamine. Reactivation of peptic ulceration has been reported.

Febrile reactions occasionally occur after the first few doses of penicillamine, and these patients seem particularly sensitive to the effect of the drug and may need only small doses for control of the disease.

Penicillamine has been shown to affect skin collagen, and there have been reports of defective wound healing and changes in skin elasticity and thickness. For this reason it has been suggested that the drug should be discontinued before elective surgery.

There have been sporadic reports invoking the drug in dermatomyositis, diffuse alveolitis, and hepatoxicity.

Careful consideration should be taken before penicillamine is given to patients with renal disease because of the risk of a superimposed nephrotic syndrome and reduction of glomerular filtration rate.

There have been reports of connective tissue defects in the fetus and, despite the fact that a number of normal pregnancies have occurred in patients taking the drug, it should be avoided in pregnancy.

Patients receiving penicillamine should be seen at least monthly, with urinalysis and a full blood count (including platelets) carried out every 3–4 weeks. Patients should also be warned to report any unexpected reactions to the physician who is supervising the treatment.

The drug is contraindicated in patients with penicillin hypersensitivity.

Penicillamine should not be co-administered with gold salts or antimalarials. The drug can safely be given with other analgesic and anti-inflammatory drugs, but it is wise to avoid using it with other drugs that affect the bone marrow (e.g. phenylbutazone, azathioprine).

6.2.4 Immunosuppressives

Although corticosteroids and antilymphocytic globulin are immunosuppressive, in this context the term refers to cytotoxic agents (cytostatic or antineoplastic drugs) and antimetabolities. Methotrexate is discussed in Section 6.4.1 in view of its particular value in psoriatic arthritis and Reiter's disease.

The immunosuppressives, particular azathioprine, cyclophosphamide and chlorambucil, first became extensively studied as a possible means of controlling rheumatoid arthritis in the early 1970s. However, there had been sporadic reports much earlier – the first report of a cytotoxic agent in the management of rheumatoid arthritis being in 1951 (Jimenez-Diaz, 1951).

The immunosuppressive agents discussed in this section have been found to be of some value in the long-term suppression of rheumatoid arthritis. In this respect they are clinically comparable with other long-term suppressives such as gold or penicillamine, and probably slightly superior in slowing the progression of radiological changes. However, immunosuppressive agents are significantly more toxic, and tend to be used only in severe disease that has failed to respond to less toxic long-term agents.

(Stevens and Willoughby, 1969; Schwartz and Gowans, 1971; Steinberg *et al.*, 1972; Parsons *et al.*, 1974; Reiner *et al.*, 1978; Barnes and Lovatt, 1982.)

(a) Azathioprine (Imuran)

Other proprietary preparations include: Imurek (Germany); Imurel (Australia, France, Sweden).

Pharmacology and pharmacokinetics
Azathioprine is 6-(1-methyl-4-nitro imidazol-5-yl-thio) purine. It is an anti-metabolite that acts by interfering with purine biosynthesis. Its action in rheumatoid arthritis is thought to be due to its immunosuppressive effect. It is generally considered to be the first choice of immunosuppressives for use in rheumatoid arthritis because it is somewhat less toxic and easier to use than alternative drugs such as cyclophosphamide or methotrexate.

Azathioprine is well absorbed when given by mouth and has a plasma half-life of about 3 hours. It is first converted in the body to 6-mercaptopurine and then to thiouric acid by xanthine oxidase. It is excreted either in this form, or in large part (50%) as unchanged 6-mercaptopurine. In view of this, the dosage of azathioprine must be reduced in patients with renal failure.

(Bertino, 1973.)

Clinical uses, preparations and dosage
The action of azathioprine in rheumatoid arthritis resembles that of penicillamine and gold. There is a gradual suppression of disease activity with relief of pain, reduction in joint swelling and other signs of inflammation. The maximal effect is achieved after 4–6 months of treatment, by which time the ESR and rheumatoid factor titre have decreased. Azathioprine is effective in about 80% of patients treated (seronegative or seropositive), but, as with other agents of this type, results are unpredictable, and there is still no way of detecting which patients belong to the responsive subgroup.

The clinical effects of azathioprine are similar to those of gold and penicillamine but, although still contentious, it is claimed that azathioprine is superior to gold in its effect on slowing radiological progression of the disease, though probably less effective in this respect than cyclophosphamide. It is probably a little less effective clinically than cyclophosphamide, but relatively less toxic.

There is no place for azathioprine (or other cytotoxic agents) in the routine management of rheumatoid arthritis. It is used, with some circumspection, as an alternative to gold and penicillamine, for patients with persistently active or progressive disease. Since response is probably not related to response to penicillamine and gold, it is a useful drug for patients unresponsive to either penicillamine or gold. It has also been used in psoriatic arthritis failing to respond to analgesic/anti-inflammatory drugs. It is used in systemic lupus erthematosus, particularly for patients needing excessive doses of corticosteroids. It is effective in Wegener's granulomatosis, and is sometimes used in polymyositis not responding to corticosteroids.

Azathioprine is available as a 50 mg tablet, and the usual dosage is 150 mg daily in two or three divided doses, or 2.5 mg kg^{-1} day^{-1}. However, trials have shown that smaller doses are equally effective in rheumatoid arthritis, and it is wise to give 100 mg daily for the first few months, increasing the dosage only if necessary. In children the daily dosage is 2.5 mg kg^{-1}.

Therapeutic studies in which azathioprine has been used are listed in Appendix 6.10.7

Side effects, precautions and contraindications
The most important toxic reactions are marrow suppression, gastrointestinal intolerance, and infections. Leucopenia is the most common haematological problem, but thrombocytopenia or pancytopenia may occur. It is imperative to perform regular blood counts, and the drug should be stopped if significant marrow suppression occurs. Usually, haematological suppression is dose related and the drug can be restarted at a lower dose.

Nausea, vomiting and diarrhoea occur in about 15% of patients, usually within days or weeks of starting treatment. In many patients, the drug must be stopped, but it is sometimes possible to treat these gastrointestinal effects with symptomatic remedies.

Superimposed infective conditions include varicella, herpes simplex, herpes zoster, warts, and sometimes more serious infections such as recurrent pneumonia. Opportunistic infections with unusual organisms or fungi (e.g. disseminated histoplasmosis) may occur and should be considered in patients who develop an unaccountable illness during treatment.

There is an increased frequency of malignancy in patients receiving azathioprine after renal transplantation, and malignancies have been reported occasionally in rheumatic patients. An increase in malig-

nancy has not yet been established in rheumatoid arthritis, and on present evidence does not appear to be a significant hazard. Occasional side effects include rash, drug fever and other hypersensitivity reactions, and alopecia. Chromosomal abnormalities have been reported, but are of doubtful clinical significance. Azoospermia does not occur. Scattered reports have implicated azathioprine as a possible cause of pancreatitis, hepatoxicity, and acute respiratory depression.

Full blood counts are necessary at least monthly in patients receiving azathioprine. The effect of azathioprine are enhanced by allopurinol and the dose should be reduced to 25% of the usual dose in patients receiving this drug. Agents which, like azathioprine, suppress the bone marrow should not be used concomitantly.

Azathioprine should be used with care in patients with liver damage or a history of liver disease. Due to its immunosuppressant action, the drug should not be given to patients with acute infections. Reduced doses may be required in patients with renal transplants.

Azathioprine should be used seldom, and only if there are most pressing indications, in young adults because of the possible effects that azathioprine might have on their offspring. It should be avoided in pregnancy. Azathioprine should be used only with extreme caution in children. It should not be used as a routine in the management of active seronegative chronic arthritis of childhood. It will need to be considered if amyloidosis (the one potentially fatal complication of juvenile chronic polyarthritis) is present, or if very serious side effects have occurred with other forms of treatment (e.g. corticosteroids, gold or penicillamine) in the presence of severe active disease (Ansell, 1980).

(b)   *Cyclophosphamide (Endoxana)*

Other proprietary names include: Cytoxan (USA); Endoxan (France, Germany, South Africa); Endoxan-Asta (Australia); Enduxon (Brazil); Genoxal (Spain); Procytox (Canada); Sendoxan (Norway, Sweden).

Pharmacology and pharmacokinetics
Cyclophosphamide is 2(di-(2-chlorethyl)-amino)-1-oxa-3 aza-2-phosphacyclohexane 2-oxide monohydrate. It is an alkylating agent which is believed to be effective in rheumatoid arthritis and other rheumatic disorders, such as systemic lupus erythematosus, because of its immunosuppressive effect. Like azathioprine it has a slow onset of action and causes improvement in extra-articular as well as articular features. In view of the serious side effects of the drug, in rheumatic disorders cyclophosphamide is best reserved for patients with states likely to prove fatal and which have failed to respond to other 'specific' agents.

Cyclophosphamide is well absorbed from the gastrointestinal tract. Peak blood levels are reached within an hour of administration, and it has a plasma half-life of $4–6\frac{1}{2}$ hours. It is not, or only slightly, bound to plasma proteins (0–10%), although its active metabolites are more protein bound (56%). It is excreted in urine and faeces either as the unchanged drug or metabolites, some with alkylating activity. The drug must be activated before it becomes effective, and this takes place in the liver.

(Lemmel *et al.*, 1971; Hurd, 1973; Strong *et al.*, 1973; Clements *et al.*, 1974.)

Clinical uses, preparations and dosage
Despite its toxicity, cyclophosphamide is undoubtedly highly effective in rheumatoid arthritis. It has a similar type of action to drugs such as penicillamine and gold, influencing extra-articular features, ESR, rheumatoid factor and X-ray changes. (Cooperating Clinics Committee of ARA, 1970; Currey *et al.*, 1974). Withdrawal of treatment is necessary in about 50% of patients, rather more than with gold and a little more often than in patients on azathioprine. Toxicity is the usual reason for stopping treatment. Because of its toxicity, cyclophosphamide should be reserved as a last resort in patients with the most severe types of disease who have failed to respond to drugs like gold, penicillamine and azathioprine, and in those with life-threatening complications. In these circumstances some clinicians prefer chlorambucil because it has fewer side effects.

Cyclophosphamide is also used in severe systemic lupus erythematosus and occasionally in some rare rheumatic diseases such as Wegener's granulomatosis. In these conditions requiring excessive levels of corticosteroids, cyclophosphamide exerts a potent steroid-sparing effect.

Cyclophosphamide is available as a 50 mg tablet. Dosage should be kept to a minimum since many side effects are dose related. The range of dosage is $1.0–1.5 \, \text{mg kg}^{-1} \, \text{day}^{-1}$ in divided doses, and most patients with rheumatoid arthritis require 50–100 mg daily. Patients should be started on 50 mg daily and dosage increased no more often than monthly.

(Fosdick *et al.*, 1968; Co-operating Clinics of ARA, 1970, 1972; Townes *et al.*, 1972; Lidsky *et al.*, 1973; Williams *et al.*, 1980.)

Side effects, precautions and contraindications
Side effects are more frequent and more severe with cyclophosphamide than with other immunosuppressive agents.

The main side effects are bone-marrow suppression, gastrointestinal effects, haemorrhagic cystitis, infections, alopecia and infertility.

Bone-marrow suppression is a direct effect and is dose related. During therapy a careful watch must be kept on haemoglobin, white count and platelets. Suppression of neutrophil count is the most common finding and this is usually reversible, responding rapidly to withdrawal of treatment. The drug can then be reintroduced at a lower dose.

Gastrointestinal side effects (anorexia, nausea, vomiting and diarrhoea) are early problems which occasionally limit the use of the drug, as may stomatitis. Anorexia, nausea and vomiting often respond to antihistamines and tranquillizers.

Haemorrhagic cystitis is a potentially serious side effect demanding immediate withdrawal of the drug. Some patients have dysuria which may require reduction in dosage. Bladder fibrosis may occur after several years of treatment and bladder carcinoma has been reported.

Alopecia, the most frequent side effect, occurs in about 20% of patients receiving 100 mg daily, and may be total. The hair regrows slowly if the drug is stopped. Patients should be warned in advance of this possibility.

Infections presumably arise because of the drug's immunosuppressive action. They vary from herpes zoster to more serious opportunistic infections with unusual organisms.

Azoospermia or amenorrhoea are common in patients receiving cyclophosphamide, and infertility is therefore also usual.

Hepatotoxicity may occur and liver function tests should be performed from time to time.

There have been reports implicating cyclophosphamide as a cause of malignancy (e.g. cervical tumour, reticulum cell sarcoma, leukaemia) in patients receiving this drug, but so far these changes have not been observed in rheumatic patients.

Occasional side effects include chromosomal abnormalities, pigmentation of the skin and nails, colitis, interstitial pulmonary fibrosis, and hypoprothrombinaemia.

Cyclophosphamide should be avoided in men and women of reproductive age, in pregnancy, and in children.

No other drug which may suppress bone marrow should be given concurrently (e.g. gold, phenylbutazone). Allopurinol increases the risk of bone-marrow suppression. Barbiturates may increase the effectiveness and toxicity of cyclophosphamide by stimulating its activation in the liver. Conversely, phenothiazines may reduce its effectiveness by inhibiting its activation in the liver.

Blood counts should be done at least once a month and patients warned to report immediately if side effects develop.

(Hutter *et al.*, 1969; Scheinman and Stamler, 1969; Struck and Hill, 1972; Pollock *et al.*, 1973.)

(c) Chlorambucil (Leukeran)

Another proprietary name is Chloraminophène (France).

Pharmacology and pharmacokinetics

Chlorambucil is γ-[p-Di(2-chloroethyl) aminophenyl] butyric acid).

Like cyclophosphamide, it is an alkylating agent which has been used in the treatment of severe rheumatic disorders. There have been fewer formal trials of chlorambucil, but there is a suggestion that it may be as effective as cyclophosphamide with fewer side effects.

It is readily absorbed with peak blood levels reached rapidly and a short plasma half-life. There are few pharmacokinetic data available.

(McClean *et al.*, 1976.)

Clinical uses, preparations and dosage

Much of the initial work on this drug in rheumatoid arthritis has come from French authors. The indications for its use are the same as those for other immunosuppressive agents. Its effect in rheumatoid arthritis compared with azathioprine or cyclophosphamide is not yet established, but it is probably comparable. There is evidence suggesting that it may be useful in children with juvenile chronic polyarthritis complicated by amyloidosis (Schnitzer and Ansell, 1977) and in patients with systemic lupus erythematosus and progressive renal disease. Behçet's syndrome has also shown an encouraging response to chlorambucil (see Section 6.3).

Chlorambucil is available as 2 and 5 mg tablets. Dosage should be kept to a minimum, and about 0.1 mg kg^{-1} day^{-1} is appropriate. Most patients with rheumatoid arthritis require between 2.5 and 7.5 mg daily. It is reasonable to start with 5 mg daily, reducing in the event of neutropenia to a lower dose. In children the dosage employed has been 0.15 mg/kg bodyweight initially, with adjustments according to regular blood monitoring (Schnitzer and Ansell, 1977).

(Snaith *et al.*, 1973; Kahn and de Seze, 1975.)

Side effects, precautions and contraindications

Side effects are similar to those of cyclophosphamide except that haemorrhagic cystitis and alopecia do not occur. The main problems are bone-marrow suppression, infections, gastrointestinal disturbances and stomatitis. The same potential hazards of oncogenesis, mutagenesis, dysmorphogenicity and infertility exist as with cyclophosphamide. The same cautions and contraindications as for cyclophosphamide apply to the use of chlorambucil.

Newer long-term suppressants

For an account of newer and still somewhat experimental suppressive agents for rheumatoid arthritis (e.g.

levamisole, dapsone, sulphasalazine) readers are referred to Chapter 12.

COMMENT

Long-term suppressive agents (remission-inducing drugs) are used in rheumatoid arthritis once it has become clear that aspirin or other analgesic/anti-inflammatory agents in full dosage are insufficient. Some clinicians, including the author, would add a small dose of corticosteroid (e.g. prednisolone 5–7.5 mg) to the non-steroidal preparation before assuming that the patient is refractory to control. Poor control (persisting disease activity with, by inference, tissue damage) can be recognized in several ways. These include clinical evidence of persisting inflammation, extra-articular manifestations, laboratory tests (e.g. raised ESR, raised serum C-reactive protein), and progressive erosive damage on bone X-rays. If some or all of these are present in spite of adequate non-specific treatment, 'specific' therapy with a long-term suppressant should be considered.

Unlike anti-inflammatory drugs, such as non-steroidal anti-inflammatories and corticosteroids, remittive agents are not immediately or directly anti-inflammatory, and hence show no short-term effect on symptoms and signs of inflammation. It is thought, however, that in varying degree they influence the progress of rheumatoid arthritis by slowing the rate at which tissues are damaged.

There is no general agreement either regarding the choice of these drugs or their details of administration. In general, the most generally used drugs are gold, penicillamine, and anti-malarials (chloroquine and hydroxychloroquine). They have each been shown to be suppressive in rheumatoid arthritis – gold and penicillamine probably being somewhat more potent than anti-malarials.

However, their main differences concern their toxic effects, each drug possessing its own complement of side effects, many of them serious. *Use of these drugs must therefore be carried out with adequate monitoring, preferably associated with units having experience of these drugs.*

Alternative suppressive agents include dapsone and sulphasalazine, but their place in the management of rheumatoid arthritis is not yet fully established (see Chapter 12).

Immunosuppressant drugs such as azathioprine, chlorambucil and cyclophosphamide have also been shown to possess remissive-inducing effects in rheumatoid arthritis. However, their toxicity and doubts concerning a possible slight risk of malignant disease demands an even more cautious approach to their use. In most special centres including the author's, this group of drugs (starting with azathioprine) is reserved for the most resistant patients, or for those with grave extra-articular problems such as vasculitis.

SYSTEMIC LUPUS ERYTHEMATOSUS

See under Sections 6.2.2–6.2.4.

6.3 SERONEGATIVE SPONDARTHRITIDES

There is evidence that psoriasis, psoriatic arthritis and, to a lesser extent, Reiter's disease may respond to immunosuppressives, particularly methotrexate. This drug may also have an application in the treatment of Behçet's syndrome.

6.3.1 Methotrexate (Methotrexate tablets; Methotrexate injection)

Another proprietary name its Ledertrexate (France).

(a) Pharmacology and pharmacokinetics

Methotrexate (amethopterin) is 4-amino-10-methylfolic acid. It is an antimetabolite that inhibits the conversion of dihydrofolic acid (formed from folic acid) to tetrahydrofolic acid by binding to dihydrofolic acid reductase. This action interferes with the synthesis of DNA. The drug is therefore active only in cells that are in a DNA-synthesizing phase.

Methotrexate is well absorbed from the gastrointestinal tract after small oral doses ($< 30\,\mathrm{mg\,m^{-2}}$), but poorly absorbed after large doses ($> 80\,\mathrm{mg\,m^{-2}}$). About a third of an oral dose undergoes metabolism by intestinal bacteria during absorption, thereby reducing bioavailability. About 50% is bound to plasma proteins. It has a plasma elimination half-life ranging from 6 to 69 hours (mean 27 hours). The drug is excreted mainly unchanged in urine, and to a lesser extent in bile. It is actively secreted in the renal tubule by the organic acid transport system. Renal clearance is correlated with endogenous creatinine clearance, and may provide a guide to dose adjustment according to renal function and age. Bound methotrexate may be retained in the body for many months.
(Kersley, 1968; Wade, 1977.)

(b) Clinical uses, preparations and dosage

Methotrexate is used for intractable psoriasis (Rees *et al.*, 1964; Haim and Alroy, 1967; Martin *et al.*, 1967; Spiro and Dennis, 1969; Baker, 1970; Nyfors and Brodthagen, 1970; Weinstein and Frost, 1971). and for psoriatic arthritis (O'Brien *et al.*, 1962; Black *et al.*, 1964; Kersley, 1964; Chaouat *et al.*, 1971; Feldges and Barnes, 1974). Its use in uncomplicated psoriasis was introduced over 30 years ago (Gubnet *et al.*, 1951), and the particular efficacy of the drug in this disease is thought to be due to holding up mitosis and cell division in a disease characterized by rapid proliferation of epidermal cells. There is an impression that methotrexate may be more effective than azathioprine for controlling psoriasis, but less effective for controlling the joint disease.

The drug has also been used in Reiter's disease (Mullins *et al.*, 1969; Owen and Cowen, 1979) and in Behçet's syndrome (Mamo and Azzam, 1970; Tricoulis, 1976).

Application of the drug has also been extended to non-spondarthritic disorders, notably polymyositis and dermatomyositis in adults (Metzger *et al.*, 1974), and dermatomyositis in children (Jacobs, 1977).

Methotrexate is available as a 2.5 mg tablet. It is probably best given in a single weekly dose of 10–25 mg before food. It can also be given by intramuscular or intravenous injection. Wright (1981) has employed the intravenous route in patients with severe psoriasis using a dose of 25 mg per week for the month after a test dose of 5 mg. Blood checks are made three days after the injection, and then every two weeks. The dosage of methotrexate must be reduced in patients with impaired renal function.

(c) Side effects, precautions and contraindications

Methotrexate may cause gastrointestinal intolerance, particularly diarrhoea, mouth ulceration, leucopenia or thrombocytopenia, suppression of ovarian and testicular function, megaloblastic anaemia, and skin changes including dermatitis, photosensitivity, alopecia and depigmentation. Cirrhosis and hepatic fibrosis have been reported in patients with psoriasis after long-term therapy. In patients treated with small dosages the extent of liver damage appears to be related to the duration of treatment. Liver function tests are not a good guide to the development of liver damage, detection of which requires liver biopsy. Renal damage, and pulmonary and neurotoxic reactions have also been documented. Chromosomal damage has not yet been reported.

Regular blood counts are essential in patients receiving methotrexate. This precaution should be combined with close observation for other side effects. Salicylates reduce the clearance rate of methotrexate and may increase the risk of toxicity. Phenylbutazone also enhances the toxicity of methotrexate, presumably by delaying renal elimination. These potential interactions with aspirin and phenylbutazone are of particular relevance in psoriatic arthropathy.

Methotrexate should be used with care in patients with depressed bone-marrow function and in the presence of hepatic and renal involvement. It should also be used cautiously in debilitated patients, alcoholics, those with infections, or those with ulcerative disorders of the gastrointestinal tract. It should not be given in early pregnancy.

(Wade, 1977.)

COMMENT

Specific therapy for members of the spondarthritis group has only relatively recently attracted attention. The most well established treatment is methotrexate in special cases of psoriatic arthritis. Reiter's disease also responds to this drug but the results are less convincing.

No long-term suppressive agent has yet been found for ankylosing spondylitis, although research continues in this direction.

6.4 GOUT

6.4.1 General comment

Although this section is largely concerned with details of drugs having a specific action in the treatment of gout, it is opportune to point out that nowadays it is possible to control both the acute attack and, on a long-term basis, the level of uric acid in the blood. In a sense, therefore, gout can now be 'cured' (controlled is more strictly correct, as the underlying genetic diathesis cannot be removed), and patients should no longer have to experience recurrences of severe acute attacks and tophus formation in the face of tedious dietary restriction.

From the point of view of drug therapy, the control of gout may be divided into: (1) control of the acute episode with colchicine, or analgesic/anti-inflammatory agents (e.g. phenylbutazone, indomethacin, naproxen); and (2) control of the level of blood uric acid, either by increasing its elimination (probenecid, sulphinpyrazone) or by decreasing its formation (allopurinol).

With the exception of colchicine, drugs used to control the acute inflammatory episode have been discussed elsewhere (see Chapter 5). Colchicine, the time-honoured remedy for the acute attack, has been included in this chapter because of its relatively specific action, not only in the management of the acute attack, but also in long-term prophylaxis. The other specific drugs used in the long-term control of gout will also be discussed in this section.

6.4.2 Drugs

(a) Colchicine (Eade's Pills contain colchicum corm; Rheumatic Dellipsoids D10 contain colchicum dry extract)

Other proprietary preparations include: Aqua-Colchin, Colcin, Colgout, Coluric (all Australia); Colchineos (France, South Africa).

Colchicine was isolated from *Colchicum autumnale* in 1820 in the great rush of phytochemical investigation of that era, and was identified as the active antigout agent of the plant.

Pharmacology and pharmacokinetics

Colchicine is an anti-inflammatory and antimitotic agent that acts by interfering with leucocyte responses (Malawista, 1968). Colchicine inhibits a variety of leucocyte functions, but its most potent inhibitory effects are on chemotaxis (Postlethwaite *et al.*, 1974) and on the random motility of leucocytes under the influence of urate (Gutman, 1966). The reduced metabolic activity of the leucocyte results in less local lactic acid formation, resulting in a reduced tendency to urate crystal formation and a lessened inflammatory response.

The drug is not an analgesic, does not relieve other types of pain, and is of no value in other types of arthritis. The dramatic pain relief resulting from colchicine in gout is attributed to its anti-inflammatory effect which tends to be largely specific to this disease, although it has been observed to reduce inflammatory manifestations of other disorders (see later in this section).

It has no effect upon urate metabolism or the concentration of urate in the serum or urine.

Oral absorption of colchicine is rapid. After intravenous administration, colchicine leaves the blood rapidly (plasma half-life 0.32 hours) and is widely distributed. The drug is concentrated in the kidney, liver, spleen and intestinal tract and has been shown to be present in leucocytes 10 days after administration of a single dose. It is partly deacetylated in the liver, and the greater part of both colchicine and its metabolities is excreted in the bile and intestinal secretions. However, up to 20% is excreted in the urine unchanged where it may be found for up to 10 days after a single intravenous dose. In renal failure, there is reduced renal excretion of colchicine, but it is not necessary to modify the dosage when the drug is used to treat the acute attack, as opposed to maintenance therapy.

(Eigsti and Dustin, 1955; Fitzgerald, 1974; Ertel *et al.*, 1976.)

Clinical uses, preparations and dosage

Colchicine is available as a tablet of 0.5 mg (it darkens

on exposure to light). An intravenous preparation (0.5 mg in 1 ml) is available and this too should be protected from light.

If colchicine is to be used in acute gout, it should be used early in the attack. The initial dose should be 1 mg orally, followed by 0.5 mg 2-hourly until gastrointestinal toxicity (usually diarrhoea or vomiting) occurs or the pain is relieved. Between 4 and 9 mg of colchicine will usually be required. As the effective dose in acute gouty arthritis is close to the toxic dose, most patients being treated for acute gout with colchicine for the first time will develop some diarrhoea and this is the sign to discontinue further doses. The dose that produces diarrhoea remains reasonably constant, so that should further attacks occur the total dose of colchicine administered can be limited to 0.5 mg less than the dose that previously caused diarrhoea.

Colchicine is effective in up to 90% of patients with acute gouty arthritis, although complete relief may be delayed until 24 hours after stopping treatment or until the development of gastrointestinal toxicity. If an intravenous preparation is available, colchicine can be given in a single dose of 2 mg well diluted in 20 ml of saline. Systemic side effects resulting from the drug administered via this route are rare, although any local extravasation may produce a necrotic slough. The lower dosages of colchicine should be used in patients with severe renal or hepatic failure.

Colchicine in low dosage is an effective prophylactic agent against acute attacks of gout (Yu and Gutman, 1961; Paulus *et al.*, 1974). Indeed, it has been used for this purpose by many clinicians for almost 50 years, particularly in the USA. However, there is still poor agreement regarding both the need for such prophylaxis and the choice between colchicine and other long-term maintenance drugs.

Such regular prophylactic use of colchicine will be associated with fewer acute attacks at times when surgery is undertaken and during maintenance therapy with urate-lowering drugs. Its effectiveness is unrelated to whether patients are hyperuricaemic or normouricaemic.

The prophylactic dose varies between 0.5 and 1.5 mg daily, 0.5 mg twice daily usually being effective. The prophylactic dose should be adjusted so as to avoid side effects. If after 12 months the serum urate has remained within the normal range, and there have been no further acute attacks, maintenance colchicine may be discontinued. Prophylactic dosage should be reduced in patients with severe renal or hepatic failure.

The manifestations of familial Mediterranean fever (recurrent polyserositis including arthritis of large joints) can be suppressed by a daily dosage of between 1 and 1.5 mg of colchicine (Goldfinger, 1972). Some response has also been reported in the arthritis as-sociated with sarcoidosis (Kaplan, 1963), erythema nodosum, calcium pyrophosphate deposition, and Behçet's syndrome.

Appendix 6.10.8 summarizes some important studies reporting the therapeutic effects of colcichine in various disorders.

Side effects, precautions and contraindications
The side effects of colchicine are usually dose related. The first symptom is most often diarrhoea with some abdominal pain. Occasional patients develop nausea and vomiting before diarrhoea. Higher dosage colchicine therapy can lead to profuse diarrhoea, gastrointestinal haemorrhage, malabsorption with mild steatorrhoea, and malabsorption of vitamin B_{12}. Rashes, renal damage, dehydration and hypotension may also occur. After prolonged treatment alopecia, peripheral neuritis, myopathy, and bone-marrow suppression have been reported. No toxic effect on testicular function has been found after prolonged therapy (Bremner and Paulsen, 1976).

Colchicine should be used with caution in patients with impaired cardiac, renal or hepatic function. Gastrointestinal symptoms are more likely to occur in patients with peptic ulcer or diseases of the colon. The drug is contraindicated in pregnancy.

(b) Anti-hyperuricaemic drugs

Probenecid (Benemid)
Other preparations include: Benacen (USA); Panuric (South Africa); Probecid (Sweden); Proben (Australia, South Africa); Probexin, Urecid (both Australia).

Pharmacology and pharmacokinetics. Probenecid, p-(dipropylsulphamoyl) benzoic acid was the first clinically useful uricosuric agent to be introduced. It lowers the serum urate by promoting its renal elimination (Kippen *et al.*, 1974) and acts as a competitive inhibitor of the renal tubular mechanism for reabsorption of urate. Probenecid also inhibits the renal tubular secretion of penicillin and was first used for this purpose. Probenecid is readily absorbed from the gastrointestinal tract and about 90% is rapidly bound to plasma proteins. Its distribution, therefore, is largely confined to the extracellular fluid. It has a plasma half-life of between 4 and 12 hours, depending on dosage. At least 80% of a given dose is rapidly metabolized in the liver, either to its acyl-monoglucuronide or by oxidation at a variety of positions on its n-propyl side chain (Dayton and Perel, 1971). The metabolites are probably also uricosuric. Excretion is by the renal route.

Clinical uses, preparations and dosage. As the increase in urinary excretion of urate is greater during the early stages of therapy, it is recommended that the first dose be small and increments gradual. The risk of uric acid crystal formation in the urine is minimized by encouraging a water diuresis. Alkalinization of the urine is desirable in the first few weeks of therapy when uricosuria is maximal. Once the serum urate has become within the normal range, the intense uricosuria subsides, although the total 24-hour excretion of uric acid on probenecid therapy is greater than before its administration. However, such an increase is relatively insignificant compared with increases due to other factors such as variation in dietary intake of purine. However, it is important to maintain a good urine volume during uricosuric therapy, preferably exceeding 2 litres per 24 hours.

The uricosuric effect of probenecid falls with impairment of glomerular filtration rate and little uricosuric response occurs at creatinine clearances of less than about 50–70 ml min^{-1}. Above this level, however, increasing the dose of probenecid may still result in a uricosuric response.

Probenecid is available as 500 mg tablets; the more recent enteric-coated preparations have been associated with a lower frequency of nausea. Very low dosage may result in urate retention in some subjects (Yu and Gutman, 1955), and the usual uricosuric dose will need to be between 1 and 3 g per day, given in two or three divided doses – 1.5–2 g per day being effective in most patients.

(Gutman, 1950, 1957; Talbott, 1964; Dayton and Perel, 1971.)

Side effects. Probenecid is generally well tolerated, although nausea, vomiting, headache, sore gums, flushing, dizziness, urinary frequency, anaemia, and rashes may occasionally occur. Rarely an anaphylactic reaction or a hypersensitivity reaction with fever, dermatitis and pruritus has occurred, and there have been reports of hepatic necrosis, the nephrotic syndrome, and aplastic anaemia. In massive overdosage probenecid causes central nervous system stimulation, with convulsions and death from respiratory failure.

Use of probenecid may precipitate an acute attack of gout in patients with gouty arthritis. Colchicine, given in the prophylactic dose of 0.5 mg once or twice daily, tends to reduce this tendency. As stressed earlier, because of the associated increased renal excretion of urate, particularly during the early stages of therapy, probenecid administration should be accompanied by a persistent water diuresis and/or alkalinization of urine. This is aimed at minimizing the risk of uric acid crystal deposition within tubules and collecting ducts or the formation of uric acid calculi.

Precautions and contraindications. Salicylates should be avoided in patients receiving probenecid (or other

Table 6.1 Effects of probenecid on the metabolism of other drugs (from Kelley, 1981)

Decreased renal excretion
p-Aminohippuric acid
Phenolsulphonphthalein
Salicylic acid and its acyl and phenolic glucuronides
Phlorizin and its glucuronide
Acetazolamide
Dapsone and its metabolites
Sulphinpyrazone and its parahydroxyl metabolite
Indomethacin
Ampicillin
Penicillin
Cephradine

Reduced volume of distribution
Ampicillin
Ancillin
Nafcillin
Cephaloridine

Impairment of hepatic intake
Sulphobromophthalein sodium
Idocyanin green
Rifampicin

Delayed metabolism
Heparin

uricosurics), as small or tolerable doses cause urate retention and also interfere with uricosuric action. Patients should be specifically warned about this and about the ubiquity of aspirin in proprietary preparations. Because of the risk of uric acid crystal formation, particular caution is needed in patients with habitually poor urine volumes. The drug should be used with caution in patients with a history of peptic ulceration. Probenecid reduces the excretion of p-aminohippuric acid (used as the sodium salt to measure renal function), some contrast media, dapsone, indomethacin, phenolsulphonphthalein, salicylates, and sulphobromophthalein sodium (used to measure liver function). It also reduces the excretion of penicillin, ampicillin and cephalothin (but not cephaloridine), an effect used to therapeutic advantage to increase serum levels of penicillin by delaying renal excretion (e.g. in infective endocarditis). A reducing substance has been found in the urine of some patients taking probenecid, and this may interfere with Benedict's tests.

A summary of the effects of probenecid on the metabolism of other drugs is given in Table 6.1.

Probenecid is contraindicated in: known hypersensitivity to probenecid; history of blood dyscrasia; uric acid renal stones. The drug should not be given to children under 2 years of age. Patients with hypoxanthine-guanine-phosphoribosyl-transferase (HGPRT) deficiency (Lesch–Nyhan syndrome) are treated with allopurinol. Its use in pregnancy requires careful balancing of expected benefits against possible hazards.

(Bozer and Strickland, 1955; Gutman and Yu, 1957; Ferris *et al.*, 1961; De Seze *et al.*, 1963; Hertz *et al.*, 1972.)

Sulphinpyrazone (sulfinpyrazone) (Anturan)

Pharmacology and pharmacokinetics. The uricosuric properties of phenylbutazone are attributable to one of its metabolites, sulphinpyrazone (1, 2-diphenyl-4-(2-phenyl-sulphinethyl)-3, 5 pyrazolidenendione) being a derivative of that metabolite. This derivative is a very potent uricosuric agent, although its anti-inflammatory effect is very mild (Emmerson, 1963). Its properties are therefore the converse of those of phenylbutazone.

Sulphinpyrazone is rapidly and completely absorbed from the gastrointestinal tract, with a peak serum concentration occurring 1 hour after oral administration. Its half-life in serum is 1–3 hours. The drug is very strongly protein bound (98%). Therefore, like probenecid, sulphinpyrazone is largely confined to the extracellular fluid. About 20–45% of the drug is excreted in the urine unchanged within 24 hours, mainly during the first 6 hours. Most of the drug is excreted as the parahydroxyl metabolite, which is also uricosuric in man. Sulphinpyrazone, on a weight basis, is 3–6 times more potent as a uricosuric than probenecid.

It is not established whether sulphinpyrazone has all the transport, excretory and metabolic effects on endogenous substances as described for probenecid, but it does suppress the excretion of aminohippuric acid and phenolsulphonphthalein.

Sulphinpyrazone has been shown to have an anti-platelet effect (e.g. reduces thrombosis in arteriovenous shunts, and prolongs platelet survival in patients with prosthetic heart valves, rheumatic heart disease, and recurrent venous thrombosis). This therapeutic effect has been attributed to inhibition of platelet prostaglandin synthesis (Ali and McDonald, 1977).

Clinical uses. Regular treatment with sulphinpyrazone will restore a normal serum urate and, as with probenecid, if this is maintained for a sufficient period, it will prevent recurrent attacks of acute gouty arthritis.

As vascular disease has been found in a significant proportion of patients with gout, the anti-platelet action of sulphinpyrazone may be beneficial to such patients, although no controlled studies have yet been done.

The uricosuric effect is reduced in renal insufficiency and is negligible at a creatinine clearance of less than 50 ml min^{-1}. However, above this value an increased

dose of sulphinpyrazone may result in a useful increase in urinary urate excretion in patients who are unable to tolerate other drugs.

Sulphinpyrazone tends to be used in patients in whom probenecid is not tolerated or has failed.

Preparations and dosage. Sulphinpyrazone is stable at room temperature and is available as 100 mg tablets. A uricosuric effect can usually be achieved at between 200 and 400 mg per day given in two doses. The dosage can be increased to 800 mg per day if necessary. As with probenecid, care concerning the maintenance of a large urine volume is essential.

(Yu *et al.*, 1958; Seegmuller and Grayzel, 1960; Persellin and Schmid, 1961; Glick, 1961.)

Side effects, precautions and contraindications. Sulphinpyrazone may cause nausea, vomiting and abdominal pain. It may aggravate peptic ulcers and may precipitate acute attacks of gout. Hypersensitivity reactions may occasionally occur. Rare instances of anaemia, agranulocytosis and thrombocytopenia have been reported. Overdosage may cause ataxia, laboured respiration, convulsions and coma.

Tolerance for sulphinpyrazone is somewhat better than for probenecid. General factors relating to toxicity, including cautions and contraindications, are as stated for probenecid with the following main differences:

1. As it is a more potent uricosuric agent than probenecid the risk of uric acid crystal formation in the renal tract might be expected to be greater. Patients on this drug should therefore be encouraged to maintain a higher urinary output (preferably $> 3 l day^{-1}$) than patients taking probenecid.

2. As sulphinpyrazole is a pyrazole derivative there is some concern about its potential for bone-marrow depression, although extensive clinical use has shown this to be only a rare association, and certainly a much less common toxic effect than occurs with phenylbutazone.

3. Patients who are hypersensitive to phenylbutazone and other pyrazole derivatives, including sulphinpyrazole, should not be given these drugs.

4. Sulphinpyrazone may aggravate or reactivate peptic ulcers and is contraindicated in patients with active peptic ulceration.

5. In addition to potentiating the effect of drugs mentioned under probenecid, sulphinpyrazone may enhance the effect of coumarin anticoagulants.

6. Interference with the results of Benedict's tests has not been reported with sulphinpyrazone, but it may invalidate renal function tests (p-aminohippuric acid, phenolsulphonphthalein).

(Yu *et al.*, 1963; Smythe *et al.*, 1965; Perel *et al.*, 1969.)

Other uricosuric drugs

The benzofuran compounds, benziodarone and benzbromarone, are very potent uricosuric drugs and appear to have an additional uricostatic effect. They are widely used on the continent of Europe but not in the UK. Benzbromarone may become available in the USA in the near future.

Many other drugs with diverse chemical structures and pharmacological properties decrease the serum urate level by enhancing renal excretion of uric acid, but are not generally used for this purpose. These drugs are summarized in Table 6.2.

Allopurinol (Zyloric)

Other proprietary names include: Bloxanth (Canada); Epidropal, Foligan, Urosin (all Germany); Zyloprim (Australia, Canada, South Africa, USA).

Pharmacology and pharmacokinetics. Allopurinol, 4-hydroxypyrazolo-(3, 4-d)-pyrimidine, an isomer of hypoxanthine, was first synthesized in 1956.

Allopurinol acts as an inhibitor of xanthine oxidase which, in man, it inhibits to about 50%. Xanthine oxidase catalyses the conversion of hypoxanthine to xanthine and of xanthine to uric acid. Inhibition of xanthine oxidase will therefore lead to both a reduction in the amount of hypoxanthine and xanthine. Thus,

Table 6.2 Drugs shown to be uricosuric in man (from Kelley, 1981)

Acetohexamide	Halofenate (MK 185)
ACTH	Iodopyracet
Ascorbic acid	Iopanoic acid
Azapropazone	Meclofenamic acid
Azauridine	Meglumine iodipamide
Benzbromarone*	Mersalyl
Benziodarone*	Metiazininic acid
Calcitonin	Niridazole
Calcium ipodate	Orotic acid
Carinamide	Outdated tetracyclines
Chlorprothixene	Phenolsulphonphthalein
Cinchophen	Phenylbutazone
Citrate	Phenylindanedione
Dicoumarol	Phenoxyisobutyric acid
Diflumidone	Probenecid and metabolites
Estrogens	Salicylates
Ethyl biscoumacetate	Sodium diatrizoate
Ethyl p-chlorophenoxy-	Sulphaethylthiadiazole
isobutyric acid	Sulphinpyrazone
Glyceryl guaiacholate	Ticrynafen
Glycine	W 2345 (5-chlorosalicylic
	acid)
Glycopyrrolate	Zoxazolamine

* Used clinically as a uricosuric agent

during allopurinol therapy, the concentration of uric acid in both serum and urine will fall, and the concentrations of hypoxanthine and xanthine will rise. The xanthine and hypoxanthine (oxypurines) are readily excreted by the kidney. After oral administration, the fall in plasma and urine uric acid occurs within 24–48 hours. Withdrawal of allopurinol results in a return towards normal values within a few days, although some of the other metabolic effects may linger for 7–10 days after drug withdrawal.

As well as diverting purine end products from uric acid to the oxypurines xanthine and hypoxanthine, allopurinol produces a reduction in total purine production. These and other metabolic effects of allopurinol are summarized in Table 6.3.

Allopurinol is well absorbed from the gastrointestinal tract and has a plasma half-life of 2–8 hours. In addition to inhibiting xanthine oxidase, it is also a substrate for this enzyme, so that much of it (about 60%) is rapidly oxidized by hepatic xanthine oxidase to its major active metabolite, oxypurinol, an analogue of xanthine. A small proportion of the oxypurinol produced is converted to the corresponding ribonucleoside and ribonucleotide. Oxypurinol has a much longer plasma half-life than allopurinol about (18–30 hours) and is probably responsible for most of the inhibition of xanthine oxidase which occurs *in vivo*. Both allopurinol and oxypurinol are distributed evenly in total body water and neither is significantly bound to plasma proteins.

Allopurinol is cleared rapidly by the kidney, probably largely by glomerular filtration. Oxypurinol is filtered at the glomerulus and reabsorbed by the tubules. It is therefore excreted much more slowly than allopurinol and its renal handling appears to be similar to that of uric acid. Probenecid accelerates the renal excretion of oxypurinol and this results in reduced efficacy of allopurinol if it is given with probenecid. If renal function is impaired there is a diminished clearance of oxypurinol, and the plasma concentration of oxypurinol becomes substantially raised if such patients are given normal doses of allopurinol.

(Wyngaarden *et al.*, 1965; Elion, 1966; Rundles *et al.*, 1966; Bardmore and Kelly, 1971; Hande *et al.*, 1978.)

Clinical uses, preparations and dosage. Allopurinol is particularly indicated, either alone or in combination with uricosuric therapy in the following:

    1. Extensive tophaceous gout.

    2. Gout where there is gross overproduction of uric acid with high urinary excretion (whether of primary origin, as in HGRPT deficiency, or secondary, as in myeloproliferative disorders).

    3. Failure of uricosuric agents to control plasma uric

Table 6.3 Metabolic effects of allopurinol (from Kelley, 1981)

Clinical effect	Mechanism	Effector
Antihyperuricemia	Xanthine oxidase inhibition	Allopurinol Oxipurinol
Decreased total purine production	Inhibition of amidophospho-ribosyltransferase	Allopurinol-1-N-ribosylphosphate; IMP
	PP-ribose-P depletion	Allopurinol
Orotidinuria	Inhibition of orotidine-5'-phosphate decarboxylase	Oxipurinol-7-N-ribosylphosphate Oxipurinol-1-N-ribosylphosphate Allopurinol-1-N-ribosylphosphate
Orotic aciduria	Inhibition of orotate phospho-ribosyltransferase	? Orotidine-5'-phosphate
	PP-ribose-P depletion	Allopurinol
Prolongation of half-life of drugs metabolized by the microsomal-oxidizing system	Inhibition of hepatic microsomal drug-metabolizing enzymes	Unknown
Apparent increased activity of orotate phosphoribosyltrans-ferase and orotidine-5'-P de-carboxylase	? Stabilization of enzymes to extraction	Unknown

acid effectively (bearing in mind that the commonest cause of this is poor compliance in taking tablets).

4. Intolerance to uricosuric agents.

5. Gout associated with severe renal failure, in which uricosuric drugs become ineffective.

6. Uric acid stone formation.

7. Acute uric acid nephropathy due to excretion of massive amounts of uric acid, as during treatment of leukaemia or reticuloses with cytotoxic drugs.

There is some evidence that allopurinol can minimize the formation of renal stones not primarily consisting of uric acid, such as calcium oxalate stones (Smith and Boyce, 1969; Coe and Kavalach, (1974).

Asymptomatic hyperuricaemia. If, as an incidental finding (often as a result of routine health screening or multi-channel biochemical investigation), or from investigation for more specific reasons, asymptomatic hyperuricaemia is found, the question arises as to how this should be managed. Opinions vary, but in the absence of any pertinent abnormalities resulting from full clinical assessment as for a patient with overt gout, it would seem reasonable to adopt a conservative approach in withholding treatment, providing hyperuricaemia is mild. With regard to higher levels of uric acid (say above 8 mg $100 \, ml^{-1}$ or $476 \, \mu mol \, l^{-1}$) opinions still vary, but, particularly if there is concomitant hyperuricosuria, patients should be given the benefit of the doubt and treated with allopurinol (Scott, 1978). The underlying reasoning in support of this approach rests on the lack of evidence to show any preventive effect (particularly regarding renal or cardiac disease) of prophylactic therapy in these patients, other than an effect on gouty arthritis or rarely (presumably) urate calculi.

Allopurinol is available as 100 and 300 mg tablets. A normal serum urate concentration can be achieved in most patients with a daily dose between 100 and 300 mg. Because of the long plasma half-life of oxypurinol (the active metabolite of allopurinol), a single daily dose of allopurinol may be as effective as a divided dose regimen. A single daily dose of 300 mg each morning is now commonly used. Smaller dosages may be indicated where there is renal impairment. If hyperuricaemia is not controlled by 300 mg daily the dosage should be increased to between 400 and 600 mg daily. Higher dosages should be used only if all other factors promoting hyperuricaemia have been corrected. Allopurinol can precipitate acute attacks of gout. The tendency for this to occur can be minimized by prophylactic colchicine therapy and by ensuring that any changes in serum rate concentration are gradual.

(Wyngaarden *et al.*, 1965; Yu, 1965; Goldfarb and Smyth, 1966; Rundles *et al.*, 1966; Loebl and Scott, 1974; Rodnan *et al.*, 1974.)

Side effects, precautions and contraindications. In over a decade of use serious complications of allopurinol therapy have been uncommon, and only about 5% of patients need to discontinue the drug. The most frequent side effect is a rash which occurs in up to 4% of patients. In the presence of renal insufficiency, however, the prevalence of skin reactions may rise to about 15% (Frisch *et al.*, 1974). In 10% of patients with a rash, this may be accompanied by severe systemic manifestations such as fever, eosinophilia and serious hypersensitivity

(Kantor, 1970; Mills, 1971). Gastric intolerance is another relatively common side effect, but this is rarely serious and can be minimized by symptomatic therapy.

Other occasional toxic effects include: toxic epidermal necrolysis, alopecia, bone-marrow suppression with leukopenia and thrombocytopenia, agranulocytosis, granulomatous hepatitis, severe jaundice, a sarcoid-like reaction, and vasculitis. At least one death has been reported (Kantor, 1970). Crystals of xanthine, hypoxanthine and oxypurinol have been observed in the skeletal muscles of gouty patients treated with allopurinol. However, this is of doubtful clinical significance because uric acid crystals have also been demonstrated by this technique in untreated gouty patients (Watts *et al.*, 1971). Other metabolic effects, some of which are at least thought to have little if any clinical significance (e.g. orotidinuria and orotic aciduria), are shown in Table 6.3, referred to previously.

Oxypurinol stones have been reported after very large oral dosage with oxypurinol (but not with allopurinol). Oxypurinol, a metabolic product of allopurinol, has been used therapeutically, particularly in patients who have shown hypersensitivity to the parent drug. There is no evidence of incorporation of allopurinol into nucleic acids (Nelson and Elion, 1975).

Provided reasonable allowance is made for side effects and interactions with other drugs, the main grounds for caution in the use of allopurinol are in patients with gross overproduction of urate. In these patients (e.g. Lesch–Nyhan syndrome) there is a potential risk of xanthine calculi or of xanthine nephropathy if the urine volume is poor. It is important that the dose be kept to a minimum in patients with renal disease, due to the decreased rate of elimination of oxypurinol, the active metabolite of allopurinol mentioned earlier.

The effect of drugs that are normally metabolized by xanthine oxidase (e.g. 6-mercaptopurine and azathioprine) is potentiated by the concomitant administration of allopurinol. Such drugs should be reduced to 25% of the usual dosage when administered with allopurinol. There is some evidence that allopurinol potentiates the action of cytotoxic drugs, especially cyclophosphamide, although the mechanism is not understood. With regard to this effect, there appears to be an increased risk of bone-marrow depression if these two drugs are given together.

An increased frequency of rash has been reported in patients receiving ampicillin together with allopurinol.

Allopurinol has also been reported to prolong the half-life of drugs which are metabolized by the hepatic microsomal enzyme oxidizing system, thus leading to possible potentiation of effect (Vessell *et al.*, 1970). This appears to apply to dicoumarol, but not warfarin. However, the clinical significance of this observation is not yet established. Prolongation of the half-life of

probenecid by allopurinol has been reported (Tjandramaga and Cucinell, 1971), but this is of doubtful significance. Similarly, marked prolongation of the half-life of chlorpropamide has been reported in some patients treated with allopurinol.

(Lidsky and Sharp, 1967; Auerbach and Orentrich, 1968; Kantor, 1970; Mills, 1971; Greenberg and Zambrano, 1972; Straitigos *et al.*, 1972; Chawla *et al.*, 1977; Swank *et al.*, 1978.)

COMMENT

Management of gout may be divided into (1) treatment of the acute attack; (2) long-term management.

Phenylbutazone or indomethacin are probably the most popular first choice anti-inflammatory drugs for using in the acute attack. They must be given in substantial dosage (i.e. phenylbutazone 200 mg four times daily or indomethacin 50 mg four times daily). Another useful preparation for the acute attack is naproxen. Colchicine, the traditional first choice, has become superseded by modern equivalents because of toxic effects, particularly diarrhoea. *Uric acid lowering drugs must not be given during the acute attack*: they may well prolong the episode.

In the treatment of early uncomplicated gout there is little to choose between uricosuric agents and allopurinol, both of which are effective in lowering the serum uric acid. However, allopurinol is the more potent drug, but long-term observation is still needed as the agent has been in use for a shorter time than have uricosurics. There are a number of circumstances calling specifically for the use of allopurinol, either alone or in combination with uricosuric therapy. These include tophi, high urinary output of uric acid, renal failure, uric acid stones, acute uric acid nephropathy, failure of uricosurics, and intolerance to uricosurics.

6.5 INFECTIOUS ARTHRITIS

6.5.1 General principles

In treating patients with septic arthritis, antibiotic selection is an important and often difficult decision. Appropriate and effective antibiotic therapy involves: (1) a high index of suspicion (particularly if the patient already has rheumatoid arthritis; (2) a careful history and physical examination; (3) identification of the infecting organism; (4) selection of the antibiotic; (5) joint drainage and surveillance; and (6) therapy to restore joint function towards normal.

6.5.2 Initial antibiotic selection

The physician's first choice of antibiotic is guided largely by the patient's age. Thus, there is a dramatic but

Table 6.4 Antibiotic selection based on patient's age and Gram stain findings (from Clarke, 1978)

Age (years)	Gram-negative bacilli	Gram-negative cocci	Gram-positive cocci	No organism seen*
$< \frac{1}{2}$	Gentamicin (Enterobacteriaceae or Pseudomonas aeruginosa)[†]	Penicillin G (*Neisseria gonorrhoeae*)	Nafcillin ‡ (Staphylococci or Streptococci)	Nafcillin and gentamicin
$\frac{1}{2}$–2	Ampicillin (*Haemophilus influenzae*)	As above	As above	Ampicillin (*Haemophilus influenzae* or Streptococci)
2–14	Gentamicin (Enterobacteriaceae or Pseudomonas aeruginosa)	As above	As above	Nafcillin
15–39	As above	As above	As above	Penicillin G (Neisseria gonorrhoeae)
>40	As above	As above	As above	Nafcillin

* Gentamicin should be added to these regimens for patients with joint trauma, malignancy, or addiction.
† Presumed identity of pathogen in parenthesis.
‡ In UK cloxacillin or flucloxacillin would be alternative penicillinase-resistant penicillins.

brief dominance of *Haemophilus influenzae* at the age of 6 months to 2 years, there is a predominance of *Neisseria gonorrhoeae* during years of increased sexual activity, and there is a slow but steady increase with age in the prevalence of *Staphylococcus aureus*. The frequency of infection due to streptococci and to gram-negative bacilli (the Enterobacteriaceae and *Pseudomonas aeruginosa*) remains relatively constant. This age–organism correlation allows the physician to base his initial therapy on the results of Gram staining (Table 6.4).

In the interval from 6 months to 2 years, Gram-negative bacilli are assumed to be *Haemophilus influenzae* and are treated with ampicillin. For any other age, Enterobacteriaceae or *Pseudomonas aeruginosa* are almost certainly the Gram-negative bacilli involved, gentamicin being the antibiotic of choice.

Gram-positive cocci are assumed to be *Staphylococcus aureus*, and are treated with a penicillinase-resistant semi-synthetic penicillin, which is also effective against the common streptococcal joint pathogens. In typical pneumococcal pneumonia complicated by septic arthritis, penicillin should be started at first.

Regardless of age, Gram-negative cocci are assumed be *Neisseria gonorrhoeae* and are treated with penicillin.

The most troublesome problem arises when no organism can be identified. In this circumstance, treatment is initially aimed at the most likely pathogen(s) for the patient's age: *Staphylococcus aureus* and coliforms in infants (cloxacillin and gentamicin); *Haemophilus influenzae* and streptococci from 6 to 24 months (ampicillin); *Staphylococcus aureus* from 2 to 14, and over 40 years of age; and *Neisseria gonorrhoeae* from 15 to 39 years. Gentamicin should be included in the regimen if there is a history of penetrating trauma, intravenous

drug abuse or malignancy (Clarke, 1978).

Much less prevalent bacterial causes of arthritis include brucellosis and syphilis.

In the world at large the most common species of brucellosis affecting man is *Brucella melitensis*, the most common cause in the USA being *Brucella abortis*. No ideal antibiotic programme has yet been established for this disease which is only infrequently associated with oligoarticular arthritis and spondylitis. A reasonably successful treatment schedule consists of tetracycline (2 g) combined with streptomycin (1–2 g) or another aminoglycoside for at least 3 weeks.

Syphilitic arthritis (due to *Treponema pallidum*) responds readily to large doses of benzathine penicillin (7.2–9 million units) in three divided doses at intervals of 7 days. An alternative regimen is aqueous penicillin, 9.6–12 million units over 2 weeks. The joint disease of primary or secondary syphilis, and in some patients the arthritis of congenital syphilis, respond well. The joint manifestations of late congenital syphilis are said to respond poorly. Bone destruction by gummata may be arrested by this therapy.

6.5.3 Definitive antibiotic selection in bacterial arthritis

(a) General comment

Although the antibiotic sensitivity of the pathogenic bacteria is the main factor in antibiotic selection, other factors include: the type of antibacterial activity, the spectrum of pathogens covered by the agent, the route of drug administration, the duration of treatment, and the patient's allergic history. Specific joint-related aspects are antibiotic penetration and antibiotic kinetics in joint fluid.

(b) Bacteriostatic and bactericidal antibiotics

Antibiotics are classed as bacteriostatic or bactericidal. Bacteriostatic agents such as tetracycline, chloramphenicol, and the sulphonamides often act by inhibiting protein synthesis. In their presence, bacterial growth is slow, but removal of the antibiotic may result in restoration of normal metabolism and growth of the micro-organism.

Bactericidal agents such as penicillin and cephalothin often work by inhibition of cell wall synthesis, and the effects of these antibiotics on the bacterium are usually irreversible.

The combination of two bacteriostatic agents such as sulphamethoxisole and trimethoprim, or of two bactericidal agents such as gentamicin and ampicillin may have a synergistic effect against specific organisms. On the other hand, the combination of a bactericidal with a bacteriostatic agent may result in antagonism. Thus, the aim should be to select a bactericidal agent rather than a bacteriostatic agent and, if more than one antibiotic is needed, to choose combinations of bactericidal agents.

(c) Broad-spectrum versus narrow-spectrum antibiotics

To minimize the risk of super-added infection a narrow-spectrum antibiotic is usually preferable. Sometimes, however, it may be advantageous to choose a broad-spectrum antibiotic that will cover the most likely infecting organism as well as other possibilities (e.g. the choice of ampicillin in a young child to treat both *Haemophilus influenzae* and streptococcal infections) (Clarke, 1978).

(d) Route of antibiotic administration

Because synovial fluid antibiotic levels are directly related to blood levels, it is important to achieve effective blood levels. Oral therapy may be complicated by irregular patient compliance and variable absorption from the gastrointestinal tract. Hence, parenteral therapy is preferred, particularly at the start of treatment. If it becomes necessary to change to oral therapy, therapeutic synovial levels should be re-checked. The parenteral route can be either intramuscular or intravenous. Intravenous therapy is used when specially indicated (e.g. inadequate muscle mass; when it is necessary to administer large volumes; the presence of excessive pain with repeated injections). Intravenous treatment should be monitored closely for malfunction of the giving set or for surrounding erythema. Steel needles are less likely to become infected than plastic cannulae. The site of intravenous therapy should be changed at least every 48–72 hours.

There has been long-standing debate as to the value (Chartier, Martin and Kelly, 1959) or not (Nelson, 1972) of intra-articular antibiotics. Advocates of the intra-articular route point to the low synovial fluid levels that were found after early low-dose antibiotic regimens, or to animal studies in which a bacteriostatic effect occurred more rapidly with intra-articular administration (Bardenheier, Morgan and Stamp, 1966). Further, it has been claimed that this route does not damage the joint, as has been argued by some workers. Also, it has been shown that intra-articular administration offers prolonged synovial fluid levels (Florey and Heatley, 1945), and less systemic toxicity from agents such as amphotericin B (Aidem, 1968).

On the other hand, it is now established that, in appropriate dosage, all the antibiotics routinely used in the therapy of septic arthritis achieve adequate synovial fluid levels. In addition, parenteral antibiotic therapy provides the advantage of treating any concurrent systemic illness as well as providing uniform levels of antibiotic in unsuspected loculated fluid pockets. Intra-articular therapy may be attended by some risk. For instance, Argen *et al.* (1966) and Drutz *et al.* (1967) noted reaccumulation of fluid and worsening of joint symptoms, and persistent sterile effusions and pleocytosis have been well documented. However, similar problems have been seen in patients not receiving intra-articular antibiotics. Many clinicians experienced in this field (e.g. Goldenberg *et al.*, 1975; Clarke, 1978) feel that, with few exceptions (e.g. the infected hip joint), uncomplicated septic arthritis should be treated by parenteral and not intra-articular therapy.

(e) Duration of antibiotic drug therapy

Recommendations for duration of therapy (Table 6.5) are arbitrary and the optimal length of treatment must be assessed for individual patients. Several factors must be considered, the type of microbial agent being the most important of these. Thus, gonococcal arthritis has been treated adequately in as little as 3 days, while tuberculosis may require at least 18 months. Other organisms lie in an intermediate range.

Host factors are also important, and patients with a foreign body or joint prosthesis, or associated osteomyelitis seem to need prolonged therapy.

Finally, some miscellaneous clinical factors may be important. An unusually slow response is seen in patients with alcoholism, diabetes mellitus or malignancy. Other associated infections such as endocarditis require prolonged treatment. Delay in starting therapy has the same effect in that treatment may have to be prolonged.

(f) Drug reactions

Allergic and toxic reactions often complicate prolonged courses of antibiotic therapy. A hypersensitivity re-

Table 6.5 Antibiotic therapy for certain forms of bacterial arthritis (from Clarke, 1978)

Organism (From Table 6.4 or cultures)	First antibiotic choice	Alternative drug choice	Duration and comments
Enterobacteriacae: includes *Escherichia coli, Salmonella, Klebsiella, Enterobacter* and *Proteus* species	Gentamicin 5 mg kg^{-1} day^{-1} in 3 doses	Tobramycin – 5 mg kg^{-1} day^{-1} Amikacin – 15 mg kg^{-1} day^{-1}	2–3 weeks; may change to or add ampicillin, carbenicillin or a cephalosporin when sensitivities are known
Pseudomonas aeruginosa	Tobramycin 5 mg kg^{-1} day^{-1} in 3 doses	Gentamicin – 5 mg kg^{-1} day^{-1} Amikacin – 15 mg kg^{-1} day^{-1}	2–3 weeks; add or change to carbenicillin – 400 mg kg^{-1} day^{-1} when confirmed
Haemophilus influenzae	Ampicillin 50 mg kg^{-1} day^{-1} in 4 doses	Chloramphenicol – 50 mg kg^{-1} day^{-1}	2 weeks; if ampicillin resistance is prevalent, chloramphenicol should be added until sensitivities are known
Neisseria gonorrhoeae	Penicillin G, 6–10 million units/day, in 3 or 4 doses	Erythromycin – 2 g/day i.v. in 4 doses for 3 days. Tetracycline-loading dose – 1·5 g, then 500 mg every 6 hours for 1 week	After response to penicillin (24–72 hours), ampicillin – 2 g/day by mouth for 1 week. Shorter therapy has been effective
Staphylococcus aureus	Nafcillin, 100–150 mg kg^{-1} day^{-1} in 4–6 doses	Cephalothin – 100 mg kg^{-1} day^{-1} Clindamycin – 30 mg kg^{-1} day^{-1} Vancomycin – 30 mg kg^{-1} day^{-1}	Parenteral therapy for a minimum of 3–4 weeks Neonatal dose of nafcillin – 25 mg kg^{-1} day^{-1}
Streptococcus pneumoniae, pyogenes and *viridans*	Penicillin G, 250 000 units kg^{-1} day^{-1}, in 2–4 doses	Same as for *Staphylococcus aureus*	

action to penicillin may require a change in drugs, and the physician should avoid chemically related compounds such as the cephalosporin antibiotics. Aminoglycosides share many toxic reactions, some of which may be cumulative. One agent used in combination with another may enhance its toxic potential by interfering with its metabolism or excretion. One example of this is the adverse effect of amphotericin B on renal function, thereby inducing 5-fluorocytosine toxicity.

(g) Passage of antibiotics into joints

Experience measuring actual synovial fluid antibiotic drug levels or antibacterial activity in septic arthritis for a large number of antibiotics has been reported in only two series (Nelson, 1971; Parker and Schmid, 1971). Many other, less comprehensive reports have given

additional information on a variety of antibiotics, for example: penicillin (Nelson, 1975); ampicillin (Howell *et al.*, 1972); carbenicillin (Chow *et al.*, 1971); cloxacillin (Newman, 1976); nafcillin (Viek, 1962); phenethicillin (Viek and Santangelo, 1962); chloramphenicol (Jocson, 1955); clindamycin and lincomycin (Feigin *et al.*, 1975); gentamicin (Marsh *et al.*, 1974); kanamycin (Baciocco and Iles, 1971). Most of these studies have been done on traumatic or rheumatoid effusions.

The following facts have emerged relating to the passage of antibiotics into joints:

1. The infective aetiology of the effusion appears to play only a small role in the penetration of antibiotics into joint fluid.

2. Antibiotic penetration into an inflamed joint may be decreased as improvement occurs.

3. Penetration of antibiotics into different joints in the

same patient appears to be similar and does not seem to be influenced by the volume of joint fluid or by repeated aspiration (Deodhar *et al.*, 1972).

4. Diffusion of antibiotics out of a joint may be greater in severely inflamed joints than in mildly inflamed joints (Herrell *et al.*, 1944).

5. It has been shown that a septic rheumatoid joint can accumulate twice as much antibiotic than a sterile rheumatoid joint. (This was demonstrated in a patient treated with nafcillin (Parker *et al.*, 1976).)

In choosing between antibiotics on a basis of maximal joint penetration, it has been suggested that molecular weight, molecular configuration, and degree of protein binding represent significant factors. The last of these is probably the most important and, other factors being equal, agents with the lowest binding have a theoretical advantage (Howell *et al.*, 1972; Parker *et al.*, 1976).

Data are incomplete regarding the kinetic relationship between blood and synovial levels of antibiotics. However, it has been shown that after parenteral administration, synovial fluid levels rise more slowly than blood levels and that the synovial level peak occurs much later than the blood peak. The synovial level remains slightly higher than the blood level after the peak has been reached and then both levels fall in parallel (Plott and Roth, 1970; Deodhar *et al.*, 1972; Parker *et al.*, 1976). Deodhar *et al.* (1972) have also shown that constant doses at regular intervals lead to fairly stable blood and synovial levels.

(h) *Pharmacology of major antibiotics*

Excellent reviews of antimicrobial therapy are available (Weinstein, 1970; Kirby and Petersdorf, 1977; Garrod and O'Grady, 1972; Clarke, 1978), and the reader is referred to these for further details.

6.5.4 Chemotherapy of mycobacterial arthritis

(a) *Tuberculous arthritis*

The antibiotic therapy of this form of tuberculosis is the same as the chemotherapy of pulmonary tuberculosis. Isoniazid therapy is continued for 2 years in conjunction with ethambutol (18–24 months) or rifampin (6–12 months). Surgery may be required in addition.

(b) *Lepromatous arthritis*

Effective treatment of leprosy is complex and for optimal results much experience is needed. As with tuberculosis, treatment must be prolonged. Sulphones (e.g. dapsone) are the drugs of choice. Other antileprotics include thiambutosine, clofazimine, and rifampicin.

6.5.5 Chemotherapy of fungal arthritis

Only two major agents, amphotericin B and 5-fluorocytosine, are available for the systemic therapy of the several types of fungal arthritis (e.g. aspergillosis, actinomycosis, blastomycosis, coccidioidomycosis, crytococcosis, histoplasmosis, sporotrichosis). Because of frequent, serious and often unpredictable toxic effects, definite confirmation of the fungal aetiology is required before a prolonged course of therapy with these drugs can be undertaken.

6.5.6 Viral arthritis

Many different viral conditions may regularly cause arthritis (e.g. hepatitis B, rubella, rubella vaccine, mumps, smallpox, epidemic polyarthritis of Australia, chikungunya, o'nyong-nyong). In some infections the association is less prominent (e.g. adenovirus type 7, varicella, infectious mononucleosis, echovirus type 3). In certain conditions the viral aetiology is only presumed (e.g. erythema infectiosum, lyme arthritis).

In these disorders no chemotherapeutic agents are available and management is symptomatic, aspirin often being helpful.

COMMENT

The treatment of septic arthritis and of other forms of joint infection should be carried out without delay, if specific treatment is available. Failure to do this may expose the patient to the hazards of systemic toxicity and progressive and often rapid joint damage.

The two main governing factors in the presumptive identification of the infecting organism are: (1) the Gram stain and (2) the patient's age (different organisms tending to affect different age groups).

In general, it is preferable to choose a bactericidal agent over a bacteriostatic agent, and, if more than one antibiotic is needed, to choose combinations of bactericidal agents.

6.6 PAGET'S DISEASE

6.6.1 General comment

Paget's disease is another condition for which specific therapy is now available. The disease is common in elderly people and causes bone and joint pain. However, most patients have no complaints and need no treatment. Many patients can be managed with analgesic and anti-inflammatory drugs alone, but those with intractable pain should be considered for specific therapy. There are three different approaches: calcitonin, disodium etidronate (EHDP), and mithramycin, and these will be considered in further detail in the following sections.

6.6.2 Calcitonin

A hormone found in the mammalian thyroid parafollicular cells and the ultimobranchial bodies in nonmammalian vertebrates. Alternatively, it may be obtained synthetically. The hormone has the property of lowering the calcium content of the blood. It is a polypeptide containing 32 amino acids. The amino acid sequence varies greatly between species.

Calcitonin (thyrocalcitonin) inhibits osteoclastic activity in bone and reduces bone turnover. Two preparations are available. Synthetic salmon calcitonin (salcatonin; calcitonin (salmon) (Calcitare)) is given in a dose of 100 international units daily for 3–6 months, then at a maintenance dose of 50 units, three times weekly. Extracted porcine calcitonin (calcitonin (pork) (Calsynar)) is given in a dose of 160 international units daily for 3–6 months, then 80 units, three times weekly. Both are given by intramuscular injection. Pain relief is achieved in about one third of all patients, although biochemical improvement is usual. Calcitonin begins to exert its effect within 2–6 weeks of starting treatment. If it achieves a response, treatment should be continued for a year, then stopped and a further course given if there is a recurrence. Side effects include anorexia and nausea. Since allergic reactions may occur, it is wise to give a test dose of intradermal calcitonin initially.

6.6.3 Disodium etidronate

Disodium etidronate (sodium etidronate, EHDP) is a diphosphonate (disodium ethane-1-hydroxy-1, 1-di phosphonate) which is thought to act by inhibiting the formation of hydroxyapatite crystals in bone. It is given in a dose of up to $20\,mg\,kg^{-1}$ EHDP a day, by mouth. Absorption is poor and, although the drug is cleared from the plasma within 24 hours of a single dose, it accumulates in bone and is only slowly removed. About 80% of patients with Paget's disease show substantial improvement in biochemical indices of the disease, but only about 50% show substantial clinical improvement (Russell *et al.*, 1974). Nausea and diarrhoea occur occasionally, raised serum phosphate levels are common, and there may be a slight increase in the frequency of fractures with prolonged high-dose treatment. Treatment should not usually be contained for longer than 6 months, but further courses can be given for recurrences.

(Russell *et al.*, 1974.)

6.6.4 Mithramycin (Mithracin)

Mithramycin (an antineoplastic antibiotic produced by the growth of *Streptomyces argillaceous, plicatus* and *tanashiensis*) is a drug that may inhibit osteoblasts and thereby new bone formation. It is given in a dose of 15 mg/kg body weight daily for 10 days by intravenous infusion over 6 hours in a solution of 5% dextrose. Serum calcium and liver function tests should be checked daily. There are few side effects, but nausea, abnormal liver function tests and hypocalcaemia may occur. Pain is often relieved within a few days of initiating treatment. Most patients respond and recurrence is unusual, at least over the first 5 years (Russell and Lentle, 1974). Biochemical abnormalities of the disease, such as raised alkaline phosphatase and increased hydroxyproline excretion, improve slowly.

(Russell and Lentle, 1974.)

COMMENT

Most patients with Paget's disease have no complaints and require no treatment. However, it is a common disorder and there must be many thousands in the UK with symptoms, most often pain.

Treatments available include (1) those which reduce symptoms and ameliorate complications; (2) those which, in addition, appear to suppress excessive bone turnover. Of the former, simple analgesics are probably more effective than analgesic/anti-inflammatory drugs. Of the latter, calcitonin and diphosphonates have attracted most interest and have both been shown to reduce the activity of Paget's disease. It is impossible to make a firm statement about the therapeutic position of these drugs, as diphosphonates have only recently become generally available. It may be that the most effective treatment will be a combination of these two types of drugs. This could produce therapeutic efficacy without the problem of abnormal mineralization seen when diphosphonates are given alone.

Mithramycin has only more recently been tried in Paget's disease. It has the disadvantage of intravenous administration and potential toxicity.

6.7 ADUVANT DRUGS

It is not intended to describe details of the drugs used as adjuvants in rheumatological management, as these are reported fully in general works. It should also be stated that although included in a chapter on specific agents in rheumatic therapy, many of these drugs are neither specific nor are they anti-rheumatic in the usual sense.

Adjuvants drugs may be classified as follows:

1. Drugs used to treat 'complications' and other problems intimately associated with rheumatic disorders. These include: muscle relaxants, psychotropic drugs (e.g. hypnotics, tranquillizers, anti-depressants), haematinics, and antibiotics.

2. Drugs used to treat co-diseases – clinical concom-

itants usually regarded as an integral feature of a rheumatic disorder (e.g. psoriasis, ulcerative colitis, uveitis, non-specific urethritis).

3. Drugs used to treat fortuitously co-existing disorders (e.g. ischaemic heart disease, chronic bronchitis, diabetes mellitus, alcoholism).

The particular importance of including adjuvant drugs in a work such as this stems from the following:

1. Rheumatological management has as much to do with problems adjacent to joints (periarticular or extra-articular disorders) and at a distance from them (systemic manifestation) as it does with the articular structures themselves.

2. The potential for interaction between adjuvant drugs and anti-rheumatic drugs is as important as the potential for interaction between anti-rheumatic drugs.

In view of the frequency with which there is a need to employ drugs in group (1), further brief comments will be made about these agents and indications for their use.

Muscle relaxants. Muscle spasm is often present in patients with rheumatic disorders, and relief of this is often achieved simply by relief of pain. However, on occasions, muscle relaxants may be useful in addition to pain-relieving drugs, preferably given as separate rather than as combined preparations. Diazepam is helpful, particularly if there is an added element of anxiety. Another useful drug is methocarbamol, which is used in the treatment of back pain.

Psychotropic drugs. Insomnia, anxiety, and depression are often present in patients with rheumatic problems. Pain relief, reassurance, empathy, and sympathy are often more valuable than psychotropic drugs in these patients. However, some patients will need hypnotics, tranquillizers or anti-depressants for varying periods during the course of their illness. It is up to clinicians to avoid unnecessarily prolonged therapy with these agents, but rather to use them to tide a patient over a difficult phase.

Haematinics. Anaemia is relatively common in patients with chronic inflammatory disorders of connective tissue. The haematological picture may be of various types but the most frequent pattern is an iron-deficiency-type of anaemia in rheumatoid patients. Although this differs from true iron deficiency, patients often respond to treatment with iron, particularly when given parenterally. With intramuscular preparations (of both iron dextran and iron sorbitol) care should be taken to avoid skin staining by giving injection deeply into muscle and by using the Z-track technique to deter iron leaking back along the needle track. Apart from being unsightly, the staining may be accompanied by tissue necrosis.

Antibiotics. Patients with rheumatoid arthritis are particularly prone to developing pyarthrosis, usually of single joints. If, therefore, one joint seems 'hotter' than the rest, synovial fluid should be aspirated and the appropriate antibiotic given if necessary (see Section 6.5).

6.8 SUMMARY AND CONCLUSIONS

This chapter has considered drugs possessing, in varying degree, a specific action against certain rheumatic disorders.

Much of the chapter has been concerned with 'specific' drugs used to treat rheumatoid arthritis. These drugs are more appropriately termed 'suppressive' or 'remission-inducing' agents, as none of them is strictly specific to rheumatoid arthritis. For example, anti-malarials are used with effect in systemic lupus erythematosus, gold in psoriatic arthritis, and immunosuppressives in both disorders. Furthermore, the value of penicillamine in disorders other than rheumatoid arthritis (e.g. Wilson's disease, cystinuria, arsenical polyneuropathy, lead and mercury poisoning) is well established. The importance of prescribing long-term rheumatoid suppressants only when more conservative therapy has failed has been stressed. Further emphasis has been placed on adequate and regular follow up to monitor therapeutic response and the appearance of toxic effects.

Long-term agents used in the management of other inflammatory arthritides such as systemic lupus erythematosus and certain spondarthritides (e.g. psoriatic arthritis) have been discussed briefly. As most of these drugs are also used in the treatment of rheumatoid arthritis, the same comments regarding lack of true specificity, careful consideration of therapeutic justification, and cautious approach to monitoring therapeutic and toxic effects also apply to the management of these non-rheumatoid disorders.

Specific drugs used in the acute attack of gout (colchicine) and in its long-term prophylaxis (i.e. uricosurics or allopurinol) have been considered. The pros and cons regarding whether or not to introduce prophylactic treatment, and the type of prophylaxis to be used (i.e. the choice between drugs which increase elimination of urate or the alternative approach using blockade of uric acid synthesis) have been presented, stress being placed on the avoidance of using long-term drugs to suppress the acute gouty episode.

The general aspects of treating infectious arthritis have been discussed in some detail. The justification for this stems from the true specificity of antimicrobial therapy and of its resulting benefits, and also because of the devastating effects on the joints if treatment of infection is delayed or inappropriate.

Patients with intractable pain from Paget's disease of bone have shown an encouraging response to long-term therapy in recent years. Results from the more tradi-tional approach, calcitonin, and those from more recently introduced agents (disodium etidronate and mithramycin) have been reported.

6.9 REFERENCES AND FURTHER READING

Rheumatoid arthritis

Gold salts

†Adams, C.H. and Cecil, R.L. (1950) Gold therapy in early rheumatoid arthritis. *Ann. Int. Med.*, **33**, 163.

*Austad, W.R. (1970) Nitroid reactions to gold treatment for arthritis. *J. Am. Med. Assoc.*, **211**, 2153.

†Bluhm, G.B. (1975) The treatment of rheumatoid arthritis with gold. *Sem. Arthr. Rheum.*, **5**, 147.

†Browning, J.S., Rice, R.M., Lee, W.V. and Baker, L.M. (1947) Gold therapy in rheumatoid arthritis. *N. Engl. J. Med.*, **237**, 428.

Campion, D.S., Olsen, R., Bohan, A. and Bluestone R. (1974) Interaction of gold sodium thiomalate (Myochrysine) with serum albumin. *J. Rheumatol.* (Suppl. 1), 116.

†Cats, A. (1976) A multicentre controlled trial of the effects of different dosage of gold therapy, followed by a maintenance dosage. *Agents and Actions*, **6**, 355.

*Cecil, R.L. (1946) The problem of dosage in the administration of gold salts for rheumatoid arthritis. *Med. Clin. N. Am.*, **30**, 545.

†Cecil, R.L., Kammerer, W.H. and DePrume, F.J. (1942) Gold salts in the treatment of rheumatoid arthritis; a study of 245 cases. *Ann. Int. Med.*, **16**, 811.

†Cohen, A., Goldman, J. and Dubbs, A.W. (1945) The treat-ment of rheumatoid arthritis with 417 courses of gold. An analysis of 259 cases. *N. Engl. J. Med.*, **233**, 199.

†Co-operating Clinics of the American Rheumatism Association (1973) A controlled trial of gold salt therapy in the treatment of rheumatoid arthritis. *Arthr. Rheum.*, **16**, 353.

†Currey, H.L.F., Harris, J., Mason, R.M. *et al.* (1974) Comparison of azathioprine, cyclophosphamide and gold in treatment of rheumatoid arthritis. *Br. Med. J.*, **iii**, 763.

*Davis, P. and Hughes, G.R.V. (1974) Significance of eosi-nophilia during gold therapy. *Arthr. Rheum.*, **17**, 964.

*Davis, P., Ezeoke, A., Munro, J. *et al.* (1973) Immunological studies on the mechanism of gold hypersensitivity reactions. *Br. Med. J.*, **iii**, 676.

*Denman, E.J. and Denman, A.M. (1968) The lymphocyte transformation test and gold hypersensitivity. *Ann. Rheum. Dis.*, **27**, 582.

*Deren, B., Masi, R., Weksler, M. and Nachman, R.L. (1974) Gold-associated thrombocytopenia. *Arch. Int. Med.*, **134**, 1012.

*Dorwart, B.B., Gall, E.P., Schumacher, H.R. and Kranser, R.E. (1978) Chrysotherapy in psoriatic arthritis. Efficacy and toxicity compared to rheumatoid arthritis. *Arthr. Rheum.*, **21**, 513.

Editorial (1974) Gold revalued. *Lancet*, **i**, 789.

Editorial (1975) Gold therapy in 1975. *Br. Med. J.*, **ii**, 156.

†Ellman, P., Lawrence, J.S. and Thorold, G.P. (1940) Gold therapy in rheumatoid arthritis. *Br. Med. J.*, **ii**, 314.

†Empire Rheumatism Council (1960) Gold therapy in rheu-matoid arthritis. Report of a multi-centre controlled trial. *Ann. Rheum. Dis.*, **19**, 95.

†Empire Rheumatism Council (1961) Gold therapy in rheu-matoid arthritis. Final report of a multi-centre controlled trial. *Ann. Rheum. Dis.*, **20**, 315.

†Forestier, J. (1935) Rheumatoid arthritis and its treatment by gold salts. The results of six years' experience. *J. Lab. Clin. Med.*, **20**, 827.

*Fraser, T.N. (1945) Gold treatment in rheumatoid arthritis. *Ann. Rheum. Dis.*, **4**, 71.

†Freyberg, R.H. (1942) Gold salts in the treatment of chronic arthritis: metabolic and clinical studies. *Proc. Staff Meetings Mayo Clin.* **17**, 534.

†Freyberg, R.H., Block, W.D. and Wells, G.S. (1942) Gold therapy for rheumatoid arthritis: considerations based upon studies of the metabolism of gold. *Clinics*, **1**, 537.

Gerber, R.C. and Paulus, H.E. (1975) Gold therapy. *Clin. Rheum. Dis.*, **1**, 307.

Gordon, M.H., Tiger, L.H. and Ehrlich, G.E. (1975) Gold reactions are *not* more common in Sjögren's syndrome. *Ann. Int. Med.*, **82**, 47.

Gottlieb, N.L. (1977) Chrysotherapy. *Bull. Rheum. Dis.*, **27**, 912.

*Gowans, J.D.C. and Salami, M. (1973) Response of rheu-matoid arthritis with leukopenia to gold salts. *N. Engl. J. Med.*, **233**, 1007.

*Grahame, J.W. and Fletcher, A.A. (1943) Gold therapy in rheumatoid arthritis. *Can. Med. Assoc. J.*, **49**, 483.

†Griffin, A.J., Gibson, T., Huston, G. and Taylor, A. (1981) Maintenance chrysotherapy in rheumatoid arthritis: a com-parison of 2 dose schedules. *Ann. Rheum. Dis.*, **40**, 250.

†Griffin, A.J., Gibson, T. and Taylor, A. (1978) Comparison of two maintenance schedules of chrysotherapy in rheumatoid arthritis: a preliminary report. *Rheumatol. Rehabil.* (Suppl: Trends in the Drug Treatment of Rheumatic Diseases), 99.

*Hanson, V., Hicks, R. and Kornreich, H. (1971) in *Eighth International Congress of Pediatrics* (ed. F. Feilhaur), Neunkirchen, Austria. pp. 169–74.

†Hartfall, S.J., Garland, H.G. and Goldie, W. (1937) Gold treatment of arthritis. A review of 900 cases. *Lancet*, **ii**, 784 and 835.

*Harth, M., Hickey, J.P., Coulter, W.K. *et al.* (1978) Gold-induced thrombocytopenia. *J. Rheumatol.*, **5**, 165.

*Hashimoto, A., Maeda, Y., Ito, H. *et al.* (1972) A clinical study in rheumatoid arthritis patients receiving gold therapy. *Arthr. Rheum.*, **15**, 309.

*Hicks, R.M., Hanson, V. and Kornreich, H.K. (1970) The use of gold in the treatment of juvenile rheumatoid arthritis. *Arthr. Rheum.*, **13**, 323 (Abstract).

†Huskisson, E.C., Gibson, T.J., Balme, H.W. *et al.* (1974) Trial comparing D-penicillamine and gold in rheumatoid arthritis. *Ann. Rheum. Dis.*, **33**, 532.

*Jalava, S., Kalimo, H., Ruuskanen, O. and Tala, E. (1979) Pulmonary reactions induced by gold therapy. *Scand. J. Rheumatol.*, **8**, 192.

Jalava, S., Luukkainen, R., Hämeenkorpi, R. *et al.* (1977) Some characteristics of RA patients with and without side effects due to gold treatment. *Scand. J. Rheumatol.*, **6**, 206.

Kean, W.F. and Anastassiades, T.P. (1979) Long term chrysotherapy. Incidence of toxicity and efficacy during sequential time periods. *Arthr. Rheum.*, **22**, 495.

*Key, J.A. Rosenfeld, H. and Tjoflat, O.E. (1939) Gold therapy in proliferative (especially atropic) arthritis. *J. Bone Joint Surg.*, **21**, 339.

*Klinefelter, H.F. (1975) Reinstitution of gold therapy in rheumatoid arthritis after muco taneous reactions. *J. Rheumatol.*, **2**, 21.

†Lawrence, J.S. (1976) Comparative toxicity of gold preparations in treatment of rheumatoid arthritis. *Ann. Rheum. Dis.*, **35**, 171.

*Lockie, L.M., Norcross, B.M. and Riordan, D.J. (1958) Gold in the treatment of rheumatoid arthritis. *J. Am. Med. Assoc.*, **167**, 1204.

†Lorber, A., Atkins C.J., Cheng, C.C. *et al.* (1973) Monitoring serum gold levels to improve chrysotherapy in rheumatoid arthritis. *Ann. Rheum. Dis.*, **32**, 133.

†Luukkainen, R., Isomaki, H. and Kajander, A. (1977a) Effect of gold treatment on the progression of erosions in RA patients. *Scand. J. Rheumatol.*, **6**, 123.

*Luukkainen, R. Isomäki, H. and Kajander, A. (1978) Gold treatment at an early stage of rheumatoid arthritis. *Rheumatol. Rehabil.* (Suppl: Trends in the Drug Treatment of Rheumatic Diseases), 94.

†Luukkainen, R., Kajander, A. and Isomäki, H. (1977b) Effect of gold on progression of erosions in rheumatoid arthritis. Better results with early treatment. *Scand. J. Rheumatol.*, **6**, 189.

†Mäkisara, P., Nissila, M., Kajander, A. *et al.* (1978) Comparison of penicillamine and gold treatment in early rheumatoid arthritis. *Scand. J. Rheumatol.*, **7**, 166.

*McCarty, D.J., Brill, J.M. and Harrop, D. (1962) Aplastic anaemia secondary to gold-salt therapy. Report of fatal case and a review of the literature. *J. Am. Med. Assoc.*, **169**, 655.

*Mettier, S.R., McBride, A. and Li, J. (1948) Thrombocytopenic purpura complicating gold therapy for rheumatoid arthritis. Report of three cases with spontaneous recovery and one case with recovery following splenectomy. *Blood*, **3**, 1105.

*Penneys, N.S., Ackerman, A.B. and Gottlieb, N.L. (1974) Gold dermatitis. A clinical and histopathological study. *Arch. Dermatol.*, **109**, 372.

*Pick, E. (1927) Versuche einer Goldbehandlung des Rheumatismus. *Wiener Klin. Wochenschr.*, **40**, 1175.

*Price, A.E. and Leichtentritt, B. (1943) Gold therapy in rheumatoid arthritis. *Ann. Int. Med.*, **19**, 70.

*Rawls, W.B., Grushin, B.J. and Ressa, A.A. (1944) Analysis of results obtained with small doses of gold salts in the treatment of rheumatoid arthritis. *Am. J. Med. Sci.*, **207**, 528.

†Research Subcommittee of the Empire Rheumatism Council (1961) Gold therapy in rheumatoid arthritis. *Ann. Rheum. Dis.*, **20**, 315.

*Richter, M.B., Kinsella, P. and Corbett, M. (1980) Gold in psoriatic arthropathy. *Ann. Rheum. Dis.*, **39**, 279.

Rothermich, N.O. (1979) in *Clinics in Rheumatic Diseases* (ed. E.C. Huskisson), Vol. 5, No. 2, Saunders, London, p. 631.

†Rothermich, N.O., Phillips, V.K., Bergen, W. and Thomas, M.H. (1976) Chrysotherapy. A prospective study. *Arthr. Rheum.*, **19**, 1321.

*Skrifvars, B.V., Törnroth, T.S. and Tallqvist, G.N. (1977) Gold-induced immune complex nephritis in seronegative rheumatoid arthritis. *Ann. Rheum. Dis.*, **36**, 549.

*Siegman-Ingra, Y., Yaron, M., Silepzki, M. *et al.* (1976) Colitis and death following gold therapy. *Rheumatol. Rehabil.*, **15**, 245.

†Sigler, J.W., Bluhm, G.B., Duncan, H. *et al.* (1974) Gold salts in the treatment of rheumatoid arthritis. *Ann. Int. Med.*, **80**, 21.

*Silverberg, D.S., Kidd, E.G., Shnitka, T.K. and Ulan, R.A. (1970) Gold nephropathy. A clinical and pathologic study. *Arthr. Rheum.*, **13**, 812.

*Smith, R.T., Peak, W.P., Kron, K.M. *et al.* (1958) Increasing the effectiveness of gold therapy in rheumatoid arthritis. *J. Am. Med. Assoc.*, **167**, 1197.

*Snorrason, E. (1952) Rheumatoid arthritis, Sanocrysin treatment and prognosis. *Acta Med. Scand.*, **142**, 249.

†Srinivasan, R., Miller, B.L. and Paulus, H.E. (1979) Long-term chrysotherapy in rheumatoid arthritis. *Arthr. Rheum.*, **22**, 105.

*Stavem, P. and Stromme, J. (1968) Immunological studies in a case of gold salt induced thrombocytopenia. *Scand. J. Haematol.*, **5**, 271.

*Sundelin, F. (1941), Goldbehandlung der chronischen Arthritis unter besonderer Berücksichtigung der Komplikationen (Academic dissertation). *Acta Med. Scand.*, Suppl., 117.

*Tannenbaum, H. and Favreau, M. (1977) *Abstracts of the XIVth International Congress of Rheumatology, San Francisco*, Abstract 292.

*Törnroth, T. and Skrifvars, B. (1974) Gold nephropathy prototype of membranous glomerulonephritis. *Am. J. Pathol.*, **75**, 573.

*Vaamonde, C.A. and Hunt, F.R. (1970) The nephrotic syndrome as a complication of gold therapy. *Arthr. Rheum.*, **13**, 826.

*Waine, H., Baker, F. and Mettier, S.R. (1947) Controlled evaluation of gold therapy in rheumatoid arthritis. *Cal. Med.*, **66**, 295.

Westwick, W.J., Allsop, J., Gumpel, J.M. and Watts, R.W.E. (1974) Studies on pyrimidine biosynthesis in the granulocytes of patients receiving gold therapy for rheumatoid arthritis. *Q. J. Med.*, *(New Ser.)*, **43**, 231.

*Williams, B.D., Lockwood, C.M. and Pussel, B.A. (1979). Inhibition of reticuloendothelial function by gold and its relation to postinjection reactions. *Br. Med. J.*, **ii**, 235.

*Winterbauer, R.H., Wilske, K.R. and Wheelis, R.F. (1976) Diffuse pulmonary injury associated with gold treatment. *N. Engl. J. Med.*, **17**, 919.

Anti-malarials

Abraham, R., Hendy, R. and Grasso, P. (1963) Formation of myeloid bodies in rat liver lysosomes after chloroquine administration. *Exp. Mol. Pathol.*, **9**, 212.

†Alving, A.S., Eichelberger, I., Craige, B. *et al.* (1948) Studies on the chronic toxicity of chloroquine. *J. Clin. Invest.*, **27** (Suppl.) 60.

*Annotation (1971) Chloroquine myopathy. *Br. Med. J.*, **iv**, 605.

*Arden, G.B. and Kolb, H. (1966) Antimalarial therapy and early retinal changes in patients with rheumatoid arthritis. *Br. Med. J.*, **i**, 270.

*Arden, G.B., Friedmann, A. and Kolby, H. (1962) Anticipation of chloroquine retinopathy. *Lancet*, **i**, 1164.

*Argov, Z. and Mastaglia, F.I. (1979) Disorders of neuromuscular transmission caused by drugs. *N. Engl. J. Med.*, **301**, 409.

†Bagnall, A.W. (1957) The value of chloroquine in rheumatoid disease. *Can. Med. Assoc. J.*, **77**, 182.

*Bartholomew, L.E. and Duff, I.F. (1963) Amopyroquin (Propoquin) in rheumatoid arthritis. *Arthr. Rheum.*, **6**, 356.

Benecze, G. and Johnson, G.D. (1965) Inhibition of anti-nuclear factor reaction by chloroquine. *Immunology*, **9**, 201.

*Berggren, I. and Rendahl, I. (1955) Quinine amblyopia. *Acta Ophthalmol.*, **33**, 217.

*Bernstein, H.N. (1967) Chloroquine ocular toxicity. *Sur. Ophthalmol.*, **12**, 415.

Bernstein, H., Zvaifler, N., Rubin, M. and Mansour, A.M. (1963) The ocular deposition of chloroquine. *Invest. Ophthalmol.*, **2**, 384.

Burns, R.P. (1966) Delayed onset of chloroquine retinopathy. *N. Engl. J. Med.*, **275**, 693.

*Buter, I. (1965) Retinopathy following the use of chloroquine and allied substances. *Ophthalmologica*, **149**, 204.

*Cann, H.M. and Verhulst, H.I. (1961) Fatal acute chloroquine poisoning in children. *Pediatrics*, **37**, 95.

Carr, R.E., Gouras, P. and Gunkel, O.D. (1966) Chloroquine retinopathy. *Arch. Ophthalmol.*, **75**, 171.

*Carr, R.E., Henkind, P., Rothfield, N. and Siegel, I.M. (1968) Ocular toxicity of antimalarial drugs: long-term follow-up. *Am. J.Ophthalmol.*, **66**, 738.

†Cohen, A.S. and Calkins, E. (1958) A controlled study of chloroquine as an antirheumatic agent. *Arthr. Rheum.*, **1**, 297.

†Cohen, S.N. and Yielding, K.I. (1964) Further studies of the mechanism of action of chloroquine: inhibition of DNA and RNA polymerase reactions. *Arthr. Rheum.*, **7**, 302.

*Crews, S.J. (1964) Chloroquine retinopathy with recovery in early stages. *Lancet*, **ii**, 436.

*Dall, J.L.C. and Keane, J.A. (1959) Disturbances of pigmentation with chloroquine. *Br. Med. J.*, **i**, 1387.

†DiMaio, V.J.M. and Henry, I.D. (1974) Chloroquine poisoning. *S. Med. J.*, **67**, 1031.

*Editorial (1964) Chloroquine and the eye. *Lancet*, **i**, 423.

*Elenius, V. and Mantyjarvi, M. (1963) Electro-oculographic and electro-retinographic evaluation of retinal function in subjects undergoing chloroquine treatment. *Acta Ophthalmol.*, **41**, 488.

†Elkington, J.R. and Huth, E.J. (1965) Letters and comments: chloroquine in rheumatoid arthritis. *Ann. Int. Med.*, **62**, 1066.

*Elman, A., Gullberg, R., Nilsson, E. *et al.* (1976) Chloroquine retinopathy in patients with rheumatoid arthritis. *Scand. J. Rheumatol.*, **5**, 161.

*Epstein, J.H. (1960) Synthetic antimalarial drug therapy in lupus erythematosus and polymorphous light eruptions. *Cal. Med.*, **92**, 135.

Fabre, J., Freundenreich, J., de, Duckert, A. *et al.* (1966) Influence of renal insufficiency on the excretion of chloroquine, phenobarbitol, phenothiazines and methacycline, *Helv. Med. Acta*, **33**, 307.

Fedorko, M. (1967) Effect of chloroquine on morphology of cytoplasmic granules in maturing human leukocytes – an ultrastructural study. *J. Clin. Invest.*, **46**, 12.

*Freedman, A. (1956) Chloroquine and rheumatoid arthritis: a short-term controlled trial. *Ann. Rheum. Dis.*, **15**, 251.

*Freedman, A. and Bach, F. (1952) Mepacrine and rheumatoid arthritis. *Lancet*, **ii**, 755.

†Freedman, A. and Steinberg, V.I. (1960) Chloroquine in rheumatoid arthritis: a double blindfold trial of treatment for one year. *Ann. Rheum. Dis.*, **19**, 243.

*Francois, J. and Maudgal, M.C. (1964) Experimental chloroquine retinopathy. *Ophthalmologica*, **148**, 442.

*Fuld, H. (1959) Retinopathy following chloroquine therapy. *Lancet*, **2**, 617 (Letter).

Gabourel, J.D. (1963) Effects of hydroxychloroquine on the growth of mammalian cells in vitro. *J. Pharmacol. Exp. Ther.*, **141**, 122.

Gerber, D.A. (1964) Effect of chloroquine on the sulfhydryl group and the denaturation of bovine serum albumin. *Arthr. Rheum.*, **7**, 193.

*Gonasun, L.M. and Potts, A.M. (1974) *In vitro* inhibition of protein synthesis in the retinal pigment epithelium by chloroquine. *Invest. Ophthalmol.*, **13**, 107.

*Good, M.I. and Shader, R.I. (1977) Behavioural toxicity and equivocal suicide associated with chloroquine and its derivatives. *Am. J. Psychiat.*, **134**, 798.

*Gregory, M.H., Rutty, D.A. and Wood, R.D. (1970) Differences in the retinotoxic action of chloroquine and phenothiazine derivatives. *J. Pathol.*, **102**, 139.

*Hamilton, E.B.D. and Scott, J.T. (1962) Hydroxychloroquine sulfate (Plaquenil) in treatment of rheumatoid arthritis. *Arthr. Rheum.*, **5**, 502.

Hart, C.W. and Naunton, R.F. (1964) The ototoxicity of chloroquine phosphate. *Arch. Otolaryngol.*, **80**, 407.

†Haydu, G.G. (1953) Rheumatoid arthritis therapy: rationale and the use of chloroquine diphosphate. *Am. J. Med. Sci.*, **225**, 71.

*Henkind, P., Carr, R.E. and Sigel, I. (1964) Early chloroquine retinopathy: clinical and functional findings. *Arch. Ophthalmol.*, **71**, 157.

*Herxheimer, A. (1971) Drugs and the fetal eye. *Lancet*, **i**, 443.

*Hobbs, S.E., Sorsby, A. and Freedman, A. (1959) Retinopathy following chloroquine therapy. *Lancet*, **ii**, 478.

Hurvitz, D. and Hirschhorn, K. (1965) Suppression of *in vitro* lymphocyte responses by chloroquine. *N. Engl. J. Med.*, **273**, 23.

*Kersley, G.D. and Palin, A.G. (1959) Amodiaquine and hydroxychloroquine in rheumatoid arthritis. *Lancet*, **ii**, 886.

†Keruzore, A., Coste, F. and Delbarre, F. (1960) The treatment

of inflammatory rheumatism by antimalarials (chloroquine and hydroxychloroquine). *Semaine de Hôpital de Paris*, **36**, 999.

†Kirsner, A.B., Sheon, R.P., Finkel, R.I. and Farber, S.J. (1979) A four-year prospective study of gold and antimalarials in rheumatoid arthritis. *Arthr. Rheum.*, **22**, 630.

*Knox, J.M. and Owens, D.W. (1966) The chloroquine mystery. *Arch. Dermatol.*, **94**, 205.

Kohno, S., Masayosh, K. and Suganuma, M. (1968) Inhibition of interferon production by chloroquine diphosphate. *Jap. J. Med. Sci. Biol.*, **21**, 239.

*Kolb, H. (1965) Electro-oculogram findings in patients treated with antimalarial drugs. *Br. J. Ophthalmol.*, **49**, 573.

*Kurtz, S.M., Kaump, D.H., Schardein, J.L. *et al.* (1967). The effect of long-term administration of amopyroquin, a 4-aminoquinoline compound, on the retina of pigmented and non-pigmented laboratory animals. *Invest. Ophthalmol.*, **6**, 420.

*Laaksonen, A.L., Koskiahde, V. and Juva, K. (1974) Dosage of antimalarial drugs for children with juvenile rheumatoid arthritis and systemic lupus erythematosus. *Scand. J. Rheumatol.* **3**, 103.

*Lanham, J. and Hughes, G.R.V. (1981) The place of antimalarials in rheumatology. *Ann. Rheum. Dis.*, **40**, 323.

*Lindquist, N.G., Sjostrand, S.E. and Ullberg, S. (1970) Accumulation of chorio-retinotoxic drugs in the fetal eye. *Acta Pharmacol. Toxicol.*, **23**, 64.

†Logan, C.E., Schmid, F.R., Kruger, S. *et al.* (1961) Double-blind study of hydroxychloroquine in rheumatoid arthritis. *Atti del X Congressa della Lega Internazionale Contro il Rheumatismo*, **2**, 1442.

†Mackenzie, A.H. (1970) An appraisal of chloroquine. *Arthr. Rheum.*, **13**, 280.

†Mackenzie, A.E. and Scherbel, A.L. (1968) A decade of chloroquine maintenance therapy: rate of administration governs incidence of retinotoxicity. *Arthr. Rheum.*, **11**, 496.

†Mackenzie, A.H. and Scherbel, A.L. (1969) Let us abandon some chloroquine dogmas. *Arthr. Rheum.*, **12**, 315 (Abstract).

*Mackenzie, A.H. and Szilagvi, P.J. (1968) Light may provide energy for retinal damage during chloroquine therapy. *Arthr. Rheum.*, **11**, 496.

*Mackenzie, A.H. and Scherbel, A.L. (1980) in *Clinics in the Rheumatic Diseases* (ed. E.C. Huskisson), Vol. 6, No. 3, Saunders, London, p. 545.

*Mainland, D. and Sutcliffe, M.I. (1962) Hydroxychloroquine sulfate in rheumatoid arthritis: a six month double blind trial. *Bull. Rheum. Dis.*, **12**, 287.

*Markowitz, H.A. and McGinley, J.M. (1964) Chloroquine poisoning in a child. *J. Am. Med. Assoc.*, **189**, 950.

†Marks, J.S. and Power, B.J. (1979) Is chloroquine obsolete in treatment of rheumatic diseases? *Lancet*, **ii**, 317.

*Mason, C.G. (1977) Ocular accumulation and toxicity of certain systemically administered drugs. *J. Toxicol. Environ. Hlt.*, **2**, 977.

*Matz, G.J. and Naunton, R.F. (1968) Ototoxicity of chloroquine. *Arch. Otolaryngol.*, **88**, 50.

McChesney, E.W., Banks, W.F. and Fabian, R.J. (1967a) Tissue distribution of chloroquine, hydroxychloroquine, and desethyl-chloroquine in the rat. *Toxicol. Appl.*

Pharmacol., **10**, 501.

McChesney, E.W., Banks, W.F. and McAuliff, J.P. (1962) Laboratory studies of the 4-aminoquinoline antimalarials: II. Plasma levels of chloroquine and hydroxychloroquine in man after various oral dosage regimens. *Antibiotics Chemother.*, **12**, 583.

McChesney, E.W., Fasco, J.J. and Banks, W.F. (1967b) The metabolism of chloroquine in man during and after repeated oral dosage. *J. Pharmacol. Exp. Ther.*, **158**, 323.

McChesney, E.W., Renselaer, N.Y. and Rothfield, N.E. (1964) Comparative metabolic studies of chloroquine and hydroxychloroquine. *Arthr. Rheum.*, **7**, 328.

*Millingen, K.S. and Suerth, E. (1966) Peripheral neuromyopathy following chloroquine therapy. *Med. J. Austr.*, **i**, 840.

*Neill, W.A., Panayi, G.S., Duthie, J.J.R. and Prescott, R.J. (1973) Action of chloroquine phosphate in rheumatoid arthritis. II. Chromosome damaging effect. *Ann. Rheum. Dis.*, **32**, 547.

*Nozik, R.A., Weinstock, F.J. and Vignos, P.J. (1964) Ocular complications of chloroquine. *Ann. J. Ophthalmol.*, **58**, 774.

*Nylander, U. (1966) Ocular damage in chloroquine therapy. *Acta Ophthalmol.*, **44**, 335.

*Okun, G., Gouras, P., Bernstein, H. and Von Sallmann, L. (1963) Chloroquine retinopathy. *Arch. Ophthalmol.*, **69**, 59.

*Page, F. (1951) Treatment of lupus erythematosus with mepacrine. *Lancet*, **ii**, 755.

†Panayi, G.S., Neill, W.A., Duthie, J.J.R. and McCormick, J.N. (1973) Action of chloroquine phosphate in rheumatoid arthritis. I. Immunosuppresive effect. *Ann. Rheum. Dis.*, **32**, 316.

*Percival, S.P.B. and Behrman, J. (1969) Ophthalmological safety of chloroquine. *Br. J. Ophthalmol.*, **53**, 101.

†Percival, S.P.B. and Meanock, I. (1968) Chloroquine: ophthalmological safety, and clinical assessment in rheumatoid arthritis. *Br. Med. J.*, **iii**, 579.

*Petrohelos, M.A. (1974) Chloroquine-induced ocular toxicity. *Am. J. Ophthalmol.*, **6**, 615.

*Popert, A.J. (1976) Chloroquine: a review. *Rheumatol. Rehabil.*, **15**, 235.

*Popert, A.J., Meijers, K.A.E., Sharp, J. and Bier, F. (1961) Chloroquine diphosphate in rheumatoid arthritis, a controlled trial. *Ann. Rheum. Dis.*, **20**, 18.

*Potts, A.M. (1966) Drug-induced macular disease. *Trans. Am. Acad. Ophthalmol. Otolaryngol.*, **70**, 1054.

Prouty, R.W. and Kuroda, K. (1958) Spectrophotometric determination and distribution of chloroquine in human tissues. *J. Lab. Clin. Med.*, **52**, 477.

Read, W.K. and Bay, W.W. (1971) Basic cellular lesion in chloroquine toxicity. *Lab. Invest.*, **24**, 246.

†Robinson, A.E., Coffer, A.I. and Camps, E.E. (1970) The distribution of chloroquine in man after fatal poisoning. *J. Pharm. Pharmacol.*, **22**, 700.

*Rosenbaum, E.E. (1979) in *Rheumatology – New Directions in Therapy*, Medical Examination Publishing, New York, pp. 20–5.

†Rothermich, N.O. (1964) Coming catastrophes with chloroquine? *Ann. Int. Med.*, **61**, 1203.

Rubin, M. and Slonicki, A. (1966) A mechanism for the toxicity of chloroquine. *Arthr. Rheum.*, **9**, 537.

*Rubin, M.L. and Thomas, W.C. (1970) Diplopia and loss of accommodation due to chloroquine. *Arthr. Rheum.*, **13**, 75.

Rubin, M., Bernstein, H.N. and Zvaifler, N.J. (1963) Studies on the pharmacology of chloroquine. *Arch. Ophthalmol.*, **70**, 474.

*Ryckewaert, A., Debeyre, N., Kahn, M.F. and de Seze, F. (1961) Essai de traitement de la polyarthrite chronique rhumatismale ou 'rhumatoide' par l'hydroxychloroquine. *Anti del X Congressa della Lega Internazionale Contro il Reumatismo*, **2**, 1439.

†Rynes, R.I., Korhel, G., Falbo, A. *et al.* (1979) Ophthalmologic safety of long-term hydroxychloroquine treatment. *Arthr. Rheum.*, **22**, 832.

*Sachs, D.D., Hoban, M.J. and Engleman, E.P. (1962) Chorioretinopathy induced by chronic administration of chloroquine phosphate. *Arthr. Rheum.*, **5**, 318.

Sams, W.M. (1967) Chloroquine, mechanism of action. *Mayo Clin. Proc.*, **42**, 300.

*Sassman, F.W., Cassidy, J.T., Alpern, M. and Maaseidvaag, F. (1970) Electroretinography in patients with connective tissue diseases treated with hydroxychloroquine. *Am. J. Ophthalmol.*, **70**, 515.

†Scherbel, A.I. (1961) in *Inflammation and Diseases of Connective Tissues* (eds I.C. Mills and J.H. Moyer), Saunders, Philadelphia, pp. 555–61.

*Scherbel, A.I., Harrison, J.W. and Atdjian, M. (1958) Further observations on the use of 4-aminoquinoline compounds in patients with rheumatoid arthritis or related diseases. *Clev. Clin. Q.*, **25**, 95.

Scherbel, A.L., Mackenzie, A.H., Nousek, J.E. and Atdjian, M. (1965) Ocular lesions in rheumatoid arthritis and related disorders with particular reference to retinopathy. *N. Engl. J. Med.*, **273**, 360.

*Scherbel, A.I., Schuchter, S.L. and Harrison, J.W. (1975) IV. Comparison of effects of two antimalarial agents. Hydroxychloroquine sulfate and chloroquine phosphate in patients with rheumatoid arthritis. *Clev. Clin. Q.*, **24**, 98.

*Schmidt, B. and Muller-Limmroth, W. (1962) Electroretinographic examinations following the application of chloroquine. *Acta Ophthalmol.*, **70** (Suppl.) 245.

*Scull, E. (1962) Chloroquine and hydroxychloroquine therapy in rheumatoid arthritis. *Arthr. Rheum.*, **5**, 30.

*Shaffer, B., Cahn, M.M. and Levy, E.J. (1958) Absorption of antimalarial drugs in human skin. *J. Invest. Dermatol.*, **30**, 341.

*Shearer, R.V. and Dubois, E.L. (1967) Ocular changes induced by long-term hydroxychloroquine (Plaquenil) therapy. *Am. J. Ophthalmol.*, **64**, 245.

*Sternberg, T.H. and Laden, E. (1959) Discoid lupus erythematosus: bilateral macular degeneration due to chloroquine. *Am. Med. Assoc. Arch. Dermatol.*, **79**, 116.

*Tuffanelli, D., Abraham, R.K. and Dubois, E.L. (1963) Pigmentation from antimalarial therapy. *Arch. Dermatol.*, **88**, 419.

*Vartanian, G.A. and Chinyanga, H.M. (1972) The mechanism of acute neuromuscular weakness induced by chloroquine. *Can. J. Physiol. Pharmacol.*, **50**, 1099.

†Voipio, H. (1966) Incidence of chloroquine retinopathy. *Acta Ophthalmol.*, **44**, 349.

*Weise, F.E. and Yannuzzi, L.A. (1974) Ring maculopathies

mimicking chloroquine retinopathy. *Am. J. Ophthalmol.*, **78**, 204.

Wetterholm, D.H. and Winter, F.C. (1964) Histopathology of chloroquine retinal toxicity. *Arch. Ophthalmol.*, **71**, 82.

Whitehouse, M.W. and Boström, H. (1965) Biochemical properties of anti-inflammatory drugs. VI. The effects of chloroquine (Resochin), mepacrine (Quinacrine) and some of their potential metabolites on cartilage metabolism and oxidative phosphorylation. *Biochem. Pharmacol.*, **14**, 1173.

Wibo, M. and Poole, B. (1974) Protein degradation in cultured cells. II. The uptake of chloroquine by rat fibroblasts and the inhibition of cellular protein degradation and cathepsin B. *J. Cell Biol.*, **63**, 430.

*Winkelmann, R.K., Merwin, C.F. and Brunsting, L.A. (1961) Antimalarial therapy in lupus erythematosus. *Ann. Int. Med.*, **55**, 772.

†Wollheim, F.A., Hanson, A. and Laurell, C.B. (1978) Chloroquine treatment in rheumatoid arthritis. *Scand. J. Rheumatol.*, **7**, 171.

Yielding, K.L. (1967) Inhibition of the replication of a bacterial DNA virus by chloroquine and other 4-aminoquinolone drugs. *Proc. Soc. Exp. Biol. Med.*, **125**, 780.

*Young, J.P. (1959) Chloroquine phosphate (Aralen) in the long-term treatment of rheumatoid arthritis. *Ann. Int. Med.*, **51**, 1159.

*Young, P., Rardin, R., Lankford, B. *et al.* (1972) The apparent elimination of chloroquine retinopathy. *Arthr. Rheum.*, **15**, 464.

Zvaifler, N.J. (1964) The subcellular localization of chloroquine and its effect on lysosomal disruption. *Arthr. Rheum.*, **7**, 760.

†Zvaifler, N.J. (1968) Antimalarial treatment of rheumatoid arthritis. *Med. Clin. N. Am.*, **52**, 759.

Penicillamine

Annotation (1973) Penicillamine in the treatment of rheumatoid arthritis. *Br. Med. J.*, **iii**, 464.

Ansell, B. and Hall, M.A. (1977) Penicillamine. *Arthr. Rheum.*, **20**, 536.

*Ansell, B.M. and Simpson, C. (1977) The effect of penicillamine on growth and height in juvenile chronic polyarthritis. *Proc. R. Soc. Med.*, **70** (Suppl. 3), 132.

*Ansell, B.M., Moran, H. and Arden, G.P. (1977) Penicillamine and wound healing in rheumatoid arthritis. *Proc. R. Soc. Med.*, **70** (Suppl. 3), 75.

*Appelbaum, T., Maubeuge, J., Unger, J. and Famaey, J.P. (1978) Cutaneous lupus induced by penicillamine. *Scand. J. Rheumatol.*, **7**, 64.

Arrigoni-Martelli, E., Braum, E. and Binderup, L. (1977) in *New Anti-Inflammatory and Anti-rheumatic Drugs* (ed. A. Bertelli), Prous, Barcelona, pp. 189–95.

Assem, E.S.K. (1974) Assay of penicillamine in blood and urine. *Curr. Med. Res. Op.*, **2**, 568.

*Bacon, P.A., Tribe, C.R., Mackenzie, J.C. *et al.* (1976) Penicillamine nephropathy in rheumatoid arthritis. *Q. J. Med., New Ser.*, **45**, 661.

*Barzilai, D., Dickstein, G., Enat, R. *et al.* (1978) Cholestatic jaundice caused by D-penicillamine. *Ann. Rheum. Dis.*, **37**, 98.

*Berry, H., Fernandes, L., Ford-Hutchinson, A.W. *et al.* (1978) Alclofenac and D-penicillamine. *Ann. Rheum. Dis.*, **37**, 93.

*Berry, H., Liyanage, S.P., Durance, R.A. *et al.* (1976) Azathioprine and penicillamine in treatment of rheumatoid arthritis: a controlled trial. *Br. Med. J.*, **i**, 1052.

Bluestone, R. and Goldberg, L.S. (1973) Effect of D-penicillamine on serum immunoglobulins and rheumatoid factor. *Ann. Rheum. Dis.*, **32**, 50.

*Bluestone, R., Grahame, R., Holloway, V. and Holt, P.J.L. (1970) Treatment of systemic sclerosis with penicillamine and a new method of observing the effect of treatment. *Ann. Rheum. Dis.*, **29**, 153.

*Bucknall, R.C. (1977) Myasthenia associated with D-penicillamine therapy in rheumatoid arthritis. *Proc. R. Soc. Med.*, **70**, (Suppl. 3), 114.

*Bucknall, R.C., Dixon, A. St. J., Glick, E.N. *et al.* (1975) Myasthenia gravis associated with penicillamine treatment for rheumatoid arthritis. *Br. Med. J.*, **i**, 600.

*Camus, J-P., Benichou, C., Guillien, P. *et al.* (1971) Traitement de la polyarthrite rhumatoïde commune par la D-penicillamine *Rev. Rhumatol.*, **38**, 809.

Chwalinska-Sadowska, H. and Baum, J. (1976) The effect of D-penicillamine on polymorphonuclear leukocyte function. *J. Clin. Invest.*, **58**, 871.

Czekalowski, J.W., Frazer, J. and Hall, D.A. (1977) A preliminary report on the effects of D-penicillamine and gold on certain proteolytic enzyme systems. *Proc. R. Soc. Med.*, **70** (Suppl. 3), 126.

*Davis, C.M. (1969) D-penicillamine for the treatment of gold dermatitis. *Am. J. Med.*, **46**, 472.

*Davison, A.M., Day, A.T., Golding, J.R. and Thomson, D. (1977) Effect of penicillamine on the kidney. *Proc. R. Soc. Med.*, **70**, (Suppl. 3), 109.

†Day, A.T., Golding, J.R., Lee, P.W. and Butterworth, A.D. (1974) Penicillamine in rheumatoid disease: a long-term study. *Br. Med. J.*, **i**, 180.

†Dippy, J.E. (1977) Penicillamine in rheumatoid arthritis – a 2 year retrospective study in 70 patients. *Br. J. Clin. Pract.*, **31**, 5.

*Dische, F.E., Swinson, D.R., Hamilton, E.D. and Parsons, V. (1976) Immunopathology of penicillamine-induced glomerular disease. *J. Rheumatol.*, **3**, 145.

*Dixon, A. St. J., Davies, J., Dormandy, T.L. (1975) Synthetic D(−) penicillamine in rheumatoid arthritis. Double-blind controlled study of a high and low dosage regimen. *Ann. Rheum. Dis.*, **34**, 416.

*Eastmond, C.J. (1976) Diffuse alveolitis as a complication of penicillamine treatment for rheumatoid arthritis. *Br. Med. J.*, **i**, 1506.

*Evans, P.H. (1977) Serum sulphydryl changes in rheumatoid coalworkers' pneumoconiosis patients treated with D-penicillamine. *Proc. R. Soc. Med.*, **70** (Suppl. 3), 95.

*Fernandes, L., Swinson, D.R. and Hamilton, E.B.D. (1977) Dermatomyositis complicating penicillamine treatment. *Ann. Rheum. Dis.*, **36**, 94.

Francis, M.J.O. and Mowat, A.G. (1974) Effects of D-penicillamine on skin collagen in man. *Postgrad. Med. J.*, **50** (Suppl. 2), 30.

†Friedman, M. (1977) Chemical basis for pharmacological and therapeutic actions of penicillamine. *Proc. R. Soc. Med.*, **70** (Suppl. 3), 50.

*Fulgham, D.D. and Katz, R. (1968) Penicillamine for scleroderma. *Acta Dermatol.*, **98**, 51.

†Gibson, T., Huskisson, E.C., Wojtewlewski, J.A. *et al.* (1976) Evidence that D-penicillamine alters the course of rheumatoid arthritis. *Rheumatol. Rehabil.*, **15**, 211.

*Golding, D.N. (1976) in *Penicillamine Research in Rheumatoid Disease* (ed. E. Munthe), Fabritius and Sonner, MSD, Oslo, pp. 282–3.

*Golding, J.R. (1968) Laboratory observations on the use of penicillamine in rheumatoid disease. *Postgrad. Med. J.* (Suppl: Symposium on Penicillamine), 40.

†Golding, J.R., Day, A.T., Tomlinson, M.R. *et al.* (1977) Rheumatoid arthritis treated with small dose of penicillamine. *Proc. R. Soc. Med.*, **70** (Suppl. 3), 131.

*Golding, J.R., Wilson, J.V. and Day, A.T. (1970) Observation on the treatment of rheumatoid disease with penicillamine. *Postgrad. Med. J.*, **46**, 599.

*Grossman, S.P. (1968) in *Drugs and Sensory Functions* (ed. H. Herxheimer), Churchill, London, pp. 101–26.

†Halverson, P.B., Kozin, F., Bernhard, G.C. and Goldman, A.L. (1978) Toxicity of penicillamine. A serious limitation to therapy in rheumatoid arthritis. *J. Am. Med. Assoc.*, **240**, 1870.

*Harris, E.D. and Sjoerdsma, A. (1966) Effect of penicillamine on human collagen and its possible application to treatment of scleroderma. *Lancet*, **ii**, 996.

*Harris, G. (1976) Leukaemia-like appearances in mice given penicillamine. *Lancet*, **ii**, 1356.

*Harrison, E.E. and Hickman, J.W. (1976) D-penicillamine and haemolytic anaemia. *Lancet*, **i** 33.

*Harvey, W., Henderson, D.R.F. and Grahame, R. (1974) Observations on *in vivo* skin elasticity and skin thickness of patients with rheumatoid arthritis treated with D-penicillamine and gold salts. *Postgrad. Med. J.*, **50**, 33.

*Henkin, R.I., Keiser, H.R., Jaffe, I.A. *et al.* (1967) Decreased taste sensitivity after D-penicillamine reversed by copper administration. *Lancet*, **ii**, 1268.

*Herbert, C.M., Lindberg, K.A., Jayson, M.I.V. and Bailey, A.J. (1974) Biosynthesis and maturation of skin collagen in scleroderma and effects of D-penicillamine. *Lancet*, **i**, 187.

Hill, H.F.H. (1974) Selection of patients with rheumatoid arthritis to be treated with penicillamine and their treatment. *Curr. Med. Res. Op.*, **2**, 573.

†Hill, H.F.H. (1977) Treatment of rheumatoid arthritis with penicillamine. *Sem. Arthr. Rheum.*, **6**, 361.

†Hill, H.F.H. and Hill, A.G.S. (1978) Penicillamine: 750 mg is not the dose. *Ann. Rheum. Dis.*, **37**, 288.

*Hill, H., Hill, A. and Davison, A.M. (1979) Resumption of treatment with penicillamine after proteinuria. *Ann. Rheum. Dis.*, **38**, 229.

†Hill, H.F.H., Hill, A.G.S., Golding, J.R. *et al.* (1979) Maintenance dose of penicillamine in rheumatoid arthritis: a comparison between a standard and a response-related flexible regimen. *Ann. Rheum. Dis.*, **38**, 429.

†Hjalmarson, D., Hanson, L.A. and Wilsson, L.A. (1977) IgA deficiency during D-penicillamine treatment. *Br. Med. J.*, **i**, 549.

†Huskisson, E.C. (1976a) Penicillamine and the rheumat-

ologist: a review. *Pharmatherapeutica*, **1**, 24.

*Huskisson, E.C. (1976b) Treatment of palindromic rheumatism with D-penicillamine. *Br. Med. J.*, **ii**, 979.

Huskisson, E.C. (1977) Is penicillamine immunostimulant? *Proc. R. Soc. Med.*, **70** (Suppl. 3), 142.

Huskisson, E.C. and Berry, H. (1974) Some immunological changes in rheumatoid arthritis among patients receiving penicillamine and gold. *Postgrad. Med. J.*, **50** (Suppl. 2), 59.

Huskisson, E.C. and Hart, F.D. (1972) Penicillamine in the treatment of rheumatoid arthritis. *Ann. Rheum. Dis.*, **31**, 402.

Huskisson, E.C., Gibson, T.J., Balme, H.W. *et al.* (1974) Trial comparing D-penicillamine and gold in rheumatoid arthritis: preliminary report. *Ann. Rheum. Dis.*, **33**, 532.

Jaffe, I.A. (1963) Comparison of the effect of plasmapheresis and penicillamine on the level of circulating rheumatoid factor. *Ann. Rheum. Dis.*, **22**, 71.

*Jaffe, I.A. (1964) Rheumatoid arthritis with arteritis. Report of a case treated with penicillamine. *Ann. Int. Med.*, **61**, 556.

Jaffe, I.A. (1965) The effect of penicillamine on the laboratory parameters in rheumatoid arthritis. *Arthr. Rheum.*, **8**, 1064.

Jaffe, I.A. (1968a) Penicillamine in rheumatoid diseases with particular reference to rheumatoid factor. *Postgrad. Med. J.* (Suppl. Symposium on Penicillamine), 34.

*Jaffe, I.A. (1968b) Effects of penicillamine on the kidney and on taste. *Postgrad. Med. J.*, **44**, 15.

†Jaffe, I.A. (1970) The treatment of rheumatoid arthritis and necrotising vasculitis with penicillamine. *Arthr. Rheum.*, **13**, 436.

*Jaffe, I.A. (1975a) Penicillamine treatment of rheumatoid arthritis: effect on immune complexes. *Ann. N. Y. Acad. Sci.*, **256**, 330.

†Jaffe, I.A. (1975b) The technique of penicillamine administration in rheumatoid arthritis. *Arthr. Rheum.*, **18**, 511.

*Jaffe, I.A. (1977) Penicillamine treatment of rheumatoid arthritis with a single daily dose of 250 g. *Proc. R. Soc. Med.*, **70** (Suppl. 3), 130.

Jaffe, I.A. (1978) D-Penicillamine. *Bull. Rheum. Dis.*, **28**, 948.

Jaffe, I.A. and Merryman, P. (1968) Effect of increased serum sulphydryl contents on titre of rheumatoid factor. *Ann. Rheum. Dis.*, **27**, 14.

*Jaffe, I.A. and Smith, R.W. (1968) Rheumatoid vasculitis. Report of a second case treated with pencillamine. *Arthr. Rheum.*, **11**, 585.

*Jaffe, I.A., Merryman, P. and Ehrenfeld, E. (1974) Further studies of the antiviral effect of D-penicillamine. *Postgrad. Med. J.*, **50**, 50.

*Jayson, M.I.V., Lovell, C., Black, C.M. and Wilson, R.S.E. (1977) Penicillamine therapy in systemic sclerosis. *Proc. R. Soc. Med.*, **70** (Suppl. 3), 82.

Jellunn, E., Aaseth, J. and Munthe, E. (1977) Is the mechanism of action during treatment of rheumatoid arthritis with penicillamine and gold thiomalate the same? *Proc. R. Soc. Med.*, **70** (Suppl. 3), 136.

*Kay, A.G.L. (1979) Myelotoxicity of D-penicillamine. *Ann. Rheum. Dis.*, **38**, 232.

*Keiser, H.R., Henkin, R.I., Bartter, F.C. and Sjoerdsma, A. (1968) Loss of taste during therapy with penicillamine. *J. Am. Med. Assoc.*, **203**, 381.

†*Leading article* (1975) D-Penicillamine in rheumatoid arthritis. *Lancet*, **i**, 1123.

†*Leading article* (1978) Penicillamine: its place in rheumatology. *Br. Med. J.*, **i**, 131.

*Leca, A.P. and Camus, J.P. (1975) Spondylarthrite ankylosante. Étude du traitement par la D-penicillamine. *Nouvelle Presse Med.*, **4**, 112.

*Lievre, J.-A., Camus, J.P., Benichou, Ch., *et al.* (1971) Traitement de la polyarthritie rhumatoïde commune par la D-penicillamine. Etude d'une serie de 22 cas. *Ann. Méd. Intern.*, **122**, 655.

*Liyange, S.P. and Currey, H.L.F. (1972) Failure of oral penicillamine to modify adjuvant arthritis or immune response in rats. *Ann. Rheum. Dis.*, **31**, 521.

*Loddo, B. and Marcialis, M.A. (1974) Characteristics of the inhibitory action of D-penicillamine on the growth of polio virus. *Postgrad. Med. J.*, **50**, 45.

Lorber, A. (1966) Penicillamine therapy for rheumatoid lung disease: effect on protein sulphydryl groups. *Nature*, **210**, 1235.

Lorber, A., Pearson, C.M., Meredith, W.L. and Goutz-Mandell, L.E. (1964) Serum sulphydryl determinations and significance in connective tissue diseases. *Ann. Int. Med.*, **61**, 423.

†Lyle, W.H. (1973) Penicillamine in rheumatoid arthritis. *Lancet*, **i**, 549.

*Lyle, W.H. (1974) Peptic ulceration and D-penicillamine. *Lancet*, **ii**, 285.

Lyle, W.H. and Kleinman, R.L. (eds) (1977) Penicillamine at 21: its place in therapeutics now. *Proc. R. Soc. Med.*, **70** (Suppl. 3), 1.

†McKenzie, J.M.M. (1975) Dosage and toxic reactions of penicillamine in the treatment of rheumatic disorders. *Scand. J. Rheumatol.* (Suppl. 8), 21.

*Mjø Lnerød, O.K. Dommerud, S.A. and Rasmussen Kand Gjeruldsen, S.T. (1971) Congenital connective tissue defect probably due to D-penicillamine treatment in pregnancy. *Lancet*, **i**, 673.

Mohammed, I., Barraclough, D., Holborrow, E.J. Ansell, B.M. (1976) Effect of penicillamine therapy on circulating immune complexes in rheumatoid arthritis. *Ann. Rheum. Dis.*, **35**, 458.

*Morris, J.J., Seifter, E., Rettura, G. *et al.* (1969) Effect of penicillamine upon healing wounds. *J. Surg. Res.*, **9**, 143.

Multicentre Trial Group (1973) Controlled trial of D-penicillamine in severe rheumatoid arthritis. *Lancet*, **i** 275.

*Nimni, M.E. (1977) Mechanism of inhibition of collagen cross linking by penicillamine. *Proc. R. Soc. Med.*, **70** (Suppl. 3), 65.

*Nimni, M.E., Deshmukh, K. and Garth, N. (1972) Collagen defect induced by penicillamine. *Nature*, **240**, 220.

*Oliver, I., Liberman, U.A. and De Vries, A. (1972) Lupus-like syndrome induced by penicillamine in cystinuria. *J. Am. Med. Assoc.*, **220**, 588.

*Pass, F., Goldfischer, S.G., Sternlieb, I. and Scheinberg, I.H. (1973) Elastosis perforans serpiginosa during penicillamine therapy for Wilson's disease. *Arch. Dermatol.*, **108**, 713.

Roath, S. and Wills, R. (1974) The effects of penicillamine on lymphocytes in culture. *Postgrad. Med. J.*, **50**, 56.

*Rosenbaum, J., Katz, W.A. and Schumacher, H.R. (1980) Hepatotoxicity associated with use of D-penicillamine in rheumatoid arthritis. *Ann. Rheum. Dis.*, **39**, 152.

Roth, S.H. (1980) *New Directions in Arthritis Therapy*, PSG Publishing Co. Inc., Littleton, Ma. p. 109.

*Schairer, H. and Stoeber, E. (1976) in *Penicillamine Research in Rheumatoid Disease* (ed. E. Munthe), Fabritius and Sønner, MSD, Oslo, pp. 279–81.

*Schrader, P.L., Peters, H.A. and Dahl, D.S. (1972) Polymyositis and penicillamine. *Arch. Neurol.*, **27**, 456.

*Soloman, L., Abrams, G., Dinner, M. and Berman, L. (1977) Neonatal abnormalities associated with D-penicillamine treatment during pregnancy. *N. Engl. J. Med.*, **296**, 54.

*Stanworth, D.R., Johns, P., Felix-Davis, D.D. *et al.* (1977) Effect of D-penicillamine treatment on certain humoral immunological parameters in clinical and experimental arthritis. *Proc. R. Soc. Med.*, **20** (Suppl. 3), 144 (Abstract).

*Tio, T.H. (1977) Penicillamine types in the sclerodermas. *Proc. R. Soc. Med.*, **70** (Suppl. 3), 78.

*Tisman, G., Herbert, V., Go., L.T. and Brenner, L. (1972) Inhibition by penicillamine of DNA and protein synthesis by human bone marrow. *Proc. Soc. Exp. Biol. Med.*, **139**, 355.

*Uitto, J., Helin, P., Rasmussen, O. and Lorenzen, I. (1970) Skin collagen in patients with scleroderma: biosynthesis and maturation *in vitro*, and the effect of D-penicillamine. *Ann. Clin. Res.*, **2**, 228.

*Zilko, P.J., Dawkins, R.L. and Cohen, M.L. (1977) Penicillamine treatment of rheumatoid arthritis: relationship of proteinuria and autoantibodies to immune status. *Proc. R. Soc. Med.*, **70**, (Suppl. 3), 118.

†Zuckner, J., Ramsey, R.H., Dorner, R.W. and Gantner, G.E. (1970) D-Penicillamine in rheumatoid arthritis. *Arthr. Rheum.*, **13**, 131.

Immunosuppressives

General

Barnes, C.G. and Lovatt, G.E. (eds) (1982) Therapeutic workshop on modifying the disease activity in rheumatoid arthritis: immunosuppression in perspective. 15th International Congress of Rheumatology, Paris, 1981. *Ann. Rheum. Dis.*, **41** (Suppl. 1), 53.

Jimenez-Diaz, C., Lopez Garcia, E., Merchante, A. and Perianes, J. (1951) Treatment of rheumatoid arthritis with nitrogen mustard. *J. Am. Med. Assoc.*, **147**, 1418.

Parsons, J.L., Strong, J.S. and Fosdick, W.M. (1974) The causes of death in patients with rheumatoid arthritis treated with cytostatic agents. *J. Rheumatol.*, **135** (Suppl. 1), 75.

Renier, J.C., Bregeon, C., Bonnette, C. *et al.* (1978) Le devenir des sujets atteints de polyarthrite rhumatoïde et traités par les immunodépresseurs entre 1965 et 1973 inclus. *Rev. Rhum. Maladies Ostéo-articul.*, **45**, 453.

Schwartz, R.S. and Gowans, J.D.C. (1971) Guidelines for the use of cytotoxic drugs in rheumatic diseases. *Arthr. Rheum.*, **14**, 134.

Steinberg, A.D., Plotz, C., Wolff, D. and Plotz, P.H. (1972) Cytotoxic drugs in treatment of nonmalignant diseases. *Ann. Int. Med.*, **76**, 619.

Stevens, J.E. and Willoughby, D.A. (1969) The anti-inflammatory effects of some immunosuppressive agents. *J. Pathol.*, **97**, 367.

Azathioprine

Ansell, B.M. (1980) *Rheumatic Disorders of Childhood*, Butterworths, London, p. 139.

Bertino, J.R. (1973) Chemical action and pharmacology of methotrexate, azathioprine and cyclophosphamide in man. *Arthr. Rheum.*, **16**, 79.

†Currey, H.L.F., Harris, J., Mason, R.M. *et al.* (1974) Comparison of azathioprine, cyclophosphamide and gold in treatment of rheumatoid arthritis. *Br. Med. J.*, **iii**, 763.

*Dale, I. (1970) Azathioprine is 'effective' in children with rheumatoid arthritis. *Med. Trib.*, **2**, 1.

*Dale, I. (1972) The treatment of juvenile rheumatoid arthritis with azathioprine. *Scand. J. Rheumatol.*, **1**, 125.

*Dodson, W.H., Holley, H.L. and Bennett, J.C. (1968) High-dose azathioprine therapy in refractory rheumatoid arthritis. *Arthr. Rheum.*, **11**, 476.

*Drinkard, J.P., Stanley, T.M., Dornfeld, L. *et al.* (1970) Azathioprine and prednisolone in the treatment of adults with lupus nephritis. *Medicine (Baltimore)*, **49**, 411.

†Dwosh, I.L., Stein, H.B., Urowitz, M.B. *et al.* (1977) Azathioprine in early rheumatoid arthritis. Comparison with gold and chloroquine. *Arthr. Rheum.*, **20**, 685.

†Ginzler, E., Sharon, E., Diamond, H. and Kaplan, D. (1975) Long-term maintenance therapy with azathioprine in systemic lupus erythematosus. *Arthr. Rheum.*, **18**, 27.

*Harris, J., Jessop, J.D. and Chaput de Saintonge, D.M. (1971) Further experience with azathioprine in rheumatoid arthritis. *Br. Med. J.*, **iv**, 463.

†Hunter, T., Urowitz, M.B., Gordon, D.A. *et al.* (1975) Azathioprine in rheumatoid arthritis, a long term follow up study. *Arthr. Rheum.*, **18**, 15.

†Kersley, G.D. (1969) Azathioprine in severe rheumatoid arthritis. *Ann. Rheum. Dis.*, **23**, 328.

*Khanna, V. and Woodbury, J.F.L. (1973) Usefulness of azathioprine in rheumatoid arthritis. *Ann. R. Coll. Phys. Surg. Can.*, **6**, 60 (Abstract).

*Levy, J., Paulus, H.E., Barnett, E.V. *et al.* (1972) A double-blind controlled evaluation of azathioprine in rheumatoid arthritis and psoriatic arthritis. *Arthr. Rheum.*, **15**, 116 (Abstract).

†Mason, M., Currey, H.L.F., Barnes, C.G. *et al.* (1969) Azathioprine in rheumatoid arthritis. *Br. Med. J.*, **i**, 420.

†Urowitz, M.B., Gordon, D.A., Smythe, H.A. *et al.* (1973) Azathioprine in rheumatoid arthritis; a double-blind, cross-over study. *Arthr. Rheum.*, **16**, 411.

Cyclophosphamide

Co-operating Clinics Committee of the American Rheumatism Association (1970) A controlled trial of cyclophosphamide in rheumatoid arthritis. *N. Engl. J. Med.*, **283**, 883.

Co-operating Clinics Committee of the American Rheumatism Association (1972) A controlled trial of high and low doses of cyclophosphamide in 82 patients with rheumatoid arthritis. *Arthr. Rheum.*, **15**, 434.

Clements, P.J., Yu, D.T., Levy, J. *et al.* (1974) Effects of cyclophosphamide on B- and T-lymphocytes in rheumatoid arthritis. *Arthr. Rheum.*, **17**, 347.

Currey, H.L.F., Harris, J., Mason, R.M. *et al.* (1974) Comparison of azathioprine, cyclophosphamide and gold in treatment of rheumatoid arthritis. *Br. Med. J.*, **iii**, 763.

Fosdick, W.M., Parsons, J.L. and Hill, D.F. (1968) Long-term cyclophosphamide therapy in rheumatoid arthritis. *Arthr. Rheum.*, **11**, 151.

Fosdick, W.M., Parsons, J.L. and Hill, D.F. (1969) Long-term cyclophosphamide therapy in rheumatoid arthritis. A progress report, six years' experience. *Arthr. Rheum.*, **12**, 663.

Hurd, E.R. (1973) Immunosuppressive and anti-inflammatory properties of cyclophosphamide, azathioprine and methotrexate. *Arthr. Rheum.*, **16**, 84.

Hutter, A.M., Bauman, A.W. and Frank, I.H. (1969) Cyclophosphamide and severe haemorrhagic cystitis. *N. Y. State J. Med.*, **69**, 305.

Lemmel, B., Hurd, E.R. and Ziff, M. (1971) Differential effects of 6MP and cyclophosphamide on the autoimmune phenomena in NZB mice. *Clin. Exp. Immunol.*, **8**, 355.

Lidsky, M.D., Sharp, J.T. and Billings, S. (1973) A double blind study of cyclophosphamide in rheumatoid arthritis. *Arthr. Rheum.*, **16**, 148.

Pollock, B.H., Barr, J.H., Stolzer, B.H. *et al.* (1973) Neoplasia and cyclophosphamide. *Arthr. Rheum.*, **16**, 524.

Scheinman, J.I. and Stamler, F.W. (1969) Cyclophosphamide and fatal varicella. *J. Pediatr.*, **74**, 117.

Strong, J.S., Bartholomew, B.A. and Smyth, C.J. (1973) Immunoresponsiveness of patients with rheumatoid arthritis receiving cyclophosphamide or gold salts. *Ann. Rheum. Dis.*, **32**, 233.

Struck, R.F. and Hill, D.L. (1972) Investigation of the synthesis of aldo-phosphamide (AP), a toxic metabolite of cyclophosphamide (CTX). *Proc. Am. Assoc. Cancer Res.*, **13** 199 (Abstract).

Townes, A.S., Sows, J.M. and Schulman, L.E. (1972) Controlled trial of cyclophosphamide in rheumatoid arthritis: an 18 month double blind crossover study. *Arthr. Rheum.*, **15**, 129.

Williams, H.J., Reading, J.C., Ward, J.R. and O'Brien, W.M. (1980) Comparison of high and low dose cyclophosphamide therapy in rheumatoid arthritis. *Arthr. Rheum.*, **23**, 521.

Chlorambucil

Bontoux, D., Kahan, A., Brouilhet, H. *et al.* (1971) Effect et mode d'action du chlorambucil dans la maladie rhumatoïde. Intérêt du test de transformation lymphoblastique. *Rev. Rhum. Maladies Ostéo-articul.*, **38**, 759.

Buriot, D., Pricur, A.M., Lebranchu, Y. *et al.* (1979) Leucemie aigue chez trois enfants atteints d'arthrite chronique juvenile traites par chlorambucil. *Arch. Francaise de Ped.*, **36**, 592.

Cayla, J. and Rondier, J. (1971) A propos du traitement de 67 polyarthrites rhumatoïdes par le chlorambucil. *Rev. Rhum. Maladies Ostéo-articul.*, **38**, 765.

Elson, L.A., Galton, D.A.G. and Till, M. (1958) The action of chlorambucil (CD 1348) – and busulphan (Myleran) on the hematopoietic organs of the rat. *Br. J. Haematol.*, **4**, 355.

Kahn, M.F. and de Seze, S. (1975) Surveillance cancerologique au long cours des patients traites par les immunodépresseurs (chlorambucil) en rhumatologie. *Scand. J. Rheumatol.*, **4** (Suppl. 8), 9.

Kahn, M.F., Bedoiseau, M., Six, B., *et al.* (1971) Le chlorambucil dans la polyarthrite rhumatoïde. *Rev. Rhum. Maladies Osteoarticul.*, **38**, 741.

Le Goff, P. (1969) *100 Cas de Polyarthrites Rhumatoïdes Traités par la Thérapeutique à Visée Immunosuppressive (Chlorambucil)*. These de Doctorat en Médecine, Paris.

McLean, A., Newell, D. and Baker, G. (1976) The metabolism of chlorambucil. *Biochem. Pharmacol.*, **25**, 2331.

Raulo, P. (1974) *Résultats à Long Terme (Au delà de 4 Ans) du Traitement de la Polyarthrite Rhumatoide par le Chlorambucil*. These de Doctorat en Médecine, Paris.

Rudd, P., Fried, J.F. and Eptein, W.V. (1975) Irreversible bone marrow failure with chlorambucil. *J. Rheumatol.*, **2**, 421.

Thorpe, P. (1976) Rheumatoid arthritis treated with chlorambucil. *Med. J. Austr.*, **ii**, 197.

Snaith, M.L., Holt, J.M., Oliver, D.O. *et al.* (1973) Treatment of patients with systemic lupus erythematosus including nephritis with chlorambucil. *Br. Med. J.*, **ii**, 197.

Schnitzer, T.J. and Ansell, B.M. (1977) Amyloidosis in juvenile chronic polyarthritis. *Arthr. Rheum.*, **20** (Suppl. 2), 245.

Seronegative spondarthritides

Baker, H. (1970) Intermittent high dose oral methotrexate in psoriasis. *Br. J. Dermatol.*, **82**, 85.

Black, R.L., O'Brien, W.M., Van Scott, E.J. *et al.* (1964) Methotrexate therapy in psoriatic arthritis – double-blind study on 21 patients. *J. Am. Med. Assoc.*, **189**, 743.

Chaouat, Y.B., Kanovitch, F.B., Grupper, C. and Borgeois-Spinasse, J. (1971) Le rhumatisme psoriatique – traitement par le méthotrexate. *Rev. Rheumatol.*, **38**, 453.

Dohl, M.G.C., Gregory, M.M. and Scheuer, P.J. (1971) Liver damage due to methotrexate in patients with psoriasis. *Br. Med. J.*, **i**, 625.

Feldges, D.H. and Barnes, C.G. (1974) Treatment of psoriatic arthropathy with either azathioprine or methotrexate. *Rheumatol. Rehabil.*, **13**, 120.

Gubner, R.S., August, S. and Grinsberg, V. (1951) Therapeutic suppression of tissue reactivity. Part 2 : Effect of aminopterin in rheumatoid arthritis and psoriasis. *Am. J. Med. Sci.*, **1**, 176.

Haim, S. and Alroy, G. (1967) Methotrexate in psoriasis. *Lancet*, **i**, 1165.

Jacobs, J.C. (1977) Methotrexate and azathioprine in the treatment of childhood dermatomyositis. *Pediatrics*, **59**, 212.

Kersley, G.D. (1968) Amethopterin (methotrexate) in connective tissue disease-psoriasis and polyarthritis. *Ann. Rheum. Dis.*, **27**, 64.

Levy, J., Paulus, H.E., Barnett, E.V. *et al.* (1972) A double-blind controlled evaluation of azathioprine in rheumatoid arthritis and psoriatic arthritis. *Arthr. Rheum.*, **15**, 11 (Abstract).

Mamo, J.G. and Azzam, S.A. (1970) Treatment of Behçet's disease with chlorambucil. *Arch. Ophthalmol.*, **84**, 446.

Martin, J.H., Gordon, M. and Wallace, R. (1967) Methotrexate in psoriasis. *Arch. Dermatol.*, **96**, 431.

Metzger, A.L., Bohan, A., Goldberg, L.S. *et al.* (1974) Polymyositis and dermatomyositis: combined methotrexate and corticosteroid therapy. *Ann. Int. Med.*, **81** 182.

Mullins, J.F., Maberry, J.D. and Stone, O.J. (1966) Reiter's syndrome treated with folic acid antagonists. *Arch. Dermatol.*, **94**, 335.

Nyfors, A. and Brodthagen, H. (1970) Methotrexate for

psoriasis in weekly oral doses without any adjunctive therapy. *Dermatologica*, **140**, 345.

O'Brien, W.B., Van Scott, E.J., Black, R.L. *et al.* (1962) Clinical trial of amethopterin (methotrexate) in psoriatic and rheumatoid arthritis. *Arthr. Rheum.*, **5**, 512.

Owen, E.T. and Cohen, M.L. (1979) Methotrexate in Reiter's disease. *Ann. Rheum. Dis.*, **38**, 48.

Rees, R.B., Bennett, J.H., Hamlin, E.M. and Marbach, H.I. (1964) Aminopterin for psoriasis. *Arch. Dermatol.* **90**, 544.

Richter, M.B., Kinsella, P. and Corbett, M. (1980) Gold in psoriatic arthropathy. *Ann. Rheum. Dis.*, **39**, 279.

Spiro, J.M. and Dennis, D.T. (1969) Treatment of psoriasis with minute divided oral doses of methotrexate. *Arch. Dermatol.*, **99**, 459.

Tricoulis, D. (1976) Treatment of Behçet's disease with chlorambucil. *Br. J. Ophthalmol.*, **60**, 55.

Wade, A. (ed.) (1977) *Martindale. The Extra Pharmacopoeia*, 27th edn. The Pharmaceutical Press, London, p. 160.

Weinstein, G.D. and Frost, P. (1971) Methotrexate for psoriasis: A new therapeutic schedule. *Arch. Dermatol.*, **103**, 33.

Wright, V. (1981) in *Textbook of Rheumatology* (eds W.N. Kelley, E.D. Harris and C.B. Sledge), Saunders, Philadelphia, p. 1060.

Gout

Colchicine

*Blomgren, S.E. (1972) Conditions associated with erythema nodosum. *N. Y. State J. Med.*, **72**, 2302.

Bremner, W.J. and Paulsen, C.A. (1976) Colchicine and testicular function in man. *N. Engl. J. Med.*, **294**, 1384.

*Cohen, A. (1936), Gout. *Am. J. Med. Sci.*, **192**, 448.

†Davis, J.S. and Bartfield, H. (1954) The effect of intravenous colchicine on acute gout. *Am. J. Med.*, **16**, 213.

Eigsti, O.J. and Dustin, P. (1955) *Colchicine in Agriculture, Medicine, Biology and Chemistry*. Iowa State College Press, Ames.

Ertel, N.H., Mittler, J.C., Akgun, S. and Wallace, S.L. (1976) Radioimmunoassay for colchicine in plasma and urine. *Science*, **193**, 233.

Fitzgerald, T.J. (1974) in *Antiinflammatory Agents: Chemistry and Pharmacology* (ed. R.A. Sherrer), Academic Press, New York, p. 295.

*Goldfinger, S.E. (1972) Colchicine for familial Mediterranean fever. *N. Engl. J. Med.*, **287**, 1302.

†Gutman, A.B. (1965) Treatment of primary gout: the present status. *Arthr. Rheum.*, **8**, 911.

Gutman, A.B. (1966) Uricosuric drugs, with special reference to probenecid and sulfinpyrazone. *Adv. Pharmacol.*, **4**, 91.

Gutman, A.B. and Yu, T.-F. (1952) Gout, a derangement of purine metabolism. *Adv. Int. Med.*, **5**, 227.

*Kaplan, H. (1963) Further experience with colchicine in the treatment of sarcoid arthritis. *N. Engl. J. Med.*, **268**, 761.

Malawista, S.E. (1968) Colchicine: a common mechanism for the anti-inflammatory and anti-mitotic effects. *Arthr. Rheum.*, **11**, 191.

*McCarty, D.J. (1963) Crystal-induced inflammation: syndromes of gout and pseudogout. *Geriatrics*, **18**, 467.

†Paulus, H.E., Schlosstein, L.H., Godfrey, R.G. *et al.* (1974) Prophylactic colchicine therapy of intercritical gout. A

placebo-controlled study of probencid-treated patients. *Arthr. Rheum.*, **17**, 609.

Postlethwaite, A.E., Gutman, R.A. and Kelley, W.N. (1974) Salicylate-mediated increase in uric acid removal during hemodialysis: evidence for urate binding *in vivo*. *Metabolism*, **23**, 771.

*Talbott, J.H. and Coombs, F.S. (1938) Metabolic studies on patients with gout. *J. Am. Med. Assoc.*, **110**, 1977.

*Zuckner, J. (1962) Colchicine therapeutic trial responses in rheumatoid arthritis. *Arthr. Rheum.*, **5**, 329 (Abstract).

*Wallace, S.L., Bernstein, D. and Diamond, H. (1967) Diagnostic value of the colchicine therapeutic trial. *J. Am. Med. Assoc.*, **199**, 525.

†Yu, T.-F. and Gutman, A.B. (1961) Efficacy of colchicine prophylaxis in gout. *Ann. Int. Med.*, **55**, 179.

Probenecid

Boger, W.P. and Strickland, S.C. (1955) Probenecid (Benemid). Its use and side-effects in 2502 patients. *Arch. Int. Med.*, **95**, 83.

Dayton, P.G. and Perel, J.M. (1971) The metabolism of probenecid in man. *Ann. N.Y. Acad. Sci.*, **179**, 399.

De Seze, S., Ryckewaert, A. and d'Anglejan, G. (1963) The treatment of gout by probenecid. (A study based on 156 cases, 68 of which were treated from 1 to 9 years). *Rev. Rhum. Maladies Ostéo-articul.*, **30**, 93.

Ferris, T.F., Morgan, W.S. and Levitin, H. (1961) Nephrotic syndrome caused by probenecid. *N. Engl. J. Med.*, **265**, 381.

Gutman, A.B. (1950) Uric acid metabolism and gout. Combined staff clinic. *Am. J. Med.*, **9**, 799.

Gutman, A.B. and Yu, T.-F. (1957) Protracted uricosuric therapy in tophaceous gout. *Lancet*, **ii**, 1256.

Hertz, P., Yager, H. and Richardson, J.A. (1972) Probenecid-induced nephrotic syndrome. *Arch. Pathol.*, **94**, 241.

Kelley, W.N. (1981) in *Textbook of Rheumatology* (eds W.N. Kelley, E.D. Harris, S. Ruddy and C.B. Sledge), Saunders Philadelphia, p. 864.

Kippen, I., Whitehouse, M.W. and Klinenberg, M.W. (1974) Pharmacology of uricosuric drugs. *Ann. Rheum. Dis.*, **33**, 391.

Talbott, J.H. (1964), *Gout*, 2nd edn, Grune and Stratton, New York, p. 206.

Yu, T.-F. and Gutman, A.B. (1955) Paradoxical retention of uric acid by uricosuric drugs in low dosages. *Proc. Soc. Exp. Biol. Med. (New York)*, **90**, 542.

Sulphinpyrazone

Ali, M. and McDonald, W.D. (1977) Effects of sulfinpyrazone on platelet prostaglandin synthesis and platelet release of serotonin. *J. Lab. Clin. Med.*, **89**, 868.

Dieterle, W., Faigle, J.W., Mory, H. *et al.* (1975) Biotransformation and pharmacokinetics of sulphinpyrazone in man. *Clin. Pharmacol.*, **9**, 135.

Emmerson, B.T. (1963) A comparison of uricosuric agents in gout with special reference to sulphinpyrazone. *Med. J. Austr.*, **i**, 839.

Glick, E.N. (1961) Sulphinpyrazone in the treatment of arthritis associated with hyperuricaemia. *Proc. R. Soc. Med.*, **54**, 423.

Perel, J.M., Dayton, P.G., Snell, M.M. *et al.* (1969) Studies of interactions among drugs in man at the renal level: probenecid and sulphinpyrazone. *Clin. Pharmacol. Ther.*, **10**, 834.

Persellin, R.H. and Schmid, F.R. (1961) The use of sulfinpyrazones in the treatment of gout reduces serum uric acid levels and diminishes severity of arthritis attacks, with freedom from significant toxicity. *J. Am. Med. Assoc.*, **175**, 471.

Seegmiller, J.E. and Grayzel, A.I. (1960) Use of the newer uricosuric agents in the management of gout. *J. Am. Med. Assoc.*, **173**, 1076.

Smythe, H.A., Ogryzlo, M.A., Murphy, E.A. and Mustard, J.F. (1965) The effect of sulphinpyrazone (Anurane) on platelet economy and blood coagulation in man. *Can. Med. Assoc. J.*, **92**, 818.

Yu, T.-F., Burns, J.J. and Gutman, A.B. (1958) Results of a clinical trial of C-28315, a sulfoxide analog of phenylbutazone, as a uricosuric agent in gout subjects. *Arthr. Rheum.*, **1**, 532.

Yu, T.-F., Dayton, P.G. and Gutman, A.B. (1963) Mutual suppression of the uricosuric effects of sulfinpyrazone and salicylate: a study in interactions between drugs. *J. Clin. Invest.*, **42**, 1330.

Other uricosuric drugs

Kelley, W.N. (1981) in *Textbook of Rheumatology* (eds W.N. Kelley, E.D. Harris, S. Ruddy and C.B. Sledge). Saunders, Philadelphia, p. 862.

Allopurinol

Auerbach, R. and Orentrich, N. (1968) Alopecia and ichthyosis secondary to allopurinol. *Arch. Dermatol.*, **98**, 104.

Bardmore, T.D. and Kelley, W.N. (1971) Mechanism of allopurinol – mediated inhibition of pyrimidine biosynthesis. *J. Lab. Clin. Med.*, **78**, 696.

Chawla, S.K., Patel, H.D., Parrino, G.R. *et al.* (1977) Allopurinol hepatotixicity. *Arthr. Rheum.*, **20**, 1546.

Coe, F.L. and Kavalach, A.G. (1974) Hypercalciuria and hyperuricosuria in patients with calcium nephrolithiasis. *N. Engl. J. Med.*, **291**, 1344.

Elion, G.B. (1966) Enzymatic and metabolic studies with allopurinol. *Ann. Rheum. Dis.*, **25**, 608.

Fox, R.M., Royce-Smith, D. and O'Sullivan, W.J. (1970) Orotidinuria induced by allopurinol. *Science*, **168**, 861.

Frisch, J.M., Lovatt, G.E., Sproit, A.R.M. and Turner, P. (1974) The adverse reaction profile of allopurinol. *Proc. 12th Intl. Congr. Int. Med.*, 412–19.

Goldfarb, E. and Smyth, C.J. (1966) Effects of allopurinol, a xanthine oxidase inhibitor, and sulfinpyrazone upon the urinary and serum urate concentrations in eight patients with tophaceous gout. *Arthr. Rheum.*, **9**, 414.

Greenberg, M.D. and Zambrano, S.S. (1972) Aplastic agranulocytosis after allopurinol therapy. *Arthr. Rheum.*, **15**, 413.

Hande, K., Reed, E. and Chabner, B. (1978) Allopurinol kinetics. *Clin. Pharmacol. Ther.*, **23**, 598.

Irby, R., Toone, E. and Owen, D. (1966) Bone marrow depression associated with allopurinol therapy. *Arthr. Rheum.*, **9**, 860 (Abstract).

Kantor, G.L. (1970) Toxic epidermal necrolysis, azotemia and death after allopurinol therapy. *J. Am. Med. Assoc.*, **212**, 478.

Kelley, W.N. (1975), Effects of drugs on uric acid in man. *Ann. Rev. Pharmacol.*, **15**, 327.

Kelley, W.N. (1981) in *Textbook of Rheumatology* (eds W.N. Kelley, E.D. Harris, S. Ruddy and C.B. Sledge), Saunders, Philadelphia, p. 868.

Lidsky, M.D. and Sharp, J.T. (1967) Jaundice with the use of 4-hydroxypyrazolo (3, 4-d) pyrimidine (4-HPP). *Arthr. Rheum.*, **10**, 294 (Abstract).

Loebl, W.Y. and Scott, J.T. (1974) Withdrawal of allopurinol in patients with gout. *Ann. Rheum. Dis.*, **33**, 304.

Mills, R.M. (1971) Severe hypersensitivity reactions associated with allopurinol. *J. Am. Med. Assoc.*, **216**, 799.

Nelson, D.J. and Elion, G.B. (1975) Metabolism of (6-^{14}C) allopurinol – lack of incorporation of allopurinol into nucleic acids. *Biochem. Pharmacol.*, **24**, 1235.

Rodnan, G., Robin, J.A. and Tolchin, S.F. (1974) in *Purine Metabolism in Man* (eds O. Sperling, A. De Vries and J.B. Wyngaarden), Plenum Press, New York, p. 571.

Rundles, R.W., Metz, E.N. and Silberman, H.R. (1966) Allopurinol in the treatment of gout. *Ann. Int. Med.*, **64**, 229.

Scott, J.T. (1978) in *Copeman's Textbook of the Rheumatic Diseases* (ed. J.T. Scott), 5th edn, Churchill Livingstone, Edinburgh, p. 683.

Simons, F., Feldman, B. and Gerely, D. (1972) Granulomatous hepatitis in a patient receiving allopurinol. *Gastroenterology*, **62**, 101.

Smith, M.J.V. and Boyce, W.E. (1969) Allopurinol and urolithiasis. *J. Urol.*, **102**, 750.

Straitigos, J.D., Bartsokas, S.K. and Capetanakis, J. (1972) Further experiences with toxic epidermal necrolysis incriminating allopurinol, pyrazolone and derivatives. *Br. J. Dermatol.*, **86**, 564.

Swank, L.E., Chejfec, G. and Nemchansky, B. (1978) Allopurinol-induced granulomatous hepatitis with cholangitis and a sarcoid-like reaction. *Arch. Int. Med.*, **138**, 997.

Tjandramaga, T.B. and Cucinell, S.A. (1971) Interaction of probenecid and allopurinol in gouty subjects. *Fed. Proc.*, **30**, 392 (Abstract 1112).

Vessell, E.S., Passananti, G.T. and Greene, F.E. (1970) Impairment of drug metabolism in man by allopurinol and nortriptyline. *N. Engl. J. Med.*, **283**, 1484.

Watts, R.W.E., Scott, J.T., Chalmers, R.A. *et al.* (1971) Microscopic studies on skeletal muscle in gout patients treated with allopurinol. *Q. J. Med.*, New Ser., **40**, 1.

Wyngaarden, J.B., Rundles, R.W. and Metz, E.N. (1965) Allopurinol in the treatment of gout. *Ann. Int. Med.*, **62**, 842.

Yu. T.-F. (1965) The effect of allopurinol in primary and secondary gout. *Arthr. Rheum.*, **8**, 907.

Infectious arthritis

Aidem, H.P. (1968) Intra-articular amphotericin B in the treatment of coccidoidal synovitis of the knee. *J. Bone Joint Surg.*, **50A**, 1663.

Argen, R.J., Wilson, C.H. and Wood, P. (1966) Suppurative arthritis: clinical features of 42 cases. *Arch. Int. Med.*, **117**, 661.

Baciocco, E.A. and Iles, R.L. (1971) Ampicillin and kanamycin concentrations in joint fluid. *Clin. Pharmacol. Ther.*, **12**, 858.

Bardenheier, J.A., Morgan, H.C. and Stamp, W.G. (1966) Treatment and sequelae of experimentally produced septic arthritis. *Surg. Gynecol. Obstet.*, **122**, 249.

Bryant, R.E. and Hammond, D. (1974) Interaction of purulent material with antibiotics used to treat *Pseudomonas* infections. *Antimicrobial Agents Chemother.*, **6**, 702.

Chow, A., Hecht, R. and Winters, R. (1971) Gentamicin and carbenicillin penetration into the septic joint. *N. Engl. J. Med.*, **285**, 178.

Chartier, Y., Martin, W.J. and Kelley, P.J. (1959) Bacterial arthritis: experiences in the treatment of 77 patients. *Ann. Int. Med.*, **50**, 1462.

Clarke, J.T. (1978) in *Clinics in the Rheumatic Diseases* (ed. F.R. Schmid), Vol. **4**, No. 1, Saunders, London, p. 133.

Deodhar, S.D., Russel, F., Dick, W.C. *et al.* (1972) Penetration of lincomycin ('Lincocin') and clindamycin ('Dalacin C') into the synovial cavity in rheumatoid arthritis. *Curr. Med. Res. Op.*, **1**, 108.

Drutz, D.J., Schaffner, W., Hillman, J.W. and Koenig, M.G. (1967) The penetration of penicillin and other antimicrobials into joint fluid. *J. Bone Joint Surg.*, **49A**, 1415.

Feigin, R.D., Pickering, L.K., Anderson, D. *et al.* (1975) Clindamycin treatment of osteomyelitis and septic arthritis in children. *Pediatrics*, **55**, 213.

Florey, M.E. and Heatley, N.G. (1945) Systemic administration of penicillin. *Lancet*, **i**, 748.

Garrod, L.P. and O'Grady, F. (1972) *Antibiotic and Chemotherapy*, 3rd edn, Williams and Wilkins, Baltimore, pp. 1–499.

Gilbaldi, M. and Schwartz, M.A. (1968) Apparent effect of probenecid on the distribution of penicillins in man. *Clin. Pharmacol. Ther.*, **9**, 345.

Goldenberg, D.D., Brandt, K.D., Cohen, A.S. and Cathcart, E.S. (1975) Treatment of septic arthritis. *Arthr. Rheum.*, **18**, 83.

Herrell, W.E., Nichols, D.R. and Heilman, D.H. (1944) Penicillin. *J. Am. Med. Assoc.*, **125**, 1003.

Howell, A., Sutherland, R. and Rolinson, G.N. (1972) Effect of protein binding on levels of ampicillin and cloxacillin in synovial fluid. *Clin. Pharmacol. Ther.*, **13**, 724.

Jocson, C.T. (1955) The diffusion of antibiotics through the synovial membrane. *J. Bone Joint Surg.*, **37A**, 107.

Kauffman, C.A., Carleton, J.A. and Frame, P.T. (1976) Simple assay for 5-fluorocytosine in the presence of amphotericin B. *Antimicrob. Agents Chemother.*, **9**, 381.

Kind, A.C., Beaty, H.N., Fenster, L.F. and Kirby, W.M.M. (1968) Inactivation of penicillins by the isolated rat liver. *J. Lab. Clin. Med.*, **70**, 728.

Kirby, W.M.M. and Petersdorf, R.G. (1977) in *Harrison's Principles of Internal Medicine* (eds G.W. Thorn, R.D. Adams, E. Braunwald *et al.*, 8th edn, McGraw-Hill, New York, pp. 775–89.

Marsh, D.C., Matthew, E.B. and Persellin, R.H. (1974) Transport of gentamicin into synovial fluid. *J. Am. Med. Assoc.*, **228**, 607.

McLaughlin, J.E. and Reeves, D.S. (1971) Clinical and laboratory evidence for inactivation of gentamicin by carbenicillin. *Lancet*, **i**, 261.

Nelson, J.D. (1971) Antibiotic concentrations in septic joint effusions. *N. Engl. J. Med.*, **284**, 349.

Nelson, J.D. (1972) The bacterial etiology and antibiotic management of septic arthritis in infants and children. *Pediatrics*, **50**, 437.

Nelson, J.D. (1975) Septic arthritis: antibiotic management. *Forum Infect.*, **1**, 1.

Newman, J.H. (1976) Review of septic arthritis throughout the antibiotic era. *Ann. Rheum. Dis.*, **35**, 198.

Parker, R.H. and Schmid, F.R. (1971) Antibacterial activity of synovial fluid during therapy of septic arthritis. *Arthr. Rheum.*, **14**, 96.

Parker, R.H., Birbara, C. and Schmid, F.R. (1976) Passage of nafcillin and ampicillin into synovial fluid. *Zentralblatt für Bakteriologie, Parasitenkunde, Infektionskrankheiten und Hygiene*, **1** (Suppl. 5), 1115.

Plott, M.A. and Roth, H. (1970) Penetration of clindamycin into synovial fluid. *Clin. Pharmacol. Ther.*, **11**, 577.

Sanders, W.E. (1976) Rifampin. *Ann. Int. Med.*, **85**, 82.

Weinstein, L. (1970) in *The Pharmacological Basis of Therapeutics* (eds L.S. Goodman and A. Gilman), 4th edn, Macmillan, New York, pp. 1154–1343.

Viek, P. (1962) in *Antimicrobial Agents and Chemotherapy (1962)* (*Proceedings 2nd Interscience Conference on Antimicrobial Agents and Chemotherapy*), American Society for Microbiology, Ann. Arbor, Michigan (1963), pp. 379–83.

Viek, P. and Santangelo, S.C. (1962) Pyarthrosis: a surgical emergency. *J. Intl. Coll. Surg.*, **37**, 88.

Paget's Disease

Doyle, F.H., Pennock, J., Greenberg, P.B. *et al.* (1974) Radiological evidence of a dose-related response to long-term treatment of Paget's disease with human calcitonin. *Br. J. Radiol.*, **47**, 1.

Grimaldi, P.M.G.B., Mohamedally, S.M. and Woodhouse, N.J.Y. (1975) Deafness in Paget's disease: effect of salmon calcitonin treatment. *Br. Med. J.*, **ii**, 726.

Kanis, J.A., Horn, D.B., Scott, R.D.M. and Strong, J.A. (1974) Treatment of Paget's disease of bone with synthetic salmon calcitonin. *Br. Med. J.*, **iii**, 727.

Moffatt, W.H., Morrow, J.D. and Simpson, N. (1974) Effect of calcitonin therapy in deafness associated with Paget's disease of bone. *Br. Med. J.*, **iv**, 203.

Raisz, L.G., An, W.Y.W. and Freidman, J. (1967) Thyrocalcitonin and bone resorption. Studies employing a tissue culture bioassay. *Am. J. Med.*, **43**, 684.

Rojanasathit, S., Rosenberg, E. and Haddad, J.G. (1974) Paget's bone disease: response to human calcitonin in patients resistant to salmon calcitonin. *Lancet*, **ii**, 1412.

De Rose, J., Singer, F.R., Avramides, A. *et al.* (1974) Response of Paget's disease to porcine and salmon calcitonins. *Am. J. Med.*, **56**, 858.

Russell, A.S. and Lentle, B.C. (1974) Mithramycin therapy in Paget's disease. *Can. Med. Assoc. J.*, **110**, 397.

Russell, R.G.G., Smith, R., Preston, C. *et al.* (1974) Diphosphonates in Paget's disease. *Lancet*, **i**, 894.

Shai, F., Baker, R.K. and Wallach, S. (1971) The clinical and metabolic effects of porcine calcitonin on Paget's disease of bone. *J. Clin. Invest.*, **50**, 1927.

Singer, F.R., Aldred, J.P., Neer, R.M. *et al.* (1972) An

evaluation of antibodies and clinical resistance to salmon calcitonin. *J. Clin. Invest.*, **51**, 2331.

Woodhouse, N.J.Y., Reinder, M., Bordier, P. *et al.* (1971) Human calcitonin in the treatment of Paget's bone disease.

Lancet, **i**, 1139.

Woodhouse, N.J.Y. (1974) Clinical applications of calcitonin. *Br. J. Hosp. Med.*, **11**, 677.

6.10 APPENDICES

6.10.1 Gold: therapeutic studies

Author(s)	Date	Disorder	Author(s)	Date	Disorder
Pick	1927	Established rheumatoid arthritis	Research Sub-committee of the ERC	1961	Established rheumatoid arthritis
Forestier	1935	Established rheumatoid arthritis	Hicks *et al.*	1970	Juvenile rheumatoid arthritis
Hartfall *et al.*	1937	Established rheumatoid arthritis	Hanson *et al.*	1971	Juvenile rheumatoid arthritis
Key *et al.*	1939	Established rheumatoid arthritis	Hashimoto *et al.*	1972	Established rheumatoid arthritis
Ellman *et al.*	1940	Established rheumatoid arthritis	Co-operating Clinics of ARA	1973	Established rheumatoid arthritis
Sundelin	1941	Established rheumatoid arthritis	Lorber *et al.*	1973	Established rheumatoid arthritis
Cecil *et al.*	1942	Established rheumatoid arthritis	Currey *et al.*	1974	Established rheumatoid arthritis
Freyberg *et al.*	1942	Established rheumatoid arthritis	Huskisson *et al.*	1974	Established rheumatoid arthritis
Grahame and Fletcher	1943	Established rheumatoid arthritis	Sigler *et al.*	1974	Established rheumatoid arthritis
Price and Leichtentritt	1943	Established rheumatoid arthritis	Bluhm	1975	Established rheumatoid arthritis
Rawls *et al.*	1944	Established rheumatoid arthritis	Cats	1976	Established rheumatoid arthritis
Cohen *et al.*	1945	Established rheumatoid arthritis	Rothermich *et al.*	1976	Established rheumatoid arthritis
Fraser	1945	Established rheumatoid arthritis	Luukkainen *et al.*	1977a	Established rheumatoid arthritis
Cecil	1946	Established rheumatoid arthritis	Luukkainen *et al.*	1977b	Established rheumatoid arthritis
Browning *et al.*	1947	Established rheumatoid arthritis	Dorwart *et al.*	1978	Psoriatic arthritis
Waine *et al.*	1947	Established rheumatoid arthritis	Griffin *et al.*	1978	Established rheumatoid arthritis
Adams and Cecil	1950	Early rheumatoid arthritis	Luukkainen *et al.*	1978	Early rheumatoid arthritis
Snorrason	1952	Established rheumatoid arthritis	Mäkisara *et al.*	1978	Early rheumatoid arthritis
Lockie *et al.*	1958	Established rheumatoid arthritis	Rothermich *et al.*	1979	Established rheumatoid arthritis
Smith *et al.*	1958	Established rheumatoid arthritis	Srinavasan *et al.*	1979	Established rheumatoid arthritis
Empire Rheumatism Council	1960	Established rheumatoid arthritis	Richter *et al.*	1980	Psoriatic arthritis
Empire Rheumatism Council	1961	Established rheumatoid arthritis	Griffin *et al.*	1981	Established rheumatoid arthritis

6.10.2 Gold: side effects

Author(s)	Date	Toxic effect	Author(s)	Date	Toxic effect
Mettier *et al.*	1948	Thrombocytopenia	Penneys *et al.*	1974	Dermatitis
McCarty *et al.*	1962	Aplastic anaemia	Törnroth and	1974	Membranous
Denman and	1968	Hypersensitivity	Skrifvars		glomerulonephritis
Denman			Klinefelter	1975	Mucocutaneous reactions
Stavem and	1968	Thrombocytopenia	Siegman-Ingra	1976	Colitis
Stromme			*et al.*		
Austad	1970	Hypersensitivity	Winterbauer	1976	Diffuse pulmonary
Silverberg *et al.*	1970	Nephropathy	*et al.*		injury
Vaamonde and	1970	Nephrotic syndrome	Skrifvars *et al.*	1977	Immune-complex
Hunt					nephritis
Davis *et al.*	1973	Hypersensitivity	Tannenbaun and	1977	Intrahepatic
Gowans and	1973	Leukopenia	Favreau		cholestasis
Salami			Harth *et al.*	1978	Thrombocytopenia
Davis and	1974	Eosinophilia	Jalava *et al.*	1979	Pulmonary reactions
Hughes			Williams *et al.*	1979	Hypersensitivity
Deren *et al.*	1974	Thrombocytopenia			

6.10.3 Antimalarials: therapeutic studies

Author(s)	Year	Disorder (with relevant drug in parenthesis)	Author(s)	Year	Disorder (with relevant drug in parenthesis)
Page	1951	Systemic lupus erythematosus (mepacrine)	Logan *et al.*	1961	Rheumatoid arthritis (hydroxychloroquine)
Freedman and Bach	1952	Rheumatoid arthritis (chloroquine)	Popert *et al.*	1961	Rheumatoid arthritis (chloroquine diphosphate)
Haydu	1953	Rheumatoid arthritis (chloroquine diphosphate)	Ryckewaert *et al.*	1961	Rheumatoid arthritis (hydroxychloroquine)
Freedman	1956	Rheumatoid arthritis (mepacrine)	Scherbel	1961	Rheumatoid arthritis (4-aminoquinoline compounds)
Bagnall	1957	Rheumatoid arthritis (chloroquine)	Winkelmann *et al.*	1961	Systemic lupus erythematosus (antimalarials)
Cohen and Calkins	1958	Rheumatoid arthritis (chloroquine)	Hamilton and Scott	1962	Rheumatoid arthritis (hydroxychloroquine sulphate)
Scherbel *et al.*	1958	Rheumatoid arthritis (4-aminoquinoline compounds)	Mainland and Sutcliffe	1962	Rheumatoid arthritis (hydroxychloroquine sulphate)
Kersley and Palin	1959	Rheumatoid arthritis (amodiaquine and hydroxychloroquine)	Scull	1962	Rheumatoid arthritis (chloroquine and hydroxy-chloroquine)
Young	1959	Rheumatoid arthritis (chloroquine phosphate)			
Epstein	1960	Systemic lupus erythematosus (mepacrine)	Bartholomew and Duff	1963	Rheumatoid arthritis (amopyroquin)
Freedman and Steinberg	1960	Rheumatoid arthritis (chloroquine)	Elkington and Huth	1965	Rheumatoid arthritis (chloroquine)
Keruzore *et al.*	1960	Rheumatoid arthritis (chloroquine and hydroxychoroquine)	Knox and Owens	1966	Rheumatoid arthritis (chloroquine)
			Zvaifler	1968	Rheumatoid arthritis (antimalarials)

Appendix 6.10.3 (*Contd.*)

Author(s)	Year	Disorder (with relevant drug in parenthesis)	Author(s)	Year	Disorder (with relevant drug in parenthesis)
Mackenzie	1970	Rheumatoid arthritis (chloroquine)	Kirsner *et al.*	1979	Rheumatoid arthritis (antimalarials)
Panayi *et al.*	1973	Rheumatoid arthritis (chloroquine phosphate)	Marks and Power	1979	Rheumatoid arthritis (chloroquine)
Laaksonen *et al.*	1974	Juvenile rheumatoid arthritis and systemic lupus erythematosus (antimalarials)	Rosenbaum	1979	Rheumatoid arthritis (chloroquine and hydroxychloroquine)
			Mackenzie and Scherbel	1980	Rheumatoid arthritis (chloroquine and hydroxychloroquine)
Scherbel *et al.*	1975	Rheumatoid arthritis (hydroxychloroquine sulphate and chloroquine phosphate)	Lanham and Hughes	1981	Rheumatoid arthritis (hydroxychloroquine and chloroquine phosphate)
Popert	1976	Rheumatoid arthritis (chloroquine)			
Wollheim *et al.*	1978	Rheumatoid arthritis (chloroquine)			

6.10.4 Antimalarials: side effects

Author(s)	Date	Feature (observed in adults unless indicated otherwise)	Author(s)	Date	Feature (observed in adults unless indicated otherwise)
Alving *et al.*	1948	General	Hart and Naunton	1964	Fetal ototoxicity and other CNS effects
Berggren and Rendahl	1955	Amblyopia	Henkind *et al.*	1964	Retinopathy
Shaffer *et al.*	1958	Skin deposition of drug	Markowitz and McGinley	1964	Poisoning in a child
Dall and Keane	1959	Skin deposition of drug	Nozik *et al.*	1964	Ocular toxicity
Hobbs *et al.*	1959	Retinopathy	Rottermich	1964	General
Sternberg and Laden	1959	Retinopathy	Wetterholm and Winter	1964	Retinopathy
Cann and Verhulst	1961	Poisoning in children	Buter	1965	Retinopathy
			Kolb	1965	Retinopathy
Arden *et al.*	1962	Retinopathy	Scherbel *et al.*	1965	Retinopathy
Sachs *et al.*	1962	Retinopathy	Arden and Kolb	1966	Retinopathy
Schmidt and Muller-Limmroth	1962	Retinopathy	Burns	1966	Retinopathy
Bernstein *et al.*	1963	Retinopathy	Carr *et al.*	1966	Retinopathy
			Millingen and Suerth	1966	Neuromyopathy
Elenius and Mantyjarvi	1963	Retinopathy	Nylander	1966	Ocular toxicity
Okun *et al.*	1963	Retinopathy	Potts	1966	Retinopathy
Tuffanelli *et al.*	1963	Pigmentation	Voipio	1966	Retinopathy
			Bernstein	1967	Ocular toxicity
Crews	1964	Retinopathy	Kurtz *et al.*	1967	Retinopathy in experimental animals
Editorial	1964	Ocular toxicity			
Francois and Mandgal	1964	Retinopathy	Shearer and Dubois	1967	Ocular toxicity

Appendix 6.10.4 (*Contd.*)

Author(s)	Date	Feature (observed in adults unless indicated otherwise)	Author(s)	Date	Feature (observed in adults unless indicated otherwise)
Carr *et al.*	1968	Ocular toxicity	Herxheimer	1971	Ocular toxicity in the fetus
Mackenzie and Scherbel	1968	General	Vartanian and Chinyanga	1972	Neuromyopathy
Mackenzie and Szilagyi	1968	Retinopathy	Young *et al.*	1972	Retinopathy
Matz and Naunton	1968	Ototoxicity	Neill *et al.*	1973	Chromosomal damage
			Di Maio and Henry	1974	Poisoning
Peroival and Meanock	1968	Ophthalmological safety	Gonasun and Potts	1974	Retinopathy
Mackenzie and Scherbel	1969	General	Petrohelos	1974	Ocular toxicity
Percival and Behrman	1969	Opthalmological safety	Weise and Yannuzzi	1974	Ocular toxicity
Gregory *et al.*	1970	Retinopathy	Elman *et al.*	1976	Ocular toxicity
Lindquist *et al.*	1970	Retinopathy in the fetus	Good and Shader	1977	Behavioural changes
Rubin and Thomas	1970	Diplopia and loss of accommodation	Mason	1977	Ocular toxicity
			Argov and Mastaglia	1979	Neutromyopathy
Sassman *et al.*	1970	Retinopathy	Rynes *et al.*	1979	Ophthalmological safety
Robinson *et al.*	1970	Poisoning			
Annotation	1971	Myopathy			

6.10.5 Penicillamine: therapeutic studies

Author(s)	Date	Disorder	Author(s)	Date	Disorder
Jaffe	1964	Rheumatoid vasculitis	Multicentre Trial Group	1973	Rheumatoid arthritis
Harris and Sjoerdsma	1966	Systemic sclerosis	Day *et al.*	1974	Rheumatoid arthritis
Lorber	1966	Rheumatoid lung disease	Herbert *et al.*	1974	Systemic sclerosis
			Hill	1974	Rheumatoid arthritis
Fulgham and Katz	1968	Systemic sclerosis	Huskisson *et al.*	1974	Rheumatoid arthritis
Golding	1968	Rheumatoid arthritis	Jaffe *et al.*	1974	Antiviral effect
Jaffe and Smith	1968	Rheumatoid vasculitis	Loddo and Moriciaty	1974	Antiviral effect
Davis	1969	Gold dermatitis	Dixon *et al.*	1975	Rheumatoid arthritis
Bluestone *et al.*	1970	Systemic sclerosis	Jaffe	1975a	Rheumatoid arthritis
Golding *et al.*	1970	Rheumatoid arthritis	Jaffe	1975b	Rheumatoid arthritis
Jaffe	1970	Rheumatoid vasculitis	Leading article	1975	Rheumatoid arthritis
Zuckner *et al.*	1970	Rheumatoid arthritis	Leca and Camus	1975	Ankylosing spondylitis
Camus *et al.*	1971	Rheumatoid arthritis			
Lievre *et al.*	1971	Rheumatoid arthritis	Berry *et al.*	1976	Rheumatoid arthritis
Huskisson and Hart	1972	Rheumatoid arthritis	Gibson *et al.*	1976	Rheumatoid arthritis
			Golding	1976	Ankylosing spondylitis Colitic arthritis Psoriatic arthritis
Liyanage and Currey	1972	Adjuvant arthritis in rats			
Schrader *et al.*	1972	Polymyositis	Huskisson	1976b	Palindromic rheumatism
Annotation	1973	Rheumatoid arthritis	Schairer and Stoeber	1976	Juvenile rheumatoid arthritis
Lyle	1973	Rheumatoid arthritis			

Appendix 6.10.5 (*Contd.*)

Author(s)	Date	Disorder	Author(s)	Date	Disorder
Ansell and Simpson	1977	Juvenile chronic polyarthritis	Jaffe	1977	Rheumatoid arthritis
			Jayson *et al.*	1977	Systemic sclerosis
			Tio	1977	Systemic sclerosis
Dippy	1977	Rheumatoid arthritis	Zilko *et al.*	1977	Rheumatoid arthritis
Evans	1977	Rheumatoid coalworkers' pneumoconiosis	Berry *et al.*	1978	Rheumatoid arthritis
			Hill and Hill	1978	Rheumatoid arthritis
Golding *et al.*	1977	Rheumatoid arthritis	Hill *et al.*	1979	Rheumatoid arthritis
Hill	1977	Rheumatoid arthritis			

6.10.6 Penicillamine: side effects

Author(s)	Date	Effect	Author(s)	Date	Effect
Henkin *et al.*	1967	Decreased taste	Bacon *et al.*	1976	Nephropathy
Grossman	1968	Decreased taste	Dische *et al.*	1976	Nephropathy
Jaffe	1968b	Nephropathy Decreased taste	Eastmond	1976	Diffuse alveolitis
Keiser *et al.*	1968	Decreased taste	Harris	1976	Leukaemia-like appearance in mice
Morris *et al.*	1969	Defective wound healing	Harrison and		
Mjø Lnerød	1971	Congenital defects	Hickman	1976	Haemolytic anaemia
Nimni *et al.*	1972	Inhibition of collagen cross linking	Ansell *et al.*	1977	Defective wound healing
			Bucknall	1977	Myasthenia
Oliver *et al.*	1972	Lupus-like syndrome	Davison *et al.*	1977	Nephropathy
Tisman *et al.*	1972	Inhibition of bone marrow, DNA and protein synthesis	Fernandes *et al.*	1977	Dermatomyositis
			Hjalmarson *et al.*	1977	IgA deficiency
			Nimni	1977	Collagen defect
Pass *et al.*	1973	Elastosis perforans serpiginosa	Soloman *et al.*	1977	Congenital defects
			Appelbaum *et al.*	1978	Cutaneous lupus
Harvey *et al.*	1974	Changes in skin elasticity and thickness	Barzilai *et al.*	1978	Cholestatic jaundice
			Halverson *et al.*	1978	General effects
Lyle	1974	Peptic ulceration	Rosenbaum *et al.*	1980	Hepatotoxicity
Bucknall *et al.*	1975	Myasthenia			

6.10.7 Azathioprine: therapeutic studies

Author(s)	Date	Disorder	Author(s)	Date	Disorder
Dodson *et al.*	1968	Rheumatoid arthritis	Levy *et al.*	1972	Rheumatoid arthritis
Kersley	1969	Rheumatoid arthritis	Khanna and Woodbury	1973	Rheumatoid arthritis
Mason *et al.*	1969	Rheumatoid arthritis	Urowitz *et al.*	1973	Rheumatoid arthritis
Dale	1970	Juvenile rheumatoid arthritis	Currey *et al.*	1974	Rheumatoid arthritis
Drinkard *et al.*	1970	Lupus nephritis	Ginzler *et al.*	1975	Systemic lupus erythematosus
Harris *et al.*	1971	Rheumatoid arthritis			
Dale	1972	Juvenile rheumatoid arthritis	Hunter *et al.*	1975	Rheumatoid arthritis
			Dwosh *et al.*	1977	Rheumatoid arthritis

6.10.8 Colchicine: therapeutic studies

Author(s)	Date	Disorder	Author(s)	Date	Disorder
Cohen	1936	Gout prophylaxis	McCarty	1963	Gout and pseudogout
Talbott and Cooms	1938	Gout prophylaxis	Gutman	1965	Gout prophylaxis
Davis and			Wallace *et al.*	1967	Acute gout (oral)
Bartfield	1954	Acute gout	Blomgren	1972	Erythema nodosum
Yu and Gutman	1961	Gout prophylaxis	Goldfinger	1972	Familial Mediterranean fever
Zuckner	1962	Rheumatoid arthritis	Paulus *et al.*	1974	Gout prophylaxis
Kaplan	1963	Sarcoid arthritis			

7
Local injection therapy

7.1 INTRODUCTORY COMMENT

Soon after the introduction of systemic corticosteroids Thorn (cited by Hollander, 1972) injected 10 mg hydrocortisone into a knee joint affected by rheumatoid arthritis with local and systemic benefit. However, the procedure did not become established until some years later when Hollander and colleagues (1951a, b) reported their findings from the University of Pennsylvania. These early findings, which demonstrated the efficacy of intra-articular injections, were further substantiated by a report a decade later (Hollander *et al.*, 1961) based on the injection of joints, bursae and tendon sheaths in a series of 4000 patients.

On the basis of Hollander's initial observations and those of his colleague (McCarty, 1972), who showed that long-lasting remissions could result from long-lasting preparations such as triamcinolone hexacetonide, the present-day practice of injection therapy for rheumatic disorders has become a routine approach in the rheumatologist's armamentarium. The treatment proved particularly useful as an adjunct to other therapeutic methods in overall management of the non-infective inflammatory arthritides (particularly rheumatoid arthritis), although in these conditions it is at best no more than a temporary palliative. However, as will be indicated later, with regard to certain soft-tissue lesions the effect may be 'curative', particularly if trauma is the triggering factor.

7.2 INJECTABLE DRUGS

7.2.1 Corticosteroids

Hydrocortisone acetate, the first intra-articular corticosteroid, is still widely used and is inexpensive. However, several other preparations are now available (Table 7.1), and these vary in potency, durability of action, solubility and cost.

Few comparative trials have been done to assess differences in efficacy and duration of action of the various injectable corticosteroid preparations, and much of present-day usage is based on personal experience. However, there is some evidence (Hollander *et al.* 1961; McCarty, 1972) that the less soluble triamcinolone hexacetonide produces the most potent and long-lasting anti-inflammatory effect.

The exact mode of action of locally injected corticosteroids is still unknown although their primary action is to suppress the local inflammatory response, whether this be in soft tissues or in the synovium.

Some clinicians prefer to mix the corticosteroid preparation with a local anaesthetic agent, partly for the anaesthetic effect, and partly to dilute a concentrated suspension to reduce the risk of soft-tissue atrophy when injecting small joints and tendons. However, care should be taken to avoid local anaesthetic agents containing preservatives (e.g. methylparaben, propylparaben, phenol) as these compounds may cause

Table 7.1 Some corticosteroid preparations used in injection therapy (after Dixon and Graber, 1978–1980)

Approved name	Proprietary name and manufacturer	Presentation
	Less prolonged acting	
Hydrocortisone (as the acetate)	Hydrocortistab (Boots)	25 mg per ml in 5 ml vial or 2 ml ampoule
Prednisolone (as the acetate)	Deltacortril (Pfizer)	25 mg per ml in multidose vial
	Deltastab (Boots)	25 mg per ml in 5 ml vial
	Prolonged acting	
Prednisolone (as the tertiarybutyl acetate)	Codelcortone (Merck Sharp & Dohme)	20 mg per ml in 5 ml vial
Prednisolone (as the pivalate)	Ultracortenol (Ciba)	50 mg per ml in 1 ml ampoule
Methylprednisolone (as the acetate)	Depo–Medrone (Upjohn)	40 mg per ml in vials, pre-filled syringe
Triamcinolone (as the acetate)	Adcortyl (Squibb)	10 mg per ml in 1 ml ampoules and 5 ml vials
Triamcinolone (as the hexacetonide)	Lederspan (Lederle)	20 mg per ml or 5 mg per ml in 5 ml vial
Prednisolone (as the sodium phosphate)	Codelsol (Merck, Sharp & Dohme)	16 mg per ml in 2 ml vial
Dexamethasone (as the sodium phosphate)	Decadron (Merck Sharp & Dohme)	4 mg per ml in 2 ml vial
	Oradexon Injection (Organon)	5 mg in 1 ml ampoule or 8 mg in 2 ml ampoule
Betamethasone (as a suspension of the sodium phosphate and acetate)	Only available outside UK (e.g. USA, Australia, South Africa as Celestone)	Betamethasone sodium equivalent to 15 mg of betamethasone + 15 mg betamethasone acetate in 5 ml vial

flocculation of the steroid. (In the UK multi-dose vials of local anaesthetic usually contain preservative, indicated on the label, but ampoules do not.)

There is no general agreement about the optimal dose of steroid that should be injected into joints of various sizes, except that the dose should be adjusted to the size of the joint – larger joints being given a higher dose than smaller joints. The doses recommended for the various joints discussed in Section 7.5 are representative of general usage but not arrived at from objective evaluation.

7.2.2 Other drugs

In view of the encouraging though relatively short-lived effect of intra-articular steroids, several other drugs have been assessed in the hope of finding a superior drug for injectable use, but so far this goal has not been attained. Salicylates were found to be too irritative (cited by Hollander, 1979) and phenylbutazone produced decreased inflammation, but only after a severe initial reaction (Neustadt and Steinbrocker, 1956). In the hope of securing a 'medical' or 'chemical synovectomy' cytotoxic agents have been injected into joints. Both nitrogen mustard (Scherbel *et al.*, 1957; Henderson and Nathan, 1969) and Thiotepa (triethylene thiophosphoramide) Flatt, 1962; Wenley and Glick, 1964; Currey, 1965) showed inflammatory suppression effects, but the

benefits were relatively short-lived and were accompanied by an initial irritant reaction. Osmic acid as an alternative agent for establishing medical synovectomy has enjoyed some popularity in recent years, notably in Scandinavia. Enthusiasm for this agent stems from its relatively non-irritant effect on the joint (Berglöf, 1959; Hurri *et al.*, 1963; Collan *et al.*, 1971; Martio *et al.*, 1972; Anttinen and Oka, 1975). Although definite long-term benefits have been noted, these have been inconsistent and side effects have included chills, fever and evidence of liver damage. 'Radiation synovectomy' has been the most recent approach, particularly for severe and chronic knee synovitis (Muller, 1962; Loevinger *et al.*, 1965; Cohen, 1970; Ingrand, 1973; Gumpel, 1973, 1974). Both radioactive gold, [198]Au (Ansell *et al.*, 1963; Makin and Robin, 1964) and radioactive yttrium, [90]Y (Oka *et al.*, 1971; Gumpel *et al.*, 1972; Rekonen *et al.*, 1972; Bayly *et al.*, 1973; Beer *et al.*, 1973; Gumpel and Stevenson, 1975) have been noted to provide reasonably long-term inflammatory suppression. The beta rays of radioactive yttrium penetrate deeper into the thickened synovium and for this reason is preferred by some workers. However, the use of radioactive isotopes for medical synovectomy is still not a universally accepted procedure, and when used is applied only to patients whose disease has been refractory to more conservative treatment. This cautious approach is all the more justified in view of disquieting reports concerning leakage from the injected joint and of danger of malignancy from such treatment (Bridgman *et al.*, 1971). To this may be added the danger and inconvenience associated with using radioactive materials.

In addition to the anti-inflammatory approach, attempts have been made to use substances as artificial lubricants in arthritic joints. So far lubricating agents (based on polymers and biopolymers) have shown disappointing results. For example, Wright *et al.* (1971), using dimethicone 300 in 40 osteoarthrotic knees, found saline to be more beneficial. Furthermore, a number of synovial reactions to the preparation were encountered. Vasilionkaitis and Matulis (1977) found more beneficial results, but no control data were reported.

At present, it would seem that for most clinicians corticosteroids remain the preferred agents for intra-articular anti-inflammatory therapy.

7.3 CLINICAL CONSIDERATIONS

7.3.1 Indications

The indications for injection therapy are as follows:

1. When one or only a few peripheral joints are inflamed.
2. When one or only a few peripheral joints are more inflamed than joints affected by more low-grade involvement.
3. When systemic therapy is contraindicated.
4. As an adjunct to systemic therapy for control of 'resistant' joints.
5. To assist mobilization and prevent deformity of joints in conjunction with a planned rehabilitation programme.
6. In certain non-articular disorders including: bursitis, tenosynovitis, 'trigger' areas, nerve entrapment syndromes.
7. Immediate analgesia.

Apart from the most frequent indication for local injection therapy – the active rheumatoid joint – the method has been readily applied to less common non-infective inflammatory arthritides. These include psoriatic arthritis, Reiter's disease, enteropathic arthropathies, ankylosing spondylitis, and juvenile chronic arthritis (see Section 7.3.3). The treatment may also be of value in pseudo-gout, in the acute phase of osteo-arthrosis, and in painful conditions due to trauma.

As stressed elsewhere, infected joints or joints in which there is a risk of infection should not be injected. Gout is not usually regarded as a clinical indication for injection therapy, although if there is no response to conventional treatment or if there is a sizeable effusion, immediate relief can be given by aspiration of the fluid (including examination for crystals) followed by intra-articular injection of a corticosteroid preparation. In these patients very special care should be taken to exclude infection as the cause of the 'hot' joint.

7.3.2 Contraindications

The relative contraindications to local injection therapy are:

1. Local infection (e.g. tuberculosis).
2. Hypersensitivity to the substance injected.
3. Bleeding diathesis.
4. Unstable joints.
5. Intra-articular fracture.
6. Essentially inaccessible joints.
7. Marked juxta-articular osteoporosis.
8. Failure to respond to previous injections.
9. Absence of a clear rationale for injection therapy.
10. Irreversible lesions which would be unlikely to respond.
11. Psychological factors may contraindicate injection therapy in view of a tendency for neurotic patients to become 'addicted' to this form of treatment.

7.3.3 Use in childhood arthritis

Local corticosteroid injections provide a useful means of regaining function in children with severe flexor tendon synovitis of the hands. Because patients are often young children needing multiple injections due to the widespread nature of the synovitis, these injections are best performed under general anaesthesia. This not only reduces the risk of performing an inaccurate injection, but is also less traumatic psychologically and physically in a child who is often frightened. For injection of a single flexor tendon sheath in an older child local anaesthesia is usually sufficient.

Other sites amenable to local injection in children are the knee, elbow and shoulder. The anxiety associated with the possibility of steroid-induced damage to the articular cartilage in children is offset by the benefits of such treatment in patients showing progressive deformity and markedly proliferative synovitis with only minimal radiological damage. In these patients Ansell (1980) recommends one injection of a long-lasting corticosteroid such as triamcinolone hexacetonide (20 mg for an elbow, 40 mg for a knee). If amelioration of symptoms does not occur the injection should not be repeated, but a surgical opinion sought. If relapse occurs after some months it is reasonable to consider a further injection after about 6 months. Local injection therapy is particularly indicated in children with pauci-articular arthritis, especially if growth problems exist.

The use of intra-articular osmic acid for the treatment of severe persistent synovitis of the knee in children has been used in Scandinavia, but is thought to have only a limited place in management (Martio *et al.*, 1972).

7.3.4 Advantages

The main benefits of local corticosteroid therapy are listed below. Some of these advantages relate purely to the arthrocentesis aspect of the procedure.

1. Synovial fluid for analysis can be obtained at the same time as injection of local corticosteroid.

2. Injections effectively reduce synovitis and relieve symptoms in most patients. In some patients the effect may last only a few days. The long-acting preparations have been shown to provide suppression of inflammation in some rheumatoid patients for over 12 months (McCarty, 1972). As with oral anti-inflammatory agents, responses between patients are very varied, and if one or two injections provide ineffective or give only transient relief it is unreasonable to persist injecting the same joint. As a 'bonus', distant joints may also benefit due to the systemic effect of the injected corticosteroid.

3. Musculoskeletal function is improved: contractures and muscular atrophy are prevented or reduced if already present, and joint laxity secondary to effusion is prevented.

4. Systemic therapy for a local problem is avoided.

5. Local injection therapy may be effectively used with other forms of therapy.

6. Local injection is associated with minimal serious toxicity/side effect/hazards.

7. The drainage of noxious fluids such as blood, pus or crystal-containing fluids usually results in immediate relief. The drainage of a 'non-specific' effusion, such as that of rheumatoid arthritis, will also relieve joint discomfort; this effect can be enhanced by irrigation, as has been shown during arthroscopy (Lindsay *et al.*, 1971; Bird and Ring, 1978).

8. Most articular and non-articular injection procedures are easy and safe to perform, and only minimal experience is needed.

9. Minimal supplies and special facilities are required and the materials are relatively inexpensive. The simplicity of the materials and method involved enables the procedure to be carried out in the patient's home.

7.3.5 Disadvantages

The main disadvantages of local corticosteroid injection are shown below. Some of these 'disadvantages' are more properly described as dangers or hazards.

1. Intra-articular injections, used adjunctively, provide only temporary relief. However, in certain soft-tissue inflammatory conditions, particularly where trauma is a precipitating factor, the disorder may be more or less permanently eradicated. (Patients should be warned that immediately after an injection a temporary return of symptoms may occur when the effect of the local anaesthetic has worn off.)

2. Apart from the risk of local osteoporosis corticosteroid injection therapy has been reported in association with destructive Charcot-like arthropathy (Chandler and Wright, 1958; Chandler *et al.*, 1959; Heinemann and Freiberger, 1960; Sweetman *et al.*, 1960; Hartnagel, 1962; Steinberg *et al.*, 1962; Boksenbaum and Mendelson, 1963; Miller and Restifo, 1966; Bentley and Goodfellow, 1969) and with tendinous (particularly the Achilles' tendon) and ligamentous rupture (Lee, 1957; Ismail *et al.*, 1969; Sweetman, 1969). The conditions predisposing to steroid-induced damage to the joint or soft tissues are still poorly understood, and there continue to be two schools of thought regarding the importance of the dangers involved in this type of therapy. Looking at the question optimistically, aseptic necrosis of the joint surface due to infarction of subchondral bone is known to occur in the hips and knees (and occasionally in other joints) of patients with severe rheumatoid arthritis who have never had corticosteroid therapy either by mouth or by local injection. Joint damage after local injection therapy may thus be coincidental, or perhaps reflects the relative increase in mobility of patients who would otherwise have become bedridden. On the other hand, McCarty and Hogan (1964) have shown in dogs that there is a migration of leucocytes into a joint after local corticosteroid injection and that the exudate was roughly proportional to the dose injected. The authors suggested that this may be a factor in increasing cartilage destruction. However, this has yet to be verified in human joints. Whatever the real significance of the damaging effects of local corticosteroids, it behoves the clinician to avoid undue frequency of injections. There is still no universal agreement as to what constitutes 'undue frequency', but an interval of 6 months between injections and avoidance of more than three injections into a single joint (particularly weight-bearing joints), as has been advocated by some clinicians, would seem to be a reasonable precaution, together with regular radiological assessment.

3. There is a risk, albeit a small one, of introducing infection into injected sites. However, the smallness of this risk has been stressed by Hollander (1979) who has reported an infection frequency of only 1 per 16 000 joint injections. This worker ascribed this low overall risk of infection to the use of disposable sterile needles and syringes – the frequency being significantly higher with boiled or autoclaved equipment.

There is also a danger of encouraging spread of infection in an already infected site. This risk is greatest when a blood-borne infection has established itself in a joint already damaged by arthritis (usually rheumatoid arthritis). These patients often show little or no sign of generalized systemic illness, and the features of bacteraemia may be further suppressed in patients treated with oral corticosteroids. The importance of microscopic examination and culture of aspirated fluid in such high-risk patients before injection of corticosteroid cannot be over stated. Often such joints feel more 'active' than neighbouring joints; the aspirated fluid often appears more opaque than usual and may be greenish and foul smelling.

4. There exists a theoretical risk of causing damage to articular cartilage by the sharp point of the needle. If this concern is a real one, it might be expected to be more significant in the hands of inexperienced practitioners who tend to advance the needle in a tentative, searching way, compared with the more confident 'single-strike' approach of the professional. (As with other intrusive bed-side procedures, there may be something to be said for encouraging the tyro to practise on a cadaver.)

5. Occasionally, local injection therapy is followed by a transient gout-like syndrome (McCarty and Hogan, 1964). This is a form of crystal synovitis due to the microcrystalline composition of some corticosteroid suspensions. The problem raises the question of post-injection sepsis in the doctor's mind, and in the patient's mind engenders some loss of confidence in a procedure that has worsened the condition. (The problem is best managed by administering a non-steroidal anti-inflammatory drug and applying a cold compress.) If the problem has not begun to settle within 24 hours, antibiotics should be started as an extra precaution.

6. Accidental encounters with nerves, vessels and viscera have been reported. A knowledge of normal anatomy, and of its many variants, is clearly a *sine qua non* to safe injection therapy.

7. Because a proportion of the injected material eventually enters the blood stream there is a possible risk of causing adrenocortical suppression. Although this risk is probably rarely, if ever of clinical significance, it should be borne in mind and checked with appropriate tests.

8. Hypersensitivity to injected material. This particularly applies to hyaluronidase, a foreign protein. This substance is added to the injection mixture by some workers to encourage more rapid spread of the corticosteroid when soft tissue areas are to be injected.

9. Intra-articular or soft-tissue haemorrhage. (The foot is particularly prone to post-injection bleeding, and it is useful to avoid dependency of the foot for a few minutes after the procedure.)

10. Leakage of the injected corticosteroid back along the needle track may cause atrophy of the overlying skin. This recedes with time.

11. Serious underlying disease, such as infection or malignancy may be marked.

12. Dependency may develop. This is most likely to occur in patients with a psychological perpetuation of symptoms.

13. Necessary surgery may be delayed.

14. Vaso-vagal syncope may occur and this tends to happen more often in the 'needle-shy'. Patients with a history of syncopal attacks associated with this or other injection procedures should be considered to be particularly at risk. If local injection therapy continues to be firmly indicated in such patients despite such a risk, maximal comfort should be provided by reassurance, local anaesthesia (spraying the skin with a refrigerant material followed by intradermal lignocaine) and if necessary sedation (e.g. intravenous diazepam, 5–10 mg).

15. A recent paper has reported two cases of separation of the metallic shaft of the hypodermic needle from its plastic hub when the needle was withdrawn after injection (Gottlieb, 1981). In each patient it was possible to extract the needle with artery forceps. A more troublesome complication has been reported during synovial biopsy of the knee during which the biopsy needles (Parker and Pearson, and Polly-Bickel) have fractured within the joint. In these cases the needle fragments could not be extracted by external manipulation and were either left in the joint cavity or removed by arthroscopy or arthrotomy (Guzman and Arinoviche, 1978; Bocanegra *et al.*, 1980).

7.4 METHODOLOGY

7.4.1 Materials

For injections to be carried out on the ward or in the clinic the various materials can be carried on a tray or trolley. For injections in the patient's home a portable case can be used (Fig. 7.1).

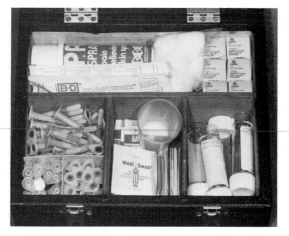

Fig. 7.1 Portable case for carrying injection materials; suitable for use on domiciliary visits.

Table 7.2 Some disposable needless* suitable for routine local injection therapy

Hub colour	Length	Bore	Use
Orange	$\frac{5}{8}$ in (15 mm)	25G	Raising skin wheal; Injecting small joints (e.g. IPs, MPs)
Orange	1 in (25 mm)	25G	
Blue	$1\frac{3}{16}$ in (30 mm)	23G	Injecting small and medium joints (e.g. MCPs, wrists, ankles)
Green	$1\frac{1}{2}$ in (40 mm)	21G	Injecting medium and large joints (e.g. wrists, elbows, shoulders, ankles, knees)
Cream	2 in (50 mm)	19G	Aspirating thick fluid (e.g. ganglion or cyst contents, inspissated knee effusions, pus etc.)

Wider gauges are available as disposable intravenous cannulae (Argyle/Medicut): effective length $1\frac{8}{10}$ in (45 mm) and bores of 18, 16 and 14G

* The disposable needles are manufactured by both Gillette and Becton, Dickinson, France, SA, and the cannulae by Sherwood Medical Industries.

The essential materials are as follows: (1) skin-cleansing agent (e.g. ether solvent or chlorhexidine in methylated spirit), and dry sterile swabs or preferably disposable swabs saturated with isopropyl alcohol (e.g. Medi Swabs, Steriswabs); (2) skin-freezing aerosol (e.g. P.R. Spray); (3) local anaesthetic (e.g. 1% lignocaine without adrenaline); (4) corticosteroid suspension (e.g. hydrocortisone acetate or triamcinolone hexacetonide); (5) a selection of disposable sterile needles (see Table 7.2); (6) a selection of disposable sterile syringes (2 ml syringe for injecting corticosteroid, 5 ml for injecting local anaesthetic or local anaesthetic/corticosteroid mixtures, and 10 ml or 20 ml for aspirating joint fluid); (7) a few gauze pads to check bleeding if necessary; (8) adhesive dressings (e.g. Band-Aids); (9)

culture tubes; (10) graduated container for measuring synovial fluid; (11) if the thumb nail is not preferred for marking the puncture site a suitable skin marker (e.g. ballpoint or felt-tip pen) should be included.

Sterile drapes and masks are optional and rubber gloves are not necessary.

Particularly for needle-shy patients or when multiple small joints are to be treated, a hypospray jet injector (Fig. 7.2(a)) may be used (Rankin and Good, 1966; Baum and Ziff, 1967).

For introducing painless intracutaneous wheals of local anaesthetic the less powerful Dermo-Jet (Fig. 7.2(b)) can be used (Steinbrocker and Neustadt, 1972), but a more convenient and much less costly expedient is to use a suitable skin-freezing aerosol (e.g. P.R. Spray).

7.4.2 Methodological principles

Local injection therapy consists of injecting painful soft-tissue structures, or synovial spaces such as a joint, tendon sheath or bursa. The general approach is similar whether solid or hollow structures are to be injected, with minor variations according to individual sites. However, confirmation that the needle has reached its target can be confirmed in the case of hollow structures lined by inflamed synovial tissue as often it is possible to aspirate fluid. This confirmation is less likely with small joints, and even in larger joints aspiration may be prevented for a number of reasons (see below). The ease with which fluid can be injected into the joint provides another valuable guide as to correct siting of the needle. For this reason it is best to confine one's experiences with injection therapy to only two or three needles and syringe sizes in order to develop the right 'feel'. This sensation involves the pressure required to depress the

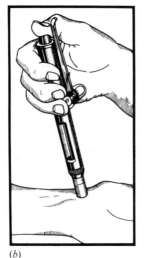

(a)   (b)

Fig. 7.2 (a) Hypospray jet injector; (b) Dermo-Jet.

plunger of the syringe and the rate at which the injected material flows through the needle.

Although a specific routine will now be outlined, it should be emphasized that there exists much variation between clinicians as to what is thought the optimal technique. For example, differences concerning the need for a local anaesthetic, the easiest and safest anatomical approach, the dosage and type of injected material, and the 'correct' dimensions of the needles needed for its delivery. Debate also exists regarding the maximal number and frequency of joint injections from the point of view of developing steroid arthropathy or other steroid-induced problems.

(a) Details of method

Before detailing the main stages involved in aspirating and injecting a joint it should be emphasized that an aseptic no-touch technique throughout the procedure is essential. Apart from the importance of thorough cleansing of the injection site mentioned below, the following points should be observed (Dixon and Graber, 1978):

1. Use only pre-packed sterilized disposable needles and syringes.

2. Use single-dose ampoules wherever available, especially for local anaesthetics.

3. Do not open any sterilized needle or syringe packs until the moment of use. Always use them direct from the pack and not from the tray or trolley via the nurse's hands.

4. Use domestically clean, *dry* hands. Formal 'scrubbing-up' is not necessary (wet hands may lead to drops running down the needle).

5. Do not guide the needle with the finger.

6. Warn the patient that he should not talk whilst the needle is exposed to the air, nor while the injection is being made. The observer should also practise what he preaches. If this rule is followed, wearing a face mask is unnecessary.

The main stages involved in aspirating and injecting a joint are as follows:

1. Choose the optimal site for inserting the needle and mark it either with a thumb nail or skin marker.

2. Cleanse the skin twice, preferably avoiding soapy solutions as these make the injection site slippery. Alcohol-containing solutions not only cleanse the skin but also ensure a dry field for injection.

3. Assess the need for local anaesthesia. Often this will not be necessary, as in the case of a large effusion in which joint puncture will be quick and easy. However, with this and all other procedures it is a kindness to the patient to numb the initial jab by freezing the skin with a suitable aerosol spray. If deeper and more prolonged anaesthesia is required 1% lignocaine (without adre-

naline) can be established after an initial skin wheal. The subcutaneous tissue and joint capsule can then be infiltrated with 2–4 ml of the solution. If a wide area is to be anaesthetized, a fan-wise technique of infiltration, using a series retractions and advances in different directions through the same puncture, can be used.

4. Insert the aspirating needle (21G usually sufficient) as quickly and confidently as possible through skin, subcutaneous tissue, capsule and synovial membrane. The necessary sleight of hand to achieve this takes a little time to acquire. Slow, ponderous, tentative advances of the needle increase the patient's discomfort, and deny the operator the correct tactile 'feedback'. For precision and delicateness of operation, the needle and syringe should be held as one would a pen or dart, rather than a grip in which the syringe rests in the palm of the hand. The tip of the needle should be freely movable if the joint space has been entered, and there may be painless grating as it encounters articular cartilage. If excess fluid is present it can then be aspirated. Distension of the synovial sac with fluid makes entry into the joint much easier than when there is no excess fluid – as one author has put it, the difference between puncturing an inflated and a deflated balloon (Copeman, 1979). Aspiration may be prevented by various factors which are summarized in Fig. 7.3. These include flaps of synovial tissue over the end of the needle creating a valve, intra-

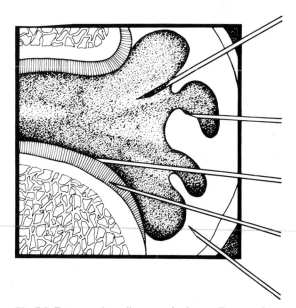

Fig. 7.3 Factors impeding aspiration. From above downwards – blockage of needle due to thickened synovial fluid, synovial flap over end of needle, tip of needle lying against articular cartilage, tip of needle embedded in articular cartilage, needle not in joint cavity.

Table 7.3 Synovial characteristics of various joint fluids (after Huskisson and Hart, 1975; and McCarty, 1979)

Feature	Normal	Non-inflammatory (e.g. osteoarthrosis, traumatic arthritis, osteochondritis dissecans, aseptic necrosis)	Inflammatory		
			Group I (e.g. rheumatoid arthritis, seronegative spondarthritides)	Group II Septic arthritis (e.g. bacterial infection, tuberculosis)	Group III Crystal synovitis (gout and pseudogout)
Volume in ml (knee)	< 4	Often > 4	Often > 4	Often > 4	Often > 4
Clarity	Clear	Clear	Often turbid	Turbid	Clear with flakes of fibrin
Colour	Clear/pale yellow	Yellow	Yellow/green	Brown/green	Yellow
Viscosity	Very high	High	Low	Very low (may be high with coagulase-positive staphylococcus)	Low
Clot formation (in heparinized fluid; avoid oxalated tubes)	No	No	Yes	Yes	Yes
Mucin clot* (supernatant of a centrifuged specimen)	Good	Fair to good	Poor to fair	Poor	Often poor
Approx. WBC count per mm³	< 150	< 3000	3–50 000	50–300 000	3–50 000
Predominant cell	Mononuclears	Mononuclears	Neutrophils	Neutrophils	Neutrophils
Crystal	No	No	No	No	Yes
Culture	Negative	Negative	Negative	Positive	Negative

* Recent effusions do not give a firm clot because of serum admixture.

articular debris, and excessive joint fluid viscosity. Blockages can usually be overcome by slight alterations in the position of the needle and/or re-injecting a little synovial fluid if some has already been aspirated. Failing this, re-puncture with a needle of wider bore may be necessary, particularly if it is felt that it is the thickness of the joint fluid that is causing the blockage. Aspiration may be facilitated by wrapping the joint, except for the site of joint puncture, with an elastic bandage to encourage the free fluid to pool into the portion of the sac to be punctured. The hand of the operator that is not supporting the needle and syringe can be used for the same purpose.

As much joint fluid as possible should be aspirated (although the value of aspiration to dryness has been questioned by some clinicians in view of the rapidity of its re-accumulation), and its physical characteristics noted (volume, colour, clarity, turbidity, blood-staining, viscosity). Some comparative details of joint-fluid differences in various disorders are summarized in Table 7.3, and further details of normal values are shown in Table 7.4. A specimen should be saved for laboratory use and divided as follows: (1) 2 ml in a tube containing EDTA for cell count and differential; (2) at least 1 ml in a sterile container for microscopy and culture – urgent Gram staining or special culture media should be requested if indicated; (3) a few drops are sufficient for examination as a wet film for crystals under polarized light.

5. Once aspiration has been completed, the aspirating syringe can be detached, leaving the needle *in situ* in the joint. A small syringe (2–5 ml for most purposes) is charged with the appropriate amount of corticosteroid suspension and then attached to the aspirating needle. The injection fluid should flow relatively freely if the needle is still in the correct place. If undue force on the

Table 7.4 Synovial fluid: some normal values (after Ropes and Bauer, 1953)

Feature	Range	Mean
pH	7·3–7·4	7·38
WBC/mm^3	13–180	63
Differential WBC (%):		
Polymorphonuclear	0–25	7
Lymphocytes	0–78	24
Monocytes	0–71	48
Clasmatocytes	0–26	10
Unclassified phagocytes	0–21	5
Synovial lining cells	0–12	4
Special cells (e.g. 'rheumatoid cells', 'LE cells', 'Rieter's cells')	0	
Erythrocytes	Absent, unless arthrocentesis traumatic	
Total protein (g/dl)	1·2–3·0	1·8
Albumin (%)	56–63	60
Globulin (%)	37–44	40
Hyaluronate (g/dl)		0·3
Fibrinogen	0	
Glucose ⎫ Non-protein nitrogen ⎬ Electrolytes ⎪ Uric acid ⎭	About the same as plasma	
Extracellular materials*	Absent	

* Extracellular materials may provide a useful clue to diagnosis, e.g. fibrillar materials (fibrin, cartilage fragments, shards of ochronotic cartilage); lipid droplets (traumatic arthritis, pancreatic fat necrosis, due to arthrocentesis); amorphous globular and irregular material (primary amyloidosis, multiple myeloma, Waldenström's macroglobulinaemia, hydroxyapatite aggregates); crystals (urate, calcium pyrophosphate); metal fragments (implant arthroplasty).

plunger is necessary the needle position should be readjusted. The suspension can be mixed with any remaining joint fluid by repeated withdrawal and re-injection (barbotage), although this is probably unnecessary.

6. The needle is then withdrawn and the injection site covered with a sterile dressing (Band-Aid). Reference has already been made to recent reports of separation of the needle shaft from the hub and of needle shaft fracture (Guzman and Arinoviche, 1978; Bocanegra *et al.*, 1980; Gottlieb, 1981). It is therefore important on withdrawing the needle to ensure that it is intact. Some bleeding may occur at the site of paracentesis due to puncture of small veins crossing the needle track. Firm pressure with a sterile swab for half a minute or so is usually sufficient to establish haemostasis.

7. Dispose of needles and syringes safely.

8. Carefully label all specimens and ensure they are dispatched to the laboratory without delay, together with an adequately filled-in form providing essential clinical details.

9. If much fluid has been aspirated from a weight-bearing joint, it is often advisable to apply an elastic bandage.

10. Joint immobilization after the injection has a steroid-potentiating effect, particularly evident when the longer acting, less-soluble crystal preparations are used. This is based on studies which have shown that the exit of material from joint cavities can be considerably slowed if the joint is splinted or rested, and increased by exercise and use of the joint. It is probably unnecessary to immobilize joints completely, but it would seem reasonable to advise against repetitive or power movements of the injected joint for 24 hours or so.

7.5 INJECTION OF SPECIFIC STRUCTURES/LESIONS

7.5.1 Head, neck and trunk

(a) Temporomandibular joint

Indications. Rheumatoid arthritis and occasionally other inflammatory arthritides such as juvenile chronic polyarthritis, ankylosing spondylitis, and psoriatic arthritis.

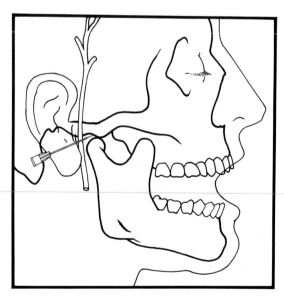

Fig. 7.4 Injection of temporomandibular joint. Note position of superficial temporal artery which is palpable somewhat posterior to the puncture site.

Technique. The patient is asked to relax in the sitting or the reclining position, with the head supported. The joint line (ascertained by asking the patient to move the lower jaw) is marked and the injection site, just below the zygomatic arch, about half an inch (1.3 cm) anterior to the tragus of the ear (Fig. 7.4) is infiltrated with 1% lignocaine before injecting 10 mg hydrocortisone acetate (or 2.5 mg triamcinolone hexacetonide), mixed with a little lignocaine, via a 23 gauge (G) injection needle $1\frac{3}{16}$ in long. The needle should be carried inwards, slightly backwards, and upwards until it has penetrated to a depth of just over half an inch (1.5 cm) and feels free in the joint.

Other comments. Check diagnosis carefully to exclude other causes of swelling in the temporomandibular joint area (e.g. enlarged preauricular lymph nodes, parotid gland swellings), and other causes of pain at this site (e.g. Costen's syndrome). Clicking of the temporomandibular joint is not in itself an indication for injection. Include X-ray of the joint in the diagnostic check. The superficial temporal artery lies somewhat posterior to the point of injection and can be palpated near the tragus with the patient's mouth closed.

Since there is a fibroarticular disc present in the joint it is often difficult to be sure the needle is properly placed. The joint may be entered more easily if the mouth is opened widely before the joint is punctured.

(b) Sternomanubrial joint

Indications. Ankylosing spondylitis, psoriatic arthritis, rheumatoid arthritis.

Technique. Locate joint by palpation. Anaesthetize area down to the fibrous covering of the joint using a small needle and, after changing syringes, inject 2 mg triamcinolone hexacetonide.

Other comments. Beware of the occurrence, albeit rare, of pyogenic arthritis of this joint. Exclude heart disease as a cause of pain in this area.

(c) Sternoclavicular joint

Indications. Inflammatory arthropathies (e.g. rheumatoid arthritis) and perhaps degenerative arthritis in its inflammatory phase.

Technique. The joint is most easily entered from a point directly in front. 15 mg hydrocortisone acetate or 7.5 mg triamcinolone hexacetonide is the usual injection dose.

Other comments. Because of its fibrocartilaginous articular disc it is rather a difficult joint to inject.

(d) Costochondral junction

Indication. Tietze's syndrome.

Technique. After infiltration of local anaesthetic, inject 10–20 mg of hydrocortisone acetate or equivalent into the swollen costochondral junction.

Other comments. Exclude other causes of swelling in the costochondral area such as neoplastic secondary deposits. Repeated infiltration may be necessary. Some clinicians find local corticosteroid injection unhelpful and use systemic corticosteroid therapy for this disorder.

(e) Apophyseal joints

Techniques exist for the injection of the apophyseal joints of the spine (particularly in the lumbar region), but these are highly specialized procedures and require careful positioning under radiographic control. They are therefore not suitable for general clinical use.

(f) Coccydynia (coccygodynia)

If coccydynia continues despite the usual conservative programme, including a coccygeal cushion, and with exclusion of demonstrable infection or injury, or specific pathology, injection of the tender area with a local anaesthetic/corticosteroid mixture using a fanwise technique, may relieve symptoms.

(g) Some other painful disorders

The following painful states may respond to infiltration with local anaesthetic with or without corticosteroid preparation.

Occipital neuralgia. A point of maximal tenderness can often be localized over the greater occipital nerve as it passes over the external occipital protuberance. The site of injection is a point just above the superior nuchal line about 2.5 cm from the mid line (Fig. 7.5). Palpation of the occipital artery lateral to the nerve serves as a further guide. A patch of scalp should be shaved to ensure a sterile injection. Entry of the needle along the line of the occipital nerve should produce paraesthesiae, indicating correct placement. 3–5 ml of 0.5–1.0% lignocaine are used. Injection may have to be repeated at 3–7-day intervals or for longer.

Tension headaches. Most so-called tension headaches are associated with increased tone of the anti-gravity muscles responsible for holding up the head, and also with increased tenderness at the insertion of these muscles (most often the sternomastoid and splenius

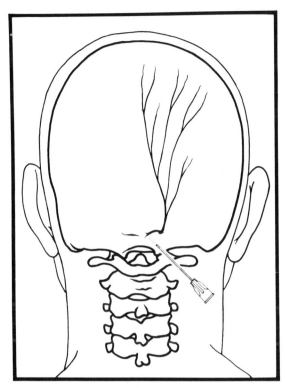

Fig. 7.5 Greater occipital nerve block.

capitis muscles) into the occipital region of the skull. Relief of pain is obtained by wide infiltration along the muscle insertion using a liberal volume of local anaesthetic/hydrocortisone mixture diluted with saline. Repeated injections at 3–7-day intervals may be needed.

'Trigger spots'. Deep lesions in the musculoskeletal system may be associated with referred pain, referred hyperalgesia, and referred spasm in the superficial muscles in the painful region. Within these areas careful palpation may reveal 'trigger spots' which often respond to injection of local anaesthetic. 'Trigger spots' are found particularly in the lower cervical and lower lumbar regions (Fig. 7.6).

Snapping scapula. This refers to the snapping or grating noise produced by certain movements of the shoulder blade. The bursa under the inferior edge of the scapula is infiltrated with local anaesthetic. However, treatment is usually by postural re-education or even removal of the bursa.

Slipping ribs. Impaction of the anterior ends of the 11th ribs on the rib cage in forward flexion or lateral flexion

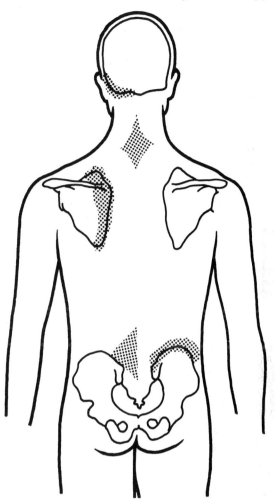

Fig. 7.6 Location of 'trigger spots' (after Dixon and Graber, 1978–80).

of the lumbar spine may be diagnosed and temporarily relieved by injection of local anaesthetic.

Costopelvic impaction. Osteoporosis sometime causes painful contact between rib margin and pelvic brim due to vertebral collapse. Local infiltration of anaesthetic will confirm the diagnosis, although treatment may require removal of part of the lower ribs.

7.5.2 Shoulder

(a) Acromioclavicular joint

Indications. Pain arising from this joint is often the result of a sports injury.

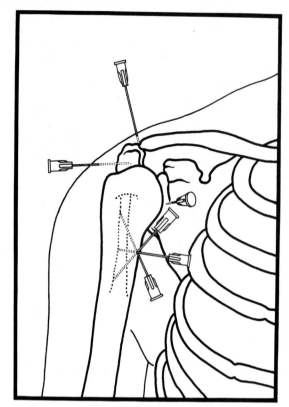

Fig. 7.7 Injection approaches to various structures in the right shoulder region: acromioclavicular joint, subacromial bursa, bicipital tendon, and glenohumeral joint.

Technique. The line of the joint is found by palpation and is entered from above and slightly anteriorly until it is felt to slide between the joint surfaces (Fig. 7.7). As the joint cavity is small it will seldom receive more than 0.5 ml of fluid. Using a fine needle 25G × $\frac{5}{8}$ in inject a mixture containing 2 mg of triamcinolone hexacetonide and 1% lignocaine.

Other comments. In lax-jointed patients the joint line may be found by lifting the clavicle up and down to produce slight subluxation of the joint. For this manoeuvre the patient should be on his or her back.

(b) Subacromial – subdeltoid bursa

Indications. Disorders associated with the painful arc sign (e.g. non-specific irritation of the subacromial bursa; lesions of the rotator cuff, such as partial rupture of the supraspinatus tendon; calcific tendinitis; other causes of synovitis, particularly rheumatoid arthritis).

Technique. The gap between the acromion and the head of the humerus is palpated and the needle aimed towards the centre of the humeral head (easily felt anteriorly) (Fig. 7.7). A 10 ml syringe fitted with a 40 × 0.8 mm gauge needle is charged with at least 5 ml of 1% lignocaine and 20–40 mg hydrocortisone acetate or 10–20 mg triamcinolone hexacetonide. If an X-ray film shows accessible calcific material a large gauge (16–18G) 2-in needle may be used to attempt aspiration of the calcific deposit, followed by instillation of the lignocaine/corticosteroid mixture.

Other comments. Bursting of any calcific nodules, with release of crystals into the subacromial bursa, causes an intensely painful reaction resembling gout. In such an event the humerus may be displaced downwards. In practice, the commonest treatable shoulder lesion in rheumatoid arthritis is subacromial rather than glenohumeral.

(c) Bicipital tendon

Indication. Bicipital tenosynovitis ('tendinitis'). This may be acute, subacute or chronic.

Technique. The bicipital tendon and the borders of its groove are nearly always palpable and the tendon can be rolled under the examiner's fingertip. The opposite (asymptomatic) side can be tested as a control and as an index of the patient's sensitivity. With the patient seated and with the arm externally rotated, needle entry is made through a skin wheal produced by local anaesthetic. The needle is brought in along the side of the tendon and is aimed at one border of the bicipital groove to produce a peritendinous infiltration. A third of the injection (3–5 ml of 1% lignocaine + 20 mg hydrocortisone acetate) is delivered at this point. The needle is then withdrawn slightly, but kept subcutaneously, redirected upward about an inch for another third of the injection. Further withdrawal and redirection downwards until the bicipital border is touched gently is carried out to complete the fan-wise operation and the rest of the injection is deposited here (Fig. 7.7). The injection may have to be repeated.

Other comments. In addition to palpable tenderness on 'rolling' the tendon, a confirmatory test (Yergason's test) may be useful. This test elicits pain along the long head of the bicipital tendon when the hand of that side, grasping the examiner's, is externally rotated (supinated) against resistance.

(d) Pain spots around the shoulder

Painful tender spots around the shoulder are often referred from the neck (usually lower cervical spondylosis), and in these patients the discomfort is unrelated to shoulder movements. 'Fibrositis' or 'deltoiditis' is sometimes used to describe this syndrome, although without pathological justification. Other painful spots may arise from muscle–bone and ligament–bone junctions (entheses) around the shoulder–anatomical sites known to be rich in pain nerve endings. In some patients, spontaneous pain or tenderness at enthesis sites probably reflects an unduly low pain threshold. If it is decided to infiltrate these painful spots with a lignocaine/corticosteroid mixture (preferably a weak mixture, e.g. hydrocortisone 10 mg diluted in 5–10 ml of 1% lignocaine), the possibility of a psychological cause should be borne in mind. The usual locations for such tender spots is at the scapular margin and along the spine of the scapula. Occasionally they can be found in the upper arm in the region of the insertion of the deltoid muscle.

(e) Glenohumeral joint (true shoulder joint)

Indications. Conditions associated with glenohumeral joint restriction (e.g. rheumatoid arthritis and other inflammatory arthropathies; adhesive capsulitis; polymyalgia rheumatica with shoulder involvement).

Technique. Aspiration of the shoulder joint is easily accomplished by anterior puncture, inserting the needle about 2.5 cm medial to the head of the humerus and about 2.5 cm below the tip of the coracoid process which is used as a valuable landmark (Fig. 7.7). The procedure may be carried out either with the patient sitting or lying supine with forearms held across the abdomen. Any tendency to hunch the shoulders should be corrected. In patients with well-developed deltoid muscles the procedure may be more difficult. Some clinicians prefer a posterior approach. The coracoid process is identified anteriorly and the joint line posteriorly with the patient in a relaxed position on the couch with the arm rotated inwards. The needle is entered pointing it towards the outer side of the coracoid process. Use a 10 ml syringe fitted with a $21G \times 1\frac{1}{2}$ in needle and charged with 10–20 mg of hydrocortisone acetate or 5–10 mg triamcinolone hexacetonide made up to 10 ml with 1% lignocaine. The facility with which fluid is discharged from the syringe provides a useful indication that the needle has been correctly placed.

Other comments. Care must be taken not to point the needle medially in the anterior approach to avoid neurovascular structures in the axilla. The anatomical relations of the shoulder joint are shown in Fig. 7.8.

7.5.3 Elbow

(a) Tennis elbow (lateral or external epicondylitis of the elbow)

Indication. Tennis elbow giving rise to significant symptoms. This is usually due to occupational trauma or sporting activities.

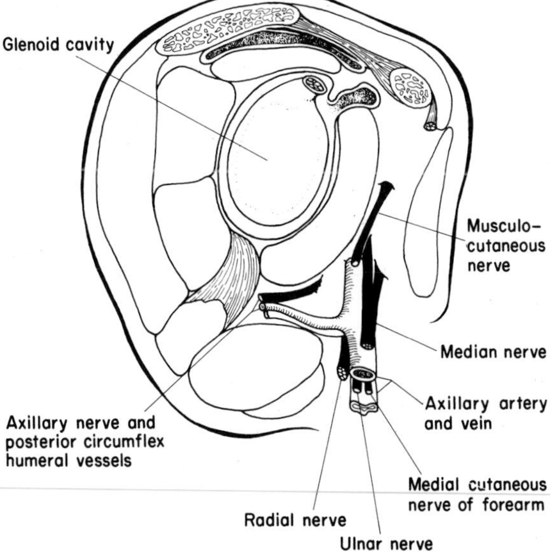

Glenoid cavity

Musculo-cutaneous nerve

Median nerve

Axillary artery and vein

Axillary nerve and posterior circumflex humeral vessels

Medial cutaneous nerve of forearm

Radial nerve

Ulnar nerve

Fig. 7.8 Cross-section showing anatomical relations of the right glenohumeral joint, looking towards the glenoid cavity.

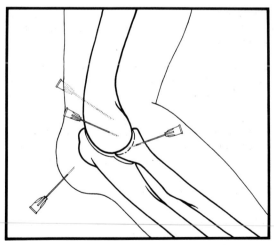

Fig. 7.9 Lateral view of right elbow region showing injection approaches to: tennis elbow, golfer's elbow, olecranon bursitis, and elbow joint.

Technique. The injection site is the point of maximal tenderness and is normally just distal to the lateral epicondyle (Fig. 7.9). (The radial head can be felt underneath the examining finger by asking the patient to rotate the forearm.) 2–5 ml of lignocaine/corticosteroid mixture (20 mg hydrocortisone acetate or 5 mg triamcinolone hexacetonide made up to 5 ml with 1% lignocaine) are injected into the junction of the forearm extensor group and its fibrous attachment to bone. Considerable pressure is needed to achieve correct delivery of the injection fluid close to the bone interface. The injection may have to be repeated, but this should be limited to two or three injections.

Other comments. Unless the needle and syringe are firmly wedged, injection fluid may burst out due to the pressure required for the injection. If the fluid enters the operator's eyes it is harmless.

(b) Golfer's elbow (medial or internal epicondylitis of the elbow)

Golfer's elbow is the medial counterpart of tennis elbow, the point of maximal tenderness being located just distal to the medial epicondyle (Fig. 7.9). Smaller volumes of fluid (1–3 ml) are used. Care should be taken to avoid injecting the ulnar nerve lying in its groove just behind the medial epicondyle (Fig. 7.10).

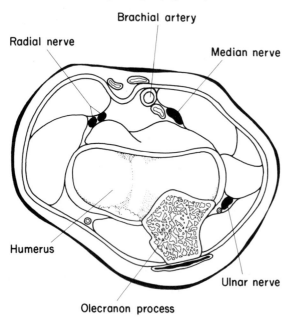

Fig. 7.10 Cross-section showing anatomical relations of right elbow joint. Note particularly the position of the ulnar nerve.

(c) Olecranon bursitis

Indications. Olecranon bursitis may be traumatic or due to non-specific inflammatory disease such as rheumatoid arthritis.

Technique. Provided there is no infection, aspirate and inject with 20 mg hydrocortisone acetate or equivalent into the apex of the bursal swelling (Fig. 7.9). Inspissated fluid may require a needle of 16 to 18G.

Other comments. As the elbow is a common site for lesions such as psoriatic plaques, rheumatoid nodules and gouty tophi, care should be taken to avoid injecting through such lesions.

(d) Elbow joint

Indications. Rheumatoid arthritis and other non-specific inflammatory arthritides. When the elbow is swollen and painful, and particularly if there is limitation of movement.

Technique. Lateral approach: With the elbow held at a right-angle, the head of the radius is palpated by getting the patient to rotate the forearm. The thumb will easily locate the joint line just below the lateral humeral epicondyle (Fig. 7.9). Inject the joint tangentially and not directly towards the centre of the joint. The ease of the injection will confirm good placement of the needle if no fluid can be aspirated.

Posterior approach: Some clinicians find this easier than the lateral approach. With the elbow held at 90° the depression in the midline at the back of the elbow is palpated. This lies between the two halves of the triceps tendon. The injection into the joint is made just above and lateral to the olecranon process and just below the lateral epicondyle.

For injections of the elbow, a mixture of 10 mg hydrocortisone acetate or 5 mg triamcinolone hexacetonide diluted in 1% lignocaine is used.

Other comments. Particularly with the posterior approach more fluid can be aspirated than is evident clinically. The joint may also be injected with the arms fully extended, a position that distends the capsule maximally. Avoid injecting medial to the olecranon in view of the proximity of the ulnar nerve (Fig. 7.10).

7.5.4 Hand and wrist

(a) Carpal tunnel syndrome

Indications. Median nerve entrapment, unless there are objective neurological signs such as sensory loss or atrophy of the thenar eminence. Some common causes of the carpal tunnel syndrome include rheumatoid arthritis (affecting the finger flexor tendon sheaths or wrist joint), other inflammatory arthropathies such as psoriatic arthritis; pregnancy; the menopause; accompanying painful shoulder syndromes; fluid-retaining drugs (e.g. phenylbutazone); after Colles' fracture. Rare causes include: hypothyroidism, acromegaly, myelomatosis, and amyloidosis. Most cases, however, are idiopathic.

Technique. The injection site lies just lateral to the midline of the flexor aspect of the wrist at the proximal skin crease (the crease lying at the junction of the forearm and hand). The median nerve lies just beneath the palmaris longus tendon (if this is present) (Fig. 7.11(a) and (b)). With the wrist dorsiflexed up to 20°, a fine-bore needle (22–24G) is directed inwards and somewhat towards the palm at an angle of about 60°. The injection mixture contains 10 mg hydrocortisone acetate or 4 mg triamcinolone hexacetonide made up to 1 ml with 1% lignocaine.

Other comments. The patient should be reassured that if there is numbness of the thumb and lateral two and a half fingers this is only temporary, but may last for 1–2 weeks. In a tissue space that readily allows advancement of the needle, care should be taken not to inject further than about 5–9 mm below the surface of the skin.

(b) De Quervain's tenosynovitis ('nappy wrist')

Indication. Stenosing tenosynovitis of extensor pollicis brevis and abductor pollicis longus which has been present for less than 6 months. More chronic De Quervain's syndrome often requires surgical decompression. The disorder is occasionally associated with rheumatoid arthritis, but more often is an occupational disorder.

Technique. After locating the tender area (usually below or over the styloid process) insert the needle tangentially alongside the tendon in a proximal direction (Fig. 7.12).

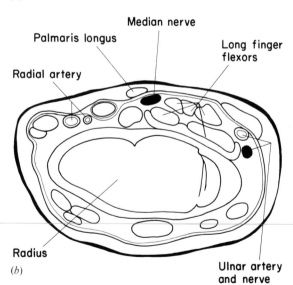

Fig. 7.11 Anatomical relations of the right median nerve as seen (*a*) from the palmar aspect and (*b*) in cross-section.

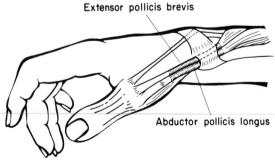

Fig. 7.12 View of right wrist to show position of tendons involved in De Quervain's syndrome (extensor pollicis brevis and abductor pollicis longus).

This is most easily achieved by supporting the patient's forearm on a pillow with the thumb grasped in the clinician's left hand. Correct placement of the needle inside the tendon sheath allows injection without much resistance and the tendon sheath can be felt to inflate along the course of the tendon. A suggested mixture for injection is 10 mg of hydrocortisone acetate or 4 mg of triamcinolone hexacetonide in 2 ml of 1% lignocaine.

Other comments. If there is doubt about correct siting of the needle, remove the syringe from the needle *in situ* and ask the patient to flex the thumb. If the needle is embedded in the tendon it will move towards the vertical.

(c) Ganglion

A ganglion on the dorsum of the wrist is a common finding. It consists of a cystic swelling containing clear jelly-like mucoid material of high density and may arise along tendon sheaths or in relation to a joint capsule. In some patients aspiration (with a large gauge needle – 18 G) and injection of corticosteroid provides relief, but often there is recurrence due to refilling from the parent synovial lining. Surgical removal is often necessary.

(d) Synovitis of the common dorsal tendon sheath

The common dorsal tendon sheath just distal to the wrist may be involved with cystic synovial swelling in rheumatoid arthritis. Although in many patients surgery becomes inevitable, temporary relief can be provided by aspiration of these fluctuant prominences, followed by instillation of a corticosteroid preparation.

(e) Tenosynovitis of digital flexor tendons ('trigger' or 'snapping' finger)

Indications. Impaction and triggering of nodules in the flexor tendons in rheumatoid arthritis; recent loss of active finger flexion due to early adhesions between the tendon and its sheath in rheumatoid arthritis and other inflammatory arthritides such as psoriatic arthritis.

Technique. Nodules can be directly infiltrated with a 50% mixture of triamcinolone hexacetonide (20 mg ml^{-1}) and 1% lignocaine. Infiltration around the nodules may also be successful. When the whole of the tendon sheath is swollen, infiltration within the tendon sheath should be carried out. With the patient seated and the palm of the hand facing upwards the injection is made in the direction of the patient's wrist. The needle is inserted slowly until flow of injection fluid proceeds without much resistance. A useful ploy is to advance the

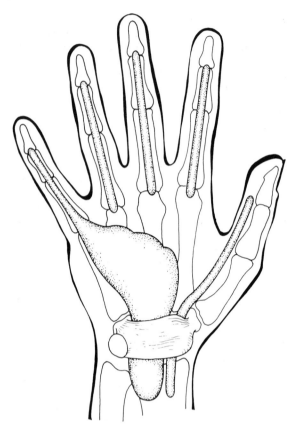

Fig. 7.13 Palmar view of right hand to show distribution of digital flexor tendon synovial sheaths.

needle disconnected from the syringe until it tilts vertically when the finger is flexed. The syringe can then be reconnected and the injection made. The above comments apply equally to the flexor sheath of the thumb.

Other comments. In the injection of individual tendon-sheath lesions the anatomical arrangement of the flexor sheath system in the hand should be borne in mind. The system is variable and adventitious bursae may develop due to disorders such as rheumatoid arthritis. Most often, the common flexor sheath (which slants an inch or so proximal to the proximal edge of the flexor retinaculum) extends to the end of the little finger. The thumb, and index, middle and ring fingers possess separate flexor sheaths (Fig. 7.13).

(f) Wrist joint

Indications. Rheumatoid arthritis and other inflammatory arthritides such as psoriatic arthritis.

Technique. This is a complex joint (Fig. 7.11(b)) and is most safely and easily aspirated dorsally. The patient's wrist should be supported, palm downwards, over a rolled bandage or small cushion. The needle should enter the joint (60° to the surface, pointing slightly towards the patient's head) just distal to the distal end of the radius and just ulnar to the 'anatomical snuffbox'. A 'T'-shaped gap between the end of the radius and the adjacent margins of the lunate and scaphoid provides a useful landmark. Correct placement of the needle is judged by easy insertion to a depth of 1–2 cm and the fact that it feels free. An ulnar approach may be used if there is synovial bulging at this site. The joint should be entered just distal to the ulnar styloid process and dorsal to the pisiform bone. Most of the small intercarpal joints have interconnecting synovial spaces and will thus be reached by injection of the main wrist joint. A suitable injection mixture is 10 mg hydrocortisone acetate or 4 mg triamcinolone hexacetonide made up to 5 ml with 1% lignocaine.

Other comments. It is preferable to support the wrist with either a bandage or light splint for 24 hours after the injection. This reduces the rate at which the injected solution enters the general circulation.

(g) Carpometacarpal joint of the thumb

Indication. Thumb-base osteoarthrosis.

Technique. The joint is entered dorsally through the palpable joint line from the radial side of the hand with the needle pointing slightly distally in the direction of the thumb. Traction on the thumb facilitates the procedure. Tensing the thumb makes it more difficult. Triamcinolone hexacetonide 2 mg made up with 1% lignocaine is usually all that a joint of this size can accept.

Other comments. Patients should be warned that there may be some increased pain for a period when the effect of the local anaesthetic has worn off.

(h) Metacarpophalangeal joint

Indication. Rheumatoid arthritis and other inflammatory arthritides.

Technique. Locate the joint line which lies about 1 cm distal to the apex of the knuckle. Apply slight traction to the patient's finger and from the lateral or medial side. Insert the needle (24 gauge) tangentially under the extensor expansion (Fig. 7.14). The digital veins provide a useful landmark and the injection should be dorsal to this vessel. Triamcinolone hexacetonide 1–2 mg in 0.5–1 ml 1% lignocaine is a usual injection dose.

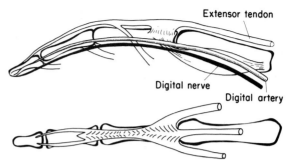

Fig. 7.14 Lateral and dorsal views of finger showing relations of the extensor tendon and its membranous expansion.

Other comments. A useful indication of correct placement of the injection is a feeling of joint distension by the clinician's index finger placed over the palmar aspect of the joint during the injection.

(i) Interphalangeal joint

The indications and technique for injecting these joints are as described for the metacarpophalangeal joint except that a slightly smaller dose of corticosteroid is used. The dose is usually little more than 1 mg of triamcinolone hexacetonide for the proximal interphalangeal joint, using a 2 ml syringe, and less for the distal interphalangeal joint, using a 1 ml syringe. The distal interphalangeal joint line may be difficult to locate, and it should be remembered that the root of the nail lies close to this joint (Fig. 7.15) and could be damaged by a misplaced injection.

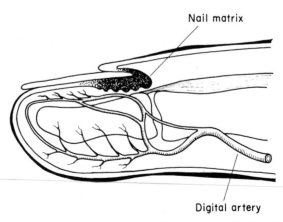

Fig. 7.15 Anatomical relationship between root of nail and distal interphalangeal joint.

7.5.5 Hip region

(a) Lesions in region of greater trochanter

Indications. Greater trochanteric bursitis; enthesitis of muscles inserted into the greater trochanter (gluteus medius, gluteus maximus). Differentiation between them is often difficult, but the method for treating pain in this area is the same.

Technique. The patient is asked to lie facing the clinician with the painful hip uppermost, flexed and adducted. This is made possible by extension of the other hip. The trochanteric prominence is then located and the point of maximal tenderness identified. The syringe (charged with 10 ml of 1% lignocaine and 40 mg of hydrocortisone acetate or 10 mg of triamcinolone hexacetonide) and needle $21G \times 1\frac{1}{2}$ in are then advanced towards the tip of the greater trochanter. If bone is encountered the area is approached more tangentially, with the aim of reaching the tough fibrous insertion of the gluteal fascia and beyond. This area is then infiltrated widely. If palpation suggests that the insertion of the gluteus maximus down the posterolateral edge of the greater trochanter is affected, this area should be infiltrated.

Other comments. In view of the several layers of muscle that have to be penetrated and other factors, precise injection of these lesions is somewhat 'blind'. However, wider infiltration with local anaesthetic/corticosteroid mixture usually achieves satisfactory results.

(b) Lesions in region of ischial tuberosity

Indications. Ischial bursitis; enthesitis of muscles attached to ischial tuberosity.

Technique. The patient is asked to lie on the couch facing away from the examiner. Using a 20 ml syringe (charged with 10 ml of 1% lignocaine and 10 mg of hydrocortisone acetate or 10 mg of triamcinolone hexacetonide) fitted with a long needle ($21G \times 1\frac{1}{2}$–2 in), the area is infiltrated widely.

Other comments. As with trochanteric lesions, it is often difficult to identify precisely the cause of pain.

(c) Meralgia paraesthetica

This is an entrapment neuropathy due to compression of the lateral cutaneous nerve of thigh as it passes through the deep fascia about 10 cm below and medial to the anterior superior iliac spine. Infiltration of this area with a mixture of 5 ml of 1% lignocaine and 5 mg of triamcinolone hexacetonide is usually successful. Care

should be taken to exclude other causes of pain in this area (e.g. incipient herpes zoster, arthritis of the hip joint, claudication of arteries in the thigh).

(d) Hip joint

Indications. Aspiration and/or injection of hip joint arthritides (e.g. rheumatoid arthritis, osteoarthrosis).

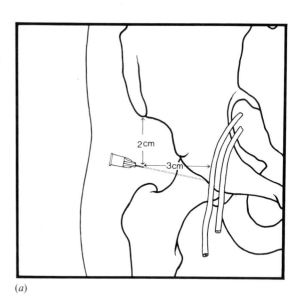

(a)

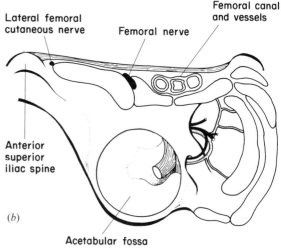

(b)

Fig. 7.16 (*a*) Anterior approach to right hip joint. Note landmarks (anterior superior iliac spine above and femoral pulse medially). (*b*) Cross-section showing anatomical relationships of right hip joint (viewed from the feet in a patient lying supine).

Technique. This joint is the most difficult to aspirate and inject because of the amount of soft tissue overlying it in all directions. The difficulty is increased by the fact that the joint space cannot be palpated, and often it is impossible to know whether the needle has entered the joint space because aspiration is hindered by blockage of the needle with either fluid that is too viscous or solid debris. Other factors increasing the difficulty of injection include obstructing osteophytes and flattening of the femoral head in osteoarthrosis, and ossification of the joint capsule in ankylosing spondylitis. It is therefore not a procedure for the inexperienced operator.

The patient lies supine with the hip in maximal extension and internal rotation. The joint may be approached anteriorly or medially. The anterior approach (usual) involves puncture 2–3 cm below the anterior superior iliac spine and 2–3 cm lateral to the femoral pulse (Fig. 7.16(a)) (depending on the size of the patient) with a long wide-bore needle (20G × 2½ in. The needle is entered at an angle of 60° to the skin, pointing posteromedially. The needle is advanced through the tough, thick capsular ligaments until bone is reached. The tip is then withdrawn slightly. After aspiration (not always possible) about 40 mg of hydrocortisone acetate or 20 mg of triamcinolone hexacetonide mixed with 2–3 ml of 1% lignocaine are injected. Injection of the hip joint by the lateral route is simpler only in that the needle follows the line of the femoral neck to the joint. A lumbar puncture needle is required for this operation. It is inserted just anterior to the greater trochanter, in a sagittal direction and is pointed towards the middle of the inguinal ligament. The needle enters the joint anteriorly, near the upper reflection of the synovial sac.

Other comments. Great care must be exercised to avoid blood vessels and nerves in this area (Fig. 7.16(b)). The question of osteonecrosis due to corticosteroid injection (steroid arthropathy) is still unresolved, but the patient should be given the benefit of the doubt and frequently repeated injections should be avoided.

7.5.6 Knee region

(a) Prepatellar bursitis (housemaid's knee, beat knee)

Prepatellar bursitis may be due to occupational causes or to religious observances involving long periods spent on the knees. Occasionally it is part of an inflammatory arthritis such as rheumatoid or psoriatic arthritis. If the injection is to be made primarily to relieve swelling (the bursitis is often not particularly painful) it should be borne in mind that aspiration often yields only a few drops of fluid due to the anatomical arrangement of the bursa. However, a small dose of hydrocortisone acetate

(about 5 mg) injected into the apex of the swelling usually causes the swelling to settle.

(b) Collateral ligaments

Valgus and varus deformities of the knees may be associated with painful medial or lateral collateral ligaments respectively. After accurate localization of the area of tenderness, an injection of 5 mg of triamcinolone hexacetonide in 0.25 ml of 1% lignocaine using a fine needle (23G × 1³⁄₁₆ in) often yields beneficial results.

(c) Patellofemoral osteoarthrosis

Localized tender spots may be elicited under the lateral edge of the patella in patellofemoral osteoarthrosis. Accurate injection in the fibrous tissue attachment of the joint capsule to the patellar edge (without actual penetration of the knee cavity) with 0.5 ml 1% lignocaine and 0.5 ml triamcinolone hexacetonide may be effective in relieving symptoms.

(d) Knee joint

Indications. Non-infective inflammatory joint disease (e.g. rheumatoid arthritis, seronegative spondarthritides, inflammatory phase of chondrocalcinosis). Corticosteroid injection of the knee joint is of limited value in osteoarthrosis (unless accompanied by an inflammatory phase) and in traumatic arthritis, and is contraindicated in gout and in haemophilia with joint

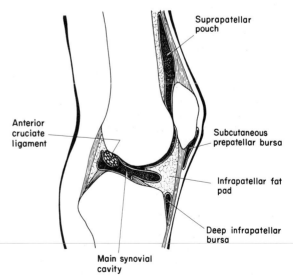

Fig. 7.17 Lateral view of right knee showing extent of synovial spaces.

involvement unless the bleeding tendency is under control.

Technique. The knee joint is the largest synovial cavity in the body (Fig. 7.17) and may yield effusions of 100 ml. It is the easiest joint to aspirate and inject. A distended knee joint can be aspirated from virtually any site over the swelling without difficulty, but the following technique is recommended for routine puncture of the joint space even if no excess fluid is present. Knee puncture is undertaken with the patient lying supine with legs as fully extended as possible. Two favoured sites of entry are just below the points where a horizontal line tangential to the upper border of the patella crosses a line parallel to the medial or lateral border of the patella.

In general, the anterolateral approach is preferred by the author as it is easier to perform – the medial approach is to some extent hampered by the presence of the other leg. This approach is particularly useful if a suprapatellar effusion is present. The needle is directed medially and downward or upward into the joint space beneath the patella, or into the greatest bulge of the effusion.

The anteromedial approach is preferred by some clinicians, and here there is a slightly larger space palpable between the patella and the femoral condyle. The needle is inserted 1–2 cm medial to the inner border of the patella in a lateral and slightly posterior direction between the posterior surface of the patella and the patellar groove of the femur. The needle tip may crepitate on the undersurface of the patella, indicating entry into the joint space. If cartilage is touched once the needle has entered the synovial space it should not be advanced further.

If the patella is ankylosed in the presence of knee joint contracture, the infrapatellar route may be used. The needle is advanced anteroposteriorly on either side of the inferior patellar tendon through or above the infrapatellar fat pad into the knee joint space between the femoral condyles. The various approaches to injecting the knee joint are shown in Fig. 7.18(a) and anatomical relationships of the joint in Fig. 7.18(b).

Puncture of the knee through the popliteal space is not advisable because of the danger of encountering the popliteal vessels (Fig. 7.18(b)). However a Baker's cyst, or posterior herniation of the knee joint capsule may be aspirated directly if superficial and distended.

A 21G, $1\frac{1}{2}$ in needle is almost always adequate for aspirating and injecting the knee joint, although if the synovial fluid is particularly viscous a wide-bore needle may be necessary. The amount of corticosteroid to be injected may vary, but a usual dose is 50 mg hydrocortisone acetate or 25 mg triamcinolone hexacetonide. This may be mixed with 1% lignocaine.

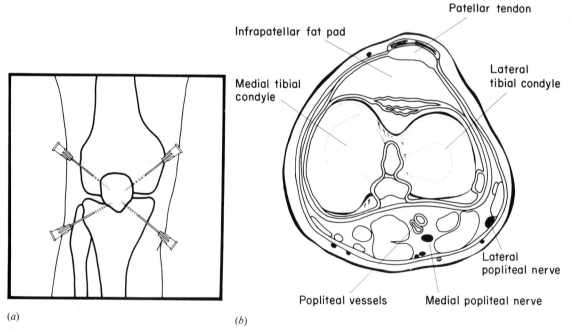

(a)   (b)

Fig. 7.18 (*a*) Anterior view of right knee showing superior and inferior anterolateral and anteromedial approaches for injecting the joint. (*b*) Cross-section showing anatomical relations of right knee.

Other comments. The value of aspirating the knee before corticosteroid injection is debatable, but most clinicians do this and there is little double that this manoeuvre alone can produce substantial, albeit brief, symptomatic relief. However, the contents of a swollen knee are in dynamic equilibrium with the blood stream, and a knee aspirated to dryness can be filled again within 48 hours.

If there is the slightest suspicion that the joint is infected, corticosteroid should *not* be injected. Infected fluid resembles pus and often smells unpleasant. Non-infected inflammatory fluid is hazy, turbid or opaque, depending on the number of cells, and it may have a greenish tinge. It is relatively non-viscous. Non-inflammatory fluid is clear and viscous (causing bubbles to rise slowly to the surface in the syringe and long threads to form when a drop of fluid is allowed to fall from the end of the syringe).

Patients are usually advised to curtail walking activities for 24 hours after the injection – active exercise after the injection encourages the corticosteroid to leave the joint more quickly.

Indications for injecting the knee in children are less than in the adult, but it can be useful in reducing the temperature of a joint affected by inflammatory arthritis. Local corticosteroid reduces acceleration of epiphyseal growth which can cause a significant difference in leg length.

(e) Acute synovial rupture of the knee

Acute synovial rupture of the knee most often occurs in the early stages of joint disease (inflammatory or degenerative) before fibrous thickening of the capsule has had time to form. In non-rheumatological circles it is often misdiagnosed as deep-vein thrombosis, with the serious consequences of anticoagulant therapy – extensive haematoma in the calf, pressure necrosis of calf muscles, and, later, flexion contracture of the ankle joint.

Treatment involves rest, elevation of the leg, diuretics, and suppressing fluid formation in the knee using a local corticosteroid preparation. If the calf cyst becomes infected, direct drainage of the cyst using a wide-bore needle or even a small incision with a scalpel blade may be necessary in addition to antibiotics.

7.5.7 Ankle and foot

(a) Achilles bursitis

Achilles bursitis may be seen in rheumatoid arthritis, as well as in HLA-B27-related disorders such as ankylosing spondylitis and Reiter's disease. It leads to calcaneal erosion. It should not be confused with Achilles tendinitis (a disorder involving the whole of the tendon and

its insertion) which, because of its diffuse nature, is not amenable to injection therapy.

It is not always easy to feel the gap between the Achilles tendon and the back of the calcaneum and reference to a lateral X-ray of the heel helps to judge the depth of the bursa. Injection is made from the lateral side of the heel slightly above the top of the calcaneum with the needle pointing medially and downwards.

5 mg triamcinolone hexacetonide or equivalent mixed with a little 1 % lignocaine is injected using a 2 ml syringe and a fine needle ($23G \times 1\frac{3}{16}$ in).

(b) Calcaneal spur (planter spur; calcaneal 'bursitis'; policeman's heel)

This is an inflammatory lesion of the insertion of the long plantar ligament into the anterior aspect of the calcaneum. It is commonly encountered in the spondarthritides, particularly ankylosing spondylitis and Reiter's disease. Painful lesions are usually associated with early spur formation. A large prominent spur seen on X-ray may be a healed lesion and may not be relevant to the patient's symptoms. Response to injection is variable but it is worth trying.

The point of maximal tenderness is identified and the needle introduced from the medial side where the heel skin is thinner. The needle ($21G \times 1\frac{1}{2}$ in) is directed laterally and slightly upwards and dorsally towards the space at the mid-point of the calcaneum. The injection is made, a drop at a time, as close as possible to bone with the aim of injecting the thick tendinous insertion. It is usually not possible to inject more than 0.5–1 ml of local anaesthetic/corticosteroid mixture (5 mg of triamcinolone hexacetonide in 1% lignocaine).

(c) Other causes of talalgia

The Achilles tendon and underside of the heel are favourite sites for rheumatoid nodules. If they are tender they may respond to injection. Other painful lesions of the heel include gouty tophi, rupture of the Achilles tendon, Ballet dancer's heel (contusion of the posterior aspect of the talus on the tibia), exostosis below the Achilles tendon insertion, bony lesions of the calcaneum (Paget's disease, secondary deposits), but treatment of these lesions does not usually include injection of corticosteroid.

(d) Tendon sheaths and ankle

Inflammation of the posterior tibial tendon sheath due to rheumatoid arthritis and other inflammatory arthritides responds well to injection therapy. The injection of the tendon sheath is made tangentially below and behind the medial malleolus (Fig. 7.19(a)) using a 2 ml

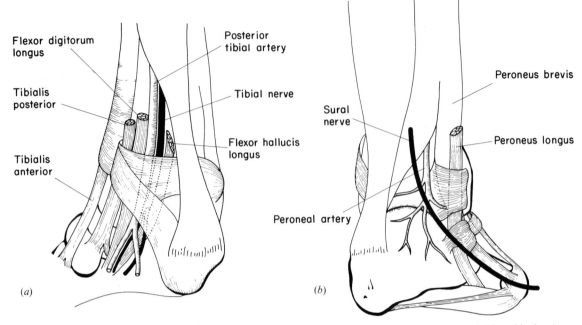

Flexor digitorum longus

Posterior tibial artery

Tibialis posterior

Tibial nerve

Tibialis anterior

Flexor hallucis longus

Peroneus brevis

Sural nerve

Peroneus longus

Peroneal artery

(a)

(b)

Fig. 7.19 (*a*) Medial aspect of right ankle showing tendons and surrounding structures. (*b*) Lateral aspect of right ankle showing tendons and surrounding structures.

syringe fitted with a $21G \times 1\frac{1}{2}$ in needle charged with 5 mg of triamcinolone hexacetonide mixed with 0·5 ml of 1% lignocaine. A correctly placed injection can be felt to spread along the tendon as the sheath is inflated. A similar technique can be used to inject the peroneal tendon sheaths behind the lateral malleolus (Fig. 7.19(b)).

(e) Ankle joint

Indications. Rheumatoid arthritis and other non-infective inflammatory arthropathies, such as those of the seronegative spondarthritis group. If the ankle joint alone is active, consider the possibility of infective arthritis, including tuberculous infection. Gout is not an indication for injecting the ankle joint.

Technique. With the foot dorsiflexed to put the tibialis anterior tendon on the stretch, the space between the tibia and talus is identified. The needle ($21G \times 1\frac{1}{2}$ in attached to a 5 ml syringe) is entered anteromedially and aimed at the tibiotalar articulation from a point 1 cm above and 1 cm lateral to the medial malleolus, just medial to the extensor hallucis longus tendon. The needle, which should enter the joint tangentially, must pass about 3 cm inwards and slightly laterally through the ligaments of the ankle joint capsule. It should then

be freely movable between the surfaces of the joint. A usual injection mixture consists of 25 mg of hydrocortisone acetate or equivalent and 1% lignocaine (up to 10 ml if the ankle is very swollen).

Sometimes signs of active inflammation are noted around the lateral aspect of the joint. Entry is then directed below the lateral malleolus.

The approach routes to the ankle joint are summarized in Fig. 7.20(a) and important anatomical relations are shown in Fig. 7.20(b).

Other comments. The commonest mistake is to inject too high or too low. If more than gentle pressure on the plunger of the syringe is required for injection, the needle tip is probably embedded in ligament or cartilage.

After the injection, the foot should be raised for a few minutes before walking as there is a tendency for bleeding to recur if the foot is in the dependent position.

(f) Posterior talocalcaneal (subtaloid) joint

This joint, relatively often involved in rheumatoid arthritis, is much more difficult to puncture than the main ankle joint, although it is often in communication with it. With the patient lying prone, the joint is approached laterally at the junction of a horizontal line

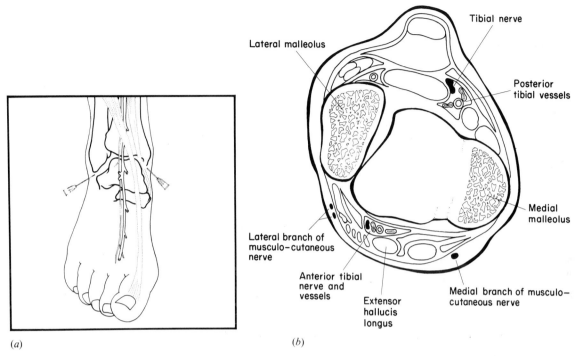

Fig. 7.20 (*a*) Anterior view of right ankle showing anteromedial and lateral approaches to ankle joint. Note position of anterior tibial artery and nerve. (*b*) Cross-section of right ankle to show important anatomical relations.

drawn 2·5 cm above the end of the lateral malleolus and a vertical line 1·0 cm from the posterior border of the shaft of the fibula. A 4 cm 21G needle is introduced at a 55° angle to the skin, with the tip aimed at the proximal end of the first metatarsal.

(g) Tarsal and tarsometatarsal joints

These joints, which only occasionally require injection, are difficult to enter. Because they lie superficial to the dorsum of the foot, these joints are best approached from this aspect rather than through the plantar surface. The needle (23G × $1\frac{3}{16}$ in) may have to be 'teased' into the space between the joint cartilage until it moves freely. 10 mg of hydrocortisone acetate or 5 mg triamcinolone hexacetonide should be sufficient for such joints.

(i) Metatarsophalangeal joints

Injecting the metatarsophalangeal joints can give substantial relief in rheumatoid arthritis. The 1st metatarsophalangeal joint is best approached from the medial side, with the needle aimed at the joint tangen-

tially under the extensor tendon. 2 mg triamcinolone hexacetonide mixed with 1% lignocaine is an acceptable mixture.

Injection of the lateral metatarsophalangeal joints, particularly in the early stage of the disease, can be helpful. The needle is introduced under the extensor tendons from the side to enter the joint as tangentially as possible. These joints cannot accept much more than 0.5 ml of the mixture of triamcinolone hexacetonide 5 mg in 0.25 ml and 1% lignocaine, 0.25 ml. A 2 ml syringe and 23G × $1\frac{3}{16}$ in needle can be used.

(j) Other lesions in region of metatarsophalangeal joints

Adventitious bursae under the metatarsal heads are usually best left alone, but if they become very tense they can be aspirated and injected with a small dose of local corticosteroid.

Morton's metatarsalgia may be due to swelling of the small bursa that lies between the metatarsal heads. If careful palpation can localize this source of pain it is worth infiltrating the area with a small amount of local anaesthetic/corticosteroid mixture.

(k) Interphalangeal joints

The interphalangeal joints of the toes may be injected in a similar fashion to the procedure outlined for injection of the corresponding joints of the fingers.

7.6 SUMMARY AND CONCLUSIONS

The materials and methodological principles involved in local injection therapy have been described and comments made on certain clinical considerations, such as indications and contraindications of such treatment. The need to exclude the presence of infection in or near a joint to be injected has been particularly emphasized.

The major part of the chapter is devoted to the indication(s), technique and problems associated with injecting specific structures/lesions, with emphasis on the importance of a knowledge of basic anatomy.

It is concluded that local injection of corticosteroid preparation is an effective and safe treatment for joint disorders and for certain extra-articular conditions as long as a careful aseptic technique and a proper knowledge of anatomical relations are applied. Over many years it has been shown that intrasynovial corticosteroid injection can give a relatively long-lasting palliation in a wide variety of non-infective inflammatory rheumatoses. It is important that the minimal effective dose of steroid should not be exceeded and that re-injection should be kept to a minimum. The importance of resting weight-bearing joints after injection has also been indicated.

Other medications such as radioisotopes, cytotoxic agents and osmic acid are still somewhat experimental.

7.7 REFERENCES AND FURTHER READING

General aspects of injection therapy

Ansell, B.M. (1980) in *Rheumatic Disorders in Childhood*, Butterworths, London, p. 143.

Baker, W.M. (1877) The formation of abnormal synovial cysts in connection with the joints. *St. Bartholomew's Hosp. Rep.*, **13**, 245.

Balch, H.W. and Jacomb, R.G. (1967) Parenteral administration of 6 α-methylprednisolone-21-acetate. Part I. Intra-articular injection: comparison with hydrocortisone acetate. *Ann. Phys. Med.*, **9**, 43.

Behrens, F., Shephard, N. and Mitchell, N. (1975) Alteration of rabbit articular cartilage by intra-articular injections of glucocorticoids. *J. Bone Joint Surg.*, **57A**, 70.

Bird, H.A. and Ring, E.F.J. (1978) Therapeutic value of arthroscopy. *Ann. Rheum. Dis.*, **37**, 78.

Boyle, A.C. (1977) in *Copeman's Textbook of Rheumatic Diseases*. (ed. J.T. Scott), 5th edn, Churchill Livingstone, Edinburgh, p. 1032.

Cohen, S.H. (1977) in *Rheumatic Diseases – Diagnosis and Management*. (ed. W.A. Katz), Lippincott, Philadelphia, p. 910.

Collins, A.J. and Cosh, J.A. (1970) Temperature and biochemical studies of joint inflammation. *Ann. Rheum. Dis.*, **29**, 386.

Corbett, M., Seifert, M.H., Hacking, C. and Webb, S. (1970) Comparison between local injections of silicone oil and hydrocortisone acetate in chronic arthritis. *Br. Med. J.*, **i**, 24.

Cyriax, J. and Russell, G. (1977) *Textbook of Orthopaedic Medicine. Treatment by Manipulation, Massage and Injection*, Volume 2. Baillière Tindall, London, pp. 234 and 328.

Haslock, I. (1976) in *Clinics in the Rheumatic Diseases* (ed. V. Wright), Vol. 2, No. 3, Saunders, London, p. 621.

Hollander, J.L. (1951a) The local effects of compound F (hydrocortisone) injected into joints. *Bull. Rheum. Dis.*, **2**, 3.

Hollander, J.L., Brown, E.J., Jessar, R.A. and Brown, C.V. (1951b) Hydrocortisone and cortisone injected into arthritic joints. *J. Am. Med. Assoc.*, **147**, 1629.

Hollander, J.L., Brown, E.M., Jessar, R.A. *et al.* (1954) Local anti-rheumatic effectiveness of higher esters and analogues of hydrocortisone. *Ann. Rheum. Dis.*, **13**, 297.

Hollander, J.L., Jessar, R.A. and Brown, E.M. (1961) Intra-synovial corticosteroid therapy: a decade of use. *Bull. Rheum. Dis.*, **11**, 239.

Hollander, J.L., Jessar, R.A., Restifo, R.A. and Fort, H.J. (1961) A new intra-articular steroid ester with longer effectiveness. *Arthr. Rheum.*, **4**, 422 (Abstract).

Huskisson, E.C. and Hart, F. (1975) *Joint Disease: All the Arthropathies*, 2nd edn, Wright, Bristol, p. x.

Jayson, M.I.V. and Dixon, A. St. J. (1968) Arthroscopy of the knee in rheumatic diseases. *Ann. Rheum. Dis.*, **27**, 503.

Jayson, M.I.V. and Dixon, A. St. J. (1970) Valvular mechanisms in juxta-articular cysts. *Ann. Rheum. Dis.*, **29**, 415.

Lewis, D.A. and Day, E.H. (1972) Biochemical factors in the action of steroids on diseased joints in rheumatoid arthritis. *Ann. Rheum. Dis.*, **31**, 374.

Lindsay, D.J., Ring, E.F.J., Coorey, P.F.J. and Jayson, M.I.V. (1971) Synovial irrigation in rheumatoid arthritis. *Acta Rheumatol. Scand.*, **17**, 169.

McCarty, D.J. (1968) A basic guide to arthrocentesis. *Hosp. Med.*, **4**, 77.

McCarty, D.J. (1972) Treatment of rheumatoid joint inflammation with triamcinolone hexacetonide. *Arthr. Rheum.*, **15**, 157.

Menkes, C.J., Aignan, M., Galmiche, B. and Le Go, A. (1972) Le traitement des rhumatismes par les synoviorthèses. Choix des malades, choix des articulations, modalités pratiques, résultats indications, contra-indications. *Rhumatologie*, **2** (Suppl. to No. 1), 61.

Miller, J.A. (1957) Joint paracentesis from an anatomic point of view. II. Hip, knee, ankle and foot. *Surgery*, **41**, 999.

Murray, R.O. (1961) Steroids and the skeleton. *Radiology*, **77**, 729.

Osler, W. (1910) *The Principles and Practice of Medicine*, 7th edn. Appleton, New York.

Steinbrocker, O. (1939) Local injections and regional analgesia with procaine solutions for intractable pain in chronic arthritis and related conditions. *Ann. Int. Med.*, **12**, 1917.

Taylor, A.R. and Rana, N.A. (1973) A valve. An explanation of the formation of popliteal cysts. *Ann. Rheum. Dis.*, **32**, 419.

Ziff, M., Contreres, V. and Schmid, T.R. (1956) Use of the hypospray jet injector for the intra-articular and local administration of hydrocortisone acetate. *Ann. Rheum. Dis.*, **15**, 227.

Local injection of non-steroidal drugs

Ansell, B.M., Crook, A., Mallard, J.R. and Bywaters, E.G.L. (1963) Evaluation of intra-articular colloidal gold [198]Au in the treatment of persistent knee effusions. *Ann. Rheum. Dis.*, **22**, 435.

Anttinen, J. and Oka, M. (1975) Intra-articular triamcinolone hexacetonide and osmic acid in persistent synovitis of the knee. *Scand. J. Rheumatol.*, **4**, 125.

Bayly, R.J., Peacegood, J.A. and Peake, S.C. (1973) Yttrium 90 ferric hydrochloric colloid. *Ann. Rheum. Dis.*, **32** (Suppl.), 10.

Beer, T.C., Crawley, J.C.W., Farran, H.E.A. and Gumpel, J.M. (1973) Preliminary assessment of ^{90}Y ferric hydrochloride colloid. *Ann. Rheum. Dis.*, **32** (Suppl.), 41.

Berglöf, F.E. (1959) Osmic acid in arthritis therapy. *Acta Rheumatol. Scand.*, **5**, 70.

Bridgman, J.F., Bruckner, F. and Bleehan, N.M. (1971) Radioactive yttrium in the treatment of rheumatoid knee effusions. *Ann. Rheum. Dis.*, **30**, 180.

Cohen, Y. (1970) in *Analytical Control of Radiopharmaceuticals*, International Atomic Energy Agency, Vienna, p. 1.

Collan, Y., Servo, C. and Winblad, I. (1971) An acute immune response to intra-articular injection of osmium tetroxide. *Acta Rheumatol. Scand.*, **17**, 236.

Currey, H.L.F. (1965) Intra-articular thiotepa in rheumatoid arthritis. *Ann. Rheum. Dis.*, **24**, 382.

Flatt, A.E. (1962) Intra-articular thio-tepa in rheumatoid disease of the hands. *Rheumatism*, **18**, 70.

Gumpel, J.M. (ed.) (1973) Symposium on radioactive colloids in the treatment of rheumatoid arthritis. *Ann. Rheum. Dis.*, **32** (Suppl.).

Gumpel, J.M. (1974) The role of radiocolloids in the treatment of arthritis. *Rheumatol. Rehabil.*, **13**, 1.

Gumpel, J.M. and Stevenson, A.C. (1975) Chromosomal damage after intra-articular injection of different colloids of yttrium 90. *Rheumatol. Rehabil.*, **14**, 7.

Gumpel, J.M., Williams, E.D. and Glass, H.I. (1972) Radio-dosimetry of [90]yttrium and its distribution through the body, following injection into the knee. *Rhumatologie*, **2** (Suppl. to No. 1), 45.

Henderson, E.O. and Nathan, F.F. (1969) Experience with injection of nitrogen mustard into joints of patients with rheumatoid arthritis. *S. Med. J.*, **62**, 1455.

Hurri, L., Sievers, K. and Oka, M. (1963) Intra-articular osmic acid in rheumatoid arthritis. *Acta Rheumatol. Scand.*, **9**, 20.

Ingrand, J. (1973) Characteristics of radio-isotopes for intra-articular therapy. *Ann. Rheum. Dis.*, **32** (Suppl.), 3.

Loevinger, R., Japha, E.M. and Brownell, G.L. (1965) *Discrete radioisotope sources in 'Radiation Dosimetry'* (eds G.H. Hine and G.L. Brownell). Academic Press, New York, p. 693.

Makin, M. and Robin, G.C. (1964) Chronic synovial effusion treated with intra-articular radioactive gold. *J. Am. Med. Assoc.*, **188**, 725.

Martio, J., Isomaki, H., Heikkola, T. and Laine, V. (1972) The effect of intra-articular osmic acid in juvenile rheumatoid arthritis. *Scand. J. Rheumatol.*, **1**, 5.

Muller, J.-H. (1962) *Radioactive Isotope Therapy with Particular Reference to the Use of Colloids*. AIEA Review, Series No. 27. International Atomic Energy Agency, Vienna.

Neustadt, D.H. and Steinbrocker, O. (1956) Observations on the effects of intra-articular phenylbutazone. *J. Lab. Clin. Med.*, **47**, 284.

Oka, M., Rekonen, A., Ruotsi, A. and Seppata, O. (1971) Intra-articular injection of Y-90 resin colloid in the treatment of rheumatoid knee joint effusions. *Acta Rheumatol. Scand.*, **17**, 148.

Rekonen, A., Oka, M. and Ruotsi, A. (1972) Intra-articularly injected ^{90}Y resin colloid. Distribution, fate, and dosimetry. *Rheumatologie*, **2** (Suppl. to No. 1), 53.

Scherbel, A.L., Schuchter, S.L. and Weyman, S.J. (1957) II. Intra-articular administration of nitrogen mustard alone and combined with a corticosteroid for rheumatoid arthritis. *Cleveland Clin. Q.*, **24**, 78.

Vasilionkaitis, V. and Matulis, A. (1977) Trials on the prevention and treatment of osteoarthritis by intra-articular use of artificial lubricants. *Proceedings of the 14th International Congress of Rheumatology, 1977*, Abstract 449, p. 113.

Wenley, W.G. and Glick, E.N. (1964) Medical synovectomy with thiotepa, *Ann. Phys. Med.*, **7**, 287.

Wright, V., Haslock, I., Dowson, E. *et al.* (1971) Evaluation of silicone as an artificial lubricant in osteoarthrotic joints. *Br. Med. J.*, **ii**, 370.

Deleterious effects of local corticosteroid therapy

Bentley, G. and Goodfellow, J.W. (1969) Disorganization of the knees following intra-articular hydrocortisone injections. *J. Bone Joint Surg.*, **51B**, 498.

Boksenbaum, M. and Mendelson, C.G. (1963) Aseptic necrosis of the femoral head associated with steroid arthropathy. *J. Am. Med. Assoc.*, **184**, 262.

Chandler, G.N. and Wright, V. (1958) Deleterious effects of intra-articular hydrocortisone. *Lancet*, **ii**, 661.

Chandler, G.N., Jones, D.T., Wright, V. and Hartfall, S.J. (1959) Charcot's arthropathy following intra-articular hydrocortisone. *Br. Med. J.*, **i**, 952.

Ismail, A.M., Balakroknan, R. and Rajakumar, M.H. (1969) Rupture of patellar ligament after steroid infiltration. *J. Bone Joint Surg.*, **51B**, 4033.

Hartnagel, E.E. (1962) Prolonged steroid therapy and accelerated joint destruction. *Am. Pract.*, **13**, 480.

Heimann, W.G. and Freiberger, R.H. (1960) Avascular necrosis of the femoral and humeral heads after high-dosage corticosteroid therapy. *N. Engl. J. Med.*, **263**, 672.

Lee, H.B. (1957) Avulsion and rupture of tendocalcaneous after injection of hydrocortisone. *Br. Med. J.*, **ii**, 395.

McCarty, D.J. and Hogan, J.M. (1964) Inflammatory reaction

after intrasynovial injection of microcrystalline adreno-corticosteroid esters. *Arthr. Rheum.*, **7**, 359.

Miller, W.T. and Restifo, R.A. (1966) Steroid arthropathy. *Radiology*, **86**, 652.

Steinberg, C.L., Duthie, R.B. and Piva, A.E. (1962) Charcot-like arthropathy following intra-articular hydrocortisone. *J. Am. Med. Assoc.*, **181**, 851.

Sweetman, R. (1969) Corticosteroid arthropathy and tendon rupture. *J. Bone Joint Surg.*, **51B**, 397.

Sweetman, D.R., Mason, R.M. and Murray, R.O. (1960) Steroid arthropathy of the hip. *Br. Med. J.*, **i**, 1392.

Methodology

Baum, J. and Ziff, M. (1967) Use of the hypospray jet injector for intra-articular injection. *Ann. Rheum. Dis.*, **26**, 143.

Bocanegra, T.S., McClelland, J.J., Germain, B.F. and Espinoza, L.R. (1980) Intraarticular fragmentation of a new Parker – Pearson synovial biopsy needle. *J. Rheumatol.*, **7**, 248.

Dixon, A. St. J. and Graber, J. (1978–80) *Local Injection Therapy (LIT) in Rheumatic Diseases (Education Separatum)*, EULAR Bulletin, Parts 1–12, Vols 7–9.

Gottlieb, N.L. (1981) Hypodermic needle separation during arthrocentesis. *Arthr. Rheum.*, **24**, 1593.

Guzman, L. and Arinoviche, R. (1978) Intraarticular fracture of synovial biopsy needle. *Arthr. Rheum.*, **21**, 742.

Hollander, J.L. (1979) in *Arthritis and Allied Conditions: A Textbook of Rheumatology*. (ed. D.J. McCarty), 9th edn, Lea and Febiger, Philadelphia, pp. 402.

Huskisson, E.C. and Hart, F.D. (1975) *Joint Diseases: All the Arthropathies*. Wright, Bristol, p. X.

McCarty, D.J. (1979) in *Arthritis and Allied Conditions; A Textbook of Rheumatology* (ed. D.J. McCarty), 9th edn, Lea and Febiger, Philadelphia, p. 51.

Owen, D.S. (1981) in *Textbook of Rheumatology*. (eds W.N. Kelley, E.D. Harris, S. Ruddy and C.B. Sledge), Saunders, Philadelphia, p. 553.

Rankin, T.J. and Good, A.E. (1966) Corticosteroid injection of small joints by hypospray. *Arthr. Rheum.*, **9**, 611.

Ropes, M.W. and Bauer, W. (1953) *Synovial Fluid Changes in Joint Disease*. Harvard University Press, Cambridge, Massachusetts.

Steinbrocker, O. and Neustadt, D.H. (1972) *Aspiration and Injection Therapy in Arthritis and Musculo-skeletal Disorders*, Harper and Row, Hagestown.

Local corticosteroid therapy of specific sites

Brown, B.B. (1978) Diagnosis and therapy of common myofascial syndromes. *J. Am. Med. Assoc.*, **239**, 646.

Clarke, A.K. and Woodland, J. (1975) Comparison of two steroid preparations used to treat tennis elbow using the hypospray. *Rheumatol. Rehabil.*, **14**, 47.

Darlington, L.G. and Coomes, E.N. (1977) The effect of local steroid injections for supaspinatus tears. *Rheumatol. Rehabil.*, **16**, 172.

Gray, R.G., Kiem, I.M. and Gottlieb, N.K. (1978) Intratendon sheath corticosteroid treatment of rheumatoid arthritis – associated and idiopathic hand flexor tenosynovitis. *Arthr. Rheum.*, **21**, 92.

Henderson, E.D. and Henderson, C.C. (1953) The use of hydrocortisone acetate (compound F acetate) in the treatment of post-traumatic bursitis of the knee and elbow. *Minnesota Med.*, **36**, 142.

Hucherson, D.C. and Freeman, G.E. (1962) Iliopectineal bursitis – a cause of hip pain frequently unrecognised. *Am. J. Orthop.*, **4**, 220.

Lapidus, P.W. and Grudotti, F.P. (1967) Report on the treatment of one hundred and two ganglions. *Bull. Hosp. Joint Dis.*, **28**, 50.

Lee, P.N., Lee, M., Haq, A.M.M.M. *et al.* (1974) Periarthritis of the shoulder: trial of treatments investigated by multivariate analysis. *Ann. Rheum. Dis.*, **33**, 116.

Miller, J.H., White, J. and Norton, T.H. (1958) The value of intra-articular injections in osteoarthritis of the knee. *J. Bone Joint Surg.*, **40B**, 636.

Myles, A.B., Casemore, V.A., Couthlard, M. *et al.* (1973) Management of the carpal tunnel syndrome with local corticosteroid injection. *Rheumatol. Rehabil.*, **12**, 205.

Rogers, M.H. (1939) Treatment of subdeltoid bursitis. *Am. J. Surg.*, **43**, 2929.

Sheldon, P. and Beer, P.C. (1973) Synovitis of the knee treated by intra-articular hydrocortisone acetate, hydrocortisone acetate plus saline, or saline alone. A double blind trial. *Rheumatol. Rehabil.*, **12**, 73.

Swartout, R. and Compere, E.L. (1974) Ischiogluteal bursitis. *J. Am. Med. Assoc.*, **227**, 551.

Symonds, G. (1975) Accurate diagnosis and treatment in painful shoulder conditions. *J. Int. Med. Res.*, **3**, 261.

Williams, M.E., Seifert, M.H., Cuddigan, J.H.P. and Wise, R.A. (1975) Treatment of capsulitis of the shoulder. *Rheumatol. Rehabil.*, **14**, 236.

8
Radiotherapy

8.1 SOME FUNDAMENTAL ASPECTS OF RADIOTHERAPY

8.1.1 Meaning of ionizing radiation

(a) Physical aspects

Electromagnetic radiation is a form of energy (other forms being potential, kinetic, electric, chemical, heat and nuclear energy) propagated by wave motion. The electromagnetic spectrum is shown in Fig. 8.1 and ranges from radio waves of long wavelength and low frequency to ionizing radiations of short wavelength and high frequency.

Radiation can be thought of as a wave passing through space, or as a discontinuous stream of discrete pockets of energy or quanta (the photons).

When the energy of photons exceeds a certain value,

ionization occurs. This is caused by high-energy photons colliding with atoms in which the binding of electrons in the outer atomic shells is overcome. The more loosely bound electrons are removed from the shells, leaving behind ionized atoms. These 'excited' atoms are chemically reactive and are chiefly responsible for radiobiological damage in living tissues.

(b) Production

Ionizing radiation is derived from: (1) X-ray machines; (2) high-energy accelerators; (3) nuclear reactors; or (4) radioisotopes.

X-rays are produced in an X-ray tube which can generate energies up to 300 kV. (The production of X-rays will be discussed in more detail in a later section.)

The linear accelerator is one of the most widely used high-energy megavoltage machines. Electrons from a gun are accelerated along a wave guide to speeds approaching that of light. The electrons can be extracted directly for treatment or they can be directed at a target to emerge as megavoltage X-rays.

Artificial radioactive isotopes may be used as radiation sources. These are contained in teletherapy units with bulky treatment heads. The most popular isotopes have been cobalt-60 and caesium-137. Large-volume radiation sources are necessary, but unfortunately these produce penumbra at the edge of the treatment field. Although this can be trimmed, the sharp definition of the linear accelerator is not possible. Cobalt-60 has a higher specific activity and lower self-absorption than caesium-137 but the shorter half-life of cobalt means that the source must be renewed every few years.

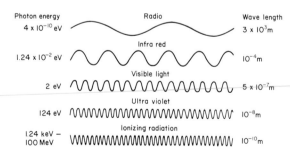

Fig. 8.1 Diagram showing the range of the electromagnetic spectrum (adapted from Lowry, 1974).

8.1.2 Production of X-rays

(a) Physical agents

X-rays are generated whenever fast electrons are slowed down in passing through matter. In a conventional X-ray tube, X-rays arise when the electron beam, which gives rise to the current through the tube, is stopped at the metal target (the anode) of the tube. The electrons, energized by the voltage applied to the tube, penetrate the target metal (tungsten) and interact with its atoms. The impinging electrons interact with the target atoms in three main ways (Walter *et al.*, 1979):

1. Most of the electrons suffer many minor deflections before coming to rest. Each deflection transfers heat to the target atom which has caused the deflection. This cools the target and is an important aspect of X-ray tube design.

2. A second type of interaction causes loss of energy from impinging electrons. This energy re-appears as photons of electromagnetic radiation and gives rise to most of the X-rays emitted from the target.

3. The remaining X-rays emitted arise from a third type of interaction (between impinging electrons and electrons in the orbital electron structure of the target atoms causing them to be ejected from the atoms). The vacant spaces created are filled by electrons in neighbouring orbits. Transfer of an electron to an inner orbit results in loss of energy which is emitted as photons of electromagnetic radiation.

(b) The X-ray set

To generate an X-ray beam for treatment purposes, it is necessary to have an evacuated tube in which the electron stream can be produced and accelerated on to a suitable target by a voltage generator. The fundamental units of an X-ray set are: (1) an evacuated tube; (2) an electron stream; (3) a target; (4) a voltage generator. A simple X-ray generator circuit and details of an X-ray tube are shown in Fig. 8.2.

The X-ray tube is an evacuated glass envelope containing two electrodes (the tungsten filament is the cathode and the other electrode, made of copper, to which the tungsten target is bonded, is the anode). The stream of electrons is produced by thermionic emission from the tungsten filament, and the number of electrons emitted is controlled by the temperature of the filament. The filament is heated by a stabilized circuit and the tube current is controlled by varying the current passing through the filament (Walter *et al.*, 1979).

8.1.3 Radiobiological effects of radiation

Most radiation damage is due to an indirect action. This is in contrast with direct radiation energy absorption by cellular molecules with resulting broken chemical bonds. Ionizing radiation dissipates its energy via ion pairs, and these changes usually occur in water where H, OH and HO_2 radicals are produced. Many of these radicals combine harmlessly to form water again. However, others interact with nearby macromolecules causing bond breakage and a general chemical change. This creates a biological system in which: (1) various 'foreign' chemicals appear; and (2) some vital constituents are destroyed. Some of this damage occurs in the DNA molecule or possibly in the nuclear membrane. These changes retard cellular metabolism but do not result in cell death unless exposed to very high doses of radiation (Lowry, 1974).

Various end-points have been used to measure radiation damage: (1) chromosome damage (most important cause of cell death); (2) mutations (occur randomly and are an insensitive index of injury at low doses); (3) delay in division; (4) loss of reproductive ability (one of the most important measurements in radiation therapy).

For further details of the radiobiological effects of radiation the reader is referred to Alexander (1965), Coggle (1971), and Duncan and Nias (1977).

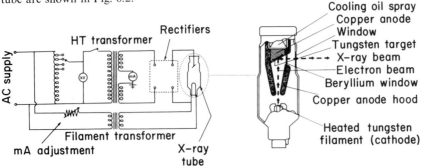

Fig. 8.2 Simple X-ray generator circuit (left) and details of an X-ray tube (right) (adapted from Walter *et al.*, 1979).

8.1.4 Radiation pathology

(a) *Effect on the skin*

Radiation damage to the skin is often the limiting factor in radiotherapy. The dose determines the amount of damage, but there is much individual variation. This depends on race, sex, age, and other factors. For example, black races can tolerate slightly higher doses than white races.

The average observed changes after single exposures of X-ray therapy are as follows:

500 rads – Temporary epilation lasting one month.
1000 rads – Temporary epilation, erythema, pigmentation.
1500 rads – Temporary epilation, erythema, pigmentation, dry desquamation.
2000 rads – Permanent epilation, erythema, moist desquamation which may lead to healing with telangiectasia.
Higher doses – Necrosis.

The histological changes in the epidermis and dermis resemble an inflammatory reaction, with repair and regeneration occurring later. The erythema, seen even after very low doses, is thought to be due to histamine release from damaged cells. An alternative explanation is that it is due to an increase in capillary blood flow and capillary permeability by proteases (Jolles and Harrison, 1966). Pigmentation is due to extravasation of iron and melanocyte migration.

(b) *Effect on blood-forming tissues*

Blood-forming tissue – mainly bone marrow and lymphoid tissue – is highly radiosensitive. The most striking effects are on the stem cells of the leucocytes, lymphocytes and platelets. Red cells are much less radiosensitive, as their life cycle is much longer (about 4 months, compared with a day or less for most types of white cells).

The effects of irradiation on blood cells depend on several factors. Particularly important is the size of the area treated and the amount of bone marrow irradiated. If only a very small part of the body is under treatment, or if therapy is superficial as for skin cancer, the blood changes will be negligible. However, during therapy involving more substantial areas and greater penetration, full blood counts will be necessary at regular intervals (weekly, sometimes even daily). As a broad guide to danger signs, white counts less than $2000\,\mathrm{mm}^{-3}$ or platelets less than $80\,000\,\mathrm{mm}^{-3}$ should be considered with particular caution.

(c) *Effect on bone and cartilage*

High dosage may result in devitalization, necrosis (early or late), and fracture. Damage to blood vessels is the main cause. In rare cases, malignant change (osteosarcoma or fibrosarcoma) has been observed years afterwards. In growing bone, damage to the epiphysis can slow growth and cause shortening of a limb or scoliosis. All the changes are aggravated or precipitated by trauma and infection (Walter *et al.*, 1979).

(d) *Effect on reproductive organs*

Males: sperm production can be halted temporarily by relatively low doses, such as 50 rads. Permanent sterility occurs after about 1000 rads. Androgenic hormone production is more resistant to the effects of radiation and is rarely of clinical significance.

Females: sterility can be induced as in the male, but hormonal effects are more obvious and are of much greater clinical importance than in the male.

Gene mutations: very low doses of radiation (too low to have any obvious effect on mitosis) are still capable of damaging the genes and these mutations are usually harmful.

Radiation in pregnancy: this is particularly undesirable as damage may be twofold – to the mother's ovaries as well as to the fetus. The fetus is particularly vulnerable in view of the rapid growth rate and immaturity of all its tissues. The first 3 months are the most hazardous, and even low-dose radiation during this period can produce such defects as hare lip, cleft palate and mental deficiency. Larger doses will kill the fetus and lead to abortion. It should be added that fetal irradiation gives rise to the further risk of childhood leukaemia.

8.2 RADIOTHERAPY AND RHEUMATIC DISEASES

8.2.1 Some early clinical observations

Soon after the therapeutic use of radiation treatment was introduced, its application to diseases of the joints started. As early as 1899 Sokolow reported improvement in four patients he had treated with X-ray therapy. In the same year Stenbeck (cited by Smyth, 1960) treated 52 patients, most of whom were 'improved'. (In these two earliest reports diagnostic details were not given.) Staunig (1925) obtained generally good results in 400 patients with 'arthritis deformans', and this report helped to pave the way for wider application of radiotherapy.

Radiotherapy was given particular prominence when

Table 8.1 Response to radiotherapy compared with physiotherapy and placebo in patients with ankylosing spondylitis (Hench, 1946)

Type of therapy	Type of assessment	Degree of improvement (%)	
		Moderate	Pronounced
Radiotherapy	Subjective	56	36
	Objective	60	8
Physiotherapy	Subjective	40	8
	Objective	32	8
Placebo	Subjective	28	9
	Objective	8	0

Smyth *et al.* reported their studies in 1940 and 1941. Their first survey (Smyth *et al.*, 1940) was based on 100 patients with different types of rheumatic disease. The results were disappointing, except in patients with ankylosing spondylitis in whom the effect of the treatment was 'significant and not temporary'. In their next paper (Smyth *et al.*, 1941) they reported 52 patients with 'rheumatoid arthritis of the spine' who had been treated with radiotherapy over a 3-year period. Seventy-two per cent of patients showed significant subjective benefit and 50% showed evidence of objective improvement.

Hench (1946) treated 25 spondylitic soldiers with radiotherapy alone, 25 with physiotherapy (deep breathing and postural exercises), and 25 with placebo therapy. The results (Table 8.1) are notably in favour of the group treated with radiotherapy.

Hemphill and Reeves (1945) pointed out the importance of early diagnosis in ankylosing spondylitis, as radiotherapy was found by them to be more effective at this stage of the disease. (This observation has since been challenged.)

Borak and Taylor (1945), in contrast to the previous experience of Smyth's group and to most clinical experience since, found radiotherapy to be beneficial in rheumatoid arthritis.

According to Leucutia (1950) radiotherapy was thought to be the treatment of choice in 'bursitis', 'tenosynovitis', and 'periarticular fibrositis', and in the acute phase of these rheumatic disorders severe pain was relieved within 48 hours.

Cipollaro and Crawford (1950) advocated radiotherapy in many non-malignant skin diseases, and, of those relevant to rheumatology, were included: psoriasis, pyoderma, 'keratosis', and sarcoidosis. They stressed the contraindication of radiotherapy in certain 'dermatological' disorders (e.g. dermatomyositis), and the importance of avoiding it in scleroderma and systemic lupus erythematosus.

Gradually the enthusiasm for radiotherapy gained momentum as a treatment in rheumatology, particularly in ankylosing spondylitis, and by the early 1950s

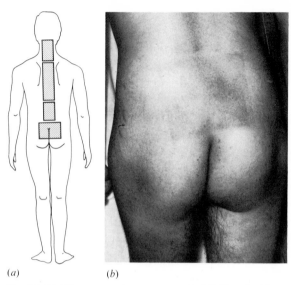

(a)　　　　　*(b)*

Fig. 8.3 (*a*) Diagram to show narrow spinal field and wider field to include both sacro-iliac joints (courtesy of Calman and Berry, 1980 and the publishers). (*b*) Residual pigmentation indicating irradiated areas in a patient with ankylosing spondylitis.

it had become the widely accepted primary treatment for this disease. Indeed, by many physicians it was accepted as the definitive treatment, and the only therapy likely to offer a cure.

Treatment with X-rays was the most popular form of therapy, although thorium X enjoyed a temporary vogue in the UK (Hernamann-Johnson, 1946), and is still in widespread use in Germany (Schales, 1969; Koch, 1969). At first, wide fields covering the entire trunk were used, but were later replaced by a narrower field (8 cm wide) to include the whole spine, and a slightly wider field to include both sacro-iliac joints (Fig. 8.3). Dosage schedules varied considerably, but a generally used regimen was to irradiate the entire spine each day (or on alternate days) to a total applied dose of 15–20 Gy (1500–2000 rads) in 2–3 weeks (Morrison, 1955). (Gy (Gray) represents a new unit of absorbed dose (1 Gy = 100 rads) named after Gray, a radiotherapeutic pioneer.)

The only treatment machines available at the time were X-ray units which emitted X-rays at 100–300 kV. As has been pointed out (Meredith, 1958; Meredith and Massey, 1972), at this energy the X-rays are differentially absorbed by bone, and the tissues within the bone such as osteoblasts and bone marrow close to the periosteum receive a relatively high dose of radiation compared with soft tissue and skin (Fig. 8.4).

This differential effect of X-rays, with blood-forming cells receiving comparatively high doses, ultimately

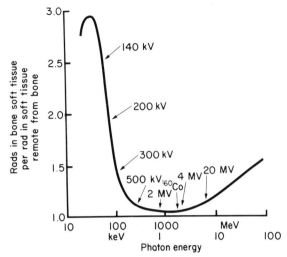

Fig. 8.4 Energy absorbed in bone from X-rays of different energies redrawn from Meredith and Massey, 1972; courtesy of Calman and Berry, 1980 and the publishers).

expressed itself in reports implicating radiotherapy as a cause of increased rates of leukaemia and aplastic anaemia in spondylitic patients (Court-Brown and Abbatt, 1955; Court-Brown and Doll, 1957; Court-Brown and Doll, 1965). The clinical concern generated by these reports rapidly led to the decline of radiotherapy as a popular treatment for ankylosing spondylitis in the late 1950s.

8.2.2 Acute effects of radiotherapy in ankylosing spondylitis

Relatively little is known about the effects of low doses of ionizing radiation on the adult skeleton. As Calman and Berry (1980) have pointed out, this is because adult bone is a non-proliferating system, and is therefore a difficult one in which to observe small amounts of radiation damage.

At high doses, such as those used to treat malignancy, the effects on the adult skeleton are probably mainly due to small blood vessel damage and changes in the central arteries of the Haversian system (Rubin and Casarett, 1968). Rosenthal and Marvin (1957) have shown irreversible damage to osteocytes after high doses of radiation, but the cells were histologically normal after small doses (single doses of 20 Gy). Osteoblasts, however, have been found to be sensitive to the lower doses of radiation used in the treatment of patients with ankylosing spondylitis (Woodward and Spiers, 1953; Regen and Wilkins, 1936), and one worker has found osteoclast activity to be retarded at even lower doses than those affecting osteoblast activity (Koch, 1969). Indeed, Schales (1969) has suggested that it is a diminution of

osteoclastic activity that arrests painful new bone formation in ankylosing spondylitis. Rubin and Casareth (1968) have shown that endochondral new bone formation is abolished at doses of radiation insufficient to cause serious vascular damage. Also, Kember (1967) has demonstrated that a single dose of 8 Gy (800 rads) is enough to reduce the proportion of proliferating chondroblasts at the bony epiphysis to 5%. However, the capacity for regeneration after radiation damage is considerable; at 50 days after a single dose of 15 Gy (1500 rads) growth in epiphyseal cartilage has completely recovered. This temporary effect of radiation emphasizes the need for repeated courses of treatment.

The biochemical changes induced by the acute phase of radiation therapy are not properly understood. Schales (1969) has suggested that ionizing radiation inhibits the pathological tendency to deposit calcium in ankylosing spondylitis. This was presumed to be through an effect on osteoclasts.

These and other aspects of the acute effects of radiotherapy are reviewed by Calman and Berry (1980).

8.2.3 Effect on the course of ankylosing spondylitis

Radiotherapy continually poses the important question concerning its influence on the natural history of the disease. This is in addition to its undoubted effect in improving the patient symptomatically. In the heyday of radiotherapy, physicians with a wide experience of this type of treatment enthusiastically believed that the spondylitic disease process could be slowed or even stopped by radiotherapy (Morrison, 1955; Turney, 1952). This therapeutic enthusiasm has not been accepted without opposition (Segal and Kellogg, 1954; Hilton, 1955; Morrison, 1957; Wilkinson and Bywaters, 1958). Even now the question is not resolved, although there are individual reports suggesting a disease-halting effect of radiotherapy. For example, Calin and Fries (1978) report a patient with ankylosing spondylitis of 30 years' duration who, many years before, had had localized radiotherapy to the T12 region which remained the only spinal area that had not become fused.

If it is to be accepted that radiotherapy can modify the natural history of the disease, what is the mechanism? Calman and Berry (1980) have, as well as previous workers (Walter and Miller, 1969), speculated on an immunosuppressive effect. The fact that immunological manifestations such as renal changes involving deposition of immunoglobulin and complement in the walls of small blood vessels (Linder and Pasternack, 1970), and other evidence showing changes in the serum and synovium of patients with ankylosing spondylitis (Castanedo and Williams, 1967; Kriegel *et al.*, 1969;

Golding, 1973; Kendall *et al.*, 1973; Veys and Van Laere, 1973; Sturrock, 1976, 1980) make this a reasonably acceptable idea, but one still needing verification.

8.2.4 Symptomatic benefit in ankylosing spondylitis

This subject has recently been fully reviewed by Calman and Berry (1980). There is much evidence (based on almost 1000 patients with ankylosing spondylitis) to support the therapeutic effect of radiotherapy in ankylosing spondylitis (Boland and Shebesta, 1946; Freyberg, 1946; Smith *et al.*, 1947; Rees *et al.*, 1948; Robinson and Lampe, 1948; Spishakoff and Low-Beer, 1949; Gelber, 1951; Richmond, 1951). Most of these reports show that radiation exerts a marked symptomatic effect, as well as a beneficial influence on objective physical findings. Such amelioration was found even in patients with advanced disease.

The symptomatic benefit is almost immediate, and in one series (Morrison, 1955) within a month of X-ray treatment two-thirds of patients had experienced substantial and even total relief of symptoms, although less than half had objective evidence of improvement.

Most of the effects of radiotherapy are temporary. For example, in the study of Wilkinson and Bywaters (1958), there was symptomatic relapse in 67% of 200 patients with ankylosing spondylitis at 1 year. The relapse rate rose to 90% after follow-up periods of more than 10 years.

Koch (1969) has treated a large series of patients with thorium-X (a particle-emitting isotope). This is almost entirely bound within the skeleton and is a more specific means of skeletal irradiation than are X-rays. Most of these patients obtained symptomatic relief and many were found to have convincing objective evidence of response. However, long-term follow-up details were not reported, nor was there a control series. Laschner (1973) reported the results of thorium-X treatment in an uncontrolled series of 133 patients. Ninety-two per cent of these patients experienced improvement in pain and increased joint mobility 1 year after treatment, 40% of whom remained in remission at 12 years. The author reported a further series of patients in which 70% improved after thorium injection treatment. (Of the 81 patients in this series, 17 (21%) had had a second course of injections, having relapsed after the first course.) In Lascher's experience thorium-X treatment gave rise to more improvement of symptoms in half his patients than any previous treatment. This observation is at variance with that of Mason (1964) who found little evidence that patients failing on drug treatment will respond to X-rays.

As far as I am aware there have been no prospective controlled trials comparing the effect of radiation therapy with the effect of anti-inflammatory drugs. However, in this context the report of Mason (1964) is of interest. Mason, reporting results from a retrospective analysis of patients treated at the London Hospital suggested that radiotherapy was less effective than anti-inflammatory drugs in achieving symptomatic or objective benefit. This survey also suggested that radiotherapy was less likely to alter the course of the disease. Thus, 35% of patients remained in remission 5 years after radiotherapy, compared with 67% still in remission after receiving anti-inflammatory agents. A further observation made by Mason concerned the optimal stage in the natural history of the disease at which to give radiotherapy. He found contrary to the generally prevalent view held at the time, that it was the patients with advanced disease with completely ossified spines who derived most benefit.

8.2.5 Effect in other rheumatic diseases and co-diseases

X-ray therapy enjoyed a particular vogue for the treatment of certain non-spondylitic rheumatic disorders in the 1940s. This practice has now been largely abandoned, but will be discussed briefly for historical interest.

Calcareous tendinitis. Radiotherapy was considered by most workers to give excellent results in acute subdeltoid bursitis, whether calcified or non-calcified. After treatment, symptoms subsided rapidly and often the calcium deposits disappeared (Smyth, 1960). Chapman (1942), in a review of 54 patients with 'bursitis of the shoulder' treated with radiotherapy, reported that when calcification was present, 'cure' was achieved in 77%, compared with 58% in patients without calcific deposits. Klein and Klemes (1941) found the average disability in 25 patients with shoulder bursitis treated with radiotherapy to be 10 days, compared with 50 days in a group treated with other types of therapy. Pohle and Morton (1947) reported satisfactory relief of symptoms in 84% of 69 patients with subdeltoid bursitis (half of whom had calcific deposits).

Rheumatoid arthritis. Smyth and colleagues used local high-voltage radiotherapy to affected joints in patients with rheumatoid arthritis and noted objective improvement in only 26%; 44% showed no subjective or objective benefit (Smyth *et al.*, 1940; Smyth *et al.*, 1941). This poor response to radiotherapy in rheumatoid patients, in contrast to the much more impressive results in ankylosing spondylitis, has been a consistent observation since the introduction of radiotherapy in the treatment of rheumatic disorders.

Osteoarthrosis. The relief of symptoms in osteoarthrosis has, in general, been as disappointing as that experienced by patients with rheumatoid arthritis, with the exception of a few favourable reports. Thus, Oppenheimer (1943) achieved pain relief in patients with acromioclavicular osteoarthrosis, and similar results were observed in hip joint disease and in cervical spondylosis (Scott, 1939). Kuhns and Morrison (1946) found marked improvement in 16%, moderate improvement in 40% and slight improvement in 29% of 118 patients with osteoarthrosis treated by radiotherapy. These results are better than those obtained by most clinicians who have employed this type of therapy. Hernamann Johnson (1949) examined the effect of hip irradiation in 100 patients with osteoarthrosis and concluded that between a quarter and a third derived 'striking benefit'. Desmarais (1952) has also noted benefit after local radiotherapy to osteoarthrotic joints and ascribed the improvement to the effect of heat.

Post-traumatic arthritis. Stoll (1957) found pain relief within 1–4 weeks in about a half of his series with post-traumatic arthritis or periarthritis.

Acute arthritis. Kahlmeter (1938) treated 5000 patients with various kinds of arthritis, including gouty, gonococcal and septic arthritis, and found the results to be 'excellent'. His results with rheumatoid arthritis, however, were less impressive.

Other forms of radiotherapy than X-rays have been applied to rheumatic disorders. For instance thorium-X was said to be useful in psoriatic arthritis as well as in ankylosing spondylitis (Smyth, 1960). Radon ointment was credited with relief of pain in most patients with 'chronic arthritis'; this involved alpha-ray therapy with a fatty carrier (neutral anhydrous lanolin) as a vehicle for the radon (Jordan, 1944). Lustig (1945) applied radon ointment to the joints of 86 patients with a variety of articular and non-articular rheumatic disorders and found its effect to be 'useful'. Kaplan (1949), on the other hand, found this form of therapy useless for arthritic conditions.

Radiotherapy has had, and still has to a limited extent, an application in rheumatic co-diseases. The co-disease of particular relevance is psoriasis in which X-rays in doses of 0.5–1 Gy (50–100 rads) will usually cause the patches to disappear. However, recurrence is common, and patients in desperation may visit unit after unit for further treatment until they develop radiation dermatitis or even malignancy.

Radiation treatment is no longer a popular treatment in psoriasis, although it may still be indicated for psoriatic problems not responsive to other forms of treatment, such as nail dystrophy and pustular psoriasis of palms and soles (Walter *et al.*, 1979).

8.3 RADIOTHERAPY AND MALIGNANCY

Radiotherapy, as a popular treatment in ankylosing spondylitis fell into disrepute in the mid 1950s after the publication of Court-Brown and Abbatt's paper which drew attention to the increased incidence of leukaemia

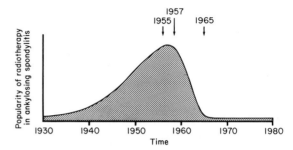

Fig. 8.5 Theoretical curve showing decline in the rheumatological use of radiotherapy since the publications of Court-Brown and colleagues (see text).

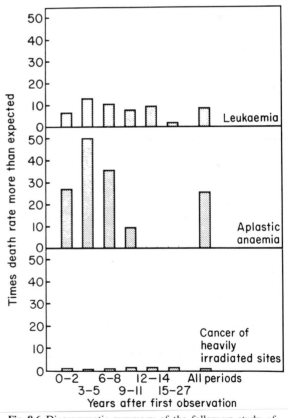

Fig. 8.6 Diagrammatic summary of the follow-up study of Court-Brown and Doll (1965) showing significant increases in death rates due to leukemia and aplastic anaemia after radiotherapy in patients with ankylosing spondylitis.

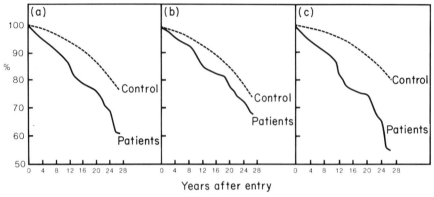

Fig. 8.7 Survival curves for male patients with ankylosing spondylitis compared with age-matched controls. (*a*) 138 patients (62 not treated with radiotherapy, 76 treated); survival decreased (p < 0.005). (*b)* 62 patients not treated with radiotherapy; survival not decreased (p > 0.5). (*c*) 76 patients treated with radiotherapy; survival decreased (p < 0.005). (Redrawn from Kaprove *et al.* 1980.)

after X-ray treatment in patients with ankylosing spondylitis (Court-Brown and Abbatt, 1955). A theoretical curve demonstrating this decline in rheumatological usage of radiotherapy is shown in Fig. 8.5. This follow-up study was later expanded 2 years later (Court-Brown and Doll, 1957), and again 10 years later (Court-Brown and Doll, 1965). At the time of this last report, an impressive total of 14 553 patients with ankylosing spondylitis who had been treated with X-rays during the period 1935–54 had been studied. The completion rate was much above average, more than 98% being traced by 1960, although less complete follow-up information was available for the subsequent 3 years. This series included nearly every spondylitic patient treated radiotherapeutically in Great Britain and Northern Ireland during a period of 20 years. The effects of irradiation were assessed by comparing the numbers of deaths observed in the study population with the numbers that would have been expected if the patients had suffered the death rates recorded in the population of England and Wales as a whole. The important findings are summarized in Fig. 8.6. Not only did this final follow-up confirm previous evidence showing significant increases in the death rates from leukaemia and aplastic anaemia, but it also revealed a significantly increased risk of developing local cancer in heavily irradiated tissues. In contrast to the last finding, the number of deaths from cancers originating in lightly irradiated tissues was not increased significantly. Court-Brown and Doll estimated that in an average follow-up period of 13 years after first treatment the excess deaths that can be attributed to the effects of ionizing radiations were 4 per 1000 patients due to leukaemia and 6 per 1000 patients due to cancers arising in heavily irradiated tissues. The authors raised the possibility that ankylosing spondylitis might itself predispose to malignancy (a

significant increase in leukaemia has been reported in rheumatoid arthritis by Isomaki *et al.*, 1979), but concluded that the blame can be left firmly with radiation treatment. In this regard, a particularly persuasive argument in support of a malignancy-inducing effect in spondylitis patients treated with radiotherapy is the type of leukaemia arising in these patients. Myeloid and myelomonocytic leukaemia are the most common types of leukaemia found in treated patients compared with untreated patients who more often develop lymphatic leukaemia. Myeloid and myelomonocytic leukaemia are also the most common types of leukaemia known to be associated with irradiation generally. Moreover, chronic lymphatic leukaemia has not been reported to be induced by radiation. Further substantiation for the dangerous effects of ionizing radiation in spondylitic patients has been reported by Abbatt and Lea (1956) and by Smith *et al.* (1977) – both groups finding no leukaemia in non-irradiated patients.

A further study of non-irradiated as well as irradiated spondylitics has been reported recently by Kaprove *et al.* (1980). The results of this survey are shown in Fig. 8.7. This demonstrates significantly (p < 0.005) lower survival curves in irradiated patients with ankylosing spondylitis than in non-irradiated patients. The curves also show a lower survival in non-irradiated spondylitics compared with the general population, but this did not reach statistical significance (p > 0.5). The causes of death which occurred more often than expected in the irradiated patients were 'leukaemia' (type not specified) and heart disease (myocardial infarction or congestive heart failure). Kaprove *et al.* found no correlation in the irradiated patients between total dose of radiation and poorer survival.

Doll and Smith (1968) showed that the risk of leukaemia from ionizing radiation is proportional to the total energy absorbed by the bone marrow, regardless of the volume of marrow irradiated. Court-Brown and Doll (1957) showed in addition that a linear dose – response relationship* for the induction of leukaemia exists and that there does not seem to be a 'threshold' dose below which leukaemia is not induced. This dose – response relationship suggested by Court-Brown and Doll is at variance with the data of Kaprove *et al.* (1980), but the latter studied a much smaller group (151 Canadian war veterans).

In support of Court-Brown and Doll are the observations of German workers (Koch, 1969; Schales, 1969) who have stressed the importance of keeping the dose of ionizing radiation to a minimum. Further, these authors prefer low-penetrating α-particles to thorium-X because of the lower dose of ionizing radiation delivered by thorium-X to the bone marrow. However, even this precaution will not abolish the induction of neoplastic changes. Thorium-X has a much shorter half life (3.64 days) than radium or thorotrast and will therefore result in less radiation reaching the skeleton. However, as Calman and Berry (1980) have pointed out in their detailed review, thorium-X has daughter products which emit relatively penetrating γ-rays having an affinity for other organs such as the liver and spleen. Clearly, therefore, bone tumours and tumours of other organs cannot be completely avoided by using low doses of thorium-X.

Mention has already been made of local cancers arising in heavily irradiated sites (Court-Brown and Doll, 1965). Sarcomas, too, have been reported in irradiated spondylitics (Edgar and Robinson, 1973; Bentley *et al.*, 1975), and malignancy has also been observed in patients treated with low doses of X-rays for other non-malignant disorders (Doll and Smith, 1968; Brinkley and Haybittle, 1969; Alderson and Jackson, 1971). The important difference between these malignancies and leukaemia is that the risk of the former appears to develop later, increases with time and shows no sign of abating.

8.4 THE PRESENT POSITION AND THE FUTURE

8.4.1 Climate of modern opinion

The climate of modern opinion can perhaps best be examined against a backcloth derived from the past. Table 8.2 shows, by means of comments culled from generally acknowledged medical texts of the period, how the enthusiasm for X-ray therapy took 40 or so

* The linear relationship between the induction of malignant bone tumours and skeletal dose has also been observed in radium watch-dial luminizers (Hems, 1967).

Table 8.2 Evolution of opinion regarding the use of X-ray therapy in ankylosing spondylitis

Year	Comment (in précis)	Reference
1910	None	Osler
1911	None	Monro
1929	None	Price
1938	X-rays not greatly used in UK for arthritis	Taylor
1955	Of all methods available for spondylitis, X-rays are the most effective	Buckley
1955	Among rheumatic diseases, X-rays are of greatest use in spondylitis	Windeyer
1960	X-ray therapy is of value in spondylitis, but should not be the only treatment	Boland
1969	X-ray therapy should only be considered, if at all, in special circumstances	Mason
1972	X-ray therapy has been abandoned by most authorities, except in the rare patient who cannot be controlled by other means	Ogryzlo
1978	X-ray therapy to the spine is reserved for special cases not responding to safer and more conventional treatment	Moll

years to get established in the UK, peaked in popularity in the early 1950s, then rapidly declined as a generally used and acceptably safe therapy when reports of marrow aplasia, malignancy, and other hazards such as transverse myelitis and amenorrhoea (Sharp and Easson, 1954; Court-Brown and Abbatt, 1955; Abbatt and Lea, 1956; Stewart and Dische, 1956; van Swaay, 1956; Court-Brown and Doll, 1957, 1965; Howard, 1957; Graham, 1958; Mason and Hayter, 1958; Cruickshank, 1960; Stjernsward *et al.*, 1972) began to be linked with irradiation. Radiotherapy has never recovered from this decline and remains in use only to treat occasional spondylitic problems which have proved refractory to safer treatments (Rechenberg, 1962; Wright and Moll, 1969; Boyle and Buchanan, 1971; Jacobs, 1973; Jayson, 1975; Moskovitz, 1975; Katz, 1977). Even those clinicians who have retained confidence in the treatment, and would be satisfied on the patients' behalf to accept the known risks, would find it difficult finding a radiotherapist willing to administer such treatment unless the clinical indications were compelling.

8.4.2 The future

From the evidence available there can be little doubt that radiotherapy, particularly for ankylosing spondylitis, provides substantial symptomatic benefit and could well influence the natural history of the disease. There is still no drug that will unequivocally alter the course of spondylitis, and for this reason alone it might be worth pursuing research into safer methods of administering radiation. Even with present dosage regimens it should be borne in mind that non-irradiated patients have a four-fold increase in deaths from peptic ulceration, 0.4% of patients dying from this cause (Radford *et al.*, 1977). This risk is of similar magnitude to that of irradiated patients dying of leukaemia.

In the future more needs to be known about the comparative effects of long-term anti-inflammatory drugs and X-ray therapy. Carefully controlled trials with prolonged follow-up to assess significant benefit, effect on the natural history of the disease, and side effects are needed. In many centres ethical objections would rightly be raised if the quality and quantity of dosage regimens closely mirrored those in the past, but the use of megavoltage X-rays which do not give a disproportionately high-energy absorption to bone might be considered to be less damaging to the bone marrow (Calman and Berry, 1980).

For the moment, however, radiotherapy will continue to be used judiciously only for the occasional patient whose spinal disease or peripheral problem (e.g. hip joint, heel) has remained uncontrolled by safer forms of treatment.

8.5 SUMMARY AND CONCLUSION

Various fundamental aspects of radiotherapy (meaning of ionizing radiation, production of X-rays, radiobiological effects of radiation, and radiation pathology) have been described. The application of radiotherapy to various rheumatological disorders, particularly ankylosing spondylitis, has been discussed, especially pinpointing its historical perspective.

Although at one time a popular form of therapy for ankylosing spondylitis in particular, despite its symptomatic and possibly disease-suppressant effects, this popularity has faded. This is due to the convincing evidence of malignancies appearing in irradiated patients. Nowadays, the use of radiotherapy in ankylosing spondylitis, if at all, is reserved for isolated peripheral structures not responding to more conservative treatment, providing there is no danger of irradiating large areas of normal tissue.

8.6 REFERENCES AND FURTHER READING

Abbatt, J.D. and Lea, A.J. (1956) The incidence of leukaemia in patients with ankylosing spondylitis treated with X-rays. *Lancet*, **ii**, 1317.

Alderson, M.R. and Jackson, S.M. (1971) Long term follow-up of patients with menorrhagia treated by irradiation. *Br. J. Radiol.*, **44**, 295.

Alexander, P. (1965) *Atomic Radiation and Life*, 2nd edn, Penguin, Harmondsworth.

Bentley, S.J., Davis, P. and Jayson, M.I.V. (1975) Neurofibrosarcoma following radiotherapy for ankylosing spondylitis. *Ann. Rheum. Dis.*, **34**, 536.

Boland, E.W. (1960) in *Arthritis and Allied Conditions. A Textbook of Rheumatology* (ed. J.L. Hollander), 6th edn, Kimpton, London, pp. 643–4.

Boland, E.W. and Shebesta, E.M. (1946) Rheumatoid spondylitis: correlation of clinical and roentgenographic features. *Radiology*, **47**, 551.

Borak, J. and Taylor, H.K. (1945) Beneficial effects of roentgen therapy in advanced cases of rheumatoid arthritis: preliminary report. *Radiology*, **45**, 377.

Boyle, J.A. and Buchanan, W.W. (1971) in *Clinical Rheumatology*, Blackwell, Oxford, p. 298.

Brinkley, D.M. and Haybittle, J.L. (1969) The late effects of artificial menopause by X-radiation. *Br. J. Radiol.*, **42**, 519.

Buckley, C.W. (1955) in *Textbook of the Rheumatic Diseases* (ed. W.S.C. Copeman), 2nd edn, Livingstone, Edinburgh, p. 341.

Calin, A. and Fries, J.F. (1978), *Ankylosing Spondylitis*, Kimpton, London, p. 86.

Calman, F.M. and Berry, H. (1980) in *Ankylosing Spondylitis* (ed. J.M.H. Moll), Churchill Livingstone, Edinburgh, p. 243.

Castanedo, J.P. and Williams, R.C. (1967) Anticomplementary activity of sera from patients with connective tissue diseases and normal subjects. *J. Lab. Clin. Med.*, **69**, 217.

Chapman, J.F. (1942) Subacromial bursitis and supraspinatus tendinitis: its roentgen treatment. *Cal. W. Med.*, **56**, 248.

Cipollaro, A.C. and Crawford, G.M. (1950) in *Clinical Therapeutic Radiology* (ed. U.V. Portmann), Nelson, New York, pp. 614–15.

Coggle, J.E. (1971) *Biological Effects of Radiation*. Wykeham, London.

Court-Brown, W.M. and Abbatt, J.D. (1955) The incidence of leukaemia in ankylosing spondylitis treated with X-rays. *Lancet*, **i**, 1283.

Court-Brown, W.M. and Doll, R. (1957) in *Special Report Series, Medical Research Council*, No. 295, HMSO, London.

Court-Brown, W.M. and Doll, R. (1965) Mortality from cancer and other causes after radiotherapy for ankylosing spondylitis. *Br. Med. J.*, **ii**, 1327.

Coutard, H. (1935) Conception of periodicity as a possible directing factor in roentgen therapy of cancer. *Proc. Inst. Med., Chicago*, **10**, 310.

Cruickshank, B. (1960) Pathology of ankylosing spondylitis. *Bull. Rheum. Dis.*, **10**, 211.

Desmarais, M.H.L. (1952) in *British Practice in Radiotherapy* (eds E.R. Carling, B.W. Windeyer, and D.W. Smithers), Butterworth, London, p. 1955.

Doll, R. and Smith, P.G. (1968) The long term effects of X-irradiation in patients treated for metropathia haemorrhagia. *Br. J. Radiol.*, **41**, 362.

Duncan, W. and Nias, A.H.W. (1977) *Clinical Radiology*, Churchill Livingstone, Edinburgh.

Edgar, M.A. and Robinson, M.P. (1973) Post-radiation sarcoma in ankylosing spondylitis. A report of five cases. *J. Bone Joint Surg.*, **55B**, 183.

Freyberg, R.H. (1946) Roentgentherapy for rheumatic diseases. *Med. Clin. N. Am.*, **30**, 603.

Gelber, L.J. (1951) A five-year summary of X-ray therapy of arthritis, bursitis and radiculitis. *Intl. Rec. Med.*, **164**, 62.

Golding, D.N. (1973) Haematology and biochemistry of ankylosing spondylitis. *Lancet*, **ii**, 663.

Graham, W. (1958) The status of phenylbutazone (Butazolidin) in the treatment of rheumatic disorders. *Can. Med. Assoc. J.*, **79**, 634.

Hemphill, J.E. and Reeves, R.J. (1945) Roentgen irradiation in treatment of Marie – Strümpell disease. *Am. J. Roentgenol.*, **54**, 282.

Hems, G. (1967) The risk of bone cancer in man from internally deposited radium. *Br. J. Radiol.*, **40**, 506.

Hench, P.S. (1946) Arthritis. *J. Am. Med. Assoc.*, **132**, 974.

Hernamann-Johnson, F. (1946) The prognosis of spondylitis in relation to treatment. *Rheumatism*, **3**, 8.

Hernamann-Johnson, F. (1949) X-ray treatment in osteoarthritis. *Rheumatism*, **5**, 44.

Hilton, G. (1955) X-ray treatment of ankylosing spondylitis. *Rheumatism*, **11**, 10.

Howard, N. (1957) The value of irradiation in ankylosing spondylitis. *Br. J. Radiol.*, **30**, 371.

Isomaki, H., Hakulinen, T. and Joutsenlahti, U. (1979) Lymphoma and rheumatoid arthritis. *Lancet*, **i**, 392.

Jacobs, B. (1973) in *Total Management of the Arthritic Patient* (ed. G.E. Erhel), Lippincott, Philadelphia, p. 156.

Jayson, M.I.V. (1975) in *Modern Medicine* (eds A.E. Read, D.W. Barritt, and R. Langton Hewer). Pitman, London, p. 31.

Jolles, B. and Harrison, R.G. (1966) Enzymic processes and vascular changes in the skin radiation reaction. *Br. J. Radiol.*, **39**, 12.

Jordan, H.H. (1944) Radon treatment in chronic arthritis. Preliminary report. *Pan-Am. Rheum. Bull.*, **A44**, 1.

Kahlmeter, G. (1938) Roentgenthérapie dans les maladies rheumatismales; expérience de plus de six ans, fondée sur environ 5,000 cas et plus de 30,000 séances. *Acta Radiol.*, **19**, 529.

Kaplan, I.I. (1949) *Clinical Radiation Therapy*, 2nd edn, Hoeber, New York, pp. 2–6.

Kaprove, R.E., Little, A.H., Graham, D.C. and Rosen, P.S. (1980) Ankylosing spondylitis. Survival in men with and without radiotherapy. *Arthr. Rheum.*, **23**, 57.

Katz, W.A. (1977) in *Rheumatic Diseases. Diagnosis and Management* (ed. W.A. Katz), Lippincott, Philadelphia, p. 535.

Kember, N.F. (1967) Cell survival and radiation damage in growth cartilage. *Br. J. Radiol.*, **40**, 496.

Kendall, M.J., Farr, M., Meynell, J.J. and Hawkins, C.F. (1973) Synovial fluid in ankylosing spondylitis. *Ann. Rheum. Dis.*, **32**, 487.

Klein, I. and Klemes, I.S. (1941) Treatment of peritendinitis calcarea in the shoulder joint. *Radiology*, **37**, 325.

Koch, W. (1969) Results of a twenty-year parenteral thorium-X treatment of Bechterew's disease. *Verhandlungen Deutschen Gesellschaft für Rheumatologie*, **1**, 132.

Kriegel, W., Burger, R., Kapp, W. and Alexopulos, J. (1969) Die immunoglobuline bei ankylosienender spondylitis *Verkandlung der Deutschen Gesellschaft für Rheumatogie*, **1**, 206.

Kuhns, J.G. and Morrison, S.L. (1946) Twelve years' experience in roentgenotherapy for chronic arthritis. *N. Engl. J. Med.*, **235**, 399.

Laschner, W. (1973) Results and complications of the treatment of Bechterew's disease with thorium-X. *Zeitschrift für Orthopaedie und ihre Grenzgebeue*, **111**, 743.

Leucutia, T. (1950) in *Clinical Therapeutic Radiology* (ed. U.V. Portmann), Nelson, New York, pp. 530–1.

Lowry, S. (1974) *Fundamentals of Radiation Therapy and Cancer Therapy*, English Universities Press, London.

Lustig, F. (1945) Radon and physical therapy. *Med. Rec.*, **158**, 225.

Mason, R.M. (1964) Spondylitis. *Proc. R. Soc. Med.*, **57**, 533.

Mason, R.M. (1969) in *Textbook of the Rheumatic Diseases* (ed. W.S.C. Copeman), 4th edn, Churchill Livingstone, Edinburgh, p. 363.

Mason, R.M. and Hayter, R.R.P. (1958) The present status of phenylbutazone therapy in rheumatic disease. *Practitioner*, **181**, 23–8.

Meredith, W.J. (1958) Some aspects of super voltage radiation therapy. *Am. J. Roentgenol.*, **79**, 57.

Meredith, W.J. and Massey, J.B. (1972) *Fundamental Physics of Radiotherapy*, 2nd edn, Wright, Bristol.

Moll, J.M.H. (1978) in *Copeman's Textbook of the Rheumatic Diseases* (ed. J.T. Scott), 5th edn, Churchill Livingstone, Edinburgh, p. 530.

Monro, T.K. (1911) *Manual of Medicine*, 3rd edn, Baillière, Tindall and Cox, London.

Morrison, R. (1955) in *British Practice in Radiotherapy* (eds E.R. Carling, B.W. Windeyer, and D.W. Smithers), Butterworth, London.

Morrison, R. (1957) Results of X-ray treatment of ankylosing spondylitis. *J. Fac. Radiol.*, **8**, 187.

Moskowitz, R.W. (1975) *Clinical Rheumatology. A Problem-Oriented Approach to Diagnosis and Management*, Lea and Febiger, Philadelphia, p. 267.

Ogryzlo, M.A. (1972) in *Arthritis and Allied Conditions* (eds J.L. Hollander and D.J. McCarty), 8th edn, Lea and Febiger, Philadelphia, p. 722.

Oppenheimer, A. (1943) Development of clinical manifestations and treatment of rheumatoid arthritis of the apophyseal intervertebral joints. *Am. J. Roentgenol.*, **49**, 49.

Osler, W. (1910) *The Principles and Practice of Medicine*, 7th edn, Appleton, New York.

Pohle, E.A. and Morton, J.A. (1947) Roentgentherapy in arthritis, bursitis and allied conditions. *Radiology*, **49**, 19.

Prasad, K.N. (1974) *Human Radiation Biology*, Harper and Row, Hagerstown, p. 4.

Price, F.W. (ed.) (1929) *A Textbook of the Practice of Medicine*. 3rd edn, Oxford University Press, London.

Radford, E.P., Doll, R. and Smith, P.G. (1977) Mortality among patients with ankylosing spondylitis not given X-ray therapy. *N. Engl. J. Med.*, **297**, 572.

Rechenberg, H.K. von (1962) *Phenylbutazone. Butazolidin*, 2nd edn, Arnold, London, p. 70.

Rees, S.E., Albers, E.A. and Nichols, G.B. (1948) Rheumatoid spondylitis: its early diagnosis and treatment. *Northwest Med.*, **47**, 260.

Regen, E.M. and Wilkins, W.E. (1936) The influence of roentgen radiation on the rate of healing of fractures and the phosphatase activity of the callus of adult bone. *J. Bone Joint Surg.*, **18**, 69.

Richmond, J.J. (1951) The importance of radiotherapy in the treatment of ankylosing spondylitis. *Proc. R. Soc. Med.*, **44**, 443.

Robinson, W.D. and Lampe, I. (1948) Long-range evaluation of radiotherapy in rheumatoid spondylitis. *Ann. Rheum. Dis.*, **7**, 245.

Rosenthal, L. and Marvin, J.F. (1957) The effect of roentgen-ray quality on bone growth and cortical bone damage. *Am. J. Roentgenol.*, **77**, 893.

Rubin, P. and Casarett, G.W. (1968) in *Clinical Radiation Pathology* (eds P. Rubin, and G.W. Casarett), Saunders, Philadelphia.

Schales, F. (1969) Radiotherapy of ankylosing spondylitis. *Zeitschrift füe Orthopaedie und ihre Grenzgebeite*, **106**, 798.

Scott, S.G. (1939) *Wide-Field X-ray Treatment*, Newnes, London.

Segal, G. and Kellogg, D.S. (1954) Osteitis condensans ilii. *Am. J. Roentgenol.*, **71**, 643.

Sharp, J. and Easson, E.C. (1954) Deep X-ray therapy in spondylitis. *Br. Med. J.*, **i**, 619.

Smith, R.T., Boland, E.W. and Hench, P.S. (1947) The effect of röntgentherapy in rheumatoid spondylitis. *Ann. Rheum. Dis.*, **6**, 114.

Smith, P.G., Doll, R. and Radford, E.P. (1977) Cancer mortality among patients with ankylosing spondylitis not given X-ray therapy. *Br. J. Radiol.*, **50**, 728.

Smyth, C.J. (1960) in *Arthritis and Allied Conditions. A Textbook of Rheumatology* (ed. J.L. Hollander), 6th edn, Kimpton, London, p. 159.

Smyth, C.J., Freyberg, R.H. and Peck, H.S. (1940) Roentgen therapy for rheumatic disease. *J. Am. Med. Assoc.*, **115**, 2209.

Smyth, C.J., Freyberg, R.H. and Lampe, I. (1941) Roentgen therapy for rheumatoid arthritis of the spine. *J. Am. Med. Assoc.*, **117**, 826.

Smyth, C.J., Bunim, J.J., Clark, W.S. *et al.* (1959) Rheumatism and arthritis: review of American and English literature of recent years. *Ann. Int. Med.*, **50**, 435.

*Sokolow (1899) Roentgenstrahlen gegen gelenk rheumatismus. *Fortsch a.d. Geb. d. Rontgenstrahlen*, **1**, 209.

Spishakoff, N.M. and Low-Beer, B.V.A. (1949) Roentgen therapy of rheumatoid spondylitis *Cal. Med.*, **70**, 1.

Staunig, K. (1925) Über Röntgentherapie der Arthritis deformans. *Strahlentherapie*, **20**, 113.

Stewart, J.W. and Dische, S. (1956) Effect of radiotherapy on bone-marrow in ankylosing spondylitis. *Lancet*, **ii**, 1063.

Stjernsward, J., Jondal, M., Vanky, F. *et al.* (1972) Lympho-penia and change in distribution of human B and T lymphocytes in peripheral blood induced by irradiation for mammary carcinoma. *Lancet*, **i**, 1352.

Stoll, B.A. (1957) X-ray therapy in post-traumatic arthritis, paraarthritis and fasciitis *Med. J. Austr.*, **i**, 868.

Sturrock, R.D. (1976) *Clinical and Immunological Studies in Ankylosing Spondylitis.* M.D. thesis, University of London.

Sturrock, R.D. (1980) in *Ankylosing Spondylitis* (ed. J.M.H. Moll), Churchill Livingstone, London.

Taylor, H.J. (1938) in *The Rheumatic Diseases* (eds L. Hill and P. Ellman), Arnold, London, p. 191.

Turney, H.F. (1952) Ankylosing spondylitis. *Proc. R. Soc. Med.*, **45**, 57.

Van Swaay, H. (1956) *Contemporary Rheumatology*, Elsevier, Amsterdam.

Veys, E.M. and Van Laere, M. (1973) Serum IgG, IgM and IgA levels in ankylosing spondylitis. *Ann. Rheum. Dis.*, **32**, 493.

Walter, J. and Miller, H. (1969) in *Short Textbook of Radiotherapy*, 3rd edn, Churchill, London.

Walter, J., Miller, H. and Bomford, C.K. (1979) *A Short Textbook of Radiotherapy. Radiation Physics, Therapy, Oncology*, 4th edn, Churchill Livingstone, Edinburgh.

Wilkinson, M. and Bywaters, E.G.L. (1958) Clinical features and course of ankylosing spondylitis. As seen in a follow-up of 222 hospital referred cases. *Ann. Rheum. Dis.*, **17**, 209.

Windeyer, B.W. (1955) in *Textbook of the Rheumatic Diseases* (ed. W.S.C. Copeman), 2nd edn, Churchill Livingstone, Edinburgh, p. 587.

Woodward, H.Q. and Spiers, F.W. (1953) The effect of X-rays of different qualities on the alkaline phosphatase of living mouse bone. *Br. J. Radiol.*, **26**, 38.

Wright, V. and Moll, J.M.H. (1969) *Seronegative Polyarthritis*, North Holland, Amsterdam, p. 417.

* The author's initials were not cited in the original publication.

9

Orthopaedic surgery

9.1 INTRODUCTION

This chapter is intended to look at the place of arthritis surgery from the physician's point of view, and will not concern itself with technical details which lie within the province of the surgeon. However, to draw a line between knowledge relevant to the physician and that relevant to the surgeon is not possible in view of the big overlap that exists between their respective responsibilities. This is a manifestation of the team approach which is pivotal to the optimal management of patients requiring surgery.

Arthritic disorders commonly encountered in rheumatological practice tend to produce similar consequences in the affected joints. Persistent pain is the primary indication for operative intervention, but loss of function, progressive damage or deformity may also be important enough to warrant surgery.

Reconstructive surgery is usually indicated to *relieve* any or all of these problems, but in some patients operative treatment may be undertaken for *preventative* reasons.

The value of surgery in the rheumatological patient on a cost – benefit basis is difficult to evaluate, and certainly with regard to patients who return to work after surgery, its worth may be questioned. However, in terms of decreased need for home help, home modifications, hospitalization or confinement to long-term care,

and in terms of release of the spouse from his/her helping role, enabling return to work, there can be little doubt about the benefits of rheumatological surgery (Jergesen *et al.*, 1978).

9.2 INDICATIONS

As stated previously, the main general (as opposed to specific) indications for surgery are persistent pain, loss of function, progressive damage/deformity, or deformity causing cosmetic dissatisfaction.

These indications are somewhat artificial in themselves as much overlap exists between them.

1. *Persistent pain.* The degree and persistence (implying continual as opposed to intermittent or migratory) of a patient's pain is often difficult to assess and is usually associated with other indications for surgery such as loss of function and/or deformity. Although some help may be gained from the findings of radiological and other objective tests, the final decision will always depend on careful clinical assessment. The latter should include a consideration of the patient's psychological make-up, particularly with regard to pain threshold, motivation and willingness to participate in the postoperative programme.

2. *Loss of function.* Functional impairment should be viewed from the standpoint of personal, sociodomestic

or occupational relevance, and not purely as an abnormality revealed by biomechanical measurement. Loss of function may be largely the effect of restricted activity due to pain or to the disruptive physical effects of the disease on the joint(s). Often clear distinction between the factors involved is not possible.

3. *Progressive damage/deformity*. This indication includes such problems as continuing flexion contracture, increasing joint laxity, or diminished joint excursion. Persistent synovial swelling (sometimes classed separately as an indication) with or without pain, deformity or loss of function constitutes another reason for surgery. The question of progressive radiological change is usually considered together with other indications, such as the presence of pain, but in the absence of pain, the justification of surgery is debatable and not generally acceptable.

4. *Cosmetic dissatisfaction*. In most patients the deterioration in appearance will be taking place gradually against a background of persisting pain and diminishing function, and there will usually be more concern about the physically incapacitating problems than with altered appearance. Surgery is therefore unusual for cosmetic reasons alone. However, some patients can be given a significant boost to their morale by improved appearance, although unfortunately, as cosmetic surgery often involves the hands, some loss of function may be the price to pay for cosmesis.

5. *Specific indications*. As opposed to the more general indications outlined above, surgery may be indicated for specific problems such as tendon rupture, persistent bursitis, removal of nodules, and nerve entrapment syndromes.

9.3 CONTRAINDICATIONS

Most operations for rheumatic patients are not essential to life, and therefore the general surgical contraindications (such as poor overall condition and advanced age), applicable to non-rheumatological as well as rheumatological problems, carry relatively more weight. However, with currently available regional anaesthesia (plexus and intravenous regional anaesthesia for the upper limb; sciatic and femoral cutaneous nerve block, and lumbar and epidural anaesthesia for the lower limb) operations can be carried out more safely than in the past.

A high degree of inflammatory activity in the target joints is not regarded as a contraindication, although surgery is usually postponed until an acute flare-up has remitted or has been brought under control by conservative measures. Generalized (polyarticular) activity is also best brought under control before a decision to operate is made in order to assess realistically the clinical significance of the changes in the joint requiring surgery.

Perhaps the most important *general* contraindication is lack of motivation on the part of the patient. Psychological inertia in the participation of intensive postoperative management can have a disastrous effect on an otherwise successful procedure.

Many questions enter into the choice and timing of an operation, and these should be answered in order to establish a reasonable operative plan, as was stressed by Wilson (1937) over 40 years ago (cited by Flatt, 1979). Some of these (1, 2, 3 and 5) have already been mentioned:

1. Is the arthritis still active?
2. Is the patient in good enough physical condition to permit extensive surgical procedures?
3. Considering the age of the patient, his physical state, and the number of operations required, is the expected gain in function from operation worth the effort?
4. Should the operation be delayed for any reason for institution of other therapy?
5. Will the patient be able to co-operate in after-care with sufficient morale and willingness to endure some pain?
6. Are the facilities necessary for successful treatment present in the hospital?
7. Will the patient be able to receive proper after-care on leaving the hospital?
8. Is the patient's financial status such that he can go through the entire treatment, or have the resources of the community been mobilized to care for such treatment? (More relevant in the USA than in the UK.)

To these considerations may be added, as Flatt (1979) has pointed out, the question regarding the patient's spontaneous wish to have the operation.

Attempts by medical advisers to 'sell' an operation should be vigorously avoided, and a useful policy, if patients are in doubt, is to introduce them to patients who have undergone a similar operation.

9.4 PREOPERATIVE ASSESSMENT AND MANAGEMENT

The success of any major surgical procedure has as much to do with careful preoperative appraisal and management as with the technical aspects of the operation itself, once the need for the operation has been decided. The main factors to be considered may be summarized as follows:

9.4.1 Psychological and sociodomestic factors

The degree of motivation and willingness of the patient to participate in the after-care programme should be assessed, and may be enhanced by ensuring adequate doctor – patient communication. This involves not only explaining to patients what is involved and what their expectations might be, but also ensuring that instructions and advice have been properly understood. Compliance is more likely to be successful if sufficient attention has been paid to communication, and there is evidence that informed patients suffer less postoperative pain than those who feel that medical explanations have been inadequate (Egbert *et al.*, 1964). In addition, it has been shown that by using structured written material preoperatively, as opposed to unstructured verbal advice, the mean length of hospital stay can be significantly reduced (Lindeman and Van Aernam, 1971).

Sociodomestic factors such as the degree of family support and the reaction of relatives to the intended operation should be carefully assessed before surgery, preferably by a home visit. Explanations regarding the likely outcome of treatment and the way in which this might affect the family can be expressed at this time, as well as questions answered regarding more personal matters which the patient may have been inhibited to raise in the clinic. Such questions might include advice regarding the effect of the operation on sexual function, childbirth, and child-rearing.

9.4.2 General medical factors

The *age* of the patient may modify decisions as to when to operate, though rarely constitutes a contraindication to surgery. Patients may be considered too young for prosthetic replacement, either because of the technical difficulty of finding a prosthesis small enough for the joint in question, or because of the limited life of the prosthesis, and the possible need for replacement later on. In these patients it may be decided to defer surgery. Advanced age on its own is not usually an influencing factor unless associated with ill health. Again, the shortened life span of patients with rheumatoid arthritis, in which life expectancy may be reduced by some 4–8 years (Uddin *et al.*, 1970), does not usually contraindicate surgery and, indeed, may be considered a reason for expediting it.

Obesity is usually more of a problem in patients with osteoarthrosis than in rheumatoid arthritis. It should be energetically treated, both to reduce unwanted stress on reconstructed weight-bearing joints and to facilitate surgery.

Anaemia – although many patients are anaemic, there is no evidence to show that there is any increased risk in operating upon patients who have adapted to haemoglobin levels as low as 10.5 g (100 ml^{-1}) (Garner *et al.*, 1973). Those with lower values are best transfused a few days before surgery.

Incidental cardiorespiratory dysfunction and pro-

blems involving other systems (e.g. renal, hepatic and endocrine disease) should be controlled if possible, even if this means substantial operative delay. Direct general medical consequences of the rheumatic disease on other systems should have a bearing on the operation. Such problems in rheumatoid patients include amyloidosis with a very low serum albumin level, vasculitis with impaired capillary blood flow, and marked osteoporosis.

The various forms of seronegative spondarthritis carry their own risks. Examples of such risks include: cardiac involvement in ankylosing spondylitis and Reiter's disease; increased risk of wound infection if incision made through a psoriatic plaque (Marples *et al.*, 1973; Aly *et al.*, 1976; Lambert and Wright, 1979); increased risk of infection in the enteropathic arthropathies (either from haematogenous seeding from a focus of bowel infection or contamination from a colostomy adjacent to the incision for hip replacement). Patients with systemic lupus erythematosus, often on large doses of corticosteroids, have a special risk of postoperative osteonecrosis and infection. In addition, lupus patients with renal involvement are more likely to have a reduced life expectancy, although prosthetic replacement may well be justified to relieve pain and to improve the quality of life for the remaining years.

Sepsis both locally and at distant sites (e.g. renal, pulmonary and dental infections) should be energetically treated in order to minimize the risk of wound infection and, more importantly, infection of the reconstructed joint.

9.4.3 Factors affecting the target structure

Factors affecting the site of surgery concern particularly the joints, as opposed to extra-articular tissues. It is unnecessary to control the activity of the local joint disease before surgery. Indeed, in the case of synovectomy of the knee, some surgeons prefer that no intra-articular injection of corticosteroids be given for at least 6 weeks before the operation, as it is easier to remove completely a thickened, readily visible synovial membrane. Deformities secondary to inflammatory (e.g. flexion deformity of the knee and elbow) should be corrected as this will simplify the surgical procedure, and the resultant improvement in the condition of surrounding muscles will hasten postoperative recovery, and is likely to improve the results of surgery.

The functional state of other joints should be included in the overall decision to operate and in the choice of the procedure to be used. Obviously correction of one joint will be wasted effort if the condition of other joints is insufficient to provide 'background support'. Conversely, an attempt should also be made to anticipate the likely effect of the operation on other joints.

Involvement of the ipsilateral hip and knee usually leads to the hip being treated first. The position of the flexed knee is used as a guide for insertion of the femoral component of the hip prosthesis. In the presence of severe knee instability and/or valgus deformity, proper positioning of the hip component will be compromised (Poss, 1979). If, due to these facts, the component is placed in retroversion, postoperative dislocation becomes more likely. Similarly, if the hip has been arthrodesed, the position of the knee components must be suitably altered, depending on the degree of abduction or adduction of the arthrodesed hip.

9.4.4 Local factors

Wound healing: the importance of eradicating septic foci has already been stressed. Other local factors of surgical significance include rashes (e.g. psoriasis) and nodules encroaching on the surgical site. Corticosteroid-induced dermal atrophy has been shown to be associated with delayed wound healing and an increase in wound infections (Garner *et al.*, 1973). The important factor identified by this study was not so much the dose level of corticosteroids (2.5–15 mg of prednisolone per day) in these patients, but the duration of treatment – patients treated for more than 3 years being particularly at risk. However, of more immediate surgical significance and concern is the importance of avoiding the application of a tight bandage before inflating the tourniquet in patients with skin damaged by corticosteroids to avoid detachment of the subcutis and deep necrosis. Mowat (1978) has summarized these and other factors which alone or in combination might be expected to influence wound healing:

1. Bacterial infection in the chest and joints.
2. Corticosteroid-induced skin thinning.
3. Leucopenia.
4. Anaemia.
5. Low serum albumin.
6. Wound haematomata secondary to aspirin and related drugs.
7. Vasculitis with skin ischaemia.
8. Reduced neutrophil leucocyte chemotactic activity.

9.4.6 Technical consideration of surgery

The choice of the operation will be based on the surgeon's personal experience and expertise, coupled with evidence from clinical studies elsewhere demonstrating its worth.

The relative amount of mobility and stability required must be assessed and the choice of surgical procedure made accordingly. Some operations may provide a greater range of movement, but with some reduction in stability. Generally, excision arthroplasty leads to less stability than prosthetic arthroplasty (particularly at the hip and elbow). This physical attribute of excision arthroplasty may have an important bearing on joints in which the removal of an infected prosthesis become necessary. Such joints are likely to be left with a good range of movement, but with considerable instability. This outcome will clearly be less acceptable for a weight-bearing joint than for an upper limb joint.

The use of a tourniquet. Unless the tourniquet is to be deflated briefly during the operation, the available time for the procedure is restricted to about $1\frac{1}{2}$ hours, with further restrictions if the patient has significant peripheral atherosclerosis or vasculitis.

Damage to the skin during surgery. Patients with rheumatoid arthritis have thinning of the skin (quite apart from corticosteroid-induced atrophy). Unless this is realized the patient may emerge from the operation covered in finger prints due to handling of the patient's face and neck by the anaesthetist and of the limbs by the surgeon and assistants. The most vulnerable area is over the shin which can be usefully covered with protective foam and bandages applied preoperatively. The delicateness of rheumatoid skin may lead the surgeon to alter his incision approach. For example, the usual parapatellar incision to open the knee may be abandoned because of thin skin over the upper tibia in favour of short medial and lateral incisions. Alternatively, a medial incision dividing vastus medialis (despite the fact that this is important for full knee extension) can be made.

Infection-biasing factors. Apart from the importance of eradicating local and distant sources of infection to avoid the catastrophe of an infected prosthesis, there are other factors that may incline a patient to be sepsis-prone. Much evidence supports the fact that patients with rheumatoid arthritis have a higher frequency of prosthetic infection than do patients with osteoarthrosis. This infection rate is also higher if the joint has been operated upon previously, regardless of whether or not a prosthesis was used (Roles, 1971; Dupoint and Charnley, 1972; Harris *et al.*, 1972).

9.4.6 Drugs

In the perioperative management of drug therapy the following should be considered (Mowat, 1978):

1. The anti-rheumatic regimen which has been stabilized preoperatively should be continued over the operative period to prevent a general flare-up of joint activity. This particularly applies to corticosteroid therapy which, although boosted by the general stimulus of surgery, should be increased parenterally to double the usual dose for 24–48 hours after surgery. Intramuscular hydrocortisone is an established means of achieving this.

2. Checks should be made to ensure that intercurrent therapy has not significantly reduced the white cell or platelet count.

3. Patients who have undergone repeated orthopaedic surgery, and consequent exposure to halothane, run a risk of developing sensitivity to this drug which may lead to hepatic damage (*Editorials*, 1974, 1975).

4. Salicylates and related anti-inflammatory agents have a direct effect on prothrombin activity and reduce platelet adhesion; this may occur even if the drugs are used in low dosage. However, wound haematoma is only a rare consequence, and the antithrombotic effects of these drugs may actually be beneficial, and may explain the relatively reduced occurrence of deep venous thrombosis in rheumatic patients who have undergone orthopaedic surgery (Salzman *et al.*, 1971).

5. Despite the findings of Salzman *et al.*, major hip and knee surgery is associated with an increased frequency of deep venous thrombosis (50%) and pulmonary embolism (2–4%), and many orthopaedic surgeons prefer to use some form of anticoagulant (Kelsey *et al.*, 1975). There is still no general agreement as to which is the superior regimen for anticoagulation in this context and the following have been employed: commarin anticoagulants; subcutaneous low-dose heparin (Nicolaides *et al.*, 1972a); low molecular weight dextran; aspirin (MRC, 1972); various mechanical devices attached to the legs (Hills *et al.*, 1972; Nicolaides *et al.*, 1972b).

A recent review published by the Drugs and Therapeutics Bulletin (Herxheimer, 1982) has pointed out that, compared with general surgery, patients who have undergone orthopaedic surgery experience less effective response to low-dose heparin in terms of reduction of deep venous thrombosis. It is recommended that for elective hip replacement dextran be used in view of the relatively poor prophylactic effects of low-dose heparin in preventing deep venous thrombosis. However, heparin could be used if dextran were contraindicated because of hypersensitivity or the risk of fluid overload.

9.4.7 Anaesthetic considerations

Rheumatic patients undergoing surgery may pose problems in handling and intubation because of the particular pattern and severity of joint involvement.

(a) Rheumatoid arthritis

Instability of the neck in rheumatoid patients with atlantoaxial subluxation, or subluxation at other levels in the cervical spine, requires very careful handling. As most of these patients are symptom free, and as those likely to be in particular jeopardy cannot be reliably screened radiographically (Smyth *et al.*, 1972), it is prudent to ensure that all rheumatoid patients enter the operating theatre wearing a soft collar. Even though this will have to be removed, it acts as a useful reminder to those involved in the preliminary handling of the patient.

(b) Ankylosing spondylitis

These patients may represent a considerable challenge to the anaesthetist for the following reasons (Cohen, 1980):

1. Difficulty in securing the airway due to anatomical distortion caused by spine involvement. Endotracheal intubation is particularly difficult in the face of fixed flexion of the head and neck, perhaps associated with some lateral distortion. An added factor may be limitation of mouth opening because of either approximation of the lower jaw to the chest wall and/or temporomandibular involvement. There are ways of overriding difficult endotracheal intubation (e.g. with specially designed laryngoscope blades), and these are preferable to the alternative of tracheostomy which is itself often precluded by the head and neck flexion deformity.

2. The severe restriction in chest wall expansion may affect the conduct of anaesthesia and its postoperative complications. Although in many patients diaphragm movement compensates well for the reduced mobility of the chest wall (Zorab, 1962), difficulty may be experienced in achieving adequate pulmonary gas exchange during anaesthesia, and considerable force may be required to establish this. (In spondylitic patients undergoing abdominal or thoracic surgery, the difficulty due to chest wall rigidity may be aggravated by limitation of diaphragm movement as a result of surgery to, or near, the diaphragm, and by the effects of retraction and packs in the abdominal cavity.)

(c) Juvenile chronic polyarthritis

Important points to consider in these patients under review for surgery are the difficulties that may arise during intubation because of apophyseal joint fusion in the cervical spine and restriction of jaw opening due to temporomandibular joint involvement (Brechner, 1968; Ornilla *et al.*, 1972; Wright and Moll, 1976). Although rare, atlantoaxial subluxation may occur in patients with juvenile ankylosing spondylitis (Reid and Hill, 1978; Ansell, 1980), and if spontaneous fusion does not occur, surgical fusion may have to be considered. These patients will need particularly careful handling preoperatively, and the comments about the importance of collar wearing applies as much to these patients as to patients with adult rheumatoid arthritis.

9.5 POSTOPERATIVE MANAGEMENT

Surgical management of patients with rheumatic disorders who have undergone reconstructive procedures includes the fundamental considerations involved in any postoperative patient, with the addition of specific factors relating to the orthopaedic procedure adopted and the rheumatic problem to which it has been applied.

General aspects such as haemostasis to minimize the potential for surgical shock and collapse, fluid/electrolyte and nutritional management, wound care, constant search for signs of local infection, the potential for respiratory failure, atelectasis, pulmonary oedema, thromboembolic disease, urinary tract infection or postoperative urinary retention must be anticipated and acted upon when necessary according to basic lines of management.

Specific considerations in postoperative management may be divided as follows:

1. Those concerned with the nature of the rheumatic disease, for example: the likelihood of postoperative flares of gout, which may be more difficult to treat than spontaneous attacks; the tendency of ectopic bone formation in patients with ankylosing spondylitis, and the question regarding the use of prophylactic agents (e.g. corticosteroids, diphosphonates) to minimize this (Francis *et al.*, 1969; Nollen and Slooff, 1973; Resnick *et al.*, 1977; Turek, 1977); the increased likelihood of wound infection in psoriatic patients; the potential for infection of the reconstruction in the enteropathic arthritides (e.g. ulcerative colitis, Crohn's disease); the susceptibility of patients needing high doses of corticosteroids (e.g. systemic lupus erythematosus) to osteonecrosis and infection.

2. Those concerned with the structure to be treated, for example various types of splintage or traction may be required, depending on the anatomical area of reconstruction (e.g. hard collar after atlantoaxial fusion; balanced suspension and traction after hip replacement). The role of physical therapy in the postoperative management of patients undergoing joint replacement surgery has not yet been clearly defined. However, there is evidence that it plays only a minimal role in patients who have undergone hip replacement (Charnley, 1979), but is much more useful in the postoperative management of hand surgery (Melvin, 1977).

3. Those concerned with the type of surgical procedure adopted. For example, radiographic evaluation is mandatory in the postoperative assessment of a new prosthetic joint to check: the position of the components of the artificial joint, the adequacy of cement fixation, and the restoration of joint alignment. The radiograph will also enable evidence of loosening to be detected.

Artificial joints also impose an increased risk from blood-borne infection (D'Ambrosia *et al.*, 1976), and it is a usual policy to institute prophylactic antibiotics in patients undergoing dental or urological procedures, and to alert these patients to the potential danger of untreated infections so that they can seek early medical attention. Details vary between surgeons but the general approaches are similar. Routine use of prophylactic antibiotics (e.g. i.v. cephalosporin) may be started about 2 hours before surgery and is continued during the operation for 48 hours (Mears, 1980).

Mention has already been made of prophylactic anticoagulation. Some surgeons use this routinely, others only in patients at high risk of thromboembolic disease, such as those with marked obesity or a past history of deep venous thrombosis or pulmonary embolism. Anticoagulants (e.g. dextran or low-dose subcutaneous heparin) are usually started preoperatively and continued for 7–10 days after the operation (Mears, 1979).

Prophylactic antibiotics and anticoagulation are also used in reconstructive surgery of the knee joint (Insall, 1981).

Most patients who undergo total hip replacement require intra or postoperative replacement of blood, even if blood loss is minimized by using the posterolateral approach to the hip joint. Some surgeons prefer to bleed patients on two occasions during the fortnight before surgery with a view to auto-transfusion.

9.6 TYPES OF SURGERY

Surgical operations used in the treatment of the rheumatic patient may be divided into articular and extra-articular surgery.

9.6.1 Articular surgery

(a) Synovectomy

Removal of some or most of the synovial lining of the joint is only considered of value in the treatment of finger, wrist, elbow and knee joints. The main indications for this type of surgery are pain and swelling of a joint unresponsive to medical therapy, preferably at an early stage of the disease before significant damage of cartilage and bone has occurred (Goldie, 1974). Earlier hope that synovectomy would confer a prophylactic effect in at least retarding the rate of joint damage in rheumatoid arthritis have not been sustained (Arthritis and Rheumatism Council/British Orthopaedic Association, 1976). Disappointing results with this surgical approach may, in part, relate to the fact that at best only 85% of the synovial tissue is excised and that the synovial lining of similar pathological type regrows within 2–3 months of surgery from existing mesenchymal elements, although it may take many more months to be clinically detectable (Taylor and Ansell 1972). However, in terms of pain relief and reduced swelling the benefits are fairly predictable and may last for 3–5 years. These benefits must be weighed against attendant problems such as the usual surgical risks, significant loss of joint mobility (particularly in finger joints), absence of prophylactic value, and the need for a relatively long period of hospitalization (3 weeks for knee synovectomy). Unfortunately, the more conservative alternative of 'medical synovectomy', using radioisotopes and other chemotherapeutic agents, has not yet been shown convincingly to be superior. In addition, these agents possess their own problems and dangers.

(b) Arthrodesis

This is performed in severe deformities which are seriously affecting function. It is best performed on a weight-bearing joint, although in the hand, arthrodesis can result in a delicate balance between stability and mobility for adequate function. Other sites amenable to surgical fusion are the wrist, the elbow, the subtalar joints, the ankle and, rarely, the hip. This surgical approach should not be dismissed as outmoded, and the benefits in terms of removing pain, increasing stability and functional amelioration of joints beyond the arthrodesis have established the operation as a useful procedure in patients who have been adequately assessed. (In order to anticipate any dissatisfaction that may arise from the loss of joint mobility, patients advised to undergo this procedure should be carefully told about this aspect of the operation beforehand.)

(c) Arthroplasty

This implies reconstituting a joint. The degree of reconstruction varies between relatively simple procedures such as resection of the damaged ends of the bone, allowing a pseudoarthrosis to develop (e.g. ulnar styloidectomy, excision of the radial head, reconstruction of metacarpophalangeal and metatarsophalangeal joints), hemiarthroplasty in which a metal insert separates part of the joint (e.g. McIntosh arthroplasty of the knee), or total joint replacement in which the entire joint is replaced by an artificial implant, with (or without) varying degrees of resection of damaged bone surfaces (e.g. total replacement of hip). The concept of total joint replacement was initiated some 20 years ago by Sir John Charnley (Charnley, 1979) and, although originally applied to the hip joint, has now been developed to cover most of the other joints.

A total joint replacement should fulfil the following desiderata (Mowat, 1978).

Clinical features
1. Relieve pain.
2. Restore movement and stability.
3. Correct deformity.

Technical and design features
1. Be chemically and physically inert in the biological environment.
2. Not generate an electrolytic current between the components.
3. Be long wearing.
4. Produce minimal wear particles (such particles should not cause cell damage, and there should be self-clearance of the particles by the device in order to minimize progressive destruction).
5. Have low friction properties.
6. Be firmly fixed to bone.
7. Be inherently stable.
8. Mimic normal joint function.

9.6.2 Extra-articular surgery

The term extra-articular procedures describes those that do not involve surgical intervention within the joint.

Osteotomy

This involves transection of a bone near to a joint, but outside the joint capsule. The operation has been used primarily to treat patients with osteoarthrosis of the hip and knee (Marmar, 1972). The success of this approach probably depends on a number of factors. The procedure allows weight to be carried through a different, largely undamaged area of the articular cartilage, and there is evidence from patients (Coventry, 1972) and from experimental animals (Bentley, 1974) that coverage of denuded areas by fibrocartilage occurs postoperatively. In addition, reduction in pain (particularly night pain) may be induced by changes in osseous venous blood flow. In rheumatoid arthritis there is less justification for osteotomy, although it may be used to correct minor deformities caused by arthritis of small joints, particularly of the feet.

Other operations that can be performed in close relation to the joint include capsulotomy to relieve flexion contracture, excision of patellar osteophytes to eliminate pain and crepitus of the knee, bursectomy, and drainage of infected calf cysts due to posterior knee rupture.

Surgical procedures involving structures less intimately associated with joints include neurolysis (relief of entrapped nerves, e.g. median and ulnar), and tendon surgery. The latter may be divided into tenotomy (surgical division of a tendon to relieve deformity), tendon repair (tenorrhaphy), tendon transfer (redirecting an intact tendon from one functional position to another), or tenolysis in which tendon action is diminished (as opposed to abolished) by cutting if there is overaction of that tendon or unopposed action from rupture of its antagonist.

9.7 REGIONAL ORTHOPAEDIC SURGERY

9.7.1 Surgery of inflammatory arthropathies

Much the most common inflammatory arthropathy requiring surgery is rheumatoid arthritis, and most of this section will be devoted to procedures relevant to this disease. Less common indications for arthritis surgery are found within the seronegative spondarthritides, for example involvement of the hips and spine in ankylosing spondylitis and foot involvement in Reiter's disease. The wisdom of operating on patients with juvenile chronic polyarthritis is still debatable, particularly operations involving bones in view of their tendency to interfere with growth. However, if the indications are sufficiently strong, there are some valuable surgical approaches in the surgical management of childhood arthritis, and these will be discussed in a later section.

(a) Rheumatoid arthritis

Upper limb – shoulder

Synovectomy. This is not a procedure appropriate to the shoulder joint as the synovial membrane is relatively inaccessible and its bulk is difficult to assess clinically.

Arthrodesis. This operation is occasionally indicated in rheumatoid arthritis when shoulder pain is severe. Scapulothoracic motion compensates fairly adequately for the loss of scapulohumeral movement, although rotary motion, so important for personal hygiene, is not regained (Neer and Hawkins, 1977).

Excision arthroplasty. This is an alternative operation to arthrodesis, and the surgical procedure and after-care are less arduous. However, the functional result, whether from humeral head resection (Jones, 1942) or glenoidectomy (Wainwright, 1976), is less acceptable than that associated with arthrodesis in view of the instability of the false joint which hampers effective abduction.

Partial replacement arthroplasty. This procedure using prosthetic replacement for the humeral head (Neer, 1953, 1955) has not been found useful in rheumatoid arthritis. Disappointing results may be related to the fact that the glenoid is usually diseased and also that the

stability resulting from this procedure is not comparable with that achieved by total replacement.

Total replacement arthroplasty. This procedure involves re-surfacing both sides of the glenohumeral joint (Kenmore, 1973; Neer *et al.*, 1977). Preliminary results have been disappointing – one survey reporting an 'unsatisfactory' result in 40% of 61 rheumatoid shoulders (Cruess, 1977).

Upper limb – elbow

Synovectomy. When there is intractable pain and the synovium is thickened, synovectomy of the elbow is occasionally useful providing there is no radiological evidence of bone damage. The procedure is often combined with radial head excision (Laine and Vainio, 1969; Wilson *et al.*, 1973; Porter *et al.*, 1974; Ferlic *et al.*, 1976).

Arthrodesis. This operation is occasionally indicated if the joint is painful and unstable. However, the difficulty of establishing fusion and the loss of mobility of the joint in the face of other involved joints makes the procedure functionally undesirable.

Excision arthroplasty. Removal of the radial head (often combined with synovectomy of the elbow joint) may increase the range of painless movement, particularly pronation and supination. Excision of the whole joint may increase mobility to a reasonable range of pain-free movement, but this is often hampered by reduced stability of the joint.

Replacement arthroplasty. Various procedures have been developed to resurface damaged parts of the joint prosthetically, but none has yet become fully established. However, it is perhaps of interest to consider some of these approaches, particularly those involving total replacement (sometimes combined with radial head excision).

As early as 1927 prosthetic hemiarthroplasty of the elbow had been performed in small numbers of patients using various materials to replace the distal humerus – rubber-covered metal (Robineau, 1927), acrylic (Tessarolo, 1952; Silva, 1967), and nylon (MacAnsland, 1954). These procedures became supplanted by methods using metal prosthesis to replace the distal humerus (Venable, 1952; Jakobsson, 1957; Lenggenhager, 1958; Barr and Eaton, 1965; Street and Stevens, 1974). Hemiarthroplasty has also been applied to the proximal part of the ulna (Johnson and Schlein, 1970; Peterson and Jones, 1971).

Procedures for total replacements of the elbow joint are summarized in Table 9.1. Many of these devices

Table 9.1 Elbow joint prostheses

Procedure	Variant	References
Fully constrained metal hinge	Dee McKee GSB Hinge	Dee (1972); Gschwend (1972); Souter (1973)
Fully constrained metal-to-plastic hinge	Stanmore Link St Georg	Devas and Shah (1977); Scales *et al.* (1977); Engelbrecht *et al.* (1978)
Semi-constrained metal-to-plastic hinge	Schlein Flexible Elbow Joint Replacement Coonrad Tri-axial GSB-New AMC; R-C Total Elbow Replacement	Gschwend (1975); Schlein (1976); Pritchard (1977); Coonrad (1978)
Semi-constrained metal-to-plastic (non-hinge)	Attenborough Dee Mayo	Attenborough (1977); Cofield *et al.* (1979)
Non-constrained metal-to-plastic	Kudo Nonblocked Liverpool Souter London Ishizuki Capitello-Condylar Elbow Arthroplasty	Cavendish (1977); Souter (1977); Ewald (1978); London (1978)

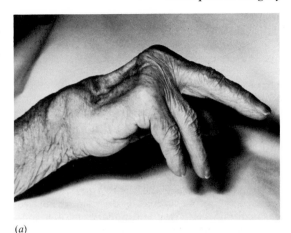

(*a*)

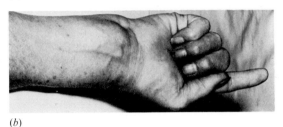

(*b*)

Fig. 9.1 (*a*) Rupture of extensor tendons of 4th and 5th digits (with inability to extend these fingers). Note the swelling on the dorsum of the wrist due to thickening of the extensor synovial sheaths and prominence of the ulnar head. (*b*) Rupture of the flexor tendon of the 2nd digit (with inability to flex this finger). Note the swelling on the palmar aspect of the wrist due to thickening of the common flexor sheath.

have not yet been evaluated, but early results are promising. Complications have included deep sepsis, recurrent dislocation, loosening of both humeral and ulnar components, fracture, rupture of triceps tendon, and transient and permanent ulnar nerve palsy (Ewald, 1981).

Upper limb – hand and wrist

Synovectomy. Metacarpophalangeal joints; radio-carpal and inferior radio-ulnar joints; extensor tendon sheaths; flexor tendon sheaths. Removal of bulky synovium before subluxation has become established may arrest this deformity. However, the relative lack of pain at the early stage necessary to achieve successful synovectomy must be balanced against the decreased

mobility that often attends synovectomy, particularly of finger joints. Synovectomy may be combined with capsular reefing to stabilize the metacarpophalangeal joints and to re-align the extensor tendons. Extensor tendons which have ruptured (Fig. 9.1(a)) may be repaired and, if necessary, their synovial sheaths removed at the same time. The same applies to the flexor tendon sheaths (Fig. 9.1(b)).

Arthrodesis. The radiocarpal joints respond particularly well to this procedure. The technique, which produces a stable, pain-free wrist with considerably improved grip, may be combined with ulnar head excision if this is dorsally dislocated. The range of pain-free supination and pronation is increased by this operation.

Excision arthroplasty. Metacarpal heads, ulnar head (see above). Although excision arthroplasty allows re-alignment of the fingers, as well as pain relief, limited mobility at the pseudoarthrosis by fibrous adhesions has prompted increasing use of total replacement arthroplasty of metacarpophalangeal joints.

Total replacement arthroplasty. Metacarpophalangeal joints, wrist. Metacarpophalangeal implants are continuing to develop. Initial attempts using a hinged metallic device (Flatt, 1963) – 'first generation' implant – led to complications such as implant fracture, bone resorption and stem perforation. 'Second generation' implants made of silicone rubber, acting as a flexible spacer between the resected bone ends, have been adopted for general use, particularly the Swanson implant (Swanson, 1968, 1972, 1973a). 'Third generation' implants (made of metal and plastic components cemented into the intramedullary canal of the resected joints) are now being used in various designs but none has replaced the flexible type.

Total replacement arthroplasty of the wrist is still in the experimental stage. Most currently available models require extensive bone resection for their insertion and the prostheses are usually cemented into place. Swanson (1973b) has had some success with a distal ulnar prosthesis which is fitted over the resected ulnar head. The prosthesis not only restores some length to the ulna but also reduces the risk of extensor tendon rupture.

Lower limb – hip

Total replacement arthroplasty has replaced other surgical procedures to treat the rheumatoid hip. The general approach to surgical management has, therefore, been relatively simplified: if the disability is trivial it should be endured, if significant the joint should be replaced. The procedures result in a painless, mobile stable hip, and the success rate is high despite some dampening of initial enthusiasm by the increasing frequency of late complications, such as loosening and infection. In 1970, Charnley (1970) reported a 96.4% success rate after a minimal follow-up of 5 years. In 1973, Charnley and Cupic (1973) reported the 9- and 10-year follow-up on these patients, the success rate being 92%. Most patients who did well initially maintained good pain relief and function. Other workers have observed success rates over 90% and a survey of the literature has shown that most surgeons obtain success rates of over 85% in terms of almost complete pain relief. A Swiss multicentre study found 96% had minor or no pain postoperatively (Debrunner and Izadpanah, 1976). Poss *et al.* (1976) reported 96% pain relief in 275 rheumatoid hips followed for an average of 35 years.

The procedures usually used for the replacement operation are all based on that developed by Charnley (Charnley, 1960, 1961, 1970, 1972a, b, 1975; Charnley and Cupic, 1973; Charnley and Halley, 1975). In this operation the surface of the acetabulum is replaced by a high-density polyethylene implant bonded to the pelvis

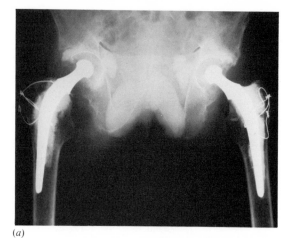

(a)

(b)

Fig. 9.2 Charnley hip prosthesis: (*a*) Radiograph showing bilateral hip replacement. (*b*) Details of prosthesis (revision specimen) showing stainless steel femoral component (right) and high-density polyethylene acetabular cup (above left) surrounded by cement. The back view (below left) shows the 'Mexican hat' component and tongues of cement which had filled the acetabular drill holes.

with polymethylmethacrylate cement (PMMA). The use of both materials was pioneered by Charnley. The femoral side of the joint is replaced by a metal prosthesis bonded to the skeleton via an intramedullary stem which is passed into the femoral shaft after resection of the head and neck of the femur (Fig. 9.2).

Two aspects of procedures conforming to the Charnley pattern have raised questions concerning possible improvement. One objection involves the resection of a functionally vital and uninvolved part of the skeleton, and, secondly, replacement by a relatively large prosthesis. Since the early 1970s a different technique has been under trial in which the femur is simply re-surfaced with a hollow metal sphere bonded with PMMA. It is still too early to assess the long-term results, but the short-term results are similar to those of the Charnley operation (Freeman, 1978). It should perhaps be mentioned that this 'new' approach was also tried by Charnley over two decades ago using a Teflon surface replacement, but was later abandoned by him because of recurrence of pain due to ischaemic necrosis of the femoral head under the Teflon cup (Charnley, 1961).

Complications are as follows:

1. *Infection.* Charnley has demonstrated that adherence to a meticulous sterile surgical technique augmented by effective air change in the operating theatre can considerably reduce infection rates (Charnley, 1972). His early infection rate was reduced 13-fold (from 0.5 to 6.6%) in this way. Later reports have shown that equally low infection rates can be achieved by using ultraviolet light and prophylactic antibiotics (Poss, 1975). There is still debate over the need for special

theatres for prosthetic surgery, although the work of Charnley has led to the widespread adoption of theatres with laminar air flow (Fig. 9.3) in which infection rates have been reduced to one-third or less compared with the infection rate found with conventional theatres (Charnley and Eftekhar, 1969). However, equally impressive results have been reported from surgeons performing total hip replacement in conventional operating rooms (Collins and Steinhaus, 1976) and in community hospitals (Mallory *et al.*, 1978).

There is evidence that patients with rheumatoid arthritis are at increased risk of developing infection (Arden *et al.*, 1970; Harris *et al.*, 1972; Todd *et al.*, 1972; Charnley and Cupic, 1973; Freeman *et al.*, 1973). However, Poss *et al.* (1976) found no difference in infection rate between rheumatoid and osteoarthrotic patients.

Revision of a previous procedure has been clearly shown to be attended by an increased infection rate (Charnley, 1972; Dupont and Charnley, 1972; Murray, 1973; Poss *et al.*, 1976). In view of this, it has been recommended that patients undergoing a revision procedure be warned of the higher risk of developing postoperative infection. Preoperative aspiration of the joint combined with arthrography may be useful in disclosing indolent sepsis (Poss and Sledge, 1981).

In the event of a prosthesis becoming infected – a serious problem attended by a 17% mortality rate and only a 12.6% chance of retaining their prosthesis without further wound infection (Hunter and Dandy, 1977) – early surgical intervention with thorough debridement and appropriate antibiotics in large dose may arrest infection and may allow the patient to retain the prosthesis. If infection is established the implant and

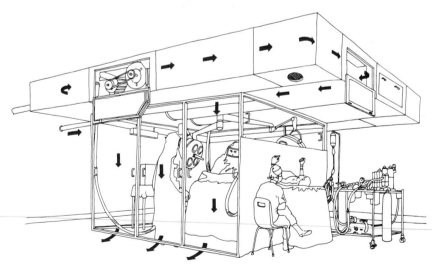

Fig. 9.3 General layout of a laminar airflow operating theatre designed to reduce sepsis.

cement should be removed as part of the debridement (Poss and Sledge, 1981).

Antibiotic-impregnated bone cement has gained cosiderable popularity in Europe, although its use in the USA has not yet been approved by the Food and Drug Administration.

It has been suggested that patients with metal implants should carry a suitable card which lists risks that they face (e.g. septic foci in nails, rheumatoid nodules, urinary tract, lungs, teeth and feet). It should also indicate from whom advice can be sought regarding prophylactic or definitive antibiotic therapy (Mowat, 1978).

2. *Wear*. The durability of high-density polyethylene has been impressive and an average rate of wear of 0.15 mm per year in patients assessed up to 10 years has been reported (Charnley and Cupic, 1973; Charnley and Halley, 1975). On this basis, if replacement is undertaken after the acetabular component has worn 5 mm, the average patient should expect the unit to last 33 years.

3. *Breakage and loosening*. Loosening is emerging as the most common long-term complication of total hip replacement. In a recent review of over 300 hips followed up for 4–7 years Beckenbaugh and Ilstrup (1978) reported radiological evidence of loosening in 24%, 8% requiring re-operation because of pain. After a 10-year follow-up Charnley and Cupic (1973) noted loosening of the acetabular component in 1% of hips. Femoral component fractures were observed in 0.23% of hips after more that $3\frac{1}{2}$ years' follow-up – the rate being 6.0% in heavy males (Charnley, 1975).

The following general observations regarding breakage and loosening have been made (Galante *et al.*, 1975; Carlsson *et al.*, 1977; Collis, 1977):

1. The frequency of acetabular and femoral component loosening may increase with time.
2. Improved positioning of the components, better cementing technique, and restoration of favourable mechanical lever arms diminish the risk of stem failure.
3. The larger, more active patients are at greater risk from these complications.
4. Loosening nearly always precedes femoral component fracture; the latter may occur as a fatigue-fracture phenomenon due to loosening of the proximal part and fixation of the distal part.

Lower limb – knee
Surgical treatment of the rheumatoid knee is varied and the choice of procedure complex. However, the trend is towards wider use of replacement surgery.

The knee joint poses a particular problem due to the superficial position of joint structures which leads to a greater risk of wound breakdown and of infection, particularly with the use of implant materials.

The rheumatoid knee presents a considerable challenge to the surgeon if all three goals of joint function are to be improved. These are freedom from pain, adequate stability, and reasonable mobility.

Synovectomy. Synovectomy of the knee joint remains a useful procedure for relief of pain and swelling, and recurrent effusion. However, earlier expectations that the procedure would confer prophylactic benefits have not been realized, and there is now a less pressing demand for early synovectomy in a joint unresponsive to medical treatment. Although in general synovectomy is unlikely to show long-lasting benefits in a joint showing significant loss of cartilage radiologically (Taylor *et al.*, 1972), there is evidence (Geens, 1969; Marmov, 1973) that operation results tend to be similar whether the operation is performed early or late based on radiological criteria. This may be related to the fact that apparently normal joints radiologically may show severe cartilage damage. Poorer results have been demonstrated in patients having widespread and active disease and with a 'dry', minimally proliferative synovium (Goldie, 1974; Ranawat and Desai, 1975). However, the correct selection of patients for synovectomy remains difficult. Results of most series show that about 80% patients report a good result at 1 year, with a steady deterioration in the success rate to about 50% at 5 years (Taylor *et al.*, 1972). The operation involves removing the anterior two-thirds of the synovium, there being little evidence to show that more radical clearance improves the results. Synovectomy is followed by regeneration of the synovium in about 50% of patients within 3 years. About 1 in 9 patients, particularly younger patients, will require postoperative manipulation to encourage the return of knee movement.

Arthrodesis. Due to the long lever arm produced by knee fusion and the stress this puts on the rheumatoid hips, this operation is not recommended in this disease except in rare circumstances.

However, on the positive side there is little doubt that an arthrodesis of the knee is the only procedure which can offer a life's guarantee in terms of pain relief and stability. Its high predictability can be most useful in patients with advanced disease in whom reliable standing stability is an important functional need. One arthrodesed knee with one mobile knee can provide useful function in these circumstances. The other use of arthrodesis is to provide an 'escape route', albeit a salvage one, in the event of total failure of any form of arthroplasty.

Osteotomy. This operation is seldom indicated for

rheumatoid arthritis, except in the infrequent case of unicompartmental disease.

The fact that osteotomy is not widely practised in rheumatoid arthritis (compared with osteoarthrosis) is somewhat surprising considering the mechanical problems resulting from the advancing rheumatoid process. The disease leads to a fixed flexion, valgus, and external rotational deformity, and it would have been thought that realignment of the femur and tibia to restore the normal weight-bearing axis would be an attractive corrective procedure. However, despite restoration of normal mechanics of the rheumatoid knee, certain factors preclude the success the procedure enjoys in osteoarthrosis (e.g. high tibial osteotomy for the varus knee deformity). These factors include: (1) the obliquity of the resulting joint line after correction of the predominantly valgus deformity, and (2) the poor tissue response fails to generate any substantial healing of the joint surfaces.

Patellectomy. Rheumatoid arthritis may severely affect the patello–femoral joint, but, surprisingly, symptoms from this compartment of the knee rarely predominate. Patellectomy as a primary procedure is therefore rarely indicated in this disorder. Occasionally the patellar is removed as part of a prosthetic operation, but the general trend now is to retain the structure whenever possible as its removal may weaken the knee by jeopardizing the quadriceps mechanism.

Replacement arthroplasty. With the impressive success and predictability of total hip replacement, hopes were high that similar success might be achieved for the knee. Unfortunately, however, this has not been borne out in practice, despite a long catalogue of endeavours, and knee replacement continues to carry a much higher morbidity rate than the hip operation.

The history of knee joint replacement arthroplasty started over 40 years ago when Campbell successfully used a moulded vitallium interposition femoral plate (Campbell, 1940). Further partial replacement implants succeeded this (McKeever, 1960; MacIntosh, 1966) and were popular in the 1960s. An alternative approach, which sacrificed the ligamentous support necessary to maintain the stability of interposition arthroplasty, was introduced in 1951 (Walldius, 1951). This prosthesis, a hinge intended to provide both stability and mobility, was followed by similar devices (Shiers, 1954; Deburge and G.U.E.P.A.R. 1976). Objections to the hinge prosthesis have been based on postoperative infection and loosening, and the fact that salvage of a failed hinge prosthesis is difficult (Bain, 1973; Moll *et al.*, 1973; Arden, 1975; Watson *et al.*, 1976). This pattern of prosthesis has now been largely replaced by metal and polyethylene surface implants. This further advance is

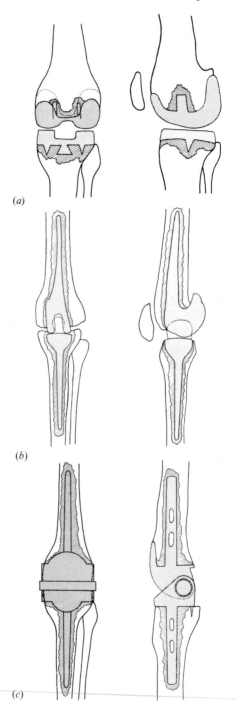

(*a*)

(*b*)

(*c*)

Fig. 9.4 diagram summarizing the three main categories of knee prosthesis. (*a*) Non-constrained. (*b*) Semi-constrained. (*c*) Constrained (hinge type).

attributable to Gunstan (1971, 1976) who was the first to employ the components which have proved so successful in total hip replacement (high-density polyethylene articulating with metal – either stainless steel or chronic cobalt alloy, bonded by methylmethacrylate cement).

Classification of currently used knee implants. It is customary to classify knee prosthesis into three categories (Fig. 9.4) (Cracchiolo, 1976).

1. *Non-constrained implants.* These are resurfacing implants, depending for stability on the integrity of existing ligaments (e.g. unicondylar, modular, polycentric and duocondylar).

2. *Semi-constrained implants.* All are non-linked but provide some inherent stability by virtue of their shape. Most are intended to substitute for cruciate ligament function. Examples are the geometric, Freeman – Swanson (ICLH), variable axis, and total condylar.

3. *Constrained implants.* These prostheses provide all the required stability and therefore both cruciate and collateral ligaments may be excised. Most experience has been with metallic hinges (Walldius, Shiers, Guepar) but this form of arthroplasty has lost popularity because of a relatively high infection (Bain, 1973; Arden, 1975) and loosening rate (Watson *et al.*, 1975), coupled with the problems of salvaging a failed hinge prosthesis. Several newer designs with metal-on-polyethylene articulations have attempted to solve these problems by allowing rotatory and gliding movements while continuing to provide the necessary stability. Examples of these newer prostheses, which are too recent to have been evaluated, are the stabilocondylar (Ranaurat), the spherocentric (Sonstegard *et al.*, 1977), and the Attenborough (Attenborough, 1976).

Non-constrained prostheses are designed for knees in which the bony architecture and ligaments are well preserved. Fully constrained prostheses are intended for severely deformed and unstable knees. The semi-constrained type occupies an intermediate position. However, the concept of a graduated system in which the prosthesis selected depends on the degree of deformity and instability is subject to a number of objections, apart from which each prosthesis involves a different surgical technique. The alternative is to use a prosthesis of the semi-constrained type for all knees, and certainly the success of the Freeman–Swanson implant supports this approach (Freeman *et al.*, 1977; Freeman, *in press*).

The profusion of knee joint designs currently available mirrors the fact that no entirely satisfactory solution has yet been found for the replacement of the arthritic knee.

Lower limb – ankle and hindfoot

Arthrodesis. Fusion of the tibiotalar joint is indicated if symptoms persist in spite of conservative measures after the other joints of the limb have been optimally aligned. However, despite 100 years of experience of ankle fusion there is still no single method that guarantees a successful result. Of the 30 or so different methods that have been described, compression arthrodesis seems to offer marginally superior results in terms of satisfactory union (Charnley, 1951; Thomas, 1969). A review of 380 attempted ankle arthrodeses by various methods has revealed a pseudoarthrosis rate of 15–23%, and an additional 1.6% required amputation to salvage complications (Johnson and Bosekar, 1968; Lance *et al.*, 1971; Said *et al.*, 1978).

Rheumatoid patients are liable to develop symptoms requiring arthrodesis of the hindfoot joints either before or after ankle fusion. A recent study of 120 ankles and hindfeet showed that hindfoot symptoms were the primary source of disability in 16% of patients, and in 42% some hindfoot symptoms were noted (King *et al.*, 1978). In this study all patients with valgus deformity had symptoms in the lateral side of the foot and many demonstrated calcaneofibular impingement. If the hindfoot deformity is incorrectable, possibly a triple arthrodesis combined with removal of appropriate wedges of bone from the respective joints will be required (Adam and Ranawat, 1976). Triple arthrodesis can be a problem in the rheumatoid hindfoot because of bone softness and the typical valgus hindfoot and abducted forefoot. These deformities will require removal of medial wedges of bone between the talus and os calcis and between the talus and the navicular bone, and metal staples should be used to maintain fixation and obviate the need for a long leg plaster.

Total replacement arthroplasty. Ankle replacement, an operation first performed in the early 1970s, has only recently started to show reliable results which, if maintained, may supplant arthrodesis as the procedure of choice in treating arthritis of the ankle joint. A recent review of 250 total ankle replacements reveals satisfactory results in 75% of patients (Buckholz *et al.*, 1973; Newton, 1975; Scholz, 1976; Evanski and Waugh, 1977; Freeman *et al.*, 1979; Stauffer, 1979). Unsatisfactory results were attributed to infection in 3.5% and loosening in 6.7%, with 15% needing revision using another ankle replacement (10%) or arthrodesis (5%). A typical ankle prosthesis (St. Georg type) is shown in Fig. 9.5.

Lower limb – toes

Synovectomy. Compared with removing the synovium of finger joints, this procedure has not been used as

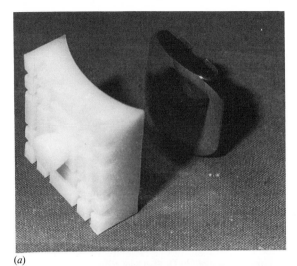

(a)

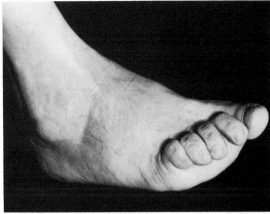

(a)

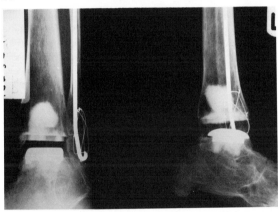

(b)

Fig. 9.5 Total replacement arthroplasty of the ankle. (*a*) Prosthesis showing polyethylene tibial component and metal talar component. (*b*) Prosthesis *in situ*. Note shadow of cement fixing both components and fibular pin.

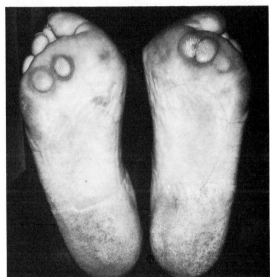

(b)

Fig. 9.6 Rheumatoid feet requiring surgery. (*a*) Lateral deviation and dorsal subluxation of the toes. (*b*) Marked hallux valgus and callosities over the metatarsal heads (imprints of elasticated metatarsal supports are also visible).

extensively for toe joints, excision arthroplasty being the method of choice to relieve the common claw-toe deformity of rheumatoid arthritis.

Excision arthroplasty. This operation is directed at the metatarsophalangeal joints where a combination of initial inflammatory changes and secondary mechanical factors give rise to the typical appearances. These include broadening and rigidity of the forefoot, hallux valgus, lateral deviation and dorsal subluxation of the other toes, and callosities over the prominent metatarsal heads in the sole (Fig. 9.6). Removal of the metatarsal heads, a procedure which may be combined with

proximal phalangectomy and division of extensor tendons, is a useful and well-established procedure that allows the toes to be re-aligned with the forefoot and successfully relieves pain under the metatarsal heads.

Several different surgical approaches have been described for the performance of a multiple metatarsal head excision. This procedure is preferred to the more radical procedure of combining this with proximal phalangectomy in view of toe instability resulting from the latter. Hoffman (1912) was the first to advocate excision of the metatarsal heads (using a plantar approach and excising the calloused skin beneath the metatarsal heads). Kats *et al.* (1967) modified this approach by excising a more proximal ellipse of the plantar skin. Larmon (1951) and Fowler (1959) advised the use of three separate longitudinal incisions, while both Aufranc (1961) and Clayton (1963) recommended a dorsal transverse incision. Either the plantar or the dorsal approach is adequate to perform the operation, and the ultimate choice depends on the degree of deformity, scars from previous surgery, and the surgeon's familiarity with the operation. In general, plantar skin heals slightly less quickly than dorsal skin, the latter being thinner and not desquamated. The second metatarsal head is usually excised first and each successive metatarsal head is trimmed slightly more proximally to create a smooth arc between the second to the fifth toe. Surgery to the great toe is performed last, resection being at the same level as the second toe. At this joint a dorsomedial approach is preferred, regardless of the approach used for the other toes.

Amputation. An alternative to excision arthroplasty for grossly deformed toes is amputation through the metatarsophalangeal joint.

Total replacement arthroplasty. Hallux valgus in the rheumatoid foot has responded well to prosthetic arthroplasty using an intramedullary silicone prosthesis. This procedure, apart from pain relief, has been found to restore stability, alignment, and motion to the great toe (Raymakers and Waugh, 1971; Whalley and Wenger, 1975; Kampner, 1978). Prosthetic arthroplasty may be combined with resection of lesser metatarsal heads.

Tarsal joints. Pain arising from the tarsal joints is preferably treated by carefully chosen footwear with appropriate insoles (see Section 10.9.2). However, occasionally arthrodesis of one of the joints (most often the talonavicular joint) is indicated; this is particularly so if the hindfoot deformity is passively correctable. A recent review of the results of talonavicular arthrodesis showed that over 90% of patients had a marked reduction in symptoms and improvement of function (Elboar *et al.*, 1976).

Cervical spine
Rheumatoid involvement of the cervical spine occasionally demands surgery. The most frequent indication is anterior atlantoaxial subluxation. Other less common structural abnormalities such as posterior atlantoaxial subluxation, downward migration of the skull due to destruction of the lateral masses of the atlas,

and subluxation in the mid-cervical spine constitute rarer indications for surgery.

Surgical fusion of the unstable atlantoaxial region is normally only considered when there are indisputable long tract signs which can be eliminated by traction. Radiological evidence of subluxation on its own is insufficient evidence for surgery. Several different techniques are available, but a posterior midline approach, with packing of bone chips between the occiput and the spines of the first three vertebrae, and wiring of the spines after correction of the subluxation, is the most popular method (Newman and Sweetman, 1969; De Andrade and MacNab, 1969). The results of the procedure are satisfactory on the whole, but fusion may fail due to the removal of bone chips by the inflammatory process before they can be incorporated into an adequate bony bar (Ferlie *et al.*, 1975).

(b) Other inflammatory arthropathies

Many of the procedures described for treating damaged joints in rheumatoid arthritis may also be applicable to other inflammatory arthropathies, for example ankylosing spondylitis, psoriatic arthritis and Reiter's disease. However, such disorders often demand special consideration, not only because of pathological differences between them and rheumatoid arthritis, but also because of the increased likelihood of the presence of an associated co-disease (e.g. psoriasis, ulcerative colitis, urinary tract infection). These considerations have been discussed fully elsewhere (Moll *et al.*, 1974; Wright and Moll, 1976; Moll, 1981), but will be outlined briefly as follows.

Ankylosing spondylitis
Most patients with established ankylosing spondylitis learn to come to terms with their moderate forward flexion deformity. However, if the deformity becomes severe, and difficulty arises with forward vision during walking or sitting at a desk, or if flexion deformity at neck, thoracic cage or abdominal level is causing encroachment on viscera or skin, surgical correction is justified. A typical patient having such an incapacitating degree of spinal deformity is shown in Fig. 9.7(a).

Flexion deformity of the spine may be corrected by posterior spinal osteotomy in the lumbar region (Fig. 9.7(b)). The technique was first described by Smith Peterson *et al.* in 1945, and several modifications of the original procedure have developed over the last 35 years (La Chapelle, 1946; Briggs *et al.*, 1947; Herbert, 1948; Adams, 1952). In recent years Simmons (1972, 1977) has written extensively on the subject, particularly concerning lumbar correction but also dorsal and cervical correction. The technical aspects and hazards associated with spinal osteotomy have recently been

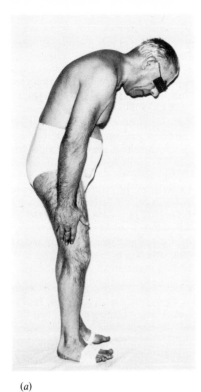
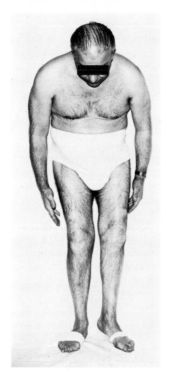

(a)

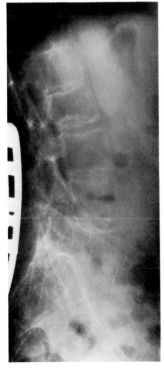
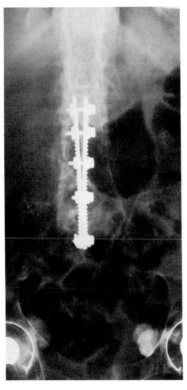

(b)

Fig. 9.7 Ankylosing spondylitis. (a) Severe flexion deformity of the spine in a patient with ankylosing spondylitis. Surgery was indicated because of restricted forward vision. (b) Lumbar osteotomy. Left: lateral view showing resected bone posteriorly and metal osteotomy plate. Right: anteroposterior view showing osteotomy plate (bilateral hip arthroplasty performed at a previous surgery are also visible).

reviewed by Owen (1980). Preoperative and anaesthetic problems (Cohen, 1980) and postoperative management (Mears, 1980) have also been considered in detail. Among the major complications in surgical straightening of the spine are gastric dilatation (due to stretching of the superior mesenteric artery over the third part of the duodenum), abdominal ileus, and aspiration of vomit. It is generally agreed that these operations should be restricted to surgeons with special experience of the procedures and performed only in patients whose problems are uncontrollable after concerted efforts by other means.

Involvement of the hips with flexion deformity unresponsive to traction and other physical measures can often be improved by arthroplasty. Cup arthroplasty (Law, 1948, 1952; Schwartzmann, 1959) was attended by a significant risk of re-ankylosis, and for some years has been superseded by total replacement arthroplasty (see details discussed under Section 9.7.1(a)). In the series of Welch and Charnley (1970), no postoperative ankylosis occurred in 35 total hip replacements, despite the fact that 23.5% of these patients had ankylosed hip joints preoperatively. However, there is no doubt that this a significant risk, and if it occurs, the new bone formation (Fig. 9.8) within the capsule and in the extracapsular layers can significantly diminish joint mobility. In Owen's experience (Owen, 1980), thorough lavage of the wound with saline and antibiotic solution to rid the operative field of bone dust has been encouraging in preventing this complication.

Psoriatic arthritis
The surgical management of patients with psoriatic arthritis has received relatively scant attention in the

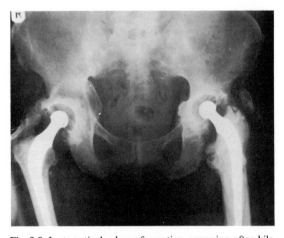

Fig. 9.8 Juxta-articular bone formation occurring after bilateral Charnley arthroplasty of the hips in ankylosing spondylitis.

literature. Generally, surgery on peripheral joints follows similar lines as reported for rheumatoid arthritis, and spondylitic involvement – of which these patients have a significant tendency (Moll, 1974) – is approached as in uncomplicated ankylosing spondylitis.

Two main considerations have a bearing on orthopaedic surgery in psoriatic patients:

1. Increased risk of deep and superficial infection (Kummerle *et al.*, 1971; Lambert and Wright, 1979), perhaps due to the fact that many psoriatic patients carry pathogenic bacteria on their normal and affected skin (Selwyn and Chalmers, 1965; Noble and Savin, 1968; *Leading Article*, 1972; Lynfield *et al.*, 1972).

In view of the risk of infection, Lynfield *et al.* (1972) have suggested the following precautions to reduce contamination of psoriatic skin by pathogenic bacteria and to reduce spreading infection to other patients:

(a) Meticulous sterilization of the surgical field. There is no need to avoid psoriatic plaques as these heal as well as normal skin. There is also no need to fear that the psoriasis will be aggravated by the surgical cleansing.
(b) The earlier after hospital admission the operation is performed the better, as patients are less liable to be carrying pathogenic bacteria on admission. It is therefore unwise to delay operation in the hope that the skin lesions will be cleared by in-patient treatment.
(c) Once the patient is known to have become a skin carrier of pathogenic organisms he should be discharged as soon as possible.

2. It might be argued that the more exuberant fibrotic reaction in psoriatic arthritis and also the tendency to osteolysis and ankylosis, might jeopardize the results of surgery in these patients, but so far this has not been reported.

Reiter's disease
Peripheral joint surgery in patients with Reiter's disease will be largely concerned with corrective procedures in the foot. The tendency to spondylitis may require surgical management along the lines discussed under 'Ankylosing spondylitis'.

As referred to previously, the significant frequency of cardiac involvement in patients with Reiter's disease should prompt careful preoperative cardiac assessment. Existing urinary tract infection should be vigorously treated and psoriasiform skin lesions should be managed as for psoriasis.

Ulcerative colitis and Crohn's disease
Surgery for the peripheral arthritis of these chronic inflammatory bowel disorders is not usually indicated as

the arthropathy tends to be a non-destructive synovitis, often affecting lower-limb joints – particularly the knees and ankles. However, the association with ankylosing spondylitis may require surgery for that condition.

Wright and Walkinson (1965, 1966) have demonstrated that patients with ulcerative colitis submitted to colectomy or ileostomy had much reduced rheumatic symptoms, although this has not been a universal experience (Fernandez-Herlihy, 1959; McEwen *et al.*, 1962). The spondylitis of patients with chronic inflammatory bowel disease, however, seems to run an independent course and does not respond to bowel surgery.

Juvenile chronic polyarthritis
Juvenile chronic polyarthritis includes juvenile rheumatoid arthritis and various forms of seronegative spondarthritis as well as the variants of Still's disease. Some of these disorders pose special problems which will be discussed under the last heading in this section.

Apart from diagnostic biopsy in monarticular disease there is no indication for surgery early in the disease (Arden and Ansell, 1978; Ansell, 1980). The management of fracture will require minimal immobilization of nearby involved joints.

Synovectomy is considered occasionally. It is especially valuable in patients with few joints involved and when overgrowth of the epiphyses or metaphyses is occurring. The most common joints to require surgery are the knees and elbows. Overall disease activity should be controlled before surgery. Synovectomy is deferred until children are old enough to co-operate in an active physiotherapeutic regimen. Remobilization is much more difficult than in adults, and many more knees have needed manipulation in children after synovectomy than in adults.

Correction of deformities
Soft-tissue releases (Granberry, 1977) are particularly valuable when there are severe flexion contractures of the hip. Surgery needs to be followed by prolonged traction and intensive physiotherapy. Flexion contractures of the knees also respond well to this procedure. If hip and knee contractures are present together they should preferably be corrected at the same operation, or one very shortly after the other.

In children with severe flexion contractures of the knees with only moderately damaged epiphyses, femoral osteotomy should be considered.

If severe valgus deformity of the knee is present at the age of 10 or 11, and growth is continuing, temporary stapling of the femoral and tibial epiphyses on the medial side of the knee may be performed. If growth is rapid, frequent postoperative examinations should be made to ensure that over-correction into a varus position does not occur. Older patients may require a tibial osteotomy to achieve a satisfactory correction.

In teenage patients, valgus deformities of the great toe may be corrected by a Mitchell's osteotomy.

Severe established deformities in adolescence will required more intensive orthopaedic management (e.g. osteotomies at different sites; fusion of carpus or tarsus in good position; lengthening of tendo Achilles or extensor tendons of the fingers; reconstructive surgery and even arthrodesis.

Arthrodesis. There is still the occasional need for arthrodesis of the knee.

Arthroplasty. Total replacement arthroplasty of the hip may require specially made small prostheses (Arden and Ansell, 1978). Some surgeons favour cup arthroplasty (Lang and Klassen, 1977). It has been suggested that in the future a double surfacing procedure may be better for young patients (Arden and Ansell, 1978).

Knee arthroplasty is still not entirely satisfactory, and at present the approach is to try to temporize with a single or double osteotomy (Benjamin-type) until more suitable replacement therapy becomes available.

Arthroplasty of other joints in children is still in the experimental stage, although Ansell's group (Ansell, 1980) have attempted shoulder and elbow replacement with reasonable success.

Special problems

Juvenile rheumatoid arthritis poses similar complications as in the adult disease. Rupture of extensor tendons at the wrist, and less often of flexor tendons (particularly of the thumb) will need repairing. Atlantoaxial subluxation may ultimately require surgical treatment. Hip arthroplasty, Fowler's procedure, and subtalar joint fusion may be indicated.

Juvenile ankylosing spondylitis. Hip arthroplasty carries a risk of postoperative re-ossification. Whenever possible therefore a prosthesis with a particularly long neck is used. In Ansell's experience (Ansell, 1980), patients with atlantoaxial subluxation have stabilized and fused with collars alone.

Anaesthesia. Intubation may be difficult because of temporomandibular joint involvement, micrognathos, and rigidity of the cervical spine. The last two features are shown in Fig. 9.9.

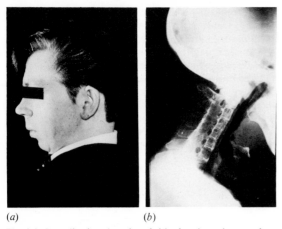

(a)   (b)

Fig. 9.9 Juvenile chronic polyarthritis showing micrognathos (*a*) and cervical spine fusion (*b*).

9.7.2 Surgery of osteoarthrosis

Comments in this section will be largely confined to the joints commonly affected by primary osteoarthrosis (hip, knee, carpometacarpal joint of thumb, and first metatarsophalangeal joint).

(a) Carpometacarpal joint of thumb

Either arthrodesis of the diseased joint or excision of the trapezium give excellent results.

(b) Toes

Not all these conditions are true osteoarthrosis but may be conveniently considered together.

(c) Hallux valgus

This is treated by excision arthroplasty of the first metatarsophalangeal joint, either by removing the base of the phalanx (Keller's operation) or the head of the first metatarsal (Mayo's operation). Medial exostoses remaining after these procedures are excised, and, if necessary, the capsule may be incised laterally and reefed medially to re-align the toe.

(d) Hallux rigidus

Arthrodesis is the treatment of choice for this condition.

(e) Claw toes

A deformity often accompanying hallux valgus, this may be treated by dorsal capsulotomy and extensor tenotomy at the metatarsophalangeal joint, together with spike arthrodesis of the proximal interphalangeal joint in an extended position.

(f) Knee

Chondromalacia patellae: The cartilage and subchondral bone have been drilled and the fibrillated cartilage shaved, but it is doubtful if these procedures are beneficial. On the assumption that a tendency to lateral subluxation of the patella is the basic underlying factor, lateral patellar retinacular release or medial transposition of the tibial tubercle have been undertaken with some success. Patellectomy should only be carried out as a last resort.

Arthrodesis used to be the treatment of choice for osteoarthrosis of the knee, but is now reserved only as a salvage procedure after total replacement arthroplasty.

Osteotomy is a useful procedure in patients in whom the range of movement is too good for replacement arthroplasty. The operation is particularly indicated if there is varus deformity (Fig. 9.10) since the opportunity can then be taken to re-align the knee. The bone to be divided is governed by the site of the major bone defect. Varus deformities are usually due to a tibial

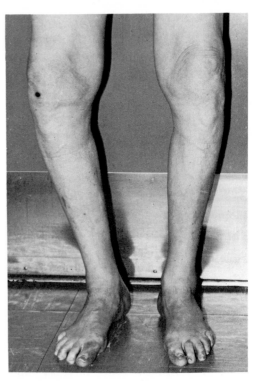

Fig. 9.10 Bilateral varus deformity of the knee due to osteoarthrosis.

defect and are therefore treated by tibial osteotomy. Valgus deformities are usually due to lateral femoral defects and are treated by supracondylar femoral osteotomy. The results of tibial osteotomy in the varus knee are superior to those of femoral osteotomy in the valgus knee.

Replacement arthroplasty is now the treatment of choice for osteoarthrosis of the knee in patients over 60. (For details see Section 9.7.1(a).)

(g) Hip

Osteoarthrosis of the hip requires surgical treatment more often than any other rheumatic disease in any other joint.

Arthrodesis is particularly applicable to secondary osteoarthrosis in young adults. Provided the spine, the other hip and the knees are mobile, gait is virtually normal after this operation. However, the significant disability imposed by a stiff hip, particularly in women, and the common occurrence of back ache by the early 40s has led to more frequent use of total replacement arthroplasty in these patients.

Osteotomy at the intertrochanteric level is indicated in patients, particularly young patients, in whom significant pain, especially at night, demands surgical relief when the range of movement is still adequate. (Seventy per cent of active flexion is taken as a rough guiding line between the need for osteotomy and arthroplasty.) Relief of pain is experienced by about 70% of patients, although there is usually no change in hip joint mobility.

Total replacement arthroplasty using implants of the Charnley type is proving as valuable in osteoarthrosis as it is in rheumatoid arthritis, and is now the standard form of treatment in osteoarthrosis of the hip. (For details see Section 9.7.1(a).)

9.7.3 Surgery of low back pain syndromes

(a) Disc herniation

The one unarguable indication for surgical removal of a disc is the cauda equina syndrome, in which midline herniation of the disc causes paralysis of the sacral roots, with bladder and bowel dysfunction, and inability to walk.

Other indications for laminectomy are marked muscular weakness and progressive neurological deficit in spite of adequate conservative treatment, including rest in bed (Macnab, 1977; Wiltse, 1977). However, there is some evidence to suggest that these indications should not be regarded as absolute. For instance, Anderson and Carlsson (1966) found that the time of onset, duration of symptoms, and surgical findings

showed no relationship to the return of motor activity in respect of foot drop. Also, there is little difference in the rate of motor return between operative and non-operative series (Weber, 1970; Hakelius, 1972), and after 1 year of follow-up the prognosis of motor return is no better after delayed surgery than with conservative therapy.

Relative indications for laminectomy are intolerable pain unrelieved by rest in bed, and recurrent episodes of incapacitating pain. In these patients it is important to exclude significant psychogenic factors (Pearce and Moll, 1967). Laminectomy for definite disc herniation has been shown by several studies to be a highly successful procedure (Hirsch and Nachemson, 1963; Hirsch, 1965; Andersson and Carlsson, 1966). The best results are obtained when a prolapsed disc can be identified, in contrast with concealed disc herniation (Hakelius, 1972; Spangfort, 1972).

(b) Spinal stenosis syndromes

Various spinal stenosis syndromes may cause root entrapment by a combination of changes, including osteophyte outgrowth and disc herniation (Macnab, 1977). Treatment of these syndromes attended by severe pain is surgical, with emphasis on adequate decompression of the entrapped roots. Wiltse et al. (1976) have reported encouraging results from this procedure.

(c) Spondylolisthesis

This indicates a separation of the pars interarticularis, allowing vertebral slipping or 'olisthesis'. There are many causes and a classification has been proposed by Wiltse et al. (1976). Management is age- and lesion-dependent. In children with more than 50% slippage, fusion is recommended regardless of symptoms. Conversely, children with persistent symptoms regardless of the degree of slippage should be advised to undergo fusion. The spine of a child less than 10 years old with a 50% slippage is often fused. Slippage will usually occur before 18 years of age, if it is going to occur; it rarely occurs after the age of 25 years. In adults of more than 40 years with painful spondylolisthesis, removing the loose posterior elements has been successful (Osterman et al., 1976). In adults without root entrapment and with only minimal slippage, Newman (1976) recommends direct repair of the defect.

9.7.4 Surgery of some 'medical orthopaedic' disorders

This section will concern itself with 'medical orthopaedic' disorders, for want of a better term. A miscellaneous collection of disorders will be considered in which 'injury' in its widest sense is often, but not always, an implicating factor. The trauma may be 'extrinsic', as in a sporting injury, or 'intrinsic' in which the trauma is related to repetitive stresses of daily activity (e.g. painting ceilings). The reader should consult more specific texts for further details (e.g. Pinals, 1979; Hazleman *et al.*, 1981).

(a) Temporomandibular joint syndrome

Conservative treatment is generally successful. This consists of reassurance, exercise to stretch spastic muscles and restore co-ordinated motion, and occasional use of tranquillizers and intra-articular corticosteroid injections. Correction of malocclusion and replacement of dentures may be appropriate in some instances. A few patients who have marked structural changes or recurrent dislocation and locking may need surgery. Operative procedures include menisectomy, arthroplasty, condylectomy, or grafts of bone and fascia.

(b) Osteitis pubis

This is usually a self-limiting condition often of those in their fourth decade. One survey (Harris and Murray, 1974) has revealed that as many as 76% of professional soccer players of one club showed radiological changes consistent with healed osteitis pubis. The condition is also seen within 2 months of delivery or after pelvic operations (e.g. prostatectomy). There is sometimes an association with pelvic sepsis. Although spontaneous remission may be expected, disabling symptoms may persist for many months. If infection is suspected, prolonged treatment with antibiotic and anti-inflammatory drugs may be tried. Occasionally surgical drainage or arthrodesis of the joint is necessary. Other treatments have included the wearing of a light pelvic belt, and radiotherapy, but there is still no general consensus as to the optimal management regimen of this condition.

(c) Entrapment neuropathies

Carpal tunnel syndrome
Median nerve compression can often be managed conservatively by splinting or local corticosteroid injection. Failing this, surgery should be undertaken and ranges from simple transection of the transverse carpal ligament, with dissection of the nerve, to volar tenosynovectomy, as in median compression due to rheumatoid arthritis (Ranawat and Straub, 1970). The operative procedures are simple and 90% effective (Marmor, 1964; Csenz *et al.*, 1966; Phalen, 1966).

Other entrapment neuropathies
Ulnar nerve compression at the elbow (Kleinert and Hayes, 1971) and the tarsal tunnel syndrome due to posterior tibial entrapment in a flexor retinaculum along the medial malleolus (Goodgold *et al.*, 1965) may also be associated with rheumatoid arthritis, although both are relatively rare. Treatment is by surgical decompression.

(d) Injuries to muscles and tendons

Tendon rupture is common in rheumatoid arthritis, especially rupture of the Achilles tendon. Otherwise tendon and ligamentous tears are usually traumatic (e.g. rupture of the rotator cuff, long head of biceps, pectoralis major, quadriceps muscle or tendon, posterior tibial tendon). Complete tears are usually treated surgically. Partial tears, such as in calf muscle tears ('tennis leg'), are treated conservatively, including adhesive strapping, followed by heat, massage and exercises.

(e) Bursitis

There are about 78 bursa on each side of the body. Inflammation of these may arise from excessive friction or direct trauma (e.g. trochanteric bursitis, olecranon bursitis, Achilles bursitis, calcaneal bursitis, prepatellar bursitis). In general, conservative treatment, including protection from irritation and trauma, appropriate padding, anti-inflammatory drugs and local corticosteroid injections are usually sufficient. However, refractory problems may need surgical excision.

(f) Rheumatoid nodules

Removal of rheumatoid nodules may be necessary: (1) if they have broken down and are discharging; (2) if they become infected, thus providing a potential source of bacteraemia; (3) if because of their size or position they have become physically irritating; (4) if they have become cosmetically unacceptable. Surgical excision should be complete, as incomplete excision may lead to a persistently discharging wound. Recurrence of nodules is common unless the mechanical factors and the underlying vasculitis can be controlled.

(g) Acute calcific tendinitis

Occasionally this condition persists despite repeating local anaesthetic/corticosteroid injections over a period of 8 weeks. This is an accepted indication for surgical intervention which may vary between simple evacuation of the calcified deposit to section of the tendon and reinsertion into bone after excising the calcified portion.

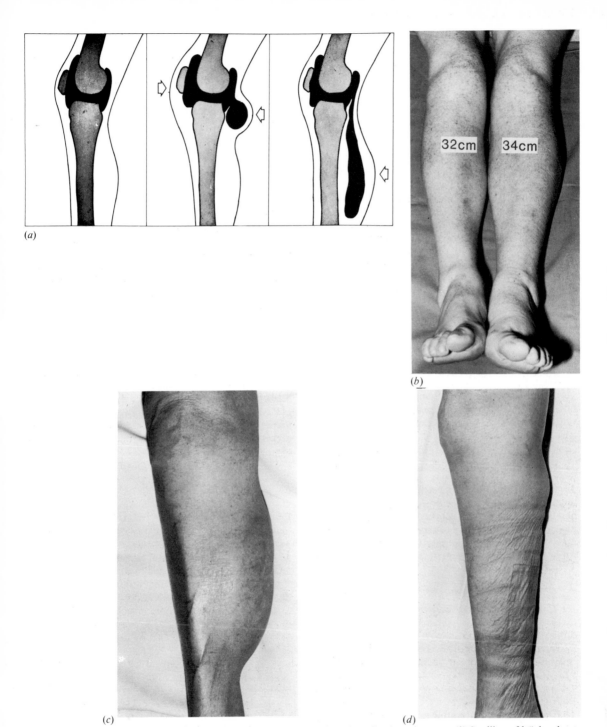

Fig. 9.11 (a) Diagram to show sequence in formation of calf cyst due to popliteal cyst rupture. (b) Swelling of left leg due to synovial fluid leakage from a ruptured popliteal cyst (often misdiagnosed as deep venous thrombosis). (c) Infected calf cyst in a patient with rheumatoid arthritis. (d) After surgical drainage of 600 ml of thick pus.

(a)

(b)

(c)

(d)

32cm 34cm

Surgery is considered more strongly indicated if the calcium deposits are large and do not respond to aspiration combined with local injection therapy.

(h) Humeral epicondylitis

Lateral involvement (tennis elbow) is more common than medial involvement (golfer's elbow). Treatment is usually conservative and includes anti-inflammatory drugs, massage, ultrasound, braces and, most commonly, local corticosteroid injection. Resistant problems may require surgery. A wide variety of operations can be performed, the most widely used being release of part of the origin of the extensor muscles. Other operations include division of the annular ligaments, excision of the synovial fringe, and radial nerve decompression.

(i) Stenosing tenovaginitis

Stenosing tenosynovitis is primarily a disorder of the fibrous wall of the tendon sheath, particularly at sites where the tendon passes through a fibrous ring. It is seen over bony prominences, such as the radial styloid and the flexor surfaces of the metacarpals. Thus, the most common locations for stenosing tenosynovitis are the thumb flexors ('snapping thumb'), thumb extensors (De Quervain's syndrome), and the finger flexors ('trigger finger'). Less common sites include the flexor carpi radialis tendon, the common peroneal sheath, and the tibialis posterior tendon.

(j) Ganglion

A ganglion is a cystic swelling near or often attached to a tendon sheath or joint capsule. A common site is on the dorsum of the hand. Ganglia may disappear spontaneously or may respond to aspiration and injection of a corticosteroid preparation. If there is recurrence surgical excision may be performed.

(k) Dupuytren's contracture

No effective treatment is known apart from operative excision of the affected palmar fascia when the condition is severe. Subcutaneous fasciotomy, limited fasciectomy, or radical fasciectomy is performed according to the extent of the deformity.

(l) Popliteal cysts (Baker's cysts)

These cysts, which in the adult are often associated with abnormalities of the knee (e.g. arthritis such as rheumatoid arthritis or osteoarthrosis, cartilage tears, osteochondromatosis), are often controlled by con-

servative treatment (e.g. rest, leg elevation, corticosteroid injection). In some patients surgery may be necessary, particularly if cysts are large or if rupture has occurred repeatedly. As cysts are due to the passage of synovial fluid from the joint to the cyst through a one-way valve (Jayson and Dixon, 1970), removal of the source of the problem by synovectomy will lead to a reduction in the size of the cyst and consequently in symptoms (Pinder, 1973). Removal of the cyst alone is rarely worth while, although if cysts are large they can be removed through a separate posterior incision at the same time as synovectomy.

Cyst rupture with leakage of synovial fluid into the calf is all too often mistaken for deep venous thrombosis. Occasionally, particularly in rheumatoid patients, calf cysts become infected and need to be drained surgically (Fig. 9.11).

Less often cyst rupture into the thigh may occur, giving rise to concern about the possibility of a malignant tumour.

(m) Tibial compartment syndromes

Anterior tibial syndrome: in the more severe types of the disorder surgery, consisting of division of the anterior fascia, may give relief. Milder forms respond to rest, elevation and massage, the provision of well-fitting rubber shoes, and the avoidance of hard surfaces.

Posterior tibial syndrome: in the early stage symptomatic treatment may help, but once the condition is established, the simplest solution is posterior tibial decompression.

9.8 SUMMARY AND CONCLUSIONS

Introductory sections have discussed the indications and contraindications for operative intervention in patients with rheumatic disorders. The importance of adequate peri-operative management has been stressed, and attention has been drawn to certain intra-operative factors of relevance to the rheumatic patient. The chapter then outlines the various types of procedure used in 'rheumatological orthopaedics', with, finally, a section on regional orthopaedic surgery.

Despite the exciting and dramatic advances in replacement surgery over the last two decades, all such procedures must still be regarded as evolutionary, and some as purely experimental. This is evident from the continuing changes in designs, surgical techniques and materials. However, there is little doubt about the success of total hip replacement and, to a lesser extent, that of total replacement of the knee.

It is concluded that although replacement procedures have much to offer patients with arthritic involvement no longer amenable to conservative management, the older and reliable procedures such as arthrodesis and osteotomy should not be forgotton (particularly in younger patients).

Whatever surgical decision is made, proper liaison between the various members of the management team should be maintained at all times to maximize long-term success of the operation.

9.9 REFERENCES AND FURTHER READING

General

Aly, R., Maibach, H.I. and Mandel, A. (1976) Bacterial flora in psoriasis. *Br. J. Dermatol.*, **95**, 603.

Ansell, B.M. (1980) in *Ankylosing Spondylitis* (ed. J.M.H. Moll), Churchill Livingstone, Edinburgh, p. 120.

Arthritis and Rheumatism Council/British Orthopaedic Association (1976) Controlled trial of synovectomy of knee and metacarpophalangeal joints in rheumatoid arthritis. *Ann. Rheum. Dis.*, **35**, 437.

Bentley, G. (1974) in *Symposium on Normal and Osteoarthritic Articular Cartilage* (eds S.Y. Ali, M.W. Elves and D.H. Leaback), Institute of Orthopaedics, London, p. 259.

Brechner, V.L. (1968) Unusual problems in the management of airways. *Anesth. Analg. Curr. Res.*, **47**, 362.

Charnley, J. (1979) *Low Friction Arthroplasty of the Hip. Theory and Practice*, Springer-Verlag, Berlin.

Cohen, M. (1980) in *Ankylosing Spondylitis* (ed. J.M.H. Moll), Churchill Livingstone, Edinburgh, p. 261.

Coventry, M.B. (1972) Surgery for arthritis of the hip. *Bull. Rheum. Dis.*, **22**, 674.

D'Ambrosia, R.D., Shoji, H. and Heater, R. (1976) Secondarily infected total joint replacements by hematogenous spread. *J. Bone Joint Sur.*, **58A**, 450.

Dupont, J.A. and Charnley, J. (1972) Low-friction arthroplasty of the hip for the failures of previous operations. *J. Bone Joint Sur.*, **54B**, 77.

Editorial (1974) Liver damage and halothane. *Br. Med. J.*, **iii**, 589.

Editorial (1975) Halothane. *Lancet*, **i**, 841.

Egbert, L.D., Battit, G.E., Welch, C.E. and Bartlett, M.K. (1964) Reduction of postoperative pain by encouragement and instruction of patients. A study of doctor-patient rapport. *N. Engl. J. Med.*, **270**, 825.

Flatt, A.E. (1979) in *Arthritis and Allied Conditions. A Textbook of Rheumatology* (ed. D.J. McCarty), Lea and Febiger, Philadelphia, 9th edn, p. 545.

Francis, D., Russell, R.G.G. and Fleisch, H. (1969) Diphosphonates inhibit the formation of calcium phosphate crystals *in vitro* and pathological calcification *in vivo*. *Science*, **165**, 1264.

Garner, R.W., Mowat, A.G. and Hazleman, B.L. (1973) Wound healing after operations on patients with rheumatoid arthritis. *J. Bone Joint Surg.*, **55B**, 134.

Goldie, I.F. (1974) Synovectomy in rheumatoid arthritis. *Sem. Arthr. Rheum.*, **3**, 219.

Harris, J., Lightowler, C.D.R. and Todd, R.C. (1972) Total hip replacement in inflammatory hip disease using the Charnley prosthesis. *Br. Med. J.*, **ii**, 750.

Herxheimer, A. (ed.) (1982) Peri-operative low-dose heparin. *Drugs Ther. Bull.*, **20**, 5. (Review: authors not specified.)

Hills, N.H., Pflug, J.J., Jeyasingh, K. *et al.* (1972) Prevention of deep venous thrombosis by intermittent pneumatic compression of calf. *Br. Med. J.*, **i**, 131.

Insall, J. (1981) in *Textbook of Rheumatology* (eds W.N. Kelley, E.D. Harris, S. Ruddy and C.B. Sledge), Saunders, Philadelphia, p. 1991.

Jergesen, H.E., Poss, R. and Sledge, C.B. (1978) Bilateral total hip and knee replacement in adults with rheumatoid arthritis. An evaluation of function. *Clin. Orthop.*, **137**, 120.

Kelsey, J.C., Wood, P.H.N. and Charnley, J. (1975) Prediction of thromboembolism following total hip replacement. *Clin. Orthop.*, **114**, 247.

Lambert, J.R. and Wright, V. (1979) Surgery in patients with psoriasis and arthritis. *Rheumatol. Rehabil.*, **18**, 35.

Lindeman, C.A. and Van Aernam, B. (1971) Nursing intervention with the presurgical patient – effects of structured and unstructured preoperative teaching. *Nurs. Res.*, **20**, 319.

Marmor, L. (1972) Surgery of osteoarthritis. *Sem. Arthr. Rheum.*, **2**, 117.

Marples, R.R., Heaton, C.L. and Kligman, A.M. (1973) Staphylococcus aureus in psoriasis. *Arch. Dermatol.*, **107**, 568.

Mears, D.C. (1979) in *Materials and Orthopaedic Surgery*, Williams and Williams, Baltimore, p. 785.

Mears, D.C. (1980) in *Ankylosing Spondylitis* (ed. J.M.H. Moll), Churchill Livingstone, Edinburgh, p. 267.

Melvin, J.L. (1977) *Rheumatic Disease: Occupational Therapy and Rehabilitation*, Davis, Philadelphia.

Mowat, A.G. (1978) in *Copeman's Textbook of the Rheumatic Diseases* (ed. J.T. Scott), Churchill Livingstone, Edinburgh, 5th edn, p. 459.

M.R.C. Trial (1972) Effect of aspirin on post-operative venous thrombosis. *Lancet*, **ii**, 441.

Nicolaides, A.N., Dupont, P.A., Desai, S. *et al.* (1972a) Small doses of subcutaneous sodium heparin in preventing deep thrombosis after major surgery. *Lancet*, **ii**, 890.

Nicolaides, A.N., Kakker, V.V., Field, E.S. and Fish, P. (1972b) Optimal electrical stimulus for preventing deep venous thrombosis. *Br. Med. J.*, **iii**, 756.

Nollen, A.J.G. and Sloof, T.J.J.H. (1973) Para-articular ossifications after total hip replacement. *Acta Orthop. Scand.*, **44**, 230.

Ornilla, E., Ansell, B.M. and Swannell, A.J. (1972) Cervical spine involvement in patients with chronic arthritis undergoing orthopaedic surgery. *Ann. Rheum. Dis.*, **31**, 364.

Poss, R. (1979) Total hip replacement in the patient with rheumatoid arthritis. *American Academy of Orthopaedic Surgery. Industrial Course Lecture* **28**, 298.

Reid, G.D. and Hill, R.H. (1978) Atlantoaxial subluxation in juvenile ankylosing spondylitis. *J. Pediatr.*, **93**, 531.

Resnick, D., Linovitz, R.J. and Feingold, M.L. (1976) Post-operative heterotopic ossification in patients with ankylosing hyperostosis of the spine (Forestier's disease). *J. Rheumatol.*, **3**, 313.

Roles, N.C. (1971) Infection in total prosthetic replacement of the hip and knee joints. *Proc. R. Soc. Med.*, **64**, 636.

Salzman, E.W., Harris, W.H. and Delanctis, R.W. (1971) Reduction in venous thromboembolism by agents affecting platelet function. *N. Engl. J. Med.*, **284**, 1287.

Smith, P., Benn, R.T. and Sharp, J. (1972) Natural history of rheumatoid cervical luxations. *Ann. Rheum. Dis.*, **32**, 431.

Taylor, A.R. and Ansell, B.M. (1972) Arthrography of the knee before and after synovectomy for rheumatoid arthritis. *J. Bone Joint Surg.*, **54B**, 110.

Turek, S.L. (1977) *Orthopaedic Principles and their Applications*, Lippincott, Philadelphia, pp. 1031, 1390.

Uddin, J., Kraus, A.S. and Kelly, H.G. (1970) Survivorship and death in rheumatoid arthritis. *Arth. Rheum.*, **13**, 125.

Wright, V. and Moll, J.M.H. (1976) in *Seronegative Polyarthritis*, North Holland, Amsterdam, p. 438.

Zorab, P.A. (1962) The lungs in ankylosing spondylitis. *Q. J. Med., New Ser.*, **31**, 267.

Shoulder

Cruess, R.L. (1977) Neer's arthroplasty of the shoulder – preliminary report (abstract). *J. Bone Joint Surg.*, **59B**, 508.

Jones, L. (1942) The shoulder joint: observations on the anatomy and physiology with an analysis of a reconstructive operation following extensive surgery. *Surg. Gynaecol. Obstet.*, **75**, 433.

Kenmore, P.I. (1973) A simple shoulder replacement. *Read at Clemson University Biomaterials Symposium*.

Neer, C.S., Brown, T.H. and McLaughlin, H.L. (1953) Fracture of the neck of the humerus with dislocation of the head fragment. *Am. J. Surg.*, **85**, 252.

Neer, C.S. (1955) Articular replacement of the humeral head. *J. Bone Joint Surg.*, **37A**, 215.

Neer, C.S. (1974) Replacement arthroplasty for glenohumeral osteoarthritis. *J. Bone Joint Surg.*, **56A**, 1.

Neer, C.S. and Hawkins, R.J. (1977) A functional analysis of shoulder fusions. *J. Bone Joint.*, **59B**, 508, Abstract.

Neer, C.S., Cruess, R.L., Sledge, C.B. and Wilde, A.H. (1977) Total shoulder replacement. A preliminary report. *J. Bone Joint. Surg.*, **1**, 244.

Wainwright, D. (1976) Glenoidectomy in the treatment of the painful arthritic shoulder. *J. Bone Joint Surg.*, **58B**, 377, Abstract.

Elbow

Attenborough, C.G. (1977) in *Joint Replacement Cement in the Upper Limb*, Mechanical Engineering Publications Ltd., London.

Barr, J.S. and Eaton, R.G. (1965) Elbow reconstruction with a new prosthesis to replace the distal end of the humerus. A case report. *J. Bone Joint Surg.*, **47A**, 1408.

Cavendish, M.E. and Elloy, M.A. (1977) in *Joint Replacement in the Upper Limb*, Mechanical Engineering Publications Ltd., London.

Cofield, R.H., Morrey, B.F. and Bryan, R.S. (1979) Total shoulder and total elbow arthroplasties: the current state of development. Part II: Total elbow arthroplasty. *J.C.E. Orthopedics*, **7**, 17.

Coonrad, R.W. (1978) Coonrad total elbow replacement. *Am. Orthop. Assoc. Meeting*, June 27.

Dee, R. (1972) Total replacement arthroplasty of the elbow for rheumatoid arthritis. *J. Bone Joint Surg.*, **54B**, 88.

Devas, M.B. and Shah, V. (1977) in *Joint Replacement in the Upper Limb*, Mechanical Engineering Publications Ltd., London.

Engelbrecht, E., Bucholz, H.W., Rottger, J. and Siegal, A. (1978) in *Joint Replacement in the Upper Limb*, Mechanical Engineering Publications Ltd., London.

Ewald, F.C. (1978) Total elbow replacement. *Am. Orth. Assoc. Meeting*, June 27.

Ewald, F.C. (1981) in *Textbook of Rheumatology* (eds W.N. Kelly, E.D. Harris, S. Ruddy and C.B. Sledge), Saunders, Philadelphia, p. 1936.

Ferlic, D.C., Clayton, M.L. and Parr, P.L. (1976) Surgery of the elbow in rheumatoid arthritis. *J. Bone Joint Surg.*, **58A**, 726.

Gschwend, N. (1972) Arthroplasty of the elbow using the GSB Prosthesis. *Proceedings of the 12th Congress of the International Society of Orthopedic Surgery and Traumatology*, Tel Aviv Oct 9–12. Excerpta Medica, Amsterdam.

Gschwend, N. (1975) Our experience of elbow arthroplasty with the GSB prosthesis. *Acta Orthop. Belg.*, **41**, 470.

Jakobsson, A. (1957) Fracture of the capitellum of the humerus in adults. Treatment with intra-articular chrome-cobalt-molybdenum prosthesis. *Acta Orthop. Scand.*, **26**, 184.

Johnson, E.W. and Schlein, A.P. (1970) Vitallium prosthesis for the olecranon and proximal part of the ulna. *J. Bone Joint. Surg.*, **52A**, 721.

Laine, V. and Vainio, K. (1969) in *Early Synovectomy in Rheumatoid Arthritis* (eds W. Hijmans, W.D. Paul and H. Herschel). Excerpta Medica Foundation, Amsterdam.

Lenggenhager, K. (1958) Zur Frage des künstlichen Ellbogengelenkes. *Helv. Chir. Acta*, **25**, 338.

London, J.T. (1978) Resurfacing total elbow arthroplasty. *Orthop. Trans.*, **2**, 217.

MacAusland, W.R. (1954) Replacement of the lower end of the humerus with a prosthesis. A report of four cases. *W. J. Surg., Gynecol. Obst.*, **62**, 557.

Peterson, L.F.A. and Jones, J.M. (1971) Surgery of rheumatoid elbow. *Orthop. Clin. N. Am.*, **2**, 667.

Porter, B.B., Richardson, C. and Vainio, K. (1974) Rheumatoid arthritis of the elbow: the results of synovectomy. *J. Bone Joint Surg.*, **56B**, 427.

Pritchard, R.W. (1977) Flexible elbow joint replacement. *Orthop. Trans.*, **1**, 109.

Robineau, R. (1927) Contribution a l'etude des prostheses osseuses. *Bull. Mém. Soc. Nat. Chir.*, **21**, 886.

Scales, J.T., Lettin, A.W.F. and Bailey, J. (1977) in *Joint Replacement in the Upper Limb*, Mechanical Engineering Publications Ltd., London.

Schlein, A.P. (1976) Semi-constrained total elbow arthroplasty. *Clin. Orthop.*, **121**, 222.

Silva, F.J. (1967) Arthroplasty of the elbow. *Singapore Med. J.*, **8**, 222.

Souter, W.A. (1973) Arthroplasty of the elbow with reference to metallic hinge arthroplasty in rheumatoid patients. *Orthop. Clin. N. Am.*, **4**, 335.

Souter, W.A. (1977) in *Joint Replacement in the Upper Limb*, Mechanical Engineering Publications Ltd., London.

Street, D.M. and Stevens, P.S. (1974) A humeral replacement prosthesis for the elbow. *J. Bone Joint Surg.*, **56A**, 1147.

Tessarolo, G. (1952) Endoprotesi acrilica articolare per il girnito. *Minerva Ortopedica*, **3**, 308.

Venable, C.S. (1952) An elbow and elbow. Case of complete loss of the lower third of the humerus. *Am. J. Surg.*, **83**, 271.

Wilson, D.W., Arden, G.P. and Ansell, B.M. (1973) Surgery of the elbow in rheumatoid arthritis. *J. Bone Joint Surg.*, **55B**, 106.

Hand/wrist

Clawson, D.K. and Convery, F.R. (1971) in *Surgery of Rheumatoid Arthritis* (eds R.L. Griess and N.S. Mitchell), Lippincott, Philadelphia, p. 135.

Flatt, A.E. (1963) *The Care of the Rheumatoid Hand*, Mosby, St. Louis.

Millender, L.H., Nalebuff, E.A., Albin, R. *et al.* (1974) Dorsal tenosynovectomy and tendon transfer in the rheumatoid hand. *J. Bone Joint Surg.*, **56A**, 601.

Millender, L.H. and Nalebuff, E.A. (1975) Reconstructive surgery in the rheumatoid hand. *Orthop. Clin. N. Am.*, **6**, 709.

Millender, L.H. and Nalebuff, E.A. (1975) Preventive surgery – tenosynovectomy and synovectomy. *Orthop. Clin. N. Am.*, **6**, 765.

Millender, L.H., Nalebuff, E.A., Hawkins, R.B. and Ennis, R. (1975) Infection after silicone prosthetic arthroplasty in the hand. *J. Bone Joint Surg.*, **57A**, 825.

Nalebuff, E.A. and Potter, T.A. (1968) Rheumatoid involvement of tendons and tendon sheaths in the hand. *Clin. Orthop.*, **59**, 147.

Nalebuff, E.A. (1969) Surgical treatment of tendon rupture in the rheumatoid hand. *Surg. Clin. N. Am.*, **49**, 811.

Nalebuff, E.A. and Millender, L.H. (1975a) Surgical treatment of the boutonnière deformity in rheumatoid arthritis. *Orthop. Clin. N. Am.*, **6**, 753.

Nalebuff, E.A. and Millender, L.H. (1975b) Surgical treatment of swan neck deformity in rheumatoid arthritis. *Orthop. Clin. N. Am.*, **6**, 733.

Neibauer, J.J. (1971) in *Symposium on the Hand* (eds L.H. Cramer and R.A. Chase), Vol. 3, Mosby St. Louis, pp. 96–105.

Straub, L.R. and Ranewat, C.S. (1969) The wrist in rheumatoid arthritis. *J. Bone Joint Surg.*, **51A**, 1.

Swanson, A.B. (1968) Silicone rubber implants for replacement of arthritic or destroyed joints in the hand. *Surg. Clin. N. Am.*, **48**, 1113.

Swanson, A.B. (1972) Flexible implant arthoplasty for arthritic finger joints. *J. Bone Joint Surg.*, **54A**, 435.

Swanson, A.B. (1973) *Flexible Implant Resection Arthroplasty in the Hand and Extremities*, Mosby, St. Louis.

Swanson, A.B. (1973b) Implant arthroplasty for disabilities of the distal radioulnar joint. Use of a silicone rubber capping implant following resection of the ulnar head. *Orthop. Clin. N. Am.*, **4**, 373.

Hip

Arden, G.P., Taylor, A.R. and Ansell, B.M. (1970) Total hip replacement using McKee–Farrar prosthesis in rheumatoid arthritis, Still's disease and ankylosing spondylitis. *Ann. Rheum. Dis.*, **29**, 1.

Beckenbaugh, R.D. and Ilstrup, D.M. (1978) Total hip arthroplasty. *J. Bone Joint Surg.*, **60A**, 306.

Carlsson, A.S., Gentz, C.F. and Stenport, J. (1977) Fracture of the femoral prosthesis in total hip replacement according to Charnley. *Acta Orthop. Scand.*, **48**, 650.

Charnley, J. (1960) Anchorage of the femoral head prosthesis to the shaft of the femur. *J. Bone Joint Surg.*, **42B**, 28.

Charnley, J. (1961) Arthroplasty of the hip: a new operation. *Lancet*, **i**, 1129.

Charnley, J. and Eftekhar, N. (1969) Post-operative infection in total prosthetic replacement arthroplasty of the hip joint. *Br. J. Surg.*, **56**, 641.

Charnley, J. (1970) Low friction arthroplasty. *Clin. Orthop. Rel. Res.*, **72**, 7.

Charnley, J. (1972a) Post-operative infection after total hip replacement with special reference to air contamination in the operating room. *Clin. Orthop.*, **87**, 167.

Charnley, J. (1972b) The long term results of low friction arthroplasty of the hip performed as a primary intervention. *J. Bone Joint Surg.*, **54B**, 61.

Charnley, J. and Cupic, F. (1973) The nine and ten year results of the low friction arthroplasty of the hip. *Clin. Orthop.*, **95**, 9.

Charnley, J. (1975) Fracture of femoral prostheses in total hip replacement. *Clin. Orthop.*, **111**, 105.

Charnley, J. and Halley, D.K. (1975) Rate of wear in total hip replacement. *Clin. Orthop.*, **112**, 17.

Collis, D.K. and Steinhaus, K. (1976) Total hip replacement without deep infection in a standard operating room. *J. Bone Joint Surg.*, **58A**, 446.

Collis, D.K. (1977) Femoral stem failure in total hip replacement. *J. Bone Joint Surg.*, **59A**, 1033.

Debrunner, H.U. and Izadpanah, M. (1976) in *Total Hip Prosthesis* (eds N. Gschwend and H.U. Debrunner), Williams and Wilkins, Baltimore, p. 27.

Dupont, J.A. and Charnley, J. (1972) Low friction arthroplasty of the hip for the failure of previous operations. *J. Bone Joint Surg.*, **54B**, 77.

Freeman, P.A., Lee, P. and Bryson, T.W. (1973) Total hip replacement in inflammatory disease using the Charnley prosthesis. *Br. Med. J.*, **ii**, 750.

Freeman, M.A.R. (ed.) (1978) Total surface replacement hip arthroplasty. *Clin. Orthop.*, **134**, 2.

Galante, J.O., Rostoker, W. and Doyle, J.M. (1975) Failed femoral stems in total hip prosthesis. *J. Bone Joint Surg.*, **57A**, 230.

Harris, J., Lightowler, C.D.R. and Todd, R.C. (1972) Total hip replacement in inflammatory disease using the Charnley prosthesis. *Br. Med. J.*, **ii**, 750.

Hunter, G. and Dandy, D. (1977) The natural history of the patient with an infected total hip replacement. *J. Bone Joint Surg.*, **59B**, 293.

Mallory, T.H., Meyer, T.L. and Bombach, J.D. (1978) Six hundred ninety total hip replacements: a comparative study. *Ohio State Med. J.*, **74**, 23.

Mowat, A.G. (1978) in *Clinics in Rheumatic Diseases* (ed. A.G. Mowat), Vol. 4, No. 2, Saunders, London, p. 260.

Murray, W.R. (1973) Results in patients with total hip replacement arthroplasty. *Clin. Orthop.*, **95**, 80.

Poss, R. (1975) Total his replacement. *Orthop. Clin. N. Am.*, **6**, 801.

Poss, R., Ewald, F.C., Thomas, W.H. and Sledge, C.B. (1976) Complications of total hip replacement arthroplasty in patients with rheumatoid arthritis. *J. Bone Joint Surg.*, **58A**, 1130..

Poss, R. and Sledge, C.B. (1981) in *Textbook of Rheumatology* (eds W.N. Kelley, E.D. Harris, S. Ruddy, and C.B. Sledge), Saunders, Philadelphia, p. 1978.

Todd, R.C., Lightowler, C.D.R. and Harris, J. (1972) Total hip replacement in osteoarthrosis using the Charnley prosthesis. *Br. Med. J.*, **ii**, 752.

Knee

Arden, G.P. (1975) Total replacement of the knee. *J. Bone Joint Surg.*, **57B**, 119.

Attenborough, C.G. (1976) Total knee replacement using the stabilized gliding prosthesis. *Ann. R. Coll. Surg. Engl.*, **57**, 283.

Bain, A.M. (1973) Replacement of the knee joint with the Walldius prosthesis using cement fixation. *Clin. Orthop.*, **94**, 65.

Campbell, W.C. (1940) Interposition of vitallium plates in arthroplasties of the knee. Preliminary report. *Am. J. Surg.*, **47**, 639.

Deburge, A. and C.U.E.P.A.R. (1976) Guepar hinge prosthesis. Complications and results with two years' follow-up. *Clin. Orthop.*, **120**, 47.

Freeman, M.A.R., Insall, J., Besser, W. *et al.* (1977) Excision of the cruciate ligaments in total knee replacement. *Clin. Orthop.*, **126**, 209.

Freeman, M.A.R. (ed.) (in press) *Arthritis of the Knee*, Springer Verlag, Heidelberg.

Geens, S. (1969) Synovectomy and debridement of the knee in rheumatoid arthritis. *J. Bone Joint Surg.*, **51A**, 617.

Goldie, I.F. (1974) Synovectomy in rheumatoid arthritis. *Sem. Arthr. Rheum.*, **3**, 219.

Gracchiolo, A. (1976) Symposium statistics of total knee replacement. *Clin. Orthop.*, **120**, 2.

Gunston, F.H. (1971) Polycentric knee arthroplasty. Prosthetic simulation of normal knee movement. *J. Bone Joint Surg.*, **53B**, 272.

Gunston, F.H. and MacKenzie, R.I. (1976) Complications of polycentric knee arthroplasty. *Clin. Orthop.*, **120**, 11.

Jayson, M.I.V. and Dixon, A. St. J. (1970) Valvular mechanisms in juxta-articular cysts. *Ann. Rheum. Dis.*, **29**, 415.

MacIntosh, D.L. (1966) Arthroplasty of the knee in rheumatoid arthritis. *J. Bone Joint Surg.*, **48B**, 179.

Marmor, L. (1973) Surgery of the rheumatoid knee. Synovectomy and dibridement. *J. Bone Joint Surg.*, **55A**, 535.

McKeever, D.C. (1960) Tibial plateau prosthesis. *Clin. Orthop.*, **18**, 86,

Moll, J.M.H., Chesterman, P.J., Meanoch, R.I. and Andrews, F.M. (1973) Walldius arthroplasty of the knee. Follow-up study of 51 operations. *Ann. Rheum. Dis.*, **32**, 397.

Pinder, I.M. (1973) Treatment of the popliteal cysts in the rheumatoid knee. *J. Bone Joint Surg.*, **55B**, 119.

Ranawat, C.S. and Desai, K. (1975) Role of early synovectomy of the knee joint in rheumatoid arthritis. *Arthr. Rheum.*, **18**, 117.

Ranawat, C.S., Brigham, L.N. and Insall, J. (1977) Stabilocondylar total knee arthroplasty. *Presented at the Annual Meeting of the American Academy of Orthopedic Surgeons, Las, Vagas, Nevada.*

Shiers, L.G.P. (1954) Arthroplasty of the knee. Preliminary report of a new method. *J. Bone Joint Surg.*, **36B**, 553.

Sonstegard, D.A., Kanfer, H. and Matthews, L.S. (1977) The spherocentric knee. Biomechanical testing and clinical trial. *J. Bone Joint Surg.*, **59A**, 602.

Taylor, A.R., Harbison, J.S. and Pepler, C. (1972) Synovectomy of the knee in rheumatoid arthritis. *Ann. Rheum. Dis.*, **31**, 159.

Walldius, B. (1957) Arthroplasty of the knee joint using endoprosthesis. *Acta Orthop. Scand.*, **24** (Suppl.), 19.

Watson, J.R., Wood, H. and Hill, R.C. (1976) The Shiers arthroplasty of the knee. *J. Bone Joint Surg.*, **58B**, 300.

Ankle and hindfoot

Adam, W. and Ranawat, C. (1976) Arthrodesis of the hindfoot in rheumatoid arthritis. *Orthop. Clin. N. Am.*, **7**, 827.

Buckholz, H.W., Engelbrecht, E. and Siegel, A. (1973) Totale sprunggelenksendoprosthese Modell 'St. Georg'. *Chirurgie*, **44**, 241.

Charnley, J. (1951) Compression arthrodesis of the ankle and shoulder. *J. Bone Joint Surg.*, **33B**, 180.

Evanski, P.M. and Waugh, T.R. (1977) Management of arthritis of the ankle. *Clin. Orthop.*, **122**, 110.

Freeman, M.A.R., Kempson, G.E., Tuke, M.D. and Samuelson, K.M. (1979) Total replacement of the ankle with the ICLH prosthesis. *Intl. Orthop.*, **2**, 327.

Johnson, E.W. and Boseker, E.H. (1968) Arthrodesis of the ankle. *Arch. Surg.*, **97**, 766.

King, J., Burke, D. and Freeman, M.A.R. (1978) The incidence of pain in the rheumatoid hindfoot and the significance of calcaneo-fibular impingement. *Intl. Orthop.*, **2**, 255.

Lance, E.M., Pavel, A., Patterson, R.L. *et al.* (1971) Arthrodesis of the ankle. *J. Bone Joint Surg.*, **53A**, 1030.

Newton, S.E. (1975) Total ankle replacement. *J. Bone Joint Surg.*, **57B**, 1033.

Said, E., Houka, L. and Siller, T.N. (1978) Where ankle fusion stands today. *J. Bone Joint Surg.*, **60A**, 211.

Scholz, K.C. (1976) in *Foot Science* (ed. J.E. Bateman), Saunders, Philadelphia, pp. 106–35.

Stauffer, R.N. (1979) Total joint arthroplasty, the ankle. *Mayo Clin. Proc.*, **54**, 570.

Thomas, F.B. (1969) Arthrodesis of the ankle. *J. Bone Joint Surg.*, **51B**, 53.

Tarsal joints

Elboar, J.E., Thomas, W.H., Weinfeld, M.S. and Potter, T.A. (1976) Talonavicular arthrodesis for rheumatoid arthritis of the hindfoot. *Orthop. Clin. N. Am.*, **7**, 821.

Toes

Aufranc, O. (1961) Reconstructive surgery of the lower extremity in rheumatoid arthritis. *AAOS Instructional Course, Miami.*

Clayton, M.L. (1963) Surgery of the lower extremity in rheumatoid arthritis. *J. Bone Joint Surg.*, **45A**, 1517.

Fowler, A.W. (1959) A method of forefoot reconstruction. *J. Bone Joint Surg.*, **41B**, 507.

Hoffman, P. (1912) An operation for severe grades of contracted clawed toes. *Am. J. Orthop. Surg.*, **9**, 441.

Kampner, S.L. (1978) Total joint replacement in bunion surgery. *Orthopedics*, **1**, 275.

Kates, A., Kessel, L. and Kay, A. (1967) Arthroplasty of the forefoot. *J. Bone Joint Surg.*, **49B**, 552.

Larmon, W. (1951) Surgical treatment of deformities of rheumatoid arthritis of the forefoot and toes. *Q. Bull. Northwestern Univ. Med. Sch.*, **25**, 37.

Raymakers, R. and Waugh, W. (1971) The treatment of metatarsalgia with hallux valgus. *J. Bone Joint Surg.*, **53B**, 684.

Whalley, R.C. and Wenger, R.J.J. (1975) Total replacement of the first metatarsophalangeal joint. *J. Bone Joint Surg.*, **57B**, 398.

Cervical spine

De Andrade, J.R. and Macnab, I. (1969) Anterior occipito-cervical fusion using an extra-pharyngeal exposure. *J. Bone Joint Surg.*, **51A**, 1621.

Ferlie, D.C., Clayton, M.L., Leidholt, J.D. and Gamble, W.E. (1975) Surgical treatment of the symptomatic unstable cervical spine in rheumatoid arthritis. *J. Bone Joint Surg.*, **57A**, 349.

Newman, P. and Sweetman, R. (1969) Occipito-cervical fusion. *J. Bone Joint Surg.*, **51B**, 423.

Other inflammatory arthritis

Adams, J.C. (1952) Technique, dangers and safeguards in osteotomy of the spine. *J. Bone Joint Surg.*, **34B**, 226.

Ansell, B.M. (1980) *Rheumatic Disorders in Childhood*, Butterworths, London, pp. 143–6.

Arden, G.P. and Ansell, B.M. (1978) *Surgical Management of Juvenile Chronic Polyarthritis*, Academic Press, London.

Briggs, H., Keats, S. and Schlesinger, P.T. (1947) Wedge osteotomy of the spine. *J. Bone Joint Surg.*, **29**, 1074.

Cohen, M. (1980) in *Ankylosing Spondylitis* (ed. J.M.H. Moll), Churchill Livingstone, Edinburgh, pp. 261–6.

Fernandez-Herliky, J.S. (1959) The articular manifestations of chronic ulcerative colitis: an analysis of 555 cases. *N. Engl. J. Med.*, **261**, 259.

Granberry, G.M. (1977) Soft tissue release in children with juvenile rheumatoid arthritis. *Arthr. Rheum.*, **20**, 565.

Herbert, J.J. (1948) Vertebral osteotomy. *J. Bone Joint Surg.*, **30A**, 680.

Kummerle, F., Wessinehage, D. and Schweikert, C.-H. (1971) Risks of alloplastic replacements in degenerative and inflammatory diseases of joints. *Acta Orthop. Belg.*, **37**, 541.

La Chappelle, E.H. (1946) Osteotomy of the lumbar spine for correction of kyphosis in a case of ankylosing spondylarthritis. *J. Bone Joint Surg.*, **28**, 851.

Lambert, J.R. and Wright, V. (1979) Surgery in patients with psoriasis and arthritis. *Rheumatol. Rehabil.*, **18**, 35.

Lang, A.G. and Klassen, R.A. (1977) Cup arthroplasties in teenagers and children. *J. Bone Joint Surg.*, **59A**, 444.

Law, W.A. (1948) Post-operative study of the vitallium mold arthroplasty of the hip joint. *J. Bone Joint Surg.*, **30B**, 76.

Law, W.A. (1952) Surgical treatment of the rheumatic diseases. *J. Bone Joint Surg.*, **34B**, 215.

Leading Article (1972) Psoriasis in the operating theatre. *Br. Med. J.*, **iv**, 62.

Mears, D.C. (1980) in *Ankylosing Spondylitis* (ed. J.M.H. Moll), Churchill Livingstone, Edinburgh, pp. 267–73.

McEwen, C., Lingg, G.C., Kirsner, J.B. and Spencer, J.A. (1962) Arthritis accompanying ulcerative colitis. *Am. J. Med.*, **33**, 923.

Moll, J.M.H. (1974) Psoriatic spondylitis: clinical, radiological and familial aspects. *Proc. R. Soc. Med.*, **67**, 46.

Moll, J.M.H., Haslock, I., Macrae, I.F. and Wright, V. (1974) Associations between ankylosing spondylitis, psoriatic arthritis, Reiter's disease, the intestinal arthropathies and Behçet's syndrome. *Medicine*, **53**, 343.

Moll, J.M.H. (ed.) (1981) *Ankylosing spondylitis*, Chapters 11, 21, 22, 23, 24, Churchill Livingstone, Edinburgh.

Noble, W.C. and Savin, J.A. (1968) Carriage of *Staphylococcus aureus* in psoriasis. *Br. Med. J.*, **i**, 417.

Owen, R. (1980) in *Ankylosing Spondylitis* (ed. J.M.H. Moll), Churchill Livingstone, Edinburgh, pp. 249–60.

Schwartzman, J.R. (1959) Arthroplasty of the hip in rheumatoid arthritis – a follow-up of sixty-eight hips. *J. Bone Joint Surg.*, **41A**, 705.

Selwyn, S. and Chalmers, D. (1965) Dispersal of bacteria from skin lesions – a hospital hazard. *Br. J. Dermatol.*, **77**, 349.

Simmons, E.H. (1972) The surgical correction of flexion deformity of the cervical spine in ankylosing spondylitis. *Clin. Orthop.*, **86**, 132.

Simmons, E.H. (1977) Kyphotic deformity of the spine in ankylosing spondylitis. *Clin. Orthop.*, **128**, 65.

Smith Petersen, N.M., Larsen, C.B. and Anfranc, O.E. (1945) Osteotomy of the spine in rheumatoid arthritis. *J. Bone Joint Surg.*, **27**, 1.

Welch, R.B. and Charnley, J. (1970) Low-friction arthroplasty of the hip in rheumatoid arthritis and ankylosing spondylitis. *Clin. Orthop.*, **72**, 22.

Wright, V. and Moll, J.M.H. (1976) in *Seronegative Polyarthritis*, North Holland, Amsterdam, pp. 411–47.

Wright, V. and Walkinson, G. (1965) The arthritis of ulcerative colitis. *Br. Med. J.*, **ii**, 670.

Wright, V. and Walkinson, G. (1966) Articular complications of ulcerative colitis. *Am. J. Proctol.*, **17**, 107.

Low back pain syndromes

Andersson, H. and Carlsson, C.A. (1966) Prognosis of operatively treated lumbar disc herniation causing foot extensor paralysis. *Acta Chir. Scand.*, **132**, 53.

Hakelius, A. (1972) Long term follow-up in sciatica. *Acta Orthop. Scand.* (Suppl.), 129.

Hirsch, C. and Nachemson, A. (1963) The reliability of lumbar disc surgery. *Clin. Orthop.*, **29**, 189.

Hirsch, C. (1965) Efficiency of surgery in low-back disorders. *J. Bone Joint Surg.*, **47A**, 991.

Macnab, I. (1977) *Backache*, Williams and Williams, Baltimore.

Newman, P.H. (1976) Surgical treatment for spondylolisthesis in the adult. *Clin. Orthop.*, **117**, 106.

Osterman, K., Lindholm, T.S. and Laurent, L.E. (1976) Late results of removal of the loose posterior element (Gill's operation) on the treatment of lumbar spondylolisthesis. *Clin. Orthop.*, **117**, 121.

Pearce, J. and Moll, J.M.H. (1967) Conservative treatment and natural history of acute lumbar disc lesions. *Neurol. Neurosurg. Psychiatr.*, **30**, 13.

Spangfort, E.V. (1972) The lumbar disc herniation. A computer-aided analysis of 2,504 operations. *Acta Orthop. Scand.* (Suppl.), 142.

Weber, H. (1970) An evaluation of conservative and surgical treatment of lumbar disc protrusion. *J. Oslo City Hosp.*, **20**, 81.

Wiltse, L.L., Kirkaldy-Willis, W.H. and McIvor, G.W.D. (1976) The treatment of spinal stenosis. *Clin. Orthop.*, **115**, 83.

Wiltse, L.L., Newman, P.H. and Macnab, I. (1976) Classification of spondylosis and spondylolisthesis. *Clin. Orthop.*, **117**, 30.

Wiltse, L.L. (1977) Surgery for intervertebral disc disease of the lumbar spine. *Clin. Orthop.*, **129**, 22.

'Medical orthopaedic' disorders

Csenz, K.A., Thomas, J.E., Lambert, E.H. *et al.* (1966) Long-term results of operation for carpal tunnel syndrome. *Proc. Mayo Clin.*, **41**, 232.

Dixon, A. St. J. and Grant, C. (1964) Acute synovial rupture in rheumatoid arthritis: clinical and experimental observations. *Lancet*, **i**, 742.

Goodgold, J., Kopell, H.P. and Spielholz, N.I. (1965) The tarsal tunnel syndrome. *N. Engl. J. Med.*, **273**, 742.

Harris, N.H. and Murray, R.G. (1974) Lesions of the symphysis pubis in arthritis. *J. Bone Joint Surg.*, **56B**, 563.

Hazleman, B.L., Laurin, C.A. and Tremblay, G.R. (1981) in *Textbook of Rheumatology* (eds W.N. Kelley, E.D. Harris, S. Ruddy and C.B. Stedge), Saunders, Philadelphia, pp. 1809–28.

Marmor, L. (1964) Median nerve compression in rheumatoid arthritis. *Arch. Surg.*, **89**, 1008.

Phalen, G.S. (1966) The carpal-tunnel syndrome: seventeen years' experience in diagnosis and treatment of six hundred and fifty-four hands. *J. Bone Joint Surg.*, **48A**, 211.

Pinals, R.S. (1979) in *Arthritis and Allied Conditions. A Textbook of Rheumatology* (ed. D.J. McCarty), 9th edn, Lea and Febiger, Philadelphia, pp. 985–1000.

Ranawat, C.S. and Straub, L.R. (1970) Volar tenosynovitis of wrist in rheumatoid arthritis. *Arthr. Rheum.*, **13**, 112.

10
Rehabilitation

10.1 INTRODUCTORY COMMENT

This chapter is largely to do with physical methods of treatment. Partly because of the inexactness of diagnosis and treatment, and partly because physical therapy represents only a part of total patient management, the term physical medicine has fallen into disrepute. 'Rheumatology' has emerged as a clinical specialty within the field of general (internal) medicine. Rehabilitation medicine is a more appropriate term to embrace the many physical, social and organizational aspects of the after-care of those patients who require more than acute and short-term definitive care.

Although the term rehabilitation has taken on several different meanings, in its widest sense it signifies the whole process of restoring a disabled person to a condition in which he is able, as early as possible, to resume a normal life (Piercy, 1956). Rehabilitation therefore is the concern of all clinicians.

For the rheumatologist, rehabilitation is used as a comprehensive term referring to the physical management of disability consisting of the maintenance of optimal functions and the promotion of patient well-being. Physiotherapy (including remedial gymnastics) and occupational therapy provide the basis for physical rehabilitation.

However, there is much more to rehabilitation than restoring ability to walk the length of the gymnasium or achieve independence in the toilet, and it must not be looked upon as a process separate from other medical care. Responsibility for its organization can often be centred on the general practitioner, but when the disorder is complex and constantly changing, the doctor with the most appropriate clinical experience must assume overall responsibility. For the rheumatic patient, this would usually be the rheumatologist, for the neurological patient, a neurologist, and so on. The special linking of rheumatology and rehabilitation, as in the UK at present, is, in my view, artificial, unnecessary, and removes the incentive for other specialties to consider properly the rehabilitation of their own chronic problems. It also hampers the development of rehabilitation services.

Patients with rheumatoid arthritis and other chronic arthritides will need periods of intermittent rehabilitation from time to time, and these should always be directed towards overcoming some intercurrent temporary change in the overall pattern of disability. The rheumatologist will wish to have access to the full range of rehabilitation services, which optimally should be closely integrated into the work of his department. When especially complex or severe problems arise, the help of a medical rehabilitationist may be sought.

Throughout this chapter I have relied heavily on the

writings of the late Dr Philip Nichols (with whom I was privileged to work), particularly concerning the sections on occupational therapy and physiotherapy.

10.2 ORGANIZATION AND PRINCIPLES OF REHABILITATION SERVICES

10.2.1 Organization

(*a*) *Rehabilitation departments*

Good rehabilitation requires careful organization, and each district general hospital should provide a comprehensive rehabilitation service.

A department of rehabilitation should:

1. Provide and organize the physical therapy services of the hospital and its dependent clinics.
2. Act as an advisory service on all problems of rehabilitation and resettlement:
   (a) By direct referral of patients to the consultant in charge of the rehabilitation department.
   (b) By referral to clinics devoted to special aspects of rehabilitation, e.g. functional assessment unit; wheelchair (and other appliances) clinics; resettlement clinics for advising and co-ordinating medical, social, industrial and training aspects of a patient's return to work.
3. Co-ordinate and correlate all services concerned with rehabilitation and resettlement in the community.
4. Provide a programme of teaching and research into problems of rehabilitation and physical handicap.

Such a department requires some beds, at least of a hostel nature, if it is to serve its purpose adequately.

(*b*) *Special rehabilitation units*

There will always be a need for some specialized units for managing the more severely disabled (e.g. very severely disabled arthritic patients, patients with head injuries, patients with spinal cord lesions), and these are likely to be organized on a regional basis, drawing patients from a group of district general hospitals. At these units, there will usually be a consultant who devotes all or most of his time to medical rehabilitation.

Apart from providing special facilities for management of the more severely disabled patients, a regional residential rehabilitation unit might be expected to provide all or some of the following facilities:

1. Short-term in-patient rehabilitation for patients unable to return home immediately because of social problems or travel difficulties.

2. Detailed functional assessment and long-term supervisory care of the severely disabled.
3. Development and manufacture of special appliances and equipment for the severely disabled.
4. Accommodation of patients needing prosthetic services, including amputees for limb-fitting and rehabilitation.
5. Facilities for assessment and training of disabled patients and their relatives.
6. Wheelchair appliance service.
7. Information service dealing with all aspects of equipment and facilities for the disabled.
8. Advice, help and training for professional workers on rehabilitation or resettlement.
9. Facilities for early industrial assessment and retraining.

(*c*) *The consultant in charge of rehabilitation services*

The clinician directing rehabilitation services should be primarily a physician. He should be able to solve problems concerning physical disorders of the locomotor system, whether rheumatological, neurological, orthopaedic or psychological. Preferably, therefore, he should have a working understanding of these specialties.

The consultant in charge of rehabilitation should provide overall guidance in the patient's management and can give the therapists the best chance of achieving the results required by:

1. Giving an accurate diagnosis.
2. Giving clear indications about the aims of treatment.
3. Giving a clear indication of the likely outcome of treatment.
4. Specifying where drug therapy, metallic surgical prostheses, or disease characteristics may require particular care in the administration of various physical treatments.

Particularly important is the realization that short, intensive periods of therapy are more likely to have a therapeutic value than the prolonged intermittent attendances for palliative treatment which rapidly become more of a social outing than a therapeutic activity.

10.2.2 Principles

Management of patients in rheumatism units has much to commend it. The remedial and social work staff of these units become particularly adept at pinpointing and reporting details which enable the rheumatologist to alter management if necessary. It is this combined approach by an experienced multidisciplinary group that results in a higher standard of patient care, decrease in morbidity, and more rapid return to independence at home and at work.

Many rheumatologists believe that a phase of intensive hospital inpatient therapy followed by careful outpatient follow up, with re-admission when necessary, will enable most patients to be maintained in a reasonable state of health for many years, or even indefinitely. With close liaison between rheumatologists, orthopaedic surgeons, and rehabilitation services, both in hospital and in the community, even the most severely disabled patients can be improved.

As Duthie (1967) has pointed out, it is important to understand the distinction between the aims of rehabilitation in the early acute stages of the disease, and those in the later chronic stages. With early diagnosis, early intensive treatment, careful instruction and training of the patient and family, and involvement of colleagues, over 60% of patients can be kept at work until retirement.

Rehabilitation in rheumatoid arthritis has five main aims: (1) relief of pain; (2) prevention of deformity; (3) correction of existing deformity; (4) improvement of functional capability; (5) control of systemic manifestations.

In order to fulfil these aims, a balance has to be maintained between rest and activity, and between medical care and surgical intervention.

It is sometimes not appreciated that rehabilitation is not a series of treatment regimens, supplemented by mechanical aids, which a remedial therapist grafts on to the final stage of the medical treatment of the patient. Rehabilitation should be interpreted in a more global sense and should embrace the total management of the patient with arthritis, aimed at restoring active life in the community.

10.3 PSYCHOSOCIAL COUNSELLING

Detailed aspects of psychosocial counselling in relation to rehabilitation are discussed in the chapter on rheumatological communication (Chapter 3).

10.4 OCCUPATIONAL THERAPY

10.4.1 Scope of occupational therapy

Occupational therapy is a service designed to help the patient to return to his or her former occupation, or, when necessary, to help adjust to an adapted or new occupation.

The term 'occupational' implies more than a person's actual work, and includes the role normally associated with it and its environment. A patient's degree of

mobility, personal independence, and psychological maturity to maintain the role of a working person are some of the associated factors encompassed by the term 'occupation'.

To achieve its goal, occupational therapy must be concerned with the assessment of the patient's physical capabilities, the exploitation of residual skills, and the planning of the re-education of patients with a permanent disability. Practical assessment should precede the final stages of rehabilitation and resettlement, and should be repeated to assess progress. Occupational therapy may therefore be regarded as a means to help the patient bridge the gap between physical disability and functional capability.

In patients of normal retirement age, or in those so severely disabled that it is impossible for work to be resumed, the emphasis will be on finding creative leisure interests (Fig. 10.1). Apart from giving personal satisfaction they will encourage contact with others, so reducing the isolation that severe handicap often brings.

Occupational therapy still carries with it the relics of an 'arts and crafts' image, and some practitioners and teachers unfortunately still place undue emphasis on diversional activities. Except in retired or severely disabled patients unable to work, these activities were never meant to be an end in themselves, but a means by which the therapist could assess and train a patient's manual skill, range of joint movement, learning ability, and work tolerance.

Although the complete functional assessment of a patient must include social, clinical, educational and domestic considerations, the patient's functional capabilities must be translated in a practical way in terms of normal activities. In view of this, an increasing number of occupational therapists are employed in domiciliary work (often attached to general practitioners) or are based in community services rather than hospital services.

(a) Occupational therapy in the district general hospital

The occupational therapy department of a district general hospital usually comprises heavy and light workshops (Fig. 10.2 (a)), a clerical section, an area for study, and a domestic unit including kitchen (Fig. 10.2 (b)), bedroom (Fig. 10.2(c)) and bathroom (Fig. 10.3), for assessing and training in activities of daily living.

A well-fitted, modern occupational therapy department is able to provide an atmosphere closely approaching that found in a normal home or at work.

The occupational therapist can provide graded activity aimed at increasing muscle power, joint range, coordination and balance. Her work complements that of the physiotherapist, and develops the use of the patient's limbs to functional activities concerned with daily

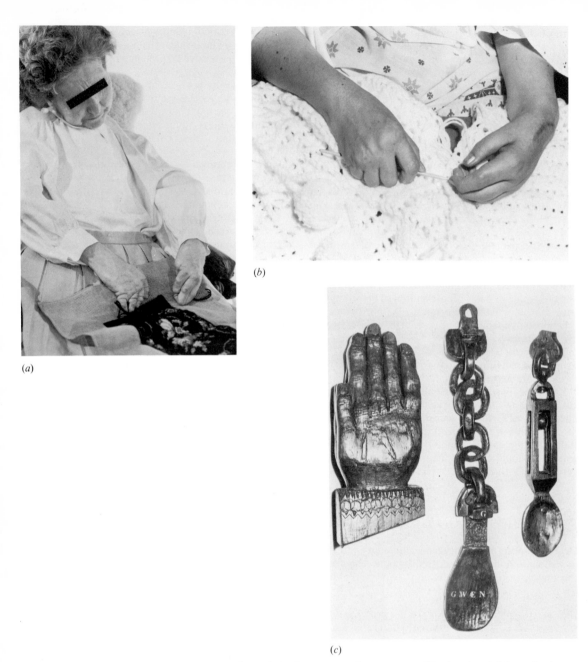

Fig. 10.1 Some creative leisure interests for the disabled. (a) Tapestry. (b) Crocheting. (c) Woodcarving (of the patient's own hand, even depicting his Heberden's nodes!).

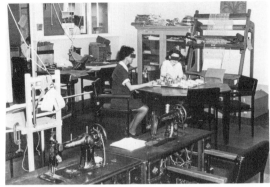

(a)

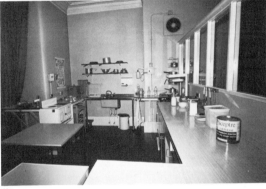

(b)

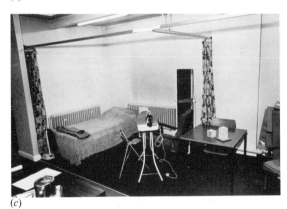

(c)

Fig. 10.2 Assessment units within an occupational therapy department of a district general hospital. (a) Light workshop. (b) Kitchen. (c) Bedroom.

living. In addition, she is able to provide a further stimulus and interest through creative activities, utilizing different aspects of motivation to achieve objectives similar to those at which the physical activities were aimed.

It is often argued that muscle strength, co-ordination and independence all improve simultaneously despite specific therapy. However, most patients do better and feel better if these activities are encouraged by specific exercises (physiotherapy) and specific functional activities (occupational therapy).

(b) Occupational therapy in the medical rehabilitation unit

Apart from management of chronic disability, another important role of the medical rehabilitation unit, whether outpatient or residential, is active restoration of function and progression to a full day's work for the patient with a temporary disability, such as an injury. In these patients the occupational therapist's role will be mainly therapeutic. This will be attained through carefully selecting for each patient appropriate activities aimed at repetitive movement of the affected part. For example, such a programme may involve progressively longer periods of standing, walking and co-ordination, and much of this activity will be supplementary and complementary to the general and specific exercises given by the physiotherapist.

(c) Domiciliary occupational therapy

Visits by the occupational therapist to the handicapped person in his/her own home are necessary to assess functional status and to identify problems in the patient's own environment.

The therapist should pass on her findings to the:

1. General practitioner.
2. Hospital – before the patient's admission, or in preparation for his return home.
3. Local authority departments concerned, including the housing department.

The therapist will be able to:

1. Continue activities of daily living training started in hospital and supply aids needed.
2. Deal with difficulties of access and mobility.
3. Assist the family and other helpers with difficulties in the care of the patient.
4. Provide educational and recreational activities for those unable to attend the day centre.

In community practice, most patients are referred to the domiciliary occupational therapist by the general practitioner and do not reach a hospital department. The domiciliary occupational therapist of the future will probably be based in a health centre, in which communication with other members of the community care team can be carried out more readily than when working in isolation.

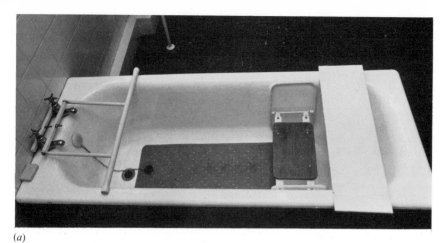

(a)

(b)

Fig. 10.3 Assessment bathroom. (*a*) Bath with aids. (*b*) Toilet with aids.

A disabled students' hostel, a residential home for the young disabled, or an old people's home should all be considered as the individual's 'home', and should receive the services of a domiciliary occupational therapist.

To patients with a locomotor disorder, life at home, at work, or in transit between the two, may be associated with hazards and discomforts. By simple changes in body posture and movements, by minor but strategic modifications in the arrangement and use of necessary home and work equipment, fittings and furniture, the occupational therapist aims to alter the patient/environment relationship in such a way that the patient's occupation and surroundings become useful in the therapeutic programme.

(d) Occupational therapy in other special units

In addition to the special role of the occupational therapist in the district general hospital, in medical rehabilitation units, and in the domiciliary field, other special areas involve their services, each with a different emphasis according to the demands of the unit concerned (e.g. industrial centre, sheltered workshop, work centre, day centre, children's assessment unit).

10.4.2 Functional assessment

The central feature of all modern occupational therapy is the functional assessment of the patient. Whereas the physiotherapist will be concerned with recording the range or strength of a movement carried out as a simple physical exercise, the occupational therapist is more concerned with the applied range, strength and co-ordination of a movement carried out in the performance of essential activities. Assessment of the patient's functional capacity cannot be considered in isolation, and must be part of a total assessment, including the clinical evaluation of status and prognosis, and a study of the patient's domestic and environmental background. Other factors, such as the patient's age, attitude of mind and social circumstances, must be taken into account.

Although most occupational therapy departments have their own assessment forms, which vary in detail, the information required to isolate the main problem areas follows a general pattern:

1. *Home conditions*: type of residence; accessibility; family and relatives or friends available for help.
2. *Mobility*: walking, use of aids and appliances; steps and other obstacles to be negotiated; use of wheelchair; need for and availability of outdoor transport.
3. *Personal care*: washing, dressing, toilet and bath; eating and drinking.
4. *Communication*: speech, telephone, writing and typing; reading; transport available; shopping.
5. *Domestic activities*: meal preparation; housework.
6. *Work*: problems of job; problems at work (including housework); schooling and education of children or training school for older children.
7. *Leisure activities*: past and present interests and problems.

During the routine part of the assessment the therapist will learn much about the patient's attitude, reactions, dependence, co-operation and adjustment to disability. These additional observations add much to the overall picture.

Functional assessment
1. Gives a base line, at any given time, from which future change in function may be measured.
2. Gives a guide to any changes that need to be made in the patient's routine or to the need for appliances, aids and equipment.
3. Gives some prognostic guide as to physical function, e.g. comparative functional assessment of a hand with and without a simple corrective splint will indicate to a surgeon whether surgical reconstruction is likely to be fruitful.
4. Gives some prognostic guide concerning the patient's motivation and ability to benefit from a programme of rehabilitation.

Specific disabilities

Tests of general functional capability, by means of activities of daily living or pre-vocational assessment activities, are non-specific and are relevant to almost all physical disabilities. However, occupational therapists have a further role in assessing specific disabilities. These assessments are used not only to ascertain the degree of specific disability. They also provide an objective evaluation of the patient as a whole, a guide concerning the effectiveness of treatment, and an indication for the need for reconstructive surgery. Rheumatological examples of such disabilities are rheumatoid arthritis and low back pain. The special factors involved in the assessment of rheumatoid disabilities merit discussion in further detail.

In patients with rheumatoid arthritis some stress on joints is inevitable during the activities of daily living, but by careful planning many unnecessary harmful stresses can be eliminated or reduced. Aids and splints can be used when it is not possible to surmount difficulties without them. For example, the use of drip-dry clothes and household linen obviates the need for ironing. A chair with a seat at an appropriate height reduces the demands made on upper limbs for pushing up from a sitting to a standing position. Appropriate grab rails in the toilet and in the bathroom will minimize the repeated weight-thrusting stress sustained in the upper limbs during toilet and bathing activities. In rheumatoid patients, particular emphasis is placed on hand function, and many occupational therapists have developed sophisticated methods to test this.

Hand function tests are usually constructed around the various types of grip.

Pin grip depends on: adequate opposition of thumb; good intrinsic control; good sensation.

Key grip depends on: strong intrinsic control; stable terminal and proximal interphalangeal joints.

Knife grip depends on: factors as for key grip; good flexion of index finger.

Handle grip or power grip depends on: adequate abduction of thumb; good finger flexion; good power in long flexors of fingers and wrist dorsiflexors.

Tests can be designed to measure the individual grips and to record their power and precision. However, hand function is only useful if the hand can be placed accurately in space. It is therefore dependent upon total upper limb function. Activities such as eating and writing must each be assessed as co-ordinated activity sequences, and can also be graded in terms of applied strength and precision. In rheumatoid arthritis, the severely involved hand rarely approaches the strength recorded in normal hands, but it is surprising what degree of precision and functional ability can be achieved (see Fig. 10.1).

Hand function tests are also of value in providing insight into the need for, and likely response to, reconstructive surgery.

10.4.3 Personal aids

(a) General

Careful assessment on admission to hospital will reveal
that many patients with temporary or permanent disability and most elderly people have some impairment
of function. Many activities of daily living (e.g. getting
in and out of bed, getting on and off the toilet, dressing,
housework and leisure activities such as gardening)
involve complex manoeuvres which are burdensome to
the elderly and arthritic. A few simple changes of
routine or a few simple aids can often make life much
easier. The provision of a home help or meals-on-wheels
may enable the patient to retain independence at home.

Proper assessment, coupled with provision of appropriate help, can contribute much to the quality of life.
Assessment must begin as soon as possible. If the patient
is in hospital, it should be initiated there, preferably in
close co-operation with the community services. Indeed,
the role of the occupational therapist should be regarded, in part, as a means of bridging the gap between
the patient's clinical care and community care.

A major sphere of activity for many occupational
therapists will therefore lie in assessing the need for aids
to daily living, in providing these aids, and in training
patients how to use them.

The aids most often required are: walking aids
(frames, sticks and crutches); bath and toilet aids;
eating aids; dressing aids; and aids for recreational
activities. (Some of these aids are shown in Fig. 10.4.)

The equipment most often required includes hoists
and wheelchairs.

All of these items need individual assessment and
practical trials. Occupational therapists are concerned
with assessing patients in all activities of daily living,

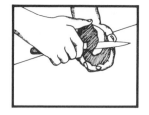
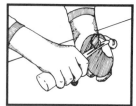
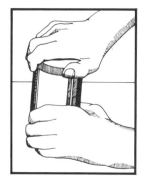
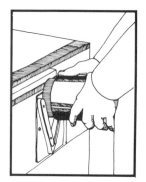
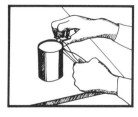
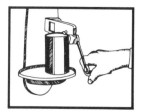

Fig. 10.5 Dos (right) and don'ts (left) in the kitchen. Top:
potato peeling. Middle: unscrewing jar lid. Bottom: opening
can.

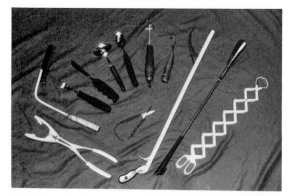

Fig. 10.4 A selection of aids. Left to right: Wexon easy-grip
tongs; long-handled comb; cutlery with padded handles; tap
turners (two designs); 'helping hand'; long-handled shoe horn;
'lazy tongs'. Centre: Stirex spring-back scissors.

determining the need for alterations to be made in the
home, demonstrating the safest routines in the kitchen
(see Figs. 10.5–10.7), helping with dressing, effecting
necessary adaptations to clothes, and helping with
problems in shopping, social and leisure activities (see
Fig. 10.8), and so on.

Patients in hospital will normally start this training in
the hospital occupational therapy department and then
continue it at home, preferably with the same occupational therapist in order to preserve continuity.

(b) Personal care activities

Toileting
Patients' self-respect will often become eroded if they
are unable to manage their excretory functions. It is

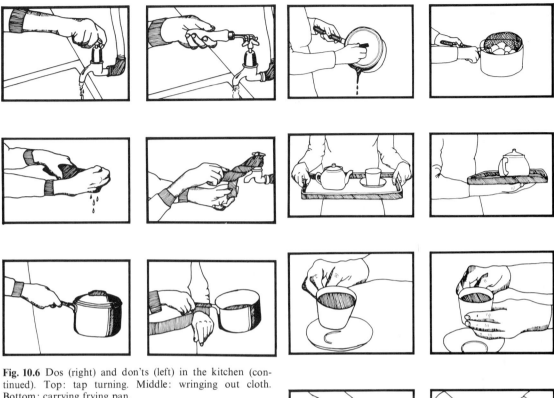

Fig. 10.6 Dos (right) and don'ts (left) in the kitchen (continued). Top: tap turning. Middle: wringing out cloth. Bottom: carrying frying pan.

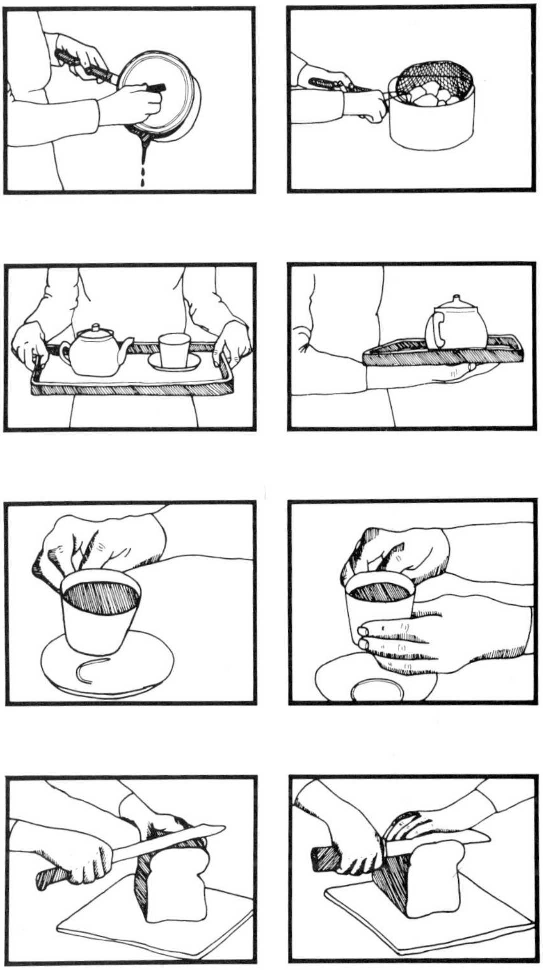

preferable that patients should open their bowels first thing in the morning so that this event will be over before they get dressed. A regular laxative may be needed to establish this routine. In other patients, defaecation may often be precipitated by an early morning cup of tea or coffee.

Many patients otherwise unable to use a lavatory pedestal may be able to do so if it is at the correct height for them, and if well-mounted grab rails are fixed around it (Fig. 10.3 (b)). Usually a seat raise of 8–15 cm is needed. This can be achieved by means of either a plastic insert for the seat, or by building a wooden commode-like structure over the pedestal. The height, spacing and diameter (3–4 cm) of the rails at the side of the pedestal may be as critical as the seat height.

Those unable to use a suitably modified lavatory or commode alone, even with assistance, can create substantial problems. Some of these patients may, in addition, have inadequate control of bowels and bladder. In these patients continuous urinary drainage (by catheter or ileal conduit in the female, and by condom drainage or catheter in the male) becomes essential. A regular bowel routine is also crucial in these patients. This may consist of a twice-weekly suppository or

Fig. 10.7 Dos (right) and don'ts (left) in the kitchen (continued). From top to bottom: straining vegetables; carrying tray; lifting cup; cutting bread.

enema followed by a period on a bedpan, commode or toilet.

Washing

Washing the upper part of the body is not usually a major difficulty. Relatively inaccessible areas such as the back can be reached with commercially available long-handled brushes or sponges. Perineal hygiene is not so easy to attain, and patients may find this a great source of embarrassment. A bidet may usefully solve such a problem.

Bathing can often be made possible by means of a board fixed securely to the wall, projecting over the side of the bath and used in conjunction with a bath seat

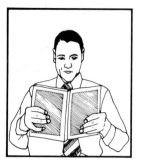 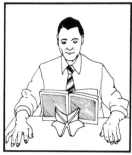

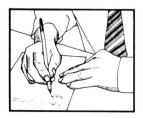 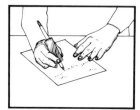

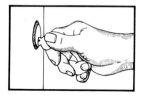 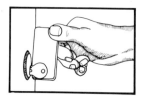

Fig. 10.8 Dos (right) and don'ts (left) concerning some social/leisure activities. Top: reading a book. Middle: writing. Bottom: key turning.

(Fig. 10.3 (a)). There must be adequate provision of grab rails, and non-slip mats must be used while getting in and out of the bath. It is often desirable that an able-bodied helper be present to assist if necessary, despite the provision of adequate aids. If accommodation for the disabled patient is to be modified or planned anew, a shower-room rather than a bathroom should be considered as a more practical alternative.

Grooming

Shaving is often simplified if the patient is prepared to use an electric razor. However, many men prefer to continue using a safety razor, and may be able to do so if they have a lightweight model or if a lengthened stem is fitted.

Application of cosmetics need not be a problem, and hair sprays in pressurized cans, long brushes, holders for eye make-up or lipstick, and long-handled combs

(Fig. 10.4) are all commercially available. However, if problems are still encountered, further help can be gained by mounting implements on wooden, perspex or aluminium handles.

Dressing

Most disabled people like to dress in the same style of clothing as their healthy fellows. A wide range of clothes is now readily available by mail order and in miltiple stores. By careful choice of commonly available clothes styles, it is often possible to keep aids and appliances to a minimum, and at the same time to give the patient fashionable and attractive clothing.

For most patients, clothing for the upper part of the body should fasten at the front; this ensures ease of access to the fastenings. If the zips present an obstacle they can be modified by inserting a curtain ring through the eyelet of the pull-tag so that the patient is able to obtain a better grip. If buttons or other small fastenings are used, Velcro provides a useful substitute. Patients with upper limb arthritis often have great difficulty in putting on clothes 'coat style' and may find it easier to use the 'over-the-head' method rather than dressing aids.

For most women, trousers are more sensible than skirts and stockings. Apart from being warmer they abolish the difficulty of putting on hosiery, and will also give more protection to legs which may have impaired sensitivity. If splints or calipers are necessary they can be hidden beneath the trousers but also readily exposed by means of a zip in the medial crease.

Shoes must be well fitting. If possible, elastic-sided footwear should be worn as they are easier to get on and off. However, if lace-up shoes need to be worn, elastic shoe laces may be helpful.

The most commonly used dressing aids are long-handled shoehorns (Fig. 10.4) and dressing sticks. Dressing sticks can be specially designed to help with specific problems such as hooking a garment around the shoulder, or they may be improvised. Wooden coat hangers, 'lazy tongs' (Fig. 10.4) or walking sticks are useful in this respect.

If possible, the number of aids should be kept to a minimum so as to avoid confusion. It is surprising how agile a determined patient can become with only one or two of them.

Feeding

Eating and drinking may be difficult for those with a poor grip and for those with weak or restricted movement of their arms. If the grip is weak, cutlery can be bought or modified so as to offer a handle of greater diameter (Fig. 10.4), and if necessary the shape of the implement may be changed. Lightweight Melaware cups and plates are also useful.

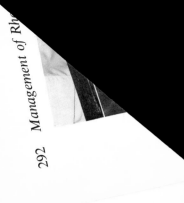

10.5 PHYSIOTHERAPY

10.5.1 General comment

The origins of physical therapy are steeped in medical history, and many forms of treatment referred to in the earliest medical records include the use of heat and hydrotherapy for the relief of discomfort from diseases of the locomotor system.

(a) Treatment evaluation

Most physical treatments involve some element of drama – electric currents, heat, light, and direct personal contact with the therapists. Such conditions favour the placebo reactor, and most would agree that the role of the physical therapist is partly to exploit the placebo response and partly to apply rational remedial therapy.

Many of the disorders traditionally treated by physical methods are degenerative, chronic and episodic. They also tend to have unpredictable remissions and exacerbations. No treatment is likely to produce dramatic results in the chronic degenerative locomoter disorders, but most patients, whatever their illness, respond to care and attention. This is what so many physiotherapy departments provide.

There is still too much that is taught and practised in physiotherapy departments that is based on tradition, personal experience and subjective patient response, and this image will probably remain until scientific evaluation becomes routinely applied to the various therapies.

(b) Trends in physiotherapy

Gradually, 'traditional' physiotherapy is becoming something of the past and the rehabilitation concept of progressive patient care is being more widely introduced.

Physiotherapy is concerned with the maintenance of total body function during acute illness, as well as with the maintenance of joint mobility and muscle power of the limbs. It is also concerned with early mobilization and short-term rehabilitation after illness or injury. For example, the physiotherapist may train the patient with rheumatoid arthritis to walk with sticks or crutches, but to the exclusion of simultaneous domestic activity such as carrying a saucepan or teapot. The occupational therapist, on the other hand, can teach the patient to be independent in the kitchen, and the patient can achieve this either by using a wheelchair which she can propel with her hands while carrying domestic equipment on a tray, or by 'paddling' with her feet, leaving the hands free. Such conflict between the use of crutches or

wheelchair can ofte[n]
than *maximal* total [

(c) Types of physiothe[rapy

It is traditional to descr[ibe
physiotherapist in term[s
cedures. Passive treatme[nt
of soothing, pain-relievin[g
use of massage, and con[
physical treatment is large[ly
from movements of single[
routines of the type used i[

(d) The physiotherapist

The art of physiotherapy rests on the selection of the appropriate technique for a particular patient at a particular time. Moreover, as Nichols (1976) has said, the quality of the physiotherapy depends almost entirely upon the quality of the physiotherapist. The quality of the physiotherapist depends upon her personality, her understanding of the patient and the disability, as well as her ability to contribute to the overall rehabilitation of the patient. In addition, the physiotherapist must have a detailed knowledge of all available techniques of physiotherapy and the use of aids and appliances, an understanding of general medical and surgical care, and an awareness of resettlement facilities provided by the statutory and voluntary bodies.

10.5.2 Passive procedures

(a) Heat

There is little doubt that for many painful conditions of the locomotor system, heat does have a palliative effect.

Heat may be applied to the body by changes in the environmental temperature, by contact with warmed substances, e.g. warm water, hot water bottles or wax baths, or by the radiation of energy into the body.

Hot water is probably the most widely used agent for conductive heating, either as warm baths, hot soaks or compresses. However, unfortunately this is too mundane a form of therapy to impress many patients (and often their physicians) as a 'special' treatment in a hospital physiotherapy department.

Wax baths (Fig. 10.9)
These are a convenient form of applying direct heat to the limbs. Paraffin wax is solid at room temperature and melts at 54°C. Once melted, it remains liquid at a temperature of about 49°C. Melting is achieved in an electrically heated bath. The wax is then applied to the skin – either by immersion of the part or by application

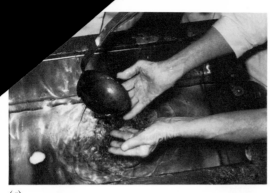

(a)

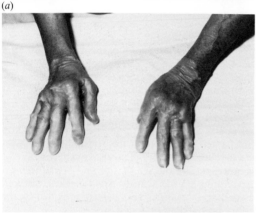

(b)

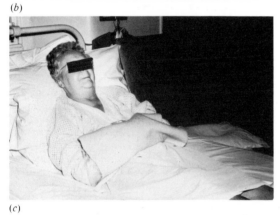

(c)

Fig. 10.9 Application of paraffin wax. (a) Molten wax being ladled onto patient's hands. (b) Hands covered with several layers of solidified wax. (c) Hands wrapped in polythene sheet (inner cover) and woolen wrap (outer cover) to retain heat.

with a brush at 48–49°C. The wax is easily peeled off after a treatment period (usually 20–30 minutes with 6 or 7 coatings of wax) and is returned to the stock for re-use. The heating effect is mainly due to the latent heat of solidification and to the specific heat of the wax. Immersion in wax is probably of no more benefit than immersion in warm water. Patients who are advised to continue this treatment at home can melt the wax in a heated pan, but it is important that this be immersed in a water bath for safety reasons (paraffin wax has a high flash-point).

Radiant heat

Infra-red rays are electromagnetic waves given off from any hot body. Electromagnetic radiations have two main properties of therapeutic relevance – in their wavelength and their intensity. In general, the hotter the source, the greater the proportion of shorter wavelength emission, and thus the greater the proportion of radiation adsorbed or dispersed. Radiant heat lamps are a convenient and relatively cheap source of superficial heat. The heat emitted is no different from that of an electric fire. Electric pads and infra-red lamps (Fig. 10.10) provide heat mainly of a longer wavelength. Their disadvantage is that they take longer to heat up – some infra-red lamps needing about 10 minutes to heat up and to reach an even temperature. This can waste time in a busy department.

From the therapeutic point of view, the value of lamps emitting radiant heat is probably two-fold. First, there is local warming of subcutaneous tissue with consequent peripheral vascular dilatation. Second, the patient has time to rest and relax during the heat treatment before the next part of the therapy.

Temperatures generated in the tissues are the product of many factors. These include the pattern of heating, the characteristics of the tissues being treated, and various biological factors associated with the organism as a whole.

Skin and fat are poor conductors of heat. The skin temperature rises rapidly when in contact with the heat source, but the underlying tissues show a temperature rise of a lesser degree. This depends partly on the heat dissipated at the skin surface (by sweat and convection) and partly on the conductivity of the subcutaneous tissue (related to the thickness of fat) and the amount of heat dissipated by the circulating blood. The temperature of muscle and joint tissue is not altered by heat conduction. However, both may show a delayed rise in temperature if a large area of the body is heated for 20–30 minutes, and this is associated with an overall rise of body temperature of 1–2°C.

Subcutaneous blood flow follows skin blood flow, and when the skin temperature is raised, skin blood flow increases by several hundred per cent. Thus both are increased by local or general heating of the body. However, surface heating is limited by the direct effect of heat on the skin tissue. A skin temperature of over 43°C is associated with pain, and a temperature of over

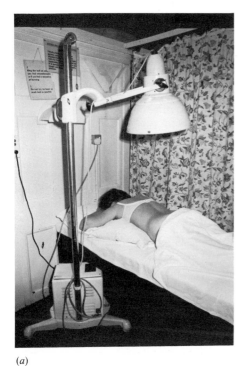

(a)

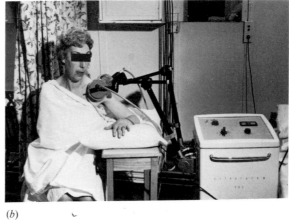

(b)

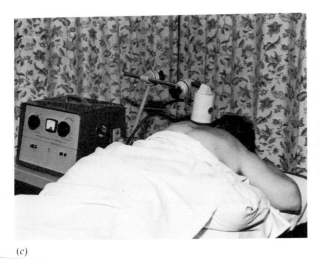

(c)

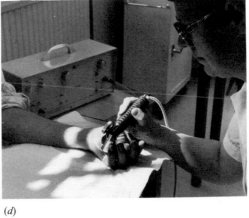

(d)

Fig. 10.10 Superficial and deep heat therapy. (*a*) Radiant heat (superficial). (*b*) Short wave diathermy (deep). (*c*) Micro-wave diathermy (deep). (*d*) Ultrasound (deep).

45° C will rapidly produce arteriolar flare and a wheal.

Because of the problems of 'conducting' heat to deeper tissues, many techniques have been devised in an attempt to produce 'deep heat', even though the value of such a therapeutic approach has yet to be proved. The only investigations on this subject show that although local and general heat will increase blood flow through skin and subcutaneous tissue, there is a much less marked and often inconstant response in deeper tissues (Nichols, 1976).

Diathermy (Deep heating)

Short-wave diathermy: There is a general belief that this form of electrical treatment (effected by short-waves: 11.0 m at 27.33 MHz) will produce deep heat (the word 'diathermy' means 'heating through').

The heating effect is achieved by placing the patient within an electric field created by a high-frequency, alternating current (Fig. 10.10). In effect, the patient forms part of the secondary circuit of a high-frequency generator. It is impossible to measure the input into the patient, and the only control of the field's intensity depends on the patient's skin sensation of heat and its level of heat tolerance. Short-wave therapy cannot produce an even heating effect in the body as tissues are not homogeneous. The highest current density will be at the surfaces, and heat here will be dissipated by circulating blood and by conduction to surrounding tissues.

These effects have been reduced by cross-fire techniques and by combining plate electrodes with conduction cables. However, studies on blood flow and radioactive isotope clearance have failed to demonstrate that short-wave diathermy has an appreciable advantage over conventional heat radiators (Nichols, 1976).

Microwave: This is another form of diathermy or deep heating by means of microwaves (12.2 cm at 2456 MHz) of electromagnetic radiations. They are directed by an antenna (Fig. 10.10) and, like short-waves, require adjustment of dosage to individual tolerance.

Ultrasound: Sound waves with a frequency of over 20 000 cycles per second are undetectable by the human ear and are referred to as ultrasonic waves or 'ultrasound'. High-frequency ultrasound (800 000–1 000 000 cycles per second), produced by applying a high-frequency current to a crystal, causing it to oscillate, is now used in many physiotherapy departments. The therapeutic machines (Fig. 10.10) produce vibrations of about 800 kHz with an output limited to 3 W cm^{-2}. The effects of the vibrations are mechanical, heating and chemical. Ultrasound appears to relieve pain and has been especially recommended for the treatment of scar tissue, bursitis, capsulitis of the shoulder and tendon lesions. However, there is no evidence that it is more effective than other modes of treatment. Furthermore, the apparatus is expensive, and the treatment is time-consuming and potentially dangerous.

Problems relating to various forms of diathermy: These include the risk of burning patients who have a poor circulation, impaired sensation or metal implants, and the assumed risk (evidence only anecdotal) of aggravating bleeding diatheses and spreading malignant tumours. Both short-wave and microwave diathermy are contraindicated in patients with cardiac pacemakers. Ultrasound can be used in the presence of metallic implants, but its safety in the presence of those embedded in methylmethacrylate has not yet been established. Ultrasound may cause spinal cord damage in the postlaminectomy patient. Testicular and lenticular damage as a consequence of the concentration of electromagnetic irradiation by metallic implants has been documented.

(b) Cold

The application of cold (e.g. as ice packs, iced baths or cold compresses) is sometimes more effective than heat in the relief of pain.

There is increasing physiological and clinical evidence (Nichols, 1976) to show that ice can decrease the spasm of spastic muscles and also produce vasodilatation in deep tissues.

Ice therapy (a typical ice-making machine is shown in Fig. 10.11) is now widely used in the mobilization of two main groups of patients:

1. Those patients with pain and oedema associated

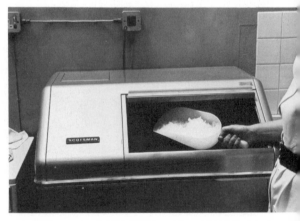

Fig. 10.11 Ice-making machine.

with recent trauma, surgery or an exacerbation of arthritis.

2. Patients with spasticity (e.g. hemiplegia, paraplegia).

(c) Electrotherapy

These days, 'electrotherapy' or 'electrical therapy' implies faradism, a term originally applied to the current obtained from a faradic coil, but now produced by electronic apparatus. Ion transfer, a form of therapy largely discarded now, ultrasonic and diapulse therapy have also been classified under this heading.

Faradism involves electrical impulses with a duration of about 1 ms repeated 50–100 times a minute. This current will stimulate motor nerves and cause a tetanic contraction of the muscle. If the current is surged a voluntary contraction can be simulated. Faradism will not stimulate denervated muscle.

Such electrical stimulation can therefore be used to produce repetitive contraction of muscle in a patient who is unable to do so because of pain or weakness. Some hypertrophy of muscle can be produced by intensive faradic stimulation if this is given several times daily, and it may be used to produce isometric contractions of the quadriceps in patients with rheumatoid arthritis or after knee surgery. It is also useful, as faradic foot baths (Fig. 10.12), in the stiff painful foot. Treatment should be used mainly in the early phase of muscle re-education to help initiate muscle action which the patient cannot at this stage perform himself.

(d) Transcutaneous nerve stimulation (TNS)

Transcutaneous nerve stimulation (TNS) (transcutaneous electrical nerve stimulation, TENS) has recently become popular as an additional means to attempt to alter pain perception by the application of an external stimulus. The technique, involving transcutaneous electrical stimulation has an historical precedent in that the early Greeks and Romans used live torpedo fish and organs of electric fish to control pain (see also Section 1.3.3), and in the late 1700s and early 1800s man-made devices replaced these natural sources of electricity.

Although the ultimate role of this therapy has not yet been established there is evidence that it can be useful in the control of certain chronic pain syndromes. The mechanism by which pain is controlled has not been delineated but theories include inhibition of pain perception via Melsack and Wall's gate-control mechanism, and activation of endogenous opiate-like substances.

Most modern devices are small, easy-to-use portable pulse generators (Fig. 10.13), but they are still mo-

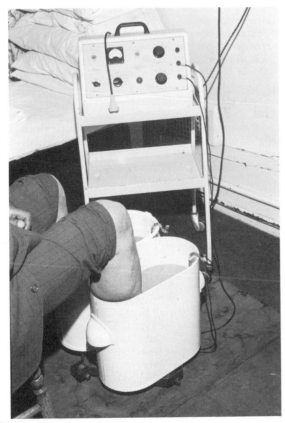

Fig. 10.12 Faradic foot baths.

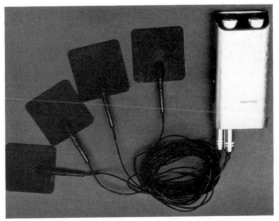

Fig. 10.13 Portable pulse generator and electrodes for administering transcutaneous nerve stimulation (TNS).

derately expensive. It is currently recommended that they be prescribed by a physician (in our unit we have found TNS of some value in cervicobrachial root syndromes). The generator can be used either by the physiotherapist or by the patient himself. Depending on the intended effect, the electrodes may be placed: (1) within or around the area of pain or tenderness; (2) at acupuncture, motor or trigger points; (3) at distant or contralateral sites; (4) on specific dermatomes or at specific spinal segmental levels; (5) over peripheral nerves.

Problems associated with TNS have been minor, and include occasional adverse reactions of the skin to the electricity, or to the tape or conducting medium between electrode and skin. The therapy is contraindicated in patients with cardiac pacemakers, over the carotid sinus, and in pregnancy.

For further details the reader is referred to a recent review published by the American Physical Therapy Association (Lister, 1979) which cites over 200 references appertaining to TNS.

10.5.3 Exercise therapy

The aims of therapeutic exercise are:

1. To mobilize stiff joints.
2. To strengthen weak muscles.
3. To prevent atrophy of bone resulting from muscular inactivity.
4. To restore and maintain function.

Successful results depend on full co-operation of the patient, as well as on adequate communication (see Chapter 3) between the physiotherapist and patient to ensure that simple instructions are properly understood. This will enable patients to continue their treatment unsupervised at home.

An important aspect of treatment is the fact that muscles do not usually act in isolation and that movement is the result of integrated activity between agonists (prime movers), antagonists (which must relax to permit agonist activity), synergists (which facilitate movement), and fixators (which stabilize the limbs and trunk).

Joint inflammation is attended by wasting and weakness of muscles acting on the joint and by further inhibition of voluntary movement due to pain and distension of the joint capsule. Rest in bed, splintage, aspiration of joint fluid, and intra-articular injection of corticosteroids, together with systemic anti-inflammatory agents, may facilitate mobilization of the joint and exercises aimed at strengthening weak muscles.

Exercises may be divided into mobilizing exercises, passive movements, muscle strengthening exercises, and proprioceptive neuromuscular facilitation. Various forms of exercise therapy are shown in Fig. 10.14.

(a) Mobilizing exercises

These can prevent a joint becoming stiff from disuse and can also increase the range of movement if this has become restricted. Such exercises should be performed under voluntary control, or, if the limb is particularly weak or painful, can be assisted by the physiotherapist, if necessary by the additional help of overhead slings or the buoyancy of water in the remedial pool.

(b) Passive movements

Stiff joints should not be forced by passive movements or manipulations, with the exception of stiff joints in the feet which are usually not possible to mobilize actively. Forced mobilization may break down intra-articular adhesions, but reactive inflammation often results in an increase in joint pain and stiffness, with the formation of further adhesions.

Traction and manipulation of the cervical and lumbar spine are sometimes included under this heading, but these will be discussed later.

(c) Muscle strengthening exercises

Muscles are strengthened by making them work repetitively against resistance such as that which can be applied by: the physiotherapist, gravity, the inertia of water, springs, weight and pulley systems, or weight-lifting techniques. Malleable putty or rubber balls are useful for strengthening grip.

As power increases, the resistance must be increased accordingly. The timing and rhythm of movements are additional factors to be considered by the physiotherapist. Excessive fatigue must be avoided and the joint must only be allowed to move within its pain-free range.

The simplest resisted exercise is static (isometric) contraction of muscle in which increase in muscle tension is not associated with a change in length. In this way, painful movement of the joint is avoided. An example of such an exercise is lifting small sandbags slung over the front of the ankle in order to strengthen the quadriceps group. This relatively mild exercise can be followed by a more taxing routine involving exercises against the resistance of springs or weights. In the more active patient, as opposed to those significantly affected by arthritis, maximal work can be provided by functional exercises in the gymnasium, including walking, stepping on and off benches, and climbing steps.

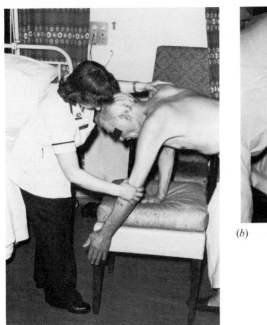

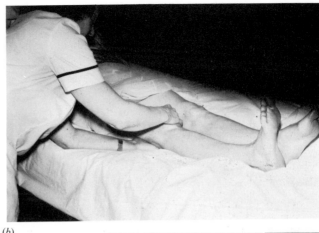

(b)

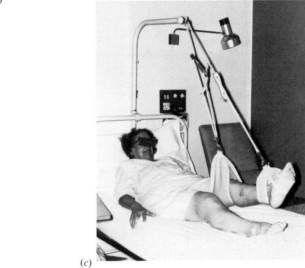

(c)

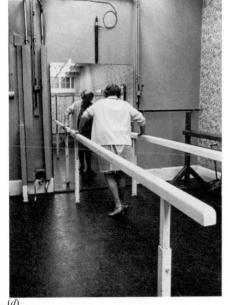

(d)

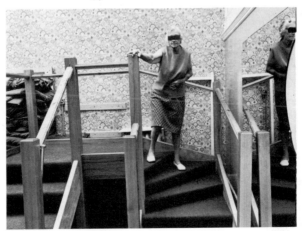

(e)

Fig. 10.14 Exercises. (*a*) Pendulum exercise for the shoulder. (*b*) Quadriceps drill. (*c*) Sling-assisted hip exercise. (*d*) Walking re-training using parallel bars. (*e*) Re-training in the use of stairs.

(d) *Proprioceptive neuromuscular facilitation (PNF)*

This technique, originally developed for the treatment of patients with neurological disease, is designed to reinforce voluntary effort (which may be impaired by pain, muscle weakness, joint stiffness, or diminished excitability of the anterior horn cell, peripheral nerve or muscle) by enhancing *reflex* muscular activity. This is brought about by stimulating sensory receptors in skin and muscle in the belief that this causes increased excitation of anterior horn cells.

The practical basis of proprioceptive neuromuscular facilitation rests on: (1) maximal resistance applied by the physiotherapist's hands; (2) proprioceptive stimuli induced before and during contractions by deep pressure, stretch before contraction, and traction and compression of the joint – all supplied by the physiotherapist's hands; (3) set movements performed in diagonal or spiral patterns; (4) the fact that the patient always just 'wins'.

The two main advantages of this method over others are that, first, movements and resistance are always under the physiotherapist's control, and secondly, no apparatus is needed.

10.5.4 Hydrotherapy

The buoyancy of water in the remedial pool supports the limbs, and the warmth of the water relieves pain and muscle spasm. When painful joints or weak leg muscles prevent the patient walking on dry land, he may be able to walk in the pool. Active exercises in the warm pool are particularly beneficial for mobilizing stiff and painful joints, e.g. in osteoarthrosis of hip, capsulitis of shoulder, ankylosing spondylitis and generalized polyarthritides.

The assistance provided by the buoyancy of the water and the resistance which it offers can be enhanced by the use of flotation devices such as inflated cushions or rubber rings attached to the arms and legs. They can also be made from buoyant materials such as polystyrene.

Flat walking areas in the pool can provide the simplest form of graduated partial weight-bearing. This is useful for re-education in walking after injuries or surgery of the lower limbs. The patient is started in relatively deep water, where most of his weight will be taken by buoyancy, and graduates to shallow water as his condition improves, finally progressing to full weight-bearing outside the pool.

In some centres, the areas of different depth are separated by internal walls or rails, whereas at others, small pools of different depths are provided as 'annexes' to the main pool.

The only contraindications to hydrotherapy, apart

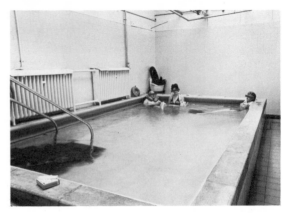

Fig. 10.15 Hydrotherapy pool: note that the edge of the pool is raised above the floor to facilitate transfers to and from wheelchairs.

from patients encased in plaster of Paris, are incontinence and open or infected wounds.

In general, the best size for a treatment pool suitable for a major rehabilitation unit or department is 40 ft × 20 ft (12.2 m × 6.1 m) (18 ft × 14 ft is the recommended minimal size). It should be kept at a temperature of 32.3–35°C. There must be easy access into the water via shallow steps, and, for the more severely disabled, appropriate hoists should be installed. Preferably, there should be graduated levels of depth from 3 ft to 4 ft 6 in (91.5 to 137.2 cm), or, if it is not possible to provide graduation, a pool of constant depth of about 2 ft 6 in to 3 ft (76 to 91.5 cm). If the edge of the pool is raised above the floor (Fig. 10.15) of the department by 2 ft to 2 ft 6 in (61 to 76 cm), transfers to and from wheelchairs are facilitated and are more easily supervised by instructors outside the pool.

There must be adequate changing-room accommodation to allow for continuous use of the pool while patients are preparing to enter the pool and for drying and dressing after treatment. Indeed, the surroundings and associated services are almost as important as the pool itself, and although they add considerably to the space and cost involved, they contribute substantially to the efficiency of the department as a whole.

Most practitioners involved in rehabilitation would agree that a well-appointed hydrotherapy unit is an indispensable feature of any physiotherapy department.

10.5.5 Traction

(a) *Spinal traction*

Traction has been used in the treatment of neck pain and backache for many years, but unfortunately there have been few scientific investigations and authenticated therapeutic trials to assess its value.

The only effects that traction can be expected to achieve are some distraction between vertebrae at the intervertebral disc and apophyseal joints – tensing the longitudinal ligaments of the spinal column (particularly the posterior common ligament), and some slight widening of the intervertebral foramina. These effects can only be expected to occur while the traction is being applied. Continuous traction may also be used to immobilize the patient in bed.

There is some evidence that acute lesions of the neck and back respond to more vigorous manipulative procedures, whereas the more chronic lesions tend to be self-limiting. Those that persist with marked general limitation of movement appear likely to respond to traction or immobilization.

It has been variously argued that traction is a *form* of manipulation, a *part* of manipulation, or a *preliminary* to manipulation. Many authorities advise a combination of treatments, particularly the use of a support (collar or lumbosacral belt) in association with traction. A well-fitting support often seems to prove beneficial after a short period (20–30 minutes) of traction. It may also prolong the symptomatic improvement achieved by traction.

(b) Manual traction (Fig. 10.16(a))

This is traction applied by the physiotherapist's hands, usually only for brief periods, often combined with lateral and rotational manoeuvres, and is really more appropriately classified as a manipulation. The best results are usually obtained in the acute phase.

(c) Continuous traction

This is applied through a harness and continued for 24 hours or longer. The forces used are relatively small and the treatment is used mainly as an in-patient procedure, and usually reserved for severe, intractable root pain.

(d) Sustained traction

This is a technique of traction usually applied for 20–30 minutes.

(e) Intermittent traction

This is similar to sustained traction but applied intermittently, the traction being alternately applied and withdrawn by various mechanical devices.

Sustained and intermittent traction are applied through harnesses. With cervical traction, the patient's

body weight provides adequate counter-weight. For lumbar traction, two sets of harnesses are usually used, providing a symmetrical pull on the torso (Fig. 10.16 (b)). In patients with a history of allergy to zinc oxide adhesive (Fig. 10.16 (c)) either a hypo-allergenic adhesive or a non-adhesive bandage (e.g. Seton, Oldham, England) should be used.

The force used may be large, from about 15–25 lb (6.8–11.3 kg) for cervical traction, to 40–50 lb (18.2–22.7 kg) for lumbar traction, but under careful control, cervical traction may be increased to 40–50 lb and lumbar traction to between 70 and 150 lb (31.7–68.1 kg).

The angle of traction, the position of the head and neck, and the weight applied are usually achieved by trial and error. Indeed, the position and weight that produce relief of pain vary from patient to patient and for each patient from day to day. Most patients with neck and arm pain respond to traction, but most also respond to simple positioning or to the application of a firm collar. However, most physiotherapists believe they can achieve optimal results by a combination of these techniques, varying their treatment according to the patient's response. It should be noted that patients with an acute lesion respond badly to sustained traction as they are particularly prone to rebound pain when traction is relaxed.

It is difficult to accept the rationale for traction in degenerative spondylosis of the cervical spine. Traction reduces the natural cervical lordosis (with a pull of 20–25 lb (9.1–11.4 kg)), and a separation between C2 and C7 of 3–14 mm can be shown at a pull of about 45 lb (20.4 kg). However, the first radiological indication of cervical spondylosis is a loss of cervical lordosis, and thus it could be argued that traction would be more likely to reproduce or exacerbate symptoms accompanying early cervical arthritis.

In the lumbar spine, traction has been demonstrated to produce a separation of about 2 mm at each disc space. However, such separations are unstable and reversible.

Therapeutic trials of traction have been inconclusive, and mostly without adequate controls. Nevertheless, there is sufficient physiotherapeutic folklore surrounding traction for it to continue as a popular mode of treatment.

Finally, traction in the treatment of skeletal pain should never be used unless bony metastases have been excluded radiologically.

10.5.6 Massage and manipulation

Massage (see also Section 11.2.21) as an effective method to induce muscle relaxation of cramped tight, tonically contracting muscles is widely accepted by the

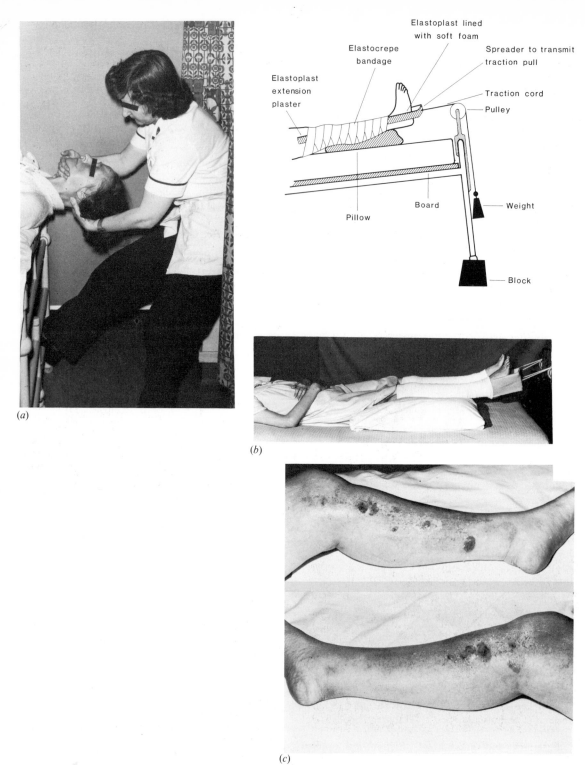

Fig. 10.16 Traction. (*a*) Manual traction of the cervical spine. (*b*) Lumbar traction applied through weights harnessed to each leg (details of the apparatus are shown in the upper diagram). (*c*) Bullous reaction due to hypersensitivity to zinc oxide adhesive used to secure leg traction.

layman, but no controlled studies of its efficacy in the management of musculoskeletal problems have yet been undertaken.

The types and indications for the commonly used massage techniques employed by physiotherapists include: stroking (effleurage), used superficially for its soothing effect and for deep muscle relaxation; compression (petrissage) (Fig. 10.17), as a kneading of tissues to stretch adhesions, mobilize oedema, and for muscle relaxation; and percussion (tapotement) as a stimulating counterirritant vibration or vigorous percussion.

Massage is expensive in terms of therapists' time and effort and should be restricted to patients in whom relaxation needed for a specific exercise cannot be obtained by simpler means such as the application of heat or cold, or by other muscle relaxation techniques.

There is much controversy about manipulative procedures most of which stems from a lack of understanding, imprecision of diagnostic terms and valueless speculation about the pathology of undefined clinical syndromes. In the generally held view, a manipulation is a passive movement restoring range of movement to a joint which is 'stuck' with intra- or periarticular adhesion, 'subluxated' or in some way limited in movement. The procedure is usually regarded as being immediate in giving relief, forceful in character and often accompanied by a 'snapping' sensation or sound. It is also widely thought that the technique can be practised by only a small group of physicians, osteopaths (Section 11.2.18) and chiropractors (Section 11.2.5). However, during recent years, many of the techniques previously restricted to such practitioners have been rationalized and are being taught to physiotherapists who are now including manipulation in their normal repertoire. In a professional physiotherapeutic sense the term 'manipulation' describes any procedure applied passively to a relaxed part of the body for the purpose of restoring joint range and functional activity. Force and flamboyance are usually unnecessary, and sudden dramatic manoeuvres are not always followed by dramatic recovery.

Radiological examination of a joint is an essential preliminary to manipulation. It should be emphasized that spinal manipulation should never be undertaken if there is evidence of vertebral fragility or instability, nor in the presence of neurological signs of cord compression or irritation.

Both 'manipulations' and 'mobilizations' are techniques to increase joint range by passive movements. The former are based on single quick movements and are often less controlled than the latter repetitive, gentler movements. It is claimed that because mobilization is more 'controlled' it can therefore be more localized, particularly in relation to spinal joints.

Although there is a considerable volume of folklore and anecdotal details of dramatic 'cures', no acceptable clinical trials, nor long-term follow-up studies of manipulation techniques have yet been undertaken.

10.6 NURSING

10.6.1 Hospital nursing

The nursing care required by any patient who suffers from a rheumatic disease is based on the following principles:

1. General care and comfort of the patient.
2. Alleviation of pain – rest, splints, drugs.
3. Prevention of deformity.
4. Careful observation.
5. Support and encouragement of the patient and the maintenance of morale.
6. A share in rehabilitation of the patient.
7. Special procedures.

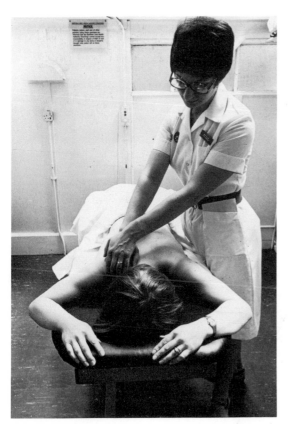

Fig. 10.17 Massage based on a compressive/kneading technique (petrissage) to encourage relaxation of muscles in the neck and shoulder region.

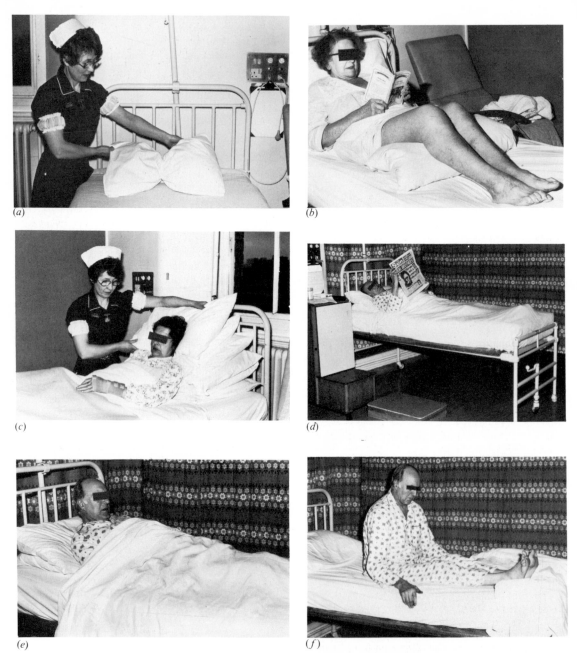

Fig. 10.18 Some aspects of rheumatological nursing. (*a*) Arranging pillow in a 'butterfly' shape for patient with a painful neck syndrome (e.g. acute cervical disc prolapse). (*b*) A pillow under the knee will encourage flexion deformity. (*c*) Too many pillows – a common cause of pain in the neck and aggravation of neurological syndromes associated with the cervical spine. (*d*) Good resting position for patient with lumbar disc lesion – note board under mattress (patients with chest disease, as in this patient, and the elderly, often find difficulty in tolerating a single pillow). (*e*) Craning of the neck should be avoided in patients with painful neck syndromes and/or associated neurological features. (*f*) 'Jack-knifing' of the trunk should be avoided in patients with lumbar disc disease.

The nurse plays her part not only during the acute phase of the disease when hospital admission is required, but also in the out-patient clinics and in the patient's home. Throughout, she is a member of a team comprising among others, doctors both in and out of hospital, physiotherapists, occupational therapists, social workers, chiropodists and members of voluntary organizations. While many of the aspects of nursing described here are especially applicable to hospital care, most of the principles involved apply equally to nursing management in the patient's home.

(a) General care

In the acute phase, the patient with arthritis is nursed at rest. The bed should have a firm mattress and fracture boards should be put under the mattress if it sags. This is particularly necessary if there are back problems. The patient must have sufficient (but not too many) pillows and must be well supported for comfort. A bed cradle will keep the weight of the bed clothes off tender, inflamed joints of the lower limb, but a thin flannelette sheet next to the patient and underneath the cradle will ensure warmth. The ill effects of rest in bed must not be forgotten. These include joint contractures, muscle wasting, thrombosis of leg veins and subsequent pulmonary embolism, osteoporosis, renal calculus and pressure sores.

However, many patients are admitted largely because of the rest under supervised conditions that hospitalization can offer. In addition to the patient with active inflammatory arthritis, this includes patients with cervical or lumber disc problems with root involvement. These patients will have to be taught how to avoid postural threats to the spine such as flexing the neck and trunk from the lying position. These and other postural aspects with which the nurse can help the patient are illustrated in Fig. 10.8.

Clothing should be light, warm and easily put on. Because much movement in this acute phase can produce pain, the nurse must handle the limbs carefully, supporting each fully so that undue and painful movement does not occur. Lifting and turning the patient must also be done slowly and carefully; any jarring of joints must be avoided. The limbs should be placed in a position as near functional as possible, and splints may be used to ensure this – preventing pain and undue deformity. Patients who require particularly careful handling are those who have been on long-term corticosteroids, since the skin is often atrophic and easily torn. Abrasions from knocking against sharp corners can readily develop into chronic ulcers. The skin over the shins may be so thin that shin guards of plastazote may be indicated.

Another patient who requires careful handling is the rheumatoid with cervical spine involvement. These patients are in constant danger of spinal cord injury and are safer nursed in a collar. Great care should be taken to avoid neck jolting when re-positioning them in bed or in transfers between bed and bedside chair.

As patients are often given drugs which encourage sweating, a daily blanket bath is essential. The patient who is sweating profusely will require additional washing. In these patients, care msut be taken to make sure that skin folds are thoroughly dried and that dusting powder is applied to prevent soreness. It is particularly important to check that the buttocks and natal cleft are kept clean and dry to prevent the development of sores. All other care, including changes of position, must be taken to prevent skin breaks.

Oedema of the legs may develop from many causes including stasis due to inactivity, poor muscle tone of the legs, and sluggish venous return in varicose veins. Pressure from knee effusions on adjacent veins has been implicated, but rarely reaches clinical reality.

Oedema may be relieved by raising the end of the bed at night. If the oedema is more intractable the legs can be raised on a frame (like half a deckchair) for half an hour, and then a Bisgaard blue-line bandage applied for the rest of the day. The elevation is repeated and the bandages are re-applied in the evening. These efforts may be supplemented in the physiotherapy department by faradism under pressure, and elastic stockings (which arthritic patients have difficulty in pulling on) may be required as a long-term measure.

(b) Diet

Patients with gout may need a low-purine diet and should avoid excess alcohol; however, strict dietary observances are less called for in patients stabilized on anti-hyperuricaemic drugs. Obese patients with arthritis of weight-bearing joints should reduce weight. Apart from these considerations, a well-balanced, nutritious diet is all that is required. Rheumatoid patients are often underweight – partly due to the systemic effect of the disease, partly to loss of appetite from disease and drugs, and partly to difficulty in making meals. Fad diets, constantly being given emphasis in quack articles addressed to patients, are to be deprecated as there is no evidence that they have any curative or beneficial effects.

(c) Alleviating pain

Rest in bed relieves pain in many patients, such as those with active rheumatoid arthritis, osteoarthrosis of weight-bearing joints, or a prolapsed intervertebral disc. The patient with chronic joint damage also benefits from an hour's rest on the bed after lunch, care being taken to encourage patients to keep the joints in a good position.

When plaster resting splints are applied, the nurse must be particularly diligent. Any signs of the plaster being too tight, such as colour changes of the limb distal to the plaster, or any signs of swelling or pain, should be reported immediately. If the plaster is too tight, it will need to be removed. Rubbing over a bony prominence or at the edge of the plaster may cause abrasion of the skin and must be avoided. A new plaster may be required, although the insertion of a small piece of sponge rubber, or dampening the edge and remoulding it, or cutting off some of the plaster, may suffice. Occasionally pressure over the region of the head of the fibula may produce a popliteal nerve palsy with foot drop.

The administration of drugs involves not only ensuring that the correct medicines are given, and in the right sequence at the right time, but also observations concerning their therapeutic and toxic effects. Although a routine of drug administration is important, drugs must not be unnecessarily withheld to fall in with 'medicine round' time. Nurses should also verse patients in drug details (see also Section 3.3), such as how to insert suppositories (see also Section 4.4.3) and how to self-administer injections (e.g. corticotrophin).

(d) Preventing deformity

The patient requires a firm mattress and the limbs must be placed gently into a good position. To ensure this, rest splints may be used for the limbs – sometimes these are worn continuously, but often they are worn only at night. These splints are usually made from plaster of Paris, but may be made from synthetic materials (e.g. Plastazote – a polyethylene foam). Splinting is particularly useful when applied to flexion deformities of the knee. For these, either serial splints or plaster of Paris or inflatable splints 'air splints' (e.g. Schuco, Williston Park, N.Y.) (Fig. 10.19) are useful. Nurses may be expected to apply splints and care must be taken to ensure that the skin is dry before the splints are fastened in position. Undue pain or soreness associated with the splint must be reported. Velcro straps are more convenient for many patients since buckles are usually too difficult for the arthritic hand to manage. Bad positioning in bed may produce deformity and must be avoided, although the patient may temporarily feel more comfortable in these positions (see Fig. 10.18 (b)).

One reason for treating patients with early rheumatoid arthritis in hospital is to familiarize them with the discipline of rest splints at night. To prevent foot drop, a foot board may be placed across the cradle at right angles to the bed.

If the patient has such fragile skin that splints cannot be tolerated, proper positioning of the legs may be obtained by sponge rubber supports. A flexion defor-

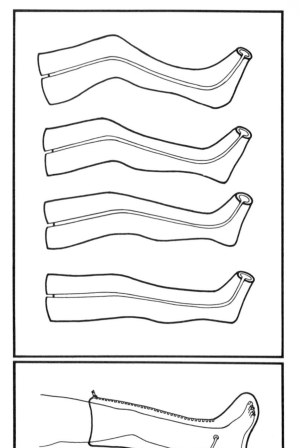

Fig. 10.19 Splinting of flexion deformity of the knee. (*a*) Serial splints made from plaster of Paris (the cut in the side of the plaster has enabled its removal). (*b*) Inflatable splint (air splint).

mity of an osteoarthrotic hip may be overcome by periods of lying prone.

(e) Observation

The patient in the acute phase of arthritis requires careful observation. Temperature, pulse and respirations should be taken regularly, although the timing of these observations will vary according to circumstances.

Increased pain and tenderness or other change in the joints should be noted whilst attending to the patient's needs.

The nurse is in a particularly good position to observe

the patients first thing in the morning when their capabilities are at their lowest. A patient whose hands are quite free by mid-morning may be unable to use them on waking and may struggle with breakfast. These problems are not usually so obvious by the time the doctor does his ward round, particularly if this is in the evening.

Urine testing is of particular importance when gold or penicillamine are given. Significant albuminuria is generally considered a contraindication to the use of either drug. Its development may also be due to a complication of the disease, such as amyloidosis in rheumatoid arthritis, or renal involvement in systemic lupus erythematosus or polyarteritis nodosa. Glycosuria may develop if steroids are taken.

(f) Patient's morale

Often patients will share anxieties about their disease and its implications with the nursing staff. In association with the physician, reassurance may be a powerful factor in treatment (see also Chapter 3). The patient may have an unjustifiable fear that he or she is going to become crippled and that there is no real hope for her condition. Moreover, anxiety about the family and about the home may dominate the patient's outlook. The help of the medical social worker may help to assuage these worries.

(g) Rehabilitation

After a period of immobility the patient may need help in establishing a proper walking pattern. The nurse often collaborates with the physiotherapist in the patient's walking re-education. The ability to take even steps and the ability to turn round may have been lost, and the patient will need to be re-taught the correct placing of the feet (and of a walking stick if this required) during these manoeuvres.

After initial rest in bed graded activity is usually prescribed. The nurse should encourage the patients to do their periods of exercise without supervision (e.g. quadriceps exercises and hand exercises).

(h) Special procedures

In addition to the normal day-to-day care of the patient, the nurse will perform or assist with a number of procedures. These include some of general application, such as dressing ulcers, postoperative care of wounds and removing stitches. Some routine procedures such as collecting mid-stream urine specimens or catheterizing female patients may be made more difficult by the restriction of joint movement in hips and knees. Both subcutaneous injections of corticotrophin and intramuscular injections of gold or iron may be given. Both these require special precautions. Injection of gold must be preceded by a urine test for albumin and enquiries regarding rash, itch or sore throat. Iron injections must be given using the Z-track technique, otherwise tattooing of the skin surface may occur due to iron oozing back along the needle track.

Intralesional injections of corticosteroid may be used in patients with such conditions as tennis elbow, tenosynovitis or carpal tunnel syndrome. The nurse will be required to assist in the same way as when joints are aspirated or injected.

Aspiration of joints may be done for diagnostic or therapeutic purposes. After appropriate hand scrubbing or sterile hand preparation, the clinician will clean the skin over the joint to be entered. Local anaesthetic is usually used, with infiltration from skin to synovium. An aspiration needle is then inserted and fluid removed. This should be collected in a sterile container for culture and other appropriate investigations. At this stage local corticosteroid may be injected. This must be of the type labelled 'for intra-articular use' and the doctor should check the label. The needle is then removed and an adhesive plaster put over the puncture site. This should be left in place for 2 days. If a weight-bearing joint has been injected the patient must rest for 2 days in order to reduce the risk of 'steroid arthropathy', if in fact this risk is significant.

A similar procedure is used for injection of radioactive isotopes such as gold or yttrium. The joint is punctured and may be aspirated. The isotope, diluted in saline, is then injected and a 'flush' of 10 ml saline is then injected to clear isotope from the needle and prevent radiation burns in the needle track. The injected limb is immobilized for 3 days after injection to prevent spread of radioactive material from the joint. No hazard exists to staff or other patients, and no special precautions are required for disposal of the patient's urine or faeces.

For further details of local injection therapy see Chapter 7.

Arthroscopy is used for viewing the inside of joints, usually the knee, and for obtaining biopsies under direct vision. This procedure is carried out in the operating theatre under general or local anaesthetic. Normal theatre procedure is used for preparing and draping the limb. The knee is aspirated and re-distended with saline either by direct intra-articular injection or by a drip inserted into the knee which runs throughout the procedure. The arthroscope is inserted in the same way as an aspiration needle and the joint viewed, photographed and biopsied through it. The limb may be wrapped in wool postoperatively, and may be swollen for 2 or 3 days. Physiotherapy, with particular stress on quadriceps exercises, should be undertaken from the first postoperative day.

10.6.2 Community nursing

The district nurse should note any drug side effects and should check that the correct dosage is being taken. Advice may be given on whether the diet is adequate, or whether help is needed with a reducing diet. She may also need to apply dressings where the skin has broken down, or after surgery. Where injections are prescribed, and the patient or a relative cannot undertake these, the district nurse may be required to give them. Gold injections, given intra-muscularly at intervals of 1 week to 1 month, should be preceded by a urine check for albumin before administering the dose. The drug should not be given if albuminuria is present, nor if the patient complains of itching or rash. Corticotrophin is given by subcutaneous injections–usually in a long-acting form two or three times a week. The anaemia of arthritic patients may warrant intramuscular injections of iron.

When bedfast the patient will need to be nursed in a light, sufficiently heated, cheerful room. If possible the bed should be near a window, allowing a view of the world outside. The patient should be encouraged with tempting meals, and depression may be lessened by endeavouring to maintain various interests (e.g. visitors, radio, reading, television). Mobility should be encouraged where the conditions allow this. Particular care must be taken with pressure areas and natural or artificial sheepskins are of value to the wasted arthritic patient. Bed cradles may be required to relieve the weight of the bed clothes. Examination of the skin should be made for infection. Personal hygiene is important and the maintenance of morale imperative.

The health visitor is another member of the nursing profession who performs a vital function in this context. She bridges the gap between home and hospital. The ideal arrangement is where the health visitor is attached to a hospital department and visits handicapped arthritic patients after discharge. In this way a planned programme of after-care can be organized in conjunction with the community services and the patient's general practitioner. The health visitor reinforces the advice given in hospital, particularly with regard to drugs, and she may liaise with the physiotherapy and occupational therapy departments after the patient has been discharged. Assessment needs to be made of the home conditions and attitudes of the patient, and of active help which is available. The health visitor and the medical social worker will then mobilize domiciliary services according to the individual patient's needs (e.g. home helps, meals-on-wheels, voluntary help with shopping and social visiting of the lonely).

The health visitor plays a supportive role at times of stress. This may be through lending a sympathetic ear, through reassurance, or in some instances through referring patients to agencies best able to cope with particular problems, for example rehousing on medical grounds, or major home adaptations such as widening the doors for wheelchairs. Arthritis, like any other handicap, may impose a strain on the marriage relationship and help may be needed from marriage guidance counsellors. Advice on family planning or on sexual problems from family planning clinics or their domiciliary services, and help in caring for children (such as play groups, nursery schools, day nurseries and child minders) may also be required. The breakdown of marriage happens all too often in these patients, and free legal aid in the case of divorce may be required. Throughout this emotionally traumatic period the patient will need much psychological support.

The burden of coping with a handicapped person may be too great at times. It is essential to identify early signs of breakdown in patients or relatives, so that relief can be given and crises avoided. With the help of the patient's general practitioner it may be possible to negotiate with the consultant physician to have the patient re-admitted on sociodomestic grounds for 2 or 3 weeks to give relatives a rest. This will also fortify them to continue the caring role when the patient returns home.

Some instruction may be required concerning weight-reducing diets, prevention of accidents due to loose stair rods or inadequate lighting, and the rearrangement of furniture to facilitate wheelchair access.

Disabled patients should realize that they are still wanted and can be useful members of society. Liaison with government rehabilitation units, employment agencies, and sheltered workshops will help to foster encouragement and help patients regain self-respect.

Interest and stimulation can be promoted by contact with charitable organizations such as the British Rheumatism Association, which gives help by providing radios, televisions, monthly social meetings, and transport for the housebound.

10.7 CHIROPODY

10.7.1 Scope of chiropody

Modern chiropodists are professionally trained. Training takes 3 years and leads to State registration. The Health Service employs only registered practitioners. Some chiropodists concentrate on the provision of moulded foot appliances, others on providing special shoes, and others on the techniques of massage, manipulation and remedial exercises for the foot. However, most of 'general practice chiropody' is concerned with the day-to-day care of the forefoot in older people – the cutting and cleaning of awkward toenails, the care and dressing of corns and callosities, the provision of pads for bunions or metatarsalgia. Most of these foot deformities are avoidable and are generally due to badly fitting shoes, weak foot muscles or excess weight.

The general treatment consists of nail cutting, removal of debris or corns in the nail sulci, and packing of nail sulci to relieve pressure. This is followed by removal of corns and calluses on the toes and foot with the application of suitable protective padding.

10.7.2 Specific problems

The main ways in which the chiropodist can help patients with arthritis of the feet are:

1. *'Ring' pads.* These take pressure off painful bony prominences by providing padding around the affected area. The most satisfactory ring pads for bunions are horseshoe-shaped and are made of thick adhesive felt. Smaller ring pads for the knuckles of the toes can be bought ready-made. Alternatively, the toes may be bound in animal wool which not only protects them but, because it is slippery, allows the sock or shoe to move over the painful area.

2. *Toe Pads.* these are put between or under the toes to 'prop' them into a better position. The painful callosities on the tips of clawed toes can often be corrected by a simple roll pad which the toes can grasp. Fig. 10.20 shows some typical uses of ring and toe pads.

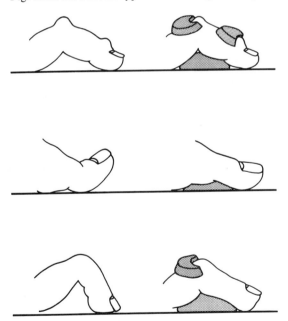

Fig. 10.20 Various types of chiropodial padding (right) and the conditions for which they are used (left). (*a*) Dorsal and plantar pads for corns. (*b*) Corrective plantar pad to proximal phalanx for big toe hyperextension. (*c*) Corrective plantar and dorsal pads for hammer toe.

3. *Moulded insoles.* Although these fall within the domain of the chiropodist, in hospital practice in the UK such appliances are usually provided by the orthotist, together with modifications to existing footwear and the manufacture of special footwear (see Section 10.9.2).

Patients presenting in the early stages with a painful 1st metatarsophalangeal joint can be helped by using fan strapping, which is fixation strapping to reduce joint stress.

All deformities (e.g. depressed metatarsal hands, retracted toes) should, where possible, be protected by the use of removable or non-adherent replaceable pads.

Patients on prolonged corticosteroid therapy present a problem in that minor abrasions tend to ulcerate rapidly, and light shoe pressure can give rise to ischaemic ulceration. Increasing the thickness of protective pads is a useful way to encourage these lesions to heal.

10.8 SOCIAL WORK

10.8.1 Scope of social work

The responsibilities of the social worker in rehabilitation are:

1. To support and help the patient to accept and live within their limitations and to provide encouragement towards independence.

2. To try to solve the patient's social and financial problems.

3. To co-operate with other members of the hospital rehabilitation team and to pass on information which may be significant to a patient's medical progress.

4. To liaise with the general practitioner, local authority services and the family to ensure continuity of care.

During rehabilitation the patient emerges from the protective environment of home or hospital to face reality. The patient has to cope not only with the physical aspects of the disability but also with a complete change in life style. The resulting social problems can have a significant effect on recovery, so that work done by the doctor and remedial therapists must be matched by the solution of practical problems concerned with finance, housing and transport, and it is principally the social worker who will be the guiding influence in achieving this.

10.8.2 Liaising function

Co-operation with the local authority, social services and with general practitioners is essential to avoid discontinuity in management between hospital, rehabilitation centre and home. The reorganization of the social services has made this easier in some areas because local authority social workers and occupational therapists can be brought in at an early stage to work with the hospital social worker and occupational therapist. It is a comfort to the patient to know before they return home that there is a friendly face, already familiar to them, who will take over. With the help of community services and the general practitioner much can be achieved in helping the disabled to live independently even in the most difficult circumstances.

10.8.3 Finance

Patients and their relatives are often confused by, and in awe of, the complexity of authorities and legislation. Many do not understand the various national insurance forms and it is not made clear enough to the public the difference in entitlement to the various benefits. The information issued to the public is often couched in governmental jargon, and tends to be vague, dull and difficult to understand. Similar difficulties are experienced in comprehending the complicated system of assessing allowances, disability pensions, earnings-related supplement, and other benefits. The Department of Health and Social Security is not obliged to release information about patients to social workers, and this is transmitted directly to the patients themselves. The Supplementary Benefits Commission is rarely permitted to pay rents direct to councils, no matter how large the rent arrears, making it difficult and time consuming to help the less intelligent and less responsible members of the community.

Financial support is an important motivating factor. Too much money can inhibit a disabled person returning to work. Our system of benefits allows the man who fractures his leg at work to draw twice as much money as the man who sustains the same injury at home or in the street. Most people are reluctant to return to work for less money than they are getting when sick. Furthermore, under the social umbrella of being 'on the sick' a patient can claim immunity from debts, prosecutions, maintenance orders and other problems.

10.8.4 Housing

Housing the disabled, single and homeless is perhaps the most taxing problem of all, and forms a hiatus in our welfare services. There is provision for the young chronic sick and for the geriatric patient, but there are few places to go if the patient is middle aged, alone and disabled. Landladies are not keen to shoulder the responsibility of a disabled person, particularly if they are not out at work all day. Some of the more enlightened and wealthy boroughs have hostels with workshops attached, but there are not many of these.

There are a few privately run residential workshops, but these require sponsorship by a local authority. Some patients end up in geriatric homes, and some find themselves uncomfortable and unwanted in lodgings or, at best, in a bed-sitting room with support from the community services.

There is a pressing need for more warden-supervized accommodation for such people, some of whom could manage a day's work, but could not look after themselves as well.

The bureaucratic intricacies of many housing departments are almost as daunting as those of the various government departments. While the shortage of council accommodation is realized, many disabled people could leave hospital earlier if housing authorities were more flexible. If a patient already lives in a council house it is difficult to get an exchange; if a patient has to start *de novo*, it is almost impossible to get a council house or flat. In some areas a supportive letter or 'phone call from the consultant in charge of the patient receives sympathetic consideration and helps to secure appropriate accommodation more quickly than could have been achieved by the patient acting alone.

10.8.5 Transport

Transport is another major problem about which patients are grateful to have help and advice. Further details about this will be discussed in Section 10.10.2.

10.9 ORTHOTICS

10.9.1 General comment

Static support for a persistently painful, unstable or permanently deformed joint can be provided by a removable device to hold the joint in a position of function. The term 'splint' is usually applied to a device made to support a main joint (or joints), such as the wrist, knee or ankle. However, in a sense, braces, foot appliances, shoes, collars and spinal corsets are also splints in that they provide some support for joints.

In the making and fitting of splintage appliances, two main principles provide the basis for sound orthotic practice:
1. The device should be fitted in the optimal position.
2. Careful thought should be applied to choosing the most suitable orthotic material for each device – preferably combining the properties of lightness, strength, durability and ease of construction and application.

10.9.2 Splintage appliances

Various suitable orthotic materials are available for making 'working' splints, including polythene, Prenyl, leather and fibre-glass, all of which combine the suitable properties mentioned in the previous section. Plastazote, although having some of these qualities, lacks the strength necessary for limb fixation, plaster of Paris is too heavy, and many of the newer plastics are unnecessarily rigid and tend to cause local sweating. Velcro or similar simple fastenings should be used, and care taken to ensure that they are positioned so that patients can use them easily.

(a) Wrist splints

For adequate immobilization a wrist splint should extent from the distal third of the forearm to the distal flexion crease of the hand, without including the thenar eminence. A position of about 10° of extension will allow optimal hand function. A useful ready-made splint is the 'Futuro' wrist splint which has adjustable Velcro fasteners, is strong and light, and contains a removable aluminium palmar support. These splints are available in three stock sizes (small, medium and large).

They can be worn throughout the day and night or at night only. If the former, removal at least once a day for gentle exercises is advisable. Plaster of Paris or Plastazote splints can be used as rest splints for patients in hospital, but for the reasons mentioned above they are not suitable for long-term wear as 'working' splints. Lively splints may be indicated in patients with extensor tendon rupture or with a dropped wrist due, for example, to rheumatoid neuropathy. There is no evidence that medial extensions of wrist splints ('ulnar deviation splints') can prevent or improve ulnar deviation of the fingers.

Fig. 10.21 summarizes the various splints mentioned here.

(b) Knee splints

A weight-bearing knee is best supported by a full cylinder, extending from upper thigh to lower leg, with the joint held in 5° of flexion, and this can be removed when the patient wishes to sit or to climb stairs. Resting splints should include the foot to the end of the toes. Working and resting and resting splints are shown in Fig. 10.22 (a). Although theoretically a knee is best supported by a hinged caliper, which allows the patient to sit easily, in practice it is difficult to produce a cosmetically acceptable device as the multiple straps and hinge mechanism cannot easily be managed by arthritic hands. Flexion deformities of the knee joint

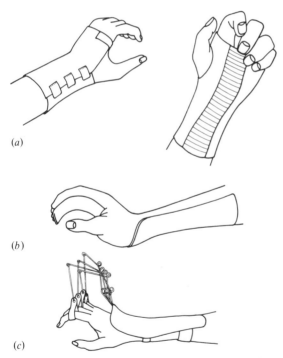

(a)

(b)

(c)

Fig. 10.21 Wrist splints. (a) Dorsal and palmar view of 'Futuro' ready-made wrist splint (note Velcro straps and palmar section containing moulded, removable aluminium strip). (b) Typical rest splint – plaster of Paris or Plastazote (note 10° angulation at wrist and extension of splint from upper forearm to end of fingers (slightly flexed)). (c) Lively splint (used for example to treat extensor tendon rupture).

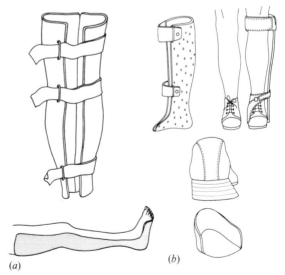

(a)

(b)

Fig. 10.22 (a) Knee splints. A bivalved working splint with Velcro straps (top) and a plaster of Paris resting splint – note inclusion of foot to end of toes and position of ankle (bottom). (b) Various devices to support the ankle. Top left: Yates'-type splint. Top right: 'T' strap and outside iron. Middle: laterally flared heel. Bottom: heel cup.

should be corrected as far as possible before supporting splints are provided (this has been discussed previously in Section 10.6.1). Otherwise uncorrected flexion deformities will tend to cause compensatory deformities at the hip and ankle joints in the same limb. Moreover, unless the inequality in leg length is corrected, similar deformities may develop in the opposite limb. Valgus deformity of the knee will generate an additional problem due to rubbing on the opposite knee.

(c) Ankle supports

Support of the ankle is often most easily achieved with boots or bootees. An alternative is to use a moulded posterior plastic or reinforced Plastazote splint extending from mid-calf to mid-tarsus and fixed with Velcro straps. This splint also fixes the sub-talar joint. Fixation of this joint or correction of the common valgus (eversion) deformity may also be achieved by a small plastic heel cup, a suitable insole or a firmly heeled shoe. An outside iron with or without a T-strap is a satisfactory but cosmetically less acceptable means of managing valgus deformity of the ankle. Flaring of the heel and other external alterations to the shoe tend to wear and hence are less practical.

The various ankle supporting devices are shown in Fig. 10.22 (b).

(d) Arch supports

These are moulded into special insoles or may be fitted to the shoe. The insoles, usually made of foam rubber or felt, are either transverse or longitudinal. Transverse (metatarsal) supports provide a useful contribution to foot care and act by taking the weight of the body off the painful metatarsophalangeal joints and transferring it further back onto the soft parts of the foot. Supports may be held on by an elastic strap, but have the disadvantage that the pad has to be removed from the strap for washing. The other type of support is in the form of an insole. It is most important that the pad or 'metatarsal button' is placed in exactly the right place. All too often the pad is put where the supplier thinks it ought to be rather than where the patient needs it. Shaped cork or composition insoles can be made to meet each individual patient's requirements.

Longitudinal (valgus) supports. These can be bought ready-made or in a form that can be easily moulded to individual requirements, or they can be custom-made out of moulded plastic. Their function is to enable the area between the heel and the big toe (the 'instep') to take some weight. They are needed only in secondary flat foot due to arthritis. However, all too often they are also supplied to young people with primary flat foot in whom they may lead to foot muscle wasting and weakness.

Preferably, valgus supports should be individually moulded and provided with a heel cup. This ensures that they are held in exactly the right position. In general, patients do not tolerate rigid supports and pads as well as supple or cushioned pads, and there is now a wide range of the latter available in modern foam plastics and microcellular rubbers. The problem with insoles or any other

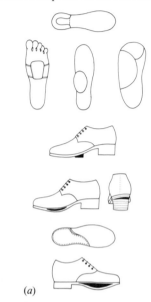

(a)

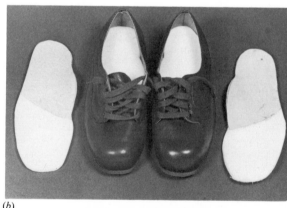

(b)

Fig. 10.23 (a) Various types of insole and modifications to footwear – heel pad (for painful heels, e.g. plantar fasciitis); domed valgus support on full-length insole (for fallen longitudinal arch, three-quarter length combined metatarsal/valgus insole (for metatarsophalangeal arthritis and fallen longitudinal arch); outside metatarsal bar (metatarsophalangeal arthritis); lateral raise (outside wedge) on sole and heel (for varus deformity of the ankle); elongation of heel (for supporting midfoot); rocker bar (for hallux rigidus). (b) surgical shoes with full-length Plastazote insole with valgus inserts.

shoe padding is that they are bulky and the shoe is often already too tight because of foot swelling. It is therefore nearly always necessary with a shaped insole in patients with arthritis to make sure that larger shoes are provided. The various types of arch support are shown in Fig. 10.23 (a).

(e) Shoes

The greatest improvement in walking may be achieved by the provision of satisfactory shoes. In the early stages of foot arthritis, wider and deeper shoes with rigid soles and good supporting heel cups, obtainable from normal retail sources, should suffice. With progression of the disease it may be necessary to provide custom-made shoes. Seamless ('space') shoes, as opposed to traditional surgical shoes, are cheaper, lighter and, in general, quicker to manufacture, but they are unsightly to many wearers and often increase sweating of the feet. However, local facilities will often govern the decision to choose a particular type of shoe, such as the speed of delivery, the accuracy of fitting and the ease of alteration. A welcome recent innovation is the 'off-the-peg' surgical shoe with compressible insole (e.g. 'Comfort', 'Radus') which are available from many surgical appliance firms at relatively reasonable cost. These are suitable for patients without gross foot deformities who have found difficulty in finding appropriate footwear in local shoe shops. Apart from the provision of special shoes for the general purpose of increasing comfort by providing more space for the foot, various special modifications can be made to the shoe. For example, where there is inequality of leg length the shoe should be raised about half the leg-length difference in young patients and about three-quarters the difference in elderly patients. Such raises should not significantly increase the weight of the shoe. Raises of over 4–5 cm ($1\frac{1}{2}$–2 in) will need to be combined with a subtalar joint support, usually a boot. Some tapering of the sole will be necessary with higher shoe raises. Other modifications include: outside metatarsal bar (for metatarsophalangeal joint arthritis); lateral raise (outside wedge) or medial raise (inside wedge) of sole and heel (for varus and valgus deformities of the ankle, respectively); flared heel, outside or inside (for varus and valgus deformities of the ankle, respectively); elongation of the heel (for supporting the mid-foot); rocker bar (for hallux rigidus).

For further details of shoes and modifications to footwear, see Fig. 10.23.

(f) Collars

These are, in effect, splints for the cervical spine. They are indicated for the stiff painful neck due to acute cervical

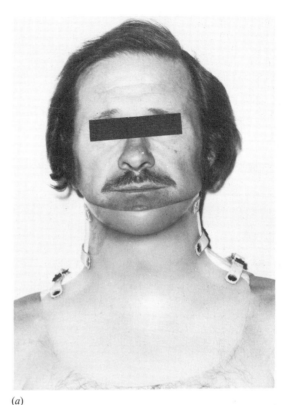

(a)

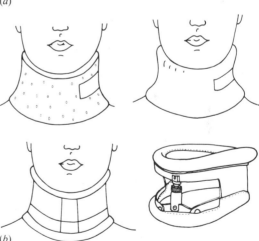

(b)

Fig. 10.24 Collars. (*a*) Moulded hard collar (polythene), to include chin, designed to immobilize neck. (*b*) Soft collars (clockwise from upper right) – soft foam with stockinette cover and Velcro fastener; 'air-flow' pattern (height adjusted by anterior screw); double-section polythene edged with soft expanded rubber trimmed with plastic (height adjusted by varying the overlap between upper and lower section); Plastazote.

disc prolapse or spondylosis, for rheumatoid atlanto-axial subluxation, and for spondylotic cervical myelopathy. In disorders requiring immobilization of the neck, a rigid collar (polythene or Plastazote reinforced with polythene) moulded to include the chin will be necessary. Otherwise soft collars, aimed at reducing rather than eliminating cervical movement should be sufficient. These are usually made of foam rubber or other foam materials such as Plastazote. Velcro straps provide useful fixation and can be easily manipulated by the patient if positioned at the front or side of the collar. Stockinette covers can be provided to facilitate laundering. Details concerning the usage of collars will vary according to the disorder for which they are prescribed.

Further detail of collars are shown in Fig. 10.24.

(g) *Spinal supports*

These are designed to splint either the lumbar or, less often, the thoracic spine. For lesions of the thoracolumbar or lower thoracic spine the support is essentially of lumbar pattern but extended to reach the mid-thoracic region. For higher lesions of the thoracic spine the extension should be to the upper thoracic spine with shoulder strap attachments. Lumbar braces vary from the light ready-made type to more robust custom-made patterns such as the Goldthwait support (Fig. 10.25). It is essential that custom-made supports should feel comfortable, and any appliance not fitting properly should be corrected, otherwise these costly devices will be rejected by the patient. As with collars, the usage of spinal supports will depend on the disorder for which they are intended.

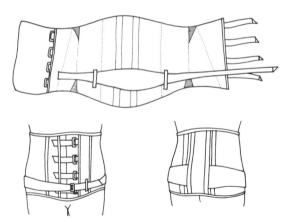

Fig. 10.25 Various views of custom-made lumbar corset (Goldthwait pattern). Note: anterior and posterior steels; leather-covered slot for moulded metal plate over lumbosacral splint; front straps with Velcro fasteners; fulcrum strap; elastic gusset. The corset is made from washable canvas.

10.10 EQUIPMENT TO ASSIST FUNCTION

10.10.1 Channels of provision

The National Health Service will provide any items that are necessary to improve an individual's functional ability. Most of these can be supplied by the local social services department, or by the workshops at the district general hospital or rheumatic centre on the recommendation of a doctor or paramedical worker. For all but the simplest devices a charge is usually made. This is usually related to the patient's financial means, but variations occur from one area to another.

The prescription of expensive and specialized equipment is limited to those with special experience in their use. Requests for remote control systems, for example, can be made only through senior administrative medical officers of regional health authorities and their authorized assessors.

Disabled people often pose complex management problems which may need to involve a team of medical and paramedical workers. Patients needing specialized assessment or advice on aids, appliances or equipment should be referred to a regional rehabilitation centre.

10.10.2 Mobility aids

Because of the frequent involvement of lower limb joints, many patients which chronic arthritis, despite the advances made recently with joint replacement surgery, will require aids for mobility at some stage of their disease. Generally, the simpler the aid the better, as they call for little manipulative skill, occupy little space, and are the least prone to mechanical failure. The progression of aids of increasing degree of substitution for normal walking may be summarized as follows:

1. Partially weight-relieving: sticks, crutches and walking frames.

2. Completely weight-relieving: patient-propelled wheelchairs, attendant-propelled wheelchairs, powered wheelchairs and outdoor vehicles.

(a) *Partial weight-relieving aids*

The simplest partial weight-relieving aid is the walking stick, either wooden or of tubular metal alloy. The walking stick can be used to relieve weight by patients with unilateral lower-limb disease. It should be held in the hand contralateral to the affected leg, although some clinicians leave the side of preference to the patient. Using two sticks enables more efficient protection of one leg by weight bearing through the sticks from 'heal-strike' to 'toe-off' of the involved leg.

Walking sticks should always be of the correct height and should be comfortable to hold. The handle of the stick should be chosen (or even designed) to suit the shape and the strength of the user's hand. A curved handle is often preferred by those with strong hands, but many patients with rheumatoid arthritis prefer a straight handle. Additional comfort can be achieved by softening and enlarging the handle with sorbo rubber, plastic foam or felt. Some sticks are available with moulded plastic handles. A walking stick must always be fitted with a removable rubber or plastic ferrule with a wide base which should be replaced when it becomes worn.

Three-legged (tripod) or four-legged (tetrapod) sticks provide greater support, but patients may find them unwieldy. However, many designs are available and it is often possible to find a walking aid that enables the patient to walk with reasonable confidence and stability.

Crutches of various types are available. The traditional underarm (axillary) crutch is suitable only for short-term use after trauma or surgery until partial weight bearing is permitted. It should not be used in the presence of joint disease of the upper limbs since it imposes much strain on all joints of the arm, particularly the shoulder. Elbow crutches are usually more suitable for the rheumatoid patient.

There are many different types of elbow crutch not all of which are satisfactory. The arm grip should be correctly aligned and well padded to avoid pressure on the ulna. The handgrip may require padding with foam or leather.

A 'gutter' crutch causes even less loading on the upper arm joints and is particularly suitable for patients with weak, painful hands and wrists. Its height should be adjustable so that the forearm rests comfortably in the horizontal gutter support when the patient is standing erect. Even more support can be provided by walking frames. These are wide based and are suitable for frail and elderly patients. Most walking frames are rigid and take up a lot of room when free-standing in the average house. However, they are stable and allow patients to get in and out of a chair and on and off the toilet, as well as being an aid for walking. However, for the patient with widespread rheumatoid disease they can be unsatisfactory because: (1) weight is borne through the hands and wrists; (2) a normal walking pattern is not possible.

A household trolley may be preferable for a disabled housewife who needs support for walking about the house and also a means of carrying domestic objects from place to place while using a walking aid.

A summary of the various walking aids discussed above is shown in Fig. 10.26.

(b) Wheelchairs

Although wheelchairs are traditionally regarded as symbols of disability, both physicians and patients

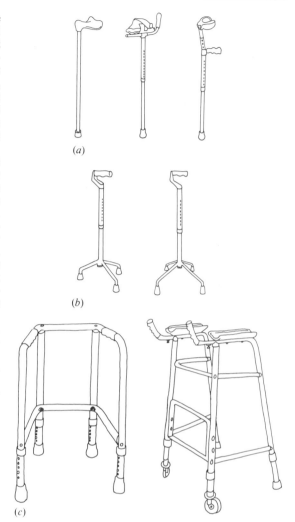

(a)

(b)

(c)

Fig. 10.26 Walking aids. (a) (Left to right): walking stick with moulded handle; gutter crutch with Velcro strap and grip; elbow crutch. (b) (Left to right): tripod; tetrapod. (c) Walking frame; walking frame with arm gutters and grip.

should realize their importance as aids to mobility and functional independence.

There are many patients with rheumatoid arthritis who can achieve or maintain independent mobility in the presence of severe disease by the judicious use of a wheelchair, whether self-propelled or powered. Furthermore, in the presence of widespread joint disease, a wheelchair will provide mobility without the stress imposed on upper limb joints by crutches. If, as in most patients which chronic arthritis who require a wheelchair, there is significant involvement of the upper limb joints, a powered indoor chair should be con-

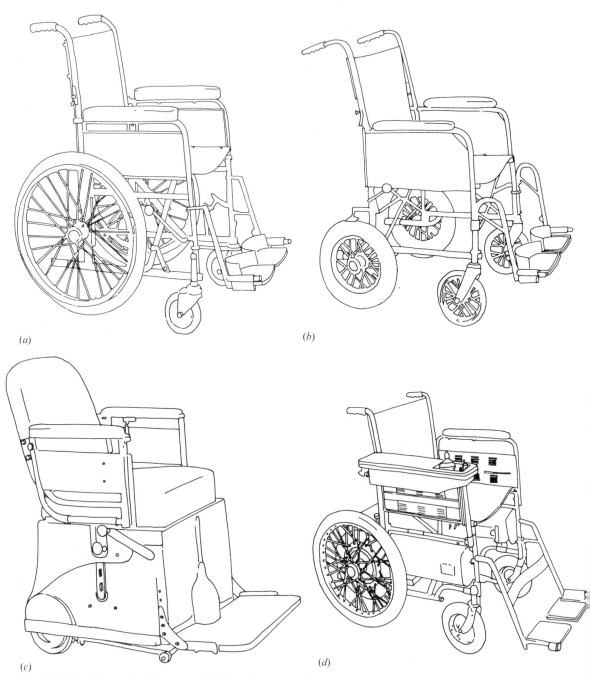

(a)

(b)

(c)

(d)

Fig. 10.27 Wheelchairs. (*a*) Lightweight, foldable self-propelling chair (DHSS 8L or 8BL pattern). (*b*) Lightweight, foldable, 'transit' chair (DHSS 9L or 9LR (with foldable back) pattern). (*c*) Standard, electrically powered chair for indoor use (DHSS EPIC Mk II). (*d*) Standard Powerdrive electrically propelled chair for outdoor use.

sidered as soon as possible in order to prevent further damage of these joints due to the work involved in operating a self-propelled wheelchair. Furthermore, although most wheelchair users propel themselves with their hands on the wheels, two sticks can be used to 'punt' the chair along, or the patient can 'walk' the chair. Such modes of propulsion can also be applied to an ordinary chair on four small universal castors.

In supplying a patient with a wheelchair a detailed functional assessment should be carried out. Factors to be considered in selecting an appropriate chair include its size, cushioning, brakes, footrests and armrests and whether additional features such as trays or head rest extensions are needed.

Most wheelchairs are supplied for use out of doors in association with transfers into a car, and are used primarily for attendants to push outside the house. The design criteria are therefore quite different for a wheelchair required for active functional use within the home. Often architectural and geographical limitations determine the choice of wheelchair. These constraints (e.g. narrow doorways and corridors, awkward access to bathroom or toilet) may enforce the patient to accept a wheelchair that is less than optimal for their disability.

A wheelchair restricts the ability to reach and to obtain access. Steps become a total barrier and doorways are often unnegotiable. Further obstacles are provided by restricted turning areas and lines of approach rather than doorway width.

In general, it is likely that the most useful wheelchair will be a standard lightweight 'transit' chair (in the UK these are the DHSS Model 9L or 9LR, the latter having a folding back). These wheelchairs (Fig. 10.27) are light and designed to enable the patient to be pushed out of doors. The 'paddling' or 'punting' technique referred to earlier can be applied to these chairs.

A small, lightweight self-propelling wheelchair (8BL) (Fig. 10.27) is often the most suitable indoor chair for housewives. Its smaller size and turning circle make it useful for use in a limited space, compared with the standard-size lightweight wheelchair (8L).

There is increasing use of electrically powered indoor and outdoor wheelchairs (Fig. 10.27) for severely disabled arthritic patients. Here, too, there are many different designs and practical tests are important to enable selection of the right chair for the right patient.

In the UK, electrically powered wheelchairs are provided through the Department of Health and Social Security for those patients who, although requiring a wheelchair, are not medically fit enough to propel themselves.

The variety of control devices for these chairs should enable even the most severely arthritic patient to be provided with an electrically powered chair.

Although a powered chair may be medically indicated, whether it will fit into the patient's home, be of real value, and be accepted by the patient is another matter. As with the prescription of many other aids and appliances, the best solution is a practical trial, preferably in the environment in which the chair will be used.

For the more severely disabled rheumatoid, especially those with cervical myelopathy, or for those with severely involved upper limbs as well as lower limbs, a powered indoor wheelchair can often bring a remarkable degree of freedom, and, in the most severely disabled, may enable him to remain at home rather than be admitted to an institution.

For further details see Goodwill (1977) and Nichols and Wilshere (1977).

(c) Transferring

This is an important aspect of independence. Provided that bed, chair and toilet are stable and of the correct height, many patients will be able to transfer by themselves, or with minimal assistance. Those requiring help when rising from a chair may find an 'ejector' seat helpful.

For those unable to stand, a polished hardwood sliding board or a hoist can be used. The hoist will usually be attendant-controlled. The type prescribed will depend mainly on the domestic environment in which it is to be used. Thus, it may be a portable hydraulic model, a fixed electric model, or an electric hoist running on a gantry or ceiling-mounted track. Whichever model is employed it is essential that the most suitable arrangement of slings is used.

(d) Hoists and other transferring methods

When the patient is so disabled as to require lifting into a wheelchair, on to the toilet, or into the bath, problems can arise for both patient and helper. If inadequately supported the patient may fall, and if the patient is heavy her helper may develop backache. A hoist can be of great value providing that both it and its sling are the most appropriate for both patient and helper, and that those who are to use it are adequately trained in its use.

Hoists may be of the following types:

1. *Overhead hoists* which are fixed to the ceiling joists or mounted on a free-standing gantry (Fig. 10.28). The lifting device may be operated electrically or manually. Running on a fixed track, their use and positioning are limited. However, with careful track positioning (i.e. bedroom to bathroom) they can be used for a number of daily living activities.

2. *Mechanical and hydraulically operated hoists* which are mobile and so can function in different places. A wide base to provide stability is essential for this type of hoist. The architectural features of many houses

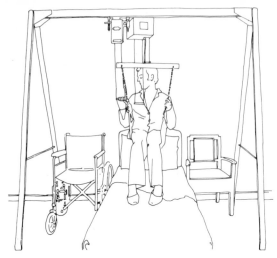

Fig. 10.28 Overhead hoist mounted on a free-standing gantry.

and the design of household fittings may not allow use of such a hoist in which case an overhead hoist would be more appropriate.

3. *Bath hoists* are operated by water pressure. Alternatively, they may be standard hoists fixed and adapted to help people in and out of an adjacent bath. Should an electric hoist be used as an aid to bathing it is necessary to install a low-voltage motor with appropriate step-down transformer and remote switches. This must be carried out by a qualified electrician.

4. *Car hoists* are available which can be fitted inside a car or on the roof. They can be operated from the car's electrical system or manually.

Most hoist users only use a hoist for getting in and out of bed. If a mobile hoist is provided, its mobility is rarely used, often from lack of space, inappropriate floor covering and awkward corners, doors and steps. In general, it is probably better to supply a hoist mounted on a gantry or fixed to the ceiling in a bedroom. This will enable the helper to get the patient in and out of bed or on and off the commode. A second track or gantry can be fixed to the ceiling in another room and the hoist easily transferred.

(e) *Outdoor transport*

For many years the Department of Health and Social Security provided an invalid tricyle (a powered three-wheeler), then it introduced the additional provision of specially adapted motorcars for disabled patients in certain categories. Now the standard provision is the Mobility Allowance and the invalid tricycle is being phased out. However, although no longer available to new applicants, current users and certain other categories will continue to be eligible for these vehicles.

In order to be eligible for a Mobility Allowance (which was increased from November 1981 to a weekly payment of £16.50) the disabled person must fall within the prescribed age limit (5–60 for women, 5–65 for men). The applicant must be unable, or virtually unable, to walk, and this inability must be likely to persist for at least 12 months, and must be such that use can be made of the allowance (i.e. the patient is able to be moved about). Eligibility is decided by an independent statutory authority after a medical examination. The allowance is intended to be spent on outdoor transport and may be used to pay for taxis, to hire a car or other vehicle, to provide holiday transport, to buy a vehicle or to pay for its adaptation (Fig. 10.29). The allowance is taxable, but is paid in addition to other social security benefits.

Recently, a further benefit – Motability – has been introduced to facilitate car purchase by patients in possession of a Mobility Allowance. The Royal Association for Disability and Rehabilitation (RADAR) is involved in assisting disabled people to solve their mobility problems and further details are available from the Disablement Research Branch of the Department of Health and Social Security.

Through the orange-badge scheme a disabled driver can obtain a car sticker from the local social services

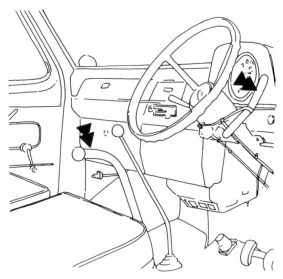

Fig. 10.29 Motor-car adaptations ('Reselco' conversion): right arrow indicates clutch and accelerator below rim of steering wheel (control is by movement towards driver): left arrow indicates brake lever (which may be detachable to allow the driver to slide from passenger to driving seat).

Table 10.1 Allowances, concessions and exemptions available to disabled people (after Roberts, 1981)

Type of benefit	Nature of benefit
Allowance	Mobility
	Travel to work
Concession	Car purchase (Motability scheme)
	Car parking
Exemption	Road tax on private cars
	Value added tax on car adaptations
	Rates on a garage

department. It entitles parking in allocated bays and on single yellow lines.

The above benefits to disabled people and other allowances, concessions, and exemptions are summarized in Table 10.1.

10.10.3 Household activities

(a) The kitchen

Work surfaces should be level and of the correct height for the patient. Activities should be planned in such a way that they can be carried out from a comfortable chair or stool of the appropriate height. Foodstuffs and cooking utensils must be easy to reach, and cupboards and drawers must have opening devices that the patient can manipulate easily.

Partly prepared foods may be of additional help to the disabled housewife, if she can open the containers. For patients wishing to prepare food in the traditional way there are many gadgets available to assist her in this.

To save the patient from lifting or carrying heavy saucepans all the working surfaces should be at the same level. Pans can then be slid to and from the stove, working surface and sink. Split-level ovens used in conjunction with a trolley of the same height will allow cooked food to be transferred without lifting.

Difficulty with water taps can be remedied by means of lever-type handles or simple tap turners.

Electricity power points in the kitchen and in the rest of the house should be fitted at the optimal height for the disabled user. Easy-to-grip plugs are readily available.

(b) Household cleaning

The more strenuous jobs will often need to be done by an able-bodied helper but lightweight long-handled brushes, mops and vacuum cleaners can often be managed by the disabled. Similarly, aerosol sprays can facilitate polishing.

A front- or top-loading washing machine may be helpful and which type is chosen will depend upon the patient's disability. Clothes are best dried on a rotary clothes line which can be adjusted in height.

Ironing can be simplified by adjusting the board to the correct height and by selecting an iron that is not too heavy.

(c) Shopping

Many patients will rely on mail-order catalogues for their clothing and furnishing requirements. Day-to-day necessities can usually be delivered by local tradesmen or brought by relatives, friends or neighbours. Those able to go to the shops may find a basket on wheels a great advantage.

Apart from advice given by medical and remedial staff patients may glean further useful information from handbooks such as *Your Home and Your Rheumatism*, published by the Arthritis and Rheumatism Council.

10.10.4 Communication and leisure activities

Social isolation among the disabled is all too common, and if the ability to communicate can be improved the patient is likely to become less dependent. Further, the ability to enjoy leisure activities will increase and the patient may be able to regain remunerative employment.

(a) Writing

For patients with a weak grip a pencil of large diameter, or a simple elastic or leather finger splint may make writing feasible. Patients with no digital power but with

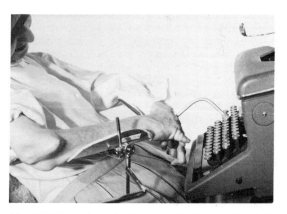

Fig. 10.30 Severely disabled patient with rheumatoid arthritis operating a manual typewriter with the help of arm rests fitted to the wheelchair and a hand-held appliance.

good wrist extension may be helped to write with a flexor hinge splint.

Typing may be found easier than writing. For the severely disabled a manual typewriter may be operated using simple adaptations and aids (Fig. 10.30), and an electric typewriter may be operated with minimal effort with a mouth-stick. A patient with such a degree of disability may be considered for the provision of a POSSUM (Patient Operated Selector Mechanism) System. This will allow remote control of up to 11 electrically operated appliances such as lights, television, curtains and front door lock.

(b) Reading

Bookrests, either free-standing or suitable for fitting to a chair, can be a great assistance, not only in rheumatoid patients but also in those with ankylosing spondylitis. Devices to help the patient to turn over the page include: (1) a stationer's rubber thimble; (2) a paper clip attached to each page enabling the patient to turn the page with a magnetic stick.

Patients with severe flexion deformity of the spine due to ankylosing spondylitis may be helped to read by using prismatic spectacles.

For those unable to read, prerecorded 'talking books' can be useful.

(c) Telephone, alarm and control systems

As well as a means of social contact and of summoning help in emergency, the telephone will, for some, provide an opportunity to become wage earning. Difficulties in dialling may be resolved either by a suitable stick or a push-button instrument. Inability to control the handpiece adequately can be rectified by a telephonist's head set or a commercially available receiver rest.

Other alarm systems have been designed, ranging from simple battery-operated signs displayed in a prominent window, through buzzers and bells, to complex habit cycles based on fixed activities (e.g. flushing the toilet).

However, the most satisfactory safeguard is the availability and co-operation of a neighbour or relative who can arrange to be telephoned at fixed intervals, have an alarm wired to their home, or be requested to visit frequently.

(d) Gardening

Much work has been done in recent years to bring this hobby within the ambit of even the severely disabled. Most patients have access to a garden or window box, and raised beds and simple modifications to readily available tools may lead to an interesting, satisfying and therapeutically beneficial hobby.

Your Garden and Your Rheumatism (Arthritis and Rheumatism Council) will be found invaluable to patients wishing to pursue their hobby in the face of disability.

(e) Vacation

With some planning and assistance it should be possible for the disabled person to enjoy a holiday away from home. For example, if mounting stairs is a difficulty, ground-floor accommodation can be sought with enquiry about obstacles such as steps leading to the front door. Blocks (or even improvised blocks such as telephone directories) can be carried with the luggage to overcome occasional steps. Entering and leaving the car can be eased by using a plastic sheet on which the patient can slide with straight legs onto the back seat. Simple expedients such as removing the glove compartment shelf can provide extra space in the passenger seat for patients with stiff straight legs.

10.10.5 Disabled mothers

Disabled mothers have doubts and uncertainties additional to those experienced by able-bodied mothers. However, physical disability need not necessarily create an obstacle to being a good mother. Indeed, the mother's reduced mobility can give the child an added sense of security through her always being there when needed.

Appendix 10.15.1 shows some methods and equipment that have been found useful to disabled mothers in various circumstances.

Within the broad compass of 'disabled mothers' might be included factors other than those strictly to do with the physical business of child rearing, such as menstruation, sexual intercourse, pregnancy and the puerperium. Some of these problems are discussed in *Marriage, Sex and Arthritis*, a handbook for patients published by the Arthritis and Rheumatism Council.

10.11 EMPLOYMENT AND TRAINING SERVICES AND THE DISABLEMENT RESETTLEMENT OFFICER (DRO)

10.11.1 Introductory comment

In 1973 Parliament passed the Employment and Training Act by which responsibility for the country's manpower services was transferred during 1974 from the Department of Employment to a public authority, the Manpower Services Commission (MSC).

The Commission has two basic tasks: (1) to help people find satisfactory jobs; (2) to help employers find suitable workers.

The Commission has a budget largely provided by the Government, and formulates its policies in conjunction with the Secretary of State for Employment. It is responsible for putting such policies into effect through its two executive agencies: the Employment Services Agency (ESA) and the Training Services Agency (TSA).

10.11.2 The Employment Service Agency (ESA)

The ESA is now responsible for over 1000 employment offices. These offices ('labour exchanges') were formerly run by the Department of Employment.

The payment of unemployment benefit is no longer the responsibility of the employment offices, many of which will be upgraded, redesigned and relocated in city centres as 'job centres'. Integration of the employment service is being facilitated by computers which store information about jobs and workers and by methods developed to circulate information rapidly through regional and area networks. Staff, which include DROs, are specially trained in interviewing and in occupational guidance.

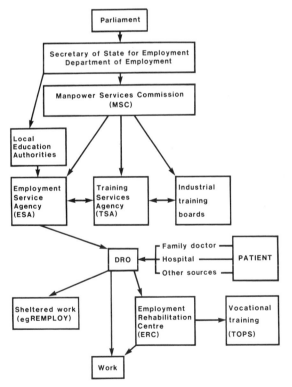

Fig. 10.31 Diagram showing central role of DRO in the rehabilitation programme (after Mattingley, 1977).

10.11.3 The new DRO service

The DRO's main function is to place disabled people in suitable work, if necessary after industrial rehabilitation or vocational training. It is essential, therefore, that he has a sound knowledge of local industry, employers and employment opportunities. He must interview individual patients in hospital, employment office or job centre, interpret medical guidance and arrange visits to employers. He must also liaise with hospital staff, general practitioners, local authorities and voluntary organizations, and establish good relations with union officials. When indicated, he will refer the patient for work assessment at an employment rehabilitation centre or make arrangements for vocational training. His central role in the rehabilitation programme is shown in Fig. 10.31.

Most DROs work from employment offices or job centres but some are based in district hospitals. Although still an experimental service, it has been shown that hospital DROs provide an effective link between medical and employment services. In-patients and out-patients can be referred to them by consultants and junior hospital doctors, nurses, social workers and remedial therapists. The hospital DRO is therefore able to initiate re-settlement at an early stage in recovery from illness, injury or surgery. He is often able to save a man's job by contacting his employer, or arrange early admission to an employment rehabilitation centre.

10.11.4 Industrial rehabilitation and the Employment Rehabilitation Centre (ERC)

The ESA is now responsible for running the 26 Employment Rehabilitation Centres (ERCs) formerly run by the Department of Employment as industrial rehabilitation units. Most are non-residential and situated in the grounds of skill centres on industrial estates in the larger towns and cities. Residential centres are available for those having difficulty in travelling. These either provide their own accommodation on the premises (Egham, Surrey), or provide lodgings or hostel accommodation (e.g. units at Coventry, Edinburgh, Garston Manor and Leicester).

An ERC is run on factory lines and is aimed at conditioning people to return to work after long unemployment because of sickness or injury. It also provides vocational guidance. The DRO is responsible for arranging admission, which, because of demand, may be delayed for several weeks.

Each rehabilitee's progress during the course (usually about 8 weeks) is reviewed at regular case-conferences, and at the end of the course a final recommendation on work or training is sent to the DRO at his local employment office for action.

The ERC does not train people for skilled jobs but will assess their suitability for training elsewhere. About 25% are in fact recommended for vocational training.

About 14 000 people pass through ERCs each year and prospects for re-employment are relatively good.

10.11.5 Vocational training and the Training Opportunities Scheme (TOPS)

Training for work is essential in any modern industrial economy and every year some 2 million people in the UK are involved in some form of systematic training. Half a million of these are released from their work for further education. In the past the bulk of industrial training was carried out by individual employers. In 1964, under the Industrial Training Act, the Government set up industrial training boards to co-ordinate that training, and by 1972 they were responsible for some 15 million workers.

This was still thought to be inadequate, and in 1972 the Department of Employment introduced the Training Opportunities Scheme (TOPS), with the aim, eventually, of providing vocational training for 100 000 people a year.

TOPS offers training not only for the unemployed, ex-servicemen and disabled workers (only a small proportion in TOPS are disabled), but also for those still in employment, subject to certain conditions such as suitability, intentions and previous education. Even housewives can apply for training if they wish to return to work. The Government pays the cost of training (more than 50 trades are taught) as well as tax-free allowances to trainees.

In addition to the skilled trades taught at government training centres (now called 'skill centres'*), limited skill training is available in engineering trades, electronics, road transport, catering and domestic heating as well as in clerical and commercial work. As with the more skilled trades, some of these trades may not be suitable for disabled people. Such courses must last a minimum of 4 weeks and not more than a year; they must be full-time and strictly vocational (i.e. the trainee is expected to go directly into employment). Details about these courses can be obtained from any job centre or employment office.

10.11.6 The Training Services Agency (TSA)

In April 1974 the Training Services Agency (TSA) assumed responsibility for co-ordinating the work of the industrial training boards and took over training ser-

---

* It is important to appreciate that TOPS training is no longer confined to skill centres and may be extended to colleges of further education and approved employers' establishments.

vices previously run by the Department of Employment. These included those provided for individuals wishing to acquire new skills, and also those available to companies for the training of instructors, supervisors and expert office staff.

10.11.7 Sheltered work

If a patient is no longer fit to work in open industry, the DRO may find him a job in a workshop run by REMPLOY or by local authorities. At present, less than 15 000 people are employed in the UK in sheltered work. The goods manufactured by REMPLOY are sold in the open market and comprise mainly furniture and luggage.

(For further details see Mattingley, 1977.)

10.12 VOLUNTARY ORGANIZATIONS

There are at least 300 voluntary bodies in the UK which deal in some way with disabled people. These organizations may be divided broadly into seven main groups. These are listed in Appendix 10.15.2 which also gives examples of specific organizations.

As far as the rheumatic patient is concerned, organizations in the UK particularly devoted to this group of diseases include the Arthritis and Rheumatism Council (ARC) and the British Rheumatism Association (BRA). The former concentrates on research funding and the education of patients and doctors, the latter more on the social aspects of the rheumatic patient, including the arrangement of holidays and social functions.

Particularly disabled patients with arthritis will also find help within organizations concerned with disability generally, both rheumatic and non-rheumatic (e.g. The Disabled Living Foundation).

10.13 SUMMARY AND CONCLUSION

The basis of good rehabilitation rests on good medicine. This includes accurate diagnosis, careful prognosis, and early, appropriate and adequate definitive care. Thereafter, in addition to the supportive role of family, friends and voluntary organizations, successful rehabilitation depends on the integrated skills of several disciplines including: physiotherapy; occupational therapy; nursing; orthotics; industrial rehabilitation; and the various aspects of the social services.

There is a need in every hospital for one consultant to be responsible for co-ordinating these services, and there is still not full agreement as to which specialty this responsibility should fall. At present, the consultant is often a rheumatologist and his role will be largely supervisory. However, in other instances, particularly where the rehabilitation service plays a large part in the hospital activities, the consultant may have rehabilitation as his special interest.

10.14 REFERENCES AND FURTHER READING

Introductory comment

Jayson, M.I.V. (1980) Viewpoint: the scope of rheumatology. *Ann. Rheum. Dis.*, **39**, 528.

Nichols, P.J.R. (1978) in *Copeman's Textbook of the Rheumatic Diseases* (ed. J.T. Scott), 5th edn, Churchill Livingstone, Edinburgh, p. 491.

Piercy, Lord (1956) *Report of the Committee of Inquiry on the Rehabilitation, Training and Resettlement of Disabled Persons*, Ministry of Labour, HMSO Cmnd 9883, London.

Organization and principles of rehabilitation services

Duthie, J.J.R. (1967) Medical management and prognosis in rheumatoid arthritis. *Scot. Med. J.*, **12**, 96.

Mattingley, S. (1968) Garston Manor: an experiment in rehabilitation. *Br. Med. J.*, **iii**, 46.

Occupational therapy

Goble, R.E.A. (1967) The role of the occupational therapist in disabled living research. *Am. J. Occup. Ther.*, **23**, 145.

Macdonald, E.M. (ed.) (1976) *Occupational Therapy in Rehabilitation*, 4th edn, Bailliére Tindall, London.

Mountford, S.W. (1965) *Towards Rehabilitation: A Study of Widening Horizons*, Churchill Livingstone, Edinburgh.

Mountford, S.W. (1971) *Introduction to Occupational Therapy*, Churchill Livingstone, Edinburgh.

Nichols, P.J.R. (1980) in *Rehabilitation Medicine*, (ed. P.J.R. Nichols), 2nd edn, Butterworths, London, pp. 32–49.

White, A.S. (1972) *Easy Path to Gardening*, Reader's Digest, London.

Physiotherapy

Bierman, W. (1954) Ultrasound in the treatment of scars. *Arch. Phys. Med. Rehabil.*, **35**, 210.

Bolton, E. and Goodwin, D. (1967) *Introduction to Pool Exercises*, 3rd edn, Churchill Livingstone, Edinburgh.

British Association of Physical Medicine (1966) Pain in the neck and arm: a multicentre trial of the effect of physiotherapy. *Br. Med. J.*, **i**, 253.

Cyriax, J.H. (1971) *Textbook of Orthopaedic Medicine*, Vols 1 and 2, 5th edn, Baillière Tindall and Cassell, London.

Davis, B.C. (1967) A technique of rehabilitation in the treatment pool. *Physiotherapy*, **53**, 57.

De Andrade, J.R., Grant, C. and Dixon, A. St. J. (1965) Joint distension and reflex muscle inhibition. *J. Bone Joint Surg.*, **47A**, 313.

Duffield, M.H.T. (1969) *Exercise and Water*, Baillière Tindall and Cassell, London.

Dyson, M. and Pond, J.M. (1970) Effect of pulsed ultrasound on tissue regeneration. *Physiotherapy*, **56**, 136.

Dyson, M. and Pond, J.M. (1973) The effects of ultrasound in the circulation, *Physiotherapy*, **59**, 284.

Gough, J.V. and Hadley, G. (1971) An investigation into the effectiveness of various forms of quadriceps exercise. *Physiotherapy*, **57**, 356.

Leach, R.E., Skyker, W.S. and Zohn, D.A. (1965) A comparative study of isometric and isotonic quadriceps exercise programmes. *J. Bone Joint Surg.*, **47A**, 1421.

Lister, M.J. (ed.) (1979) *Transcutaneous Electrical Nerve Stimulation*, American Physical Therapy Association, Washington.

Maitland, G.D. (1964) *Vertebral Manipulation*, Butterworths, London.

Maitland, G.D. (1970) *Peripheral Manipulation*, Butterworths, London.

Matthews, J.A. (1968) Dynamic discography. A study of lumbar traction. *Ann. Phys. Med.*, **9**, 275.

Nichols, P.J.R. and Howell, B. (1968) Routine pre- and post-operative physiotherapy: results of a questionnaire. *Ann. Phys. Med.*, **9**, 264.

Nichols, P.J.R. (1980) in *Rehabilitation Medicine* (ed. P.J.R. Nichols), 2nd edn, Butterworths, London, pp. 11–31.

Powell, M. (1970) *Orthopaedic Nursing*, 6th edn, Churchill Livingstone, London.

Salter, N. (1967) Exercise therapy. *Ann. Phys. Med.*, **4**, 81.

Stoddard, A. (1959) *Manual of Osteopathic Techniques*, Hutchinson, London.

Summer, W. and Patrick, M.K. (1964) *Ultrasonic Therapy*, Elsevier, Amsterdam.

Yates, D.A.H. (1972) Indications and contraindications for spinal traction, *Physiotherapy*, **58**, 2, 55.

Nursing

Bowden, S.A. (1976) New surgery for arthritic hands. *Nursing*, **6**, 8.

Brassell, M.P., Rossky, E., Schaal, F. and Spergel, P. (1972) Helping patients adjust to arthritis. *Nursing*, **10**, 11.

Brassell, M.P. (1977) in *Rheumatic Diseases, Diagnosis and Management*, Lippincott, Philadelphia, p. 1000.

Elliott, M. (1979) *Nursing Rheumatic Disease*, Churchill Livingstone, Edinburgh.

Firth, D., Roberts, M., Wright, J.G. *et al.* (1973) The value of health visitors in a rehabilitation unit. *Rheumatol. Rehabil.*, **12**, 143.

Hastings, J.B. (1973) Nurses play many vital roles. *Nursing*, **3**, 7.

Kerr, A. (1969) *Orthopedic Nursing Procedures*, Springer–Verlag, New York.

Larson, C. B. and Gould, M. (1974) *Orthopedic Nursing*, 8th edn, C. V. Mosby, St. Louis.

Olson, E. and Johnson, B.J. (1967) Hazards of immobility. *Am. J. Nurs.*, **67**, 781.

Pigg, J. (1974) Fifty helpful hints for active arthritis patients. *Nursing*, **4**, 40.

Vignos, P.J. (1973) in *Total Management of the Arthritic Patient*, Lippincott, Philadelphia, p. 117.

Walker, K.A. (1971) in *Pressure Sores. Prevention and Treatment* (ed. W.E. Broome), Nursing in Depth Series, Butterworths, London.

Wright, V., Haslock, I. and Champney, B. (1977) in *Rheumatism for Nurses and Remedial Therapists*, Heinemann, London.

Chiropody

Bunting, E.G.V. (1928) *Practical Chiropody*, 3rd edn, Faber and Gwyer, London.

Jayson, M.I.V. and Dixon, A. St. J. (1974) in *Rheumatism and Arthritis*, Pan, London, p. 227.

Social work

Broome, M. and McMullan, J.J. (1977) in *Rehabilitation Today* (ed. S. Mattingley), Update, London, p. 33.

Orthotics

Aids and Splintmaking – Catalogue (1978) Handicraft Ltd., Nottingham.

Aids and Splintmaking – Catalogue (1979) Handicraft Ltd., Nottingham.

Bennett, R.L. (1965) Orthotic devices to prevent deformities of the hand in rheumatoid arthritis. *Arthr. Rheum.*, **8**, 1006.

Bennett, R.L. (1969) in *Arthritis and Physical Medicine* (ed. S. Licht), Waverly Press, Baltimore, p. 482.

British Medical Association Planning Unit No. 2 (1968) *Report of the Working Party on Aids for the Disabled*, British Medical Association, London.

Campbell, J.W. and Inman, V.T. (1974) Treatment of plantar fasciitis and calcaneal spurs with the UC-BL shoe insert. *Clin. Orthop.*, **103**, 57.

Cervical and Spinal Orthoses – Catalogue (Undated), S.H. Camp Co. Ltd., Andover.

Deaver, G.G. (1966) in *Orthotics Etcetera* (eds S. Licht and H. Kamenetz), E. Licht, New Haven, pp. 249, 266.

Futuro Adjustable Wrist Brace – Leaflet (Undated), Ling Products, Inc., Cincinnati, Ohio.

Harris, R. (1966) in *Orthotics Etcetcera* (eds S. Licht and H. Kamenetz), E. Licht, New Haven, p. 336.

Hinders–Leslie Met–Brace – Appliance instructions (Undated), Hinders–Leslie Ltd., London.

Lehmann, J.F. and Warren, C.G. (1976) Restraining forces in various designs of knee ankle orthoses: their placement and effect on the anatomical knee joint. *Arch. Phys. Med. Rehabil.*, **57**, 430.

Lehneis, H.R., Bergofsky, E. and Frisina, W. (1976) Energy expenditure with advanced lower limb orthoses and with conventional braces. *Arch. Phys. Med. Rehabil.*, **57**, 20.

Long, C. (1966) in *Orthotics Etcetera* (eds S. Licht and H. Kamenetz), E. Licht, New Haven, p. 152.

Malick, M.H. (1972) *Manual on Static Hand Splinting*. Harmarville Rehabilitation Centre, Pittsburgh.

Malick, M.H. (1974) *Manual on Dynamic Hand Splinting with Thermoplastic Materials*. Harmarville Rehabilitation Centre, Pittsburgh.

Nichols, P. (1973) *Living with a Handicap*, Priory Press, London.

Nichols, P.J.R. and Mowat, A.G. (1971) Splints, walking aids and appliances for the arthritic patient. *Reports on the Rheumatic Diseases*, Arthritis and Rheumatism Council, London, p. 158.

Nichols, P.J.R. and Mowat, A.G. (1972) Splints, walking aids and appliances for the arthritic patient, *Rep. Rheum. Dis.*, No. 48, Arthritis and Rheumatism Council, London.

Nichols, P.J.R. and Williams, E. (1977) in *Rehabilitation Today* (ed. S. Mattingley), Update, London, p. 74.

Norton, P.L. and Brown, T. (1957) The immobilizing efficiency of back braces. *J. Bone Joint Surg.*, **39A**, 111.

Orthopaedic Catalogue (Undated) The Medical Supply Association Limited, Dundee.

Orthotic Appliances Illustrated Supplement (1974) Department of Health and Social Security, London.

Prenyl – Leaflet (undated) Ortho Industries Inc., New Rochelle, New York.

Roaf, R. and Hodkinson, L.J. (1971) *Textbook of Orthopaedic Nursing*, Blackwell, Oxford.

Rizzo, F., Hamilton, B.B. and Keagy, R.D. (1975) Orthotics research evaluation framework. *Arch. Phys. Med. Rehabil.*, **56**, 304.

Rotstein, J. (1965) Use of splints in conservation management of acutely inflamed joints in rheumatoid arthritis. *Arch. Phys. Med.*, **46**, 198.

Schuco First Aid Air Splints – Appliance instructions (undated), American Caduceus Industries, Inc., Williston Parky, New York.

Standard Supports – Catalogue (undated), Spencer Ltd., Banbury.

Stewart, J.D.M. (1975) *Traction and Orthopaedic Appliances*, Churchill Livingstone, Edinburgh.

Swezey, R.L. (1975) Below-knee weight-bearing brace for the arthritic foot. *Arch. Phys. Med. Rehabil.*, **56**, 176.

Swezey, R.L. (1978) in *Arthritis: Rational Therapy and Rehabilitation*, Saunders, Philadelphia, p. 103.

Zamosky, I. and Licht, S. (1966) in *Orthotics Etcetera* (eds S. Licht and H. Kamenetz), E. Licht, New Haven, p. 403.

Equipment to assist function

Cuniffe, T. (1974) *The application of cryonomics to the design of wheelchairs*, Thesis submitted to Loughborough University of Technology.

Goodwill, C.J. (1977) in *Rehabilitation Today* (ed. S. Mattingley), Update, London, p. 82.

Hawker, M.B. (1974) Wheelchair. *Mod. Geriatr.*, **4**, 503.

Hollings, E.M. and McCay, G. (1966) Adaptations to wheelchairs. *Physiotherapy*, **52**, 151.

Kamenetz, H.L. (1969) *The Wheelchair Book*, Thomas, Springfield, Illinois.

McCay, G., Hollings, E.M. and Nichols, P.J.R. (1969) Problems of living on wheels: a synopsis. *Physiotherapy*, **55**, 447.

Mowat, A.G. and Nichols, P.J.R. (1975) Aids and appliances for the disabled. *Medicine*, 2nd Ser., No. 16, part 2, 760.

Nichols, P.J.R. and Wilshere, E.R. (1977) *Equipment for the Disabled: Wheelchairs*, 4th edn, Oxford Regional Health Authority.

Nichols, P.J.R. (1978) in *Copeman's Textbook of the Rheumatic Diseases* (ed. J.T. Scott), Churchill Livingstone, Edinburgh, p. 501.

Roberts, G.S. (1981) Helping disabled people with travelling costs. *Br. Med. J.*, **283**, 480.

Sperryn, P.N. (1974) Two years in a wheelchair clinic. *Rheumatol. Rehabil.*, **13**, 184.

Walking Aids and Rehabilitation Equipment (1979) Remploy, London.

White, A.S. (1972) *The Easy Path to Gardening*, Reader's Digest, London.

Wilshere, E.R., Hollings, E.M., Nichols, P.J.R. and Rostance, B.H. (eds) (1973) *Equipment for the Disabled: No. 4. Disabled Mothers*, National Fund for Research into Crippling Diseases, Horsham.

Wilshere, E.R., Hollings, E.M. and Nichols, P.J.R. (eds) (1974) *Equipment for the Disabled: No. 8. Hoists, Walking Aids*, National Fund for Research into Crippling Diseases, Horsham.

Winyard, G.P., Luker, C. and Nichols, P.J.R. (1976) The uses and usefulness of electrically powered indoor chairs. *Rheumatol. Rehabil.*, **15**, 254.

Employment and Training Services and the DRO

Mattingley, S. (1977) in *Rehabilitation Today* (ed. S. Mattingley), Update, London, p. 42.

Voluntary Organizations

Sommerville, J.G. (1977) in *Rehabilitation Today* (ed. S. Mattingley) Update, London, p. 36.

10.15 APPENDICES

10.15.1 Some problem-solving suggestions for disabled mothers (from Wilshere *et al.*, 1973–abbreviated.)

Activity	Disability	Suggestion
Lifting: general points	All disabilities	(1) Have table, cot, chair, bath at the same height. Collect all necessary equipment beforehand. (2) Utilize the natural instinct of a baby to cling to the mother and to clamber up. (3) During the day the child should be as free of clothing as possible so that his arms are not hampered in their efforts to hold and cling. Many babies adapt to the parental method of handling.
Feeding	Wheelchair user	(1) Use screw-on teats. (2) Prepare one feed at a time. Keep all requisites, feed, electric kettle, bottle in Milton (or equivalent) ready in one place so that there is no need to move wheelchair and dirty the hands. Wash hands in Phisohex before preparation. (3) 24 hours' food can be made at a time and kept in the fridge if preferred.
Bathing from standing position	Limited movement of all joints	(1) Arrange tea-trolley and pram by sink to make three sides of a square, mother being on the fourth side. Soap baby on trolley, rinse in sink, lift on to draining board to dry, powder, etc., thence to pram. (2) Sink can still be used for a child up to 4 to 5 years on occasions. Or have bath on a chair or table, fill from saucepan or jug, soap baby in chair or on the table first, rinse in bath and dry.
Bathing from sitting position	Wheelchair user with weakness of upper limbs	(1) Blanket bath baby using table, chair, bed or trolley padded with blankets, protected by plastic sheeting with towelling on top, or use Top-'n'-Tail mattress. (2) Keep trolley or bag to hold all requirements close by. (3) Use baby bath on trolley, chair or table at correct height. It is probably easier to have chair sideways on. (4) Bath may be filled from bucket or smaller container, or by hose on the tap. When preparing bath, allow for water cooling while equipment is being collected and baby undressed. (5) Make a stand or trolley specially to take a baby bath with a drainage hole in it, and have a bucket underneath for easy emptying.
Dressing: choice of clothing	Poor hand function	(1) Avoid ribbons, small buttons, open-ended zips. Use big buttons and toggles. Use stretch-type all-in-one garments with press fasteners. (2) If child is to be lifted by the clothes make sure that fasteners are strong enough to take the strain. If necessary replace by hooks and eyes. (3) Use woollen nighties which open out flat. (4) Teach the child to dress himself early. (5) Use envelope-neck vests and pullovers. (6) Avoid nylon dresses because they are slippery. (7) When crawling use dungarees with press fasteners on inner leg seam.

10.15.1 Appendix (*Contd.*)

Activity	Disability	Suggestion
Nappy changing: General points	All disabilities	(1) Change on Top-'n'-Tail mattress on table, trolley, convenient height chair with closed-in arms, or on the lap wearing a plastic apron with a towel over it. Or change nappy in pram for safety. (2) Cover mattress with a waterproof fitted cover and use a plastic sheet under a draw-sheet on the bed. (3) Use an apron with a divided pocket, one side lined with waterproof material or containing a polythene bag, to take wet nappies, dirty cotton wool, etc.
Nappy changing: Fastening	Poor hand function	(1) Avoid fastenings; use plastic pants with a disposable nappy inside terry pants. (2) Sew Velcro on fitted nappies. (3) Tie ends of nappy in knot. This will hold under plastic pants. (4) Pin one side of nappy first, then slip baby's leg in, pull nappy up and pin other side. (5) Use plastic pants which open out flat and are fastened by press fasteners.
Potty training: supporting child on potty	Wheelchair user	(1) Use firm-based potty on a chair, on the lap, or on the floor. (2) Put potty in pram and prop up the child with cushions. (3) A trainer seat over the lavatory is usually at a convenient height for a wheelchair mother to hold steady if there is enough room for her chair by the lavatory.
Pram	Ambulant user	(1) Have heavy pram, fairly high, which will not tip. (2) Baby should be strapped in at all times.
	Wheelchair user	(1) To let pram into garden, tie rope or strap round axle and pay it out allowing pram to run down ramp. It can be pulled back to give baby attention from time to time. (2) Baby should be strapped in at all times.
Crawling	Wheelchair user	(1) A playpen may be helpful; one with a gate allows easy access. A floor in the pen raises the baby but makes the playpen heavy, and it may take up too much space for a wheelchair mother.
Toddling	Wheelchair user	(1) When child able to toddle a rein can be used, longer in safer areas, shorter on pavement or in shops. The child can climb back onto mother's lap and its harness can be clipped to her chair again when the child is tired. (2) The child can push a baby walker while fastened by rein to mother's chair. (3) A child may safely be left on a swing if a harness is used and clipped on to it.
Games and play activities	All disabilities with mobility problems	(1) Mother can share in many games and play-interests with children including Lego, playing records and 'Play School'. Mother can read to them and draw with them. They can go for outings wearing the harness on a rein. (2) A 'stable' door enables mother to keep an eye on the child while he or she is safely enclosed in an adjoining room.

10.15.2 Voluntary organizations dealing with the disabled (after Sommerville, 1977.)

Voluntary organization	Examples
1. Catalytic groups that try to co-ordinate the efforts required to deal with the problems	The British Council for the Rehabilitation of the Disabled The Central Council for the Disabled The British Red Cross Society.
2. Groups that deal with a particular disability	British Rheumatism Association (BRA) The Royal National Institute for the Blind
3. Pressure groups that try to mobilize support and legislation to further their aims in relation to helping the disabled	Disabled Income Group (DIG) League of Friends of Hospitals The Disabled Drivers' Association
4. Groups that are involved in providing training for the disabled, or organizing sporting activities, convalescent holidays, leisure groups and sheltered workshops	The Queen Elizabeth's Foundation for the Disabled The Thistle Foundation The Greater London Association for the Disabled
5. Objective groups that tackle in a realistic manner the problems of disabled people, and publish literature, provide fixed and mobile exhibitions, encourage local authorities and departments of the Government to improve facilities for disabled people and, in particular, to make certain that such facilities are accessible to disabled people	The Disabled Living Foundation The Horder Centre for Arthritics, Crowborough, Sussex The Winged Fellowship Trust
6. Groups that are entirely involved in research in relation to the disabled, and will give grants to universities, technical colleges, hospitals and individuals, to undertake specific research programmes	Arthritis and Rheumatism Council The National Fund for Research into Crippling Diseases The Imperial Cancer Research Fund The Wolfson Foundation
7. Self-perpetuating groups. These are organizations that originally had a good reason for existence, but this reason has either partially or completely disappeared in that it has been overtaken by events or met by enlightened legislation	Examples purposely not quoted

11
Heterodox
procedures

11.1 GENERAL INTRODUCTION

11.1.1 Introductory comment

This chapter is neither a condemnation nor a recommendation. It has been included to provide those with an interest in treating rheumatic patients with some background information about remedies other than orthodox therapies about which patients so often seek advice. Many doctors feel that they are too unversed in this field to answer these questions satisfactorily, and it is hoped that the following account will to some extent fill this gap.

It should be stressed at the outset that an original intention to approach the subject throughout with vigorous criticality was often thwarted by a dearth of facts upon which to base such an approach.

11.1.2 The meaning of heterodoxy

The term 'heterodox' used in the title of this chapter could equally have been 'unorthodox', 'natural', 'alternative' or 'fringe' medicine to describe those therapeutic approaches that do not fall within allopathic medicine. 'Heterodox' or 'unorthodox' are terms most popularly used by medical practitioners, while the terms 'natural', 'alternative' or 'fringe' medicine tend to be used by the lay population. International differences may also confuse the picture. The Americans prefer 'Alternative Medicine', the Italians 'The Other Medicine', and the French 'Biotherapy'. The World Health Organization has settled for 'Traditional Medicine' (Inglis, 1979). 'Fringe Medicine' seems to have become replaced by 'Natural Medicine' in the UK. To the author's knowledge, no one has yet coined the phrase 'Paramedicine', although the British Department of Health refers to 'paramedical practitioners'.

Whatever term is used none is perfectly apt. The term heterodox rather than unorthodox was chosen by the present author because of the semantic implication of 'hetero' suggesting 'different from' as opposed to 'un' implying 'not' (orthodox). Heterodox carries a less punitive sense, and would appear to be more appropriate, considering the lack of proof that many of these therapies are useless. The kinder terms 'fringe' and 'alternative' emphasize different aspects of the heterodox movement – 'fringe' stressing the close position of these therapies to the edge or border of orthodox medicine, 'alternative', wrongly in the author's opinion, stressing the mutually inclusive characteristic of the two approaches. Stanway (1980) has recently emphasized the supplementary role of heterodox medicine, and it would seem to the present author that 'supplementary medicine' would be a more realistic lay term than 'alternative medicine'.

That no term is entirely suitable is obvious from the fact that some heterodox procedures, such as herbalism, have counterparts deeply embedded in 'respectable' medicine (valuable drugs of plant origin such as colchicine and digitalis), and some orthodox procedures, such as manipulation, have counterparts within heterodox medicine (chiropractic and osteopathy).

To distinguish between orthodox and heterodox medicine is not as easy as it might seem. In Britain, once qualified, a doctor may practise any form of medicine he likes and would not be prevented from employing any of the methods commonly associated with heterodox practice, although in so doing his promotion in the medical hierarchy and reputation might suffer. However, (as the General Medical Council advises) 'any medical practitioner... who knowingly enables or assists a person not registered as a medical practitioner to practise medicine... is liable to erasure'. It is important to stress that this reputation does not restrict 'the legitimate employment of nurses, midwives, physiotherapists, dispensers and other persons trained to perform specialized functions relevant to medicine, surgery and midwifery, provided that the medical practitioners so employed *exercise effective supervision over any person so employed and retain personal responsibility for the treatment of the patient'.

Herein lies the crucial pointer to the difference between orthodox and heterodox practitioners, one relying on differences in responsibility rather than differences in technique. For example, manipulation by a physiotherapist working under the supervision of a medical practitioner is orthodox, whereas manipulation by an osteopath, who claims to be able to diagnose and treat patients in his own right, is heterodox because there is no official link with a registered medical practitioner.

Another criterion to decide between orthodoxy and heterodoxy is whether or not the particular discipline is taught in the standard medical curriculum. A feature common to all the main fringe theories is that medical students are not taught anything about them before they qualify. They are, of course, free to study them, but they must do this in their own time or after qualification. Fringe methods vary in the degree to which they satisfy this criterion. Homœopathy, for example, although now part of the medical establishment (homœopathic treatment and drugs are available on the National Health Service, and there are a few hospitals now devoted entirely to homœopathy) is still not taught in medical schools. Psychotherapy, on the other hand, has acquired some acceptance in the medical profession, and the subject is now being taught at a handful of medical schools. These and other points of differentiation are discussed by Inglis and the reader is referred to his books for further details (Inglis, 1964; 1979).

The US Consumer's Union (Editors of Consumer Reports Books, 1980) has recently published a useful list of characteristic features of the quack therapist in order to help the lay public to recognize these practitioners more easily. The features listed are as follows:

1. He may offer a 'special' or 'secret' formula or device for 'curing' arthritis.
2. He advertises and uses case histories and testimonials from satisfied patients.
3. He may promise (or imply) a quick or easy cure.
4. He may claim to know the cause of arthritis and may talk about 'cleansing' your body of 'poisons' and 'pepping up' your health.
5. He may say surgery, X-rays and drugs prescribed by a physician are unnecessary.
6. He may accuse the medical establishment of deliberately thwarting progress or of persecuting him.
7. He does not let his method be tested in tried and proved ways.

11.1.3 The present position

It has been estimated that in Britain alone there are about 20 000 people practising without any official medical qualification or approval. About a quarter of them make a full-time living from their various therapies (Eagle, 1978a). The extent of the heterodox movement will be appreciated from Appendices 11.5.1 and 11.5.2 which respectively list the various types of heterodox procedures, the associations and societies, and training centres concerned with heterodox practice, and some products relevant to heterodox medicine. Appendix 11.5.3 provides a list of health farms in the UK (for further details, see Hulke, 1978).

Patients seeking help from these practitioners have barely no means of establishing whether their therapies are genuine, dangerous or useless, and all too often they are seduced by the persuasive literature provided by many heterodox associations. These invariably contain impressive claims which have not been subjected to scientific scrutiny.

The question regarding heterodoxy versus orthodoxy is more complex than might appear from these and often literary castigations, no matter how realistic many of these criticisms may be. First, there is little doubt that confusion arises from lumping together the various heterodox procedures, as some lie remarkably close to orthodox practice, while others can be regarded as totally alien to scientific medical thinking. Secondly, though not necessarily a recommendation, most heterodox therapies can be regarded as harmless, unless because of them patients delay seeking orthodox advice concerning a potentially treatable disease. Thirdly, indirect support for the heterodox system derives from the high rate of iatrogenic diseases which arise from orthodox practice. For instance, as Eagle (1978a) has pointed out, it is estimated that more than one in eight patients in hospital has an iatrogenic disease (i.e. diseases caused by doctors or drugs). In the USA the figure is reported to be as high as 30% in some states.

Further evidence comes from Canada which has shown that of over 700 hospital patients in a general medical unit, 26% suffered from the adverse consequences of drug therapy.

These alarming figures from orthodox practice will, in the minds of many physicians, generate a hope for safer medicine. Moreover, they may provide some justification for investigating heterodox procedures using the rigorous scientific approaches which have already been applied to orthodox medicine, in the hope of pinpointing heterodox treatments of real value.

11.2 SOME HETERODOX PROCEDURES USED TO TREAT RHEUMATIC DISORDERS

11.2.1 Introductory comment

The following account does not claim to present a comprehensive list of all known heterodox procedures used to treat rheumatic disorders, merely a selection of the more common procedures. Some practitioners would quibble about the inclusion of some therapies on the grounds that they represent 'self-help' rather than 'alternative medicine'. As these definitions are by no means yet established, and also the fact that the broad terms 'heterodox' or 'unorthodox' medicine, 'fringe medicine' or 'alternative medicine' are themselves unclear, no such distinction was felt justified here.

Each type of therapy will be explained briefly, and where it exists evidence to support it will be given. As might be anticipated, however, fulfilment of the second criterion has not often been possible.

For convenience, the therapies have been presented in alphabetical order, although an alternative presentation based on the general target area (body, mind or spirit) at which individual therapies are aimed was considered. However, this idea was rejected in view of the difficulty in isolating the intended target area in some therapies, and in others because the considerable overlap between target areas would have posed problems.

It should be pointed out at this stage that although the therapeutic procedures are presented as separate entities, there are common threads running through many of them. For example, naturopathy often includes homœopathic treatment; the health food approach may include medicated bee venom therapy; vegetarians often do yoga, and so on.

11.2.2 Acupuncture

In view of the current scepticism surrounding acupuncture, it is perhaps of interest to record a comment made by the eminent physician Sir William Osler in the 7th edition of his *Principles and Practice of Medicine* (1910):

> For lumbago, acupuncture is in acute cases the most efficient treatment. Needles from three to four inches in length, ordinary bonnet needles, sterilized, will do. They are thrusted into the lumbar muscles at the seat of pain, and withdrawn after five to ten minutes. In many instances the relief is immediate, and I can confirm fully the statements of Ringer, who taught me this practice, as to its extraordinary and prompt efficacy in many instances.

At the time this statement was written, acupuncture had already been in regular use in Britain and in the USA for several decades, and was thought to have been introduced into Europe from China by French Jesuit priests.

The widespread disappearance of acupuncture from European and American medical practice until its recent re-introduction on a smaller scale is not properly understood, but has been attributed by some to the introduction of aspirin in 1899.

Acupuncture, introduced by the Chinese over 2500 years ago, is based on the ancient Chinese belief that a life force flows through all things. This life force, Chi (also spelt Chhi, Ki, Qi, Ch'i) is supposed to be influenced by the forces of Yin and Yang, two polar principles which roughly correspond to our idea of negative and positive, or female and male. The concept of Yin and Yang defies precise translation, but certain foods, substances and even places are said to be Yin, while others are Yang.

For a body to be healthy, the Chinese claimed that Yin and Yang must be in a state of balance, and acupuncture was the means by which disequilibrium could be restored. Acupuncture was not only aimed at 'curing' disease but also at preventing it.

According to classical acupuncture theory, Chi flows around the body along channels – meridians. It is claimed that there are 12 major meridians, six for Yin organs (liver, heart, spleen, kidney, lung and pericardium) and six for Yang organs (stomach, gall bladder, urinary bladder, large intestine, small intestine and 'triple warmer'). In addition to these 12 meridians there are two other important ones – the conception vessel (which runs up the front of the body from perineum to chin) and the governing vessel (which runs down the spine).

The classical acupuncturist assesses his patient by feeling the pulses of each meridian – six pulses on the left radial artery and six on the right. Up to 27 different characteristics are sought, in contrast to the more modest sign-searching of the western physician based on assessing pulse rate, rhythm, volume, and wave pattern.

One of the most popular explanations for the origin of acupuncture stems from reports that hunters and

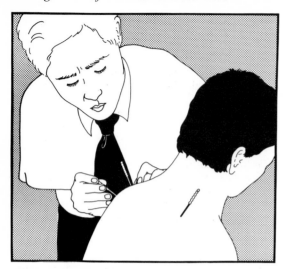

Fig. 11.1 Acupuncture: insertion of modern steel needles.

soldiers injured by arrows subsequently recovered from diseases which had previously afflicted them.

The earliest non-mythical records (inscribed on tortoise shell) of acupuncture date from Stone Age China. These explain how flint needles were used to cure diseases. Later, jade and bamboo became popular, and subsequently iron, bronze, silver and gold needles were introduced. Silver was regarded as Yin and was thus used for its sedative effect, while gold was Yang and accordingly used for increasing the 'tone' of the system. Today, needles are still most often used (Fig. 11.1), and Yin/Yang balance is achieved by twisting the needles (usually steel) clockwise or anticlockwise respectively. Moxibustion (burning small cones of the dried herb *artemesia* on the acupuncture point) is sometimes used as an alternative to needling.

The evidence for meridians is steeped in doubt and controversy. Meridians have variously been ascribed to anatomical channels (subsequently shown to be more likely the result of overenthusiastic cadaveric dissection and the use of dyes), to lines of reduced electrical resistance, and to an image resulting from psychic vision. More likely is the proposal that meridian charts represent a map of lymphangitis resulting from the unsterile approach to acupuncture in the old days.

While it is likely that the meridians that appear on classical charts bear no more relevance to the foundations of acupuncture than a vestige of dirty practice, there have been several interesting speculations as to how acupuncture works. These have been reviewed by Eagle (1978a).

One idea, supported by the doyen of British medical acupuncturists, Dr Felix Mann (Mann, 1971a) im-

plicates the nervous reflex, and claims that acupuncture can be explained in terms of conventional physiology.

Another idea, at present popular, has been proposed by Melzack and Wall (1965, 1968). These workers have proposed a hypothetical 'gate' in the spinal cord which can prevent pain signals from reaching the brain. Briefly, stimulation of certain small nerve fibres opens the gate, while stimulation of larger nerve fibres closes the gate.

The idea of chemical mediation of the pain relief of acupuncture has also acquired some popularity recently, the proposal being that acupuncture needling leads to a slow but definite accumulation of endorphins, substances pharmacologically but not chemically similar to opiates. Of further interest in this respect is the observation that the anti-narcotic drug, naloxone, which is used to reverse the effects of opiates, can also abolish the analgesia induced by acupuncture.

Yet another explanation for the analgesic effect of acupuncture involves hypnosis. However, there are major differences between hypnosis-induced analgesia and acupuncture-induced analgesia. First, patients can be hypnotized in about 1 min and can successfully undergo surgery without pain-killing drugs. To achieve this degree of analgesia with acupuncture, 30 min or so of twiddling or electrical stimulation through needles is required. Secondly, as referred to earlier, acupuncture analgesia can be blocked by naloxone, whereas hypnosis-induced analgesia cannot. Thirdly, acupuncture analgesia can be abolished in experimental animals if the dorsolateral tract of the spinal cord is interrupted. This effect does not occur in hypnotized animals.

Melzack (1978) has recently reviewed ideas on the mechanism of acupuncture pain relief. He points out that short-acting local anaesthetic blocks of trigger points often give rise to prolonged and sometimes permanent relief of certain forms of myofascial or visceral pain (Livingstone, 1943; Travell and Rinzler, 1952; Bonica, 1953). Dry needling or intense cold (Travell and Rinzler, 1952), injection of normal saline (Sola and Williams, 1956), and transcutaneous electrical stimulation (Melzack, 1978) may also relieve these pains for days. Melzack has also found that acupuncture and transcutaneous electrical stimulation were equally effective in relieving chronic low-back pain. Hyperstimulation analgesia is the term that has been recently applied to this type of intense stimulation resembling the effect of acupuncture (Melzack, 1973). Controlled work has shown that intense stimulation of trigger points produces significantly greater pain relief than placebo (Anderson *et al.*, 1974).

Further observations from Melzack's unit have revealed a high degree (71%) of correspondence between trigger points and acupuncture points for pain, a correlation suggesting that both kinds of points, though labelled differently, can be explained by the same neural mechanisms. Godfrey and Morgan (1978) have recently reported work that lends further support to the 'demystification' of acupuncture. Pain was reduced in 60% of their patients whether appropriate and inappropriate acupuncture points were stimulated. This led to the conclusion that the sensory input is more important than the exact point stimulated.

Melzack (1978) admits that the relief of pain by brief, intense stimulation of distant trigger points is still a major puzzle. He feels that the most likely explanation is that the brain-stem areas that are known to exert a powerful inhibitory control over transmission in the pain signalling system may be involved. These areas, which he calls the 'central biasing mechanism', receive input from diverse parts of the spinal cord and brain. The stimulation of particular nerves or tissues by needles could increase input to the central biasing mechanism and close the gate to input from selected body areas. The cells of the midbrain reticular formation are known to have large receptive fields (Rossi and Zanchetti, 1957) and the electrical stimulation of points within the reticular formation can produce analgesia in discrete areas of the body (Balagura and Ralph, 1973). It is possible, therefore, that particular body areas may project especially strongly to some reticular areas, and these, in turn, could block input from particular parts of the body.

How successful is acupuncture? First, the point should be made that modern thinking supports its success as an analgesic but not as a cure. However, even the former is probably not as impressive as demonstrations by Chinese doctors in the early 1970s led us to believe. Since then the Chinese have surveyed 80 000 operations in which the patient was given acupuncture. Only 37% responded strongly enough to feel no pain. A further 38% experienced slight pain, but not without an occasional groan. One patient in 12 responded so poorly that he had to be given a general anaesthetic. Experience in Britain has cast further doubt on the efficacy of acupuncture in surgical analgesia, and one study suggested that analgesia was adequate in only 10% of patients.

Table 11.1 Results of stimulating appropriate and inappropriate acupuncture points. Number of patients showing reduction of pain after third and fifth treatments (from Godfrey and Morgan, 1978)

| | Site stimulated | | | |
| | Appropriate | | Inappropriate | |
Pain	3rd treatment	5th treatment	3rd treatment	5th treatment
Reduced	60	53	48	45
Same or worse	28	31	37	39
Total	88	84	85	84
% Reduced	68·2	63·1	56·5	53·6

Table 11.2 Results of acupuncture in various disorders (after Turban and Urlich, 1978)

Diagnoses	No. of patients	Success level* 1	2	3	4	5
Migraine headaches	26	38·46	38·46	15·38	3·85	3·85
Cephalgia	21	23·81	52·38	14·29	0	9·52
Cervical ligamentous strain	26	19·23	53·85	15·38	3·85	7·69
Osteoarthritis	169	16·57	49·11	16·57	8·28	9·47
Sciatic neuralgia	54	16·67	46·30	12·96	18·52	3·70
Rheumatoid arthritis	29	6·90	55·17	10·34	6·90	20·69
Lumbosacral sprain	29	17·24	31·03	20·69	17·24	13·79
Nerve deafness	28	7·14	7·14	7·14	39·20	39·20
Loss of hearing	11	9·09	0	27·27	27·27	36·36

* 1 = no symptoms; 2 = significant improvement; 3 = improvement; 4 = slight improvement; 5 = no change.

However, despite these poor results, there has recently been some renewed enthusiasm for acupuncture in this field.

Most patients who consult a medical acupuncturist are suffering from painful conditions, and a 70% success has been claimed in treating arthritis, migraine, sinusitis, and menstrual pains. The response of back pain to acupuncture has been variable, but is claimed to be comparable with conventional drug or orthopaedic therapy (Eagle, 1978). This figure has recently been supported by the work of Godfrey and Morgan (1978) to which reference has already been made. This showed that among 193 patients with painful conditions due to a variety of rheumatic disorders (degenerative disc disease, osteoarthrosis, lumbosacral pain, cervical strain, tennis elbow, bursitis) a roughly similar proportion (68.2% for appropriate stimulation; 56.5% for inappropriate stimulation) had reduced pain after three treatments, regardless of whether the place stimulated corresponded to a classical acupuncture point (Table 11.1). The success level in another series of subjects with mixed diagnoses is shown in Table 11.2 (Turban and Urlich, 1978). In the rheumatic subjects 'success' was based on the patients' judgements.

Details of acupuncture points claimed to be of value in rheumatic diseases are summarized in Table 11.3.

The problems associated with acupuncture include:

1. The camouflaging of potentially treatable diseases by pain relief induced by a lay acupuncturist.
2. Advice to patients by lay acupuncturists that all drugs should be stopped while acupuncture treatment is in progress. Clearly sudden withdrawal of some drugs such as corticosteroids or anticonvulsants could be dangerous.
3. The more ambitious acupuncturists may cause damage by using needles that are too long (some are as much as a foot long) or malpositioned (pneumothorax has been reported).
4. If needles are not sterilized, hepatitis may be transmitted between patients.

Some distinction should be made between lay and medical practitioners. Lay practitioners are often members of the Acupuncture Association, most of whom are osteopaths or naturopaths. They may sport impressive titles such as 'Doctor of Acupuncture' or even 'professorships' conferred by institutions in Taiwan and Hong Kong, but these are not recognized by British universities. On the other hand, medical practitioners are qualified doctors who have partially or fully turned to acupuncture. Their association, the Medical Acupuncture Association (70 members), whose founder and president is Dr Felix Mann, runs courses for doctors interested in acupuncture.

In other parts of Europe acupuncture is in more widespread use. In France about 1500 doctors use acupuncture, and as many as ten French hospitals have departments of acupuncture. In the Soviet Union acupuncture is taught in medical schools.

Further research is needed before acupuncture can enjoy a firmer grip on conventional medicine in the UK. However, this form of treatment has already gained some respectability (particularly as a possible alternative to traditional methods of establishing analgesia/anaesthesia), and it could find itself as a more frequently used therapy in the rheumatological armoury in the not too distant future. Currently, however, its use in orthodox medicine is more or less confined to pain clinics.

Table 11.3 Some acupuncture points claimed to be useful in rheumatic disorders (Mann, 1974)*

Acute and chronic rheumatoid arthritis
Gv14 B11 Li15 Li11 T5 Li4
Plus local points 3–6 cm away from pain

Muscular rheumatism
In loin B22 B24 B46 B31 B54 or B23 B25 B47 B32 S36
In neck G20 B10 Si15 Si14 T10 Si4
In scapular and interscapular area B36 B13 B39 B15 B40 B42 or B37 B12 B38 B14 B41 B18
In shoulders Li16 T15 Li15 Li14 T13 T14
Of pectoralis major and minor S13 S15 Sp20 G23 Li10 G34 or S14 S16 Sp19 Sp21 Li11 S36

Arthritis of knee
S33 Liv8 Liv7 XL2 G34 Sp6 Sp9

Gout
B23 B24 B19 Cv4 Sp6
Plus local points

* For further details see Mann (1971a, 1974).
Key: B = bladder; G = gall bladder; Gr = girdle vessel; Li = large intestine; Si = small intestine; S = stomach; Sp = spleen; Liv = liver; T = triple warmer.

11.2.3 Aromathérapie

Aromathérapie is an ancient therapeutic method based on the use of essential oils and essences extracted from flowers, plants, resins and other substances.

The use of essential oils as an aid to good health and in cosmetology formed a large part of traditional medicine in Tibet, India, China, and the Middle East. Moreover, ancient Egyptian medicine going back as far as 4500 BC was almost entirely based on the use of aromatic substances which now form the basis of modern aromathérapie.

Present-day aromathérapie was evolved in Europe by the late Marguerite Maury who, working in France with her husband, was able to modify the traditional methods into a form thought to be more suitable for countering the pressures and life-style of modern times. This new method was published as *The Secret of Life and Youth* in 1962 (cited by Ryman, 1978). Although the early work of the Maurys was aimed at 'rejuvenation', later a wider potential for this therapy was conceived. This was based on an assumption that the essential oils penetrating the skin would be rapidly distributed around the body with a direct stimulating or healing effect on the internal organs and muscle. It was thought that the essential oils act not only by a chemical process alone but also 'through the odoriferous molecules which are composed of free electrons'.

The natural essential oil used in aromathérapie includes the following: from flowers – carnation, rose, neroli, jasmin, lotus and lilac; from aromatic plants – cinnamon, cardamom, camomile, angelica, tonka beans and violet leaves; from resins – rosewood, galbanum, styrax and sandalwood.

In order to retain the properties of the essential oil, the method of extraction is thought to be important, and it is claimed that distillation produced an oil less effective than one produced by 'enfleurage', a process involving slow diffusion of odoriferous molecules into an oil and subsequent separation of the aromatic essence from the oil by a volatile process.

Each essence is thought to possess a different health-promoting property. For instance, cinnamon is alleged to stimulate the respiratory and cardiovascular systems, lavender the nervous system, and angelica the digestive system. Ryman (1978) states that subjects with 'rheumatism' have been treated with success, but no further details are given.

The treatment embodies a mixture of different and doubtless psychologically stimulating phases as follows. Patients have an initial consultation at which a specimen of blood is taken and 'analysed' to discover the essential oil needed. Radiesthesia is sometimes used for this analysis. An oil tailored to the needs of the patient is prepared and consists of a mixture derived from a pool of 250 oils. This oil is then applied during a massage which concentrates on the spine using the method of German soft-tissue massage and acupressure points. Patients are advised to take a course consisting of 6–10 treatments, 2 or 3 times a year as required.

11.2.4 Biofeedback

Biofeedback may be regarded as a modern variant of yoga. It stems from a principle based on body control by means of an awareness (feedback) of how the body is functioning.

Its main application, supposedly by promoting para-sympathetic as opposed to sympathetic activity, has been in reducing stress as a potent aggravating factor in hypertension, migraine, and tension headache. A possible rheumatological application concerns the potential value of biofeedback in re-training muscles and in posture control.

Feedback may be provided electroencephalographically, electromyographically or by means of measuring electrical skin resistance. Patients are given initial instruction by the practitioner about what to look for in the instrumental traces and what ultimately to achieve. It is claimed that, in time, total relaxation may be achieved without the aid of instrumental feedback, and a state of self-induced freedom from stress 'willed' spontaneously (Blundell, 1977a, b; Eagle, 1978).

11.2.5 Chiropractic

Literally meaning 'done by hand' (combining the two Greek words 'cheiro' and 'praktikos', chiropractic is one form of manipulation. It differs from osteopathy in depending for its effect more on thrusts than on leverage. It also differs in its basic tenet which reasons that joint manipulation restores health by re-establishing a normal nerve supply to the affected parts. However, there is a school which recognizes the close parallels that exist between chiropractic and osteopathy, and these practitioners prefer to use the term 'osteopractic'.

Chiropractic was discovered in 1895 by Daniel David Palmer in Davenport, Iowa, USA. Palmer's interests chiefly concerned healing, which in those days centred on medical practices of blood-letting, use of chemicals, necromancy and potions.

Palmer's first patient was his janitor who had apparently become deaf after dislocating his neck. Palmer corrected his dislocation and restored the janitor's hearing.

The aspect of chiropractic which generates particular concern among orthodox medical manipulators, such as Cyriax, has to do with the diagnostic assumptions of the therapy rather than with its physical effect on the patient. For instance, chiropractic (and osteopathy) readily ascribe disease in distant organs and systems to spinal malfunction; even diseases such as diabetes mellitus and thyroid disturbances can be attributed to vertebral disease. This is a line of thinking substantially at variance with that of orthodox medical manipulators who usually stray no further than from simple diagnostic assumptions based on disc derangement and its attendant lumbago and sciatica. However, there are some chiropractic diagnoses which have just enough plausibility to persuade even the most sceptic of orthodox practitioners. For instance, it is difficult not to accept that some truth might underlie the suggestion that there is a link between flat foot and headache which the chiropractor explains in terms of the following flow of events: flat foot – leg shortening – spinal curvature – head tilting – compensatory muscle contraction – headache.

In Britain, chiropractors are outnumbered by osteopaths, which differs from most other countries where alternative practitioners flourish. It has been said (Hewitt and Wood, 1975) that chiropractors are perhaps more conscious of their public image and attempt to proselytize through such bodies as pro-chiropractic associations and the Back Pain Association. Chiropractors appear to make more use of radiography and, compared with osteopaths, their higher throughput often permits the charging of lower fees. Like osteopathy, chiropractic requires two 'A' levels and a 4-year training which covers most subjects featuring in a conventional medical school syllabus, with the difference that much of the knowledge is derived from text books as opposed to clinical experience. For those with a registrable medical qualification a 1-year course is available.

With the exception of Breen's study (Breen, 1977), surprisingly little work has been done to examine the size and success of chiropractic therapy in the UK. Breen undertook a survey of British chiropractors and their practices and found that most patients attended for back pain. This has been confirmed in another study (Table 11.4). The average age of patients was 47 years, the sex ratio was equal, and most had had their complaints for more than 3 months. Patients were

Table 11.4 Preponderance of back complaints among 2987 patients seeking chiropractic treatment (from Doran and Newell, 1975)

Site of presenting complaint	Patients presenting with complaint in particular site (not exclusive)	
	Number	Proportion (%)
Lower back	1598	53·4
Neck	615	20·5
Lower leg	595	19·9
Thigh and knee	523	17·5
Head	379	12·7
Shoulder	368	12·3
Hip and buttock	324	10·8
Thorax	284	9·5
Upper arm and elbow	250	8·4
Ankle and foot	204	6·8
Wrist and hand	126	4·2
Abdomen and groin	106	3.5
Lower arm	76	2·5
Not specifically located (probably emotional)	40	1·3

Table 11.5 Benefit obtained in patients with low-back pain (from Doran and Newell, 1975)

Outcome of treatment	Patients	
	Number	Proportion (%)
Worse	11	1·0
No change	49	4·6
Some temporary improvement	191	17·8
Some lasting improvement	384	35·7
Temporary remission*	355	33·0
Lasting remission	85	7·9
Inadequate record of outcome	523	32·7
All patients	1598	100·0

* This outcome was inferred for patients in whom remission was recorded without a return visit after 6 months to assess progress.

largely housewives and persons from executive and managerial occupations. Treatment was mostly manual and directed at the spinal column. The benefit obtained, as assessed by the chiropractors, was comparable with that reported in studies of 'orthodox' manipulation, such as that of Doran and Newell (1975), and are shown in Table 11.5.

Another study (Kane *et al.*, 1974), which compared back problems treated by a chiropractor (122 patients) with those treated by a physician using various types of treatment (drugs, neck braces, exercises) (110 patients), showed little difference between the two groups. Table 11.6 shows the patients' satisfaction according to which type of practitioner they saw. The only significant difference was the superior ability of chiropractors to explain to patients the nature of the problem and of its treatment.

11.2.6 Copper

The use of copper, usually as a copper bangle (Fig. 11.2), to ease rheumatic pains has been known for centuries. Much of the justification for this 'therapy' comes from the old wives' tale that copper removes electricity from the body. Associated with this 'electrical theory' is the claim by many patients that rheumatic problems are due to wearing shoes which insulate the feet from the ground, thus encouraging the retention of electricity within the body. Some patients are so convinced by this theory that they attach one end of a wire to the leg and trail the other end on the ground behind in order to discharge this build-up of electricity. I have also heard patients draw a parallel between the success of

Table 11.6 Measures of patient satisfaction in patients treated by a physician and by a chiropractor (from Kane *et al.*, 1974)

Therapeutic variable	Patients treated by physician		Patients treated by chiropractor	
	Satisfied	Dissatisfied	Satisfied	Dissatisfied
Ability of practitioner to return patient to previous functional level	101 (91·7%)	9 (8·3%)	115 (94·0%)	7 (6·0%)
Ability of practitioner to make patient feel welcome*	103 (93·5%)	7 (6·5%)	122 (100%)	0
Ability of practitioner to gain confidence of patient	105 (95·4%)	5 (4·6%)	116 (94·8%)	6 (5·2%)
Ability of practitioner to explain problem and treatment*	93 (84·3%)	17 (15·7%)	116 (94·8%)	6 (5·2%)

* Differences between physician-treated and chiropractor-treated patients significant at $p < 0.05$ (χ^2 test).

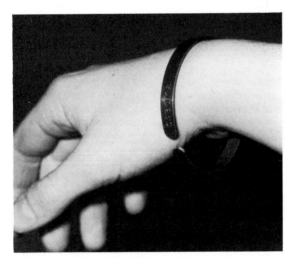

Fig. 11.2 Copper bangle.

copper wire in preventing rising damp and of its success in preventing rheumatic complaints on this basis!

Rather more scientifically serious are the theories that justify the use of copper on the grounds of a copper deficiency, particularly in rheumatoid arthritis. However, there is little consistent evidence to support this, although there are some data pointing to *raised* levels of copper in the serum and synovial fluid of rheumatoid patients (Niedermeier *et al.*, 1962; Koskelo *et al.*, 1966; West, 1970; Scudder *et al.*, 1978a, b; Brown *et al.*, 1979).

11.2.7 Cupping

Cupping was used 5000 years ago by the ancient Egyptians to treat various diseases. Hippocrates appreciated its benefits and Alexander Tralianus, a contemporary of the Emperor Justinian, and writer of an extensive textbook on medicine, employed it for treating certain forms of arthritis and rheumatism.

There are two types of cupping, dry and wet. In dry cupping, a cupping glass or a thick glass tumbler can be used. A few drops of methylated spirit are placed on a swab of cotton-wool or a fragment of blotting paper, ignited, and put in the glass, the mouth of which is placed firmly on the area to be treated. A vacuum is created causing the skin to swell into the glass, as blood is displaced into smaller blood vessels. The process is repeated up to eight times on different parts of the body and relies on a 'massage' effect generated by the vacuum. This type of cupping has been used to treat multiple sclerosis and to promote the healing of scars, but convincing evidence to support any therapeutic effect is lacking.

Wet cupping involves shallow scarification of an area treated by dry cupping, with further application of the cupping glass to draw blood. Again, as far as the author is aware, there is no evidence to support any claims as to the efficacy of this therapy.

11.2.8 Flower healing

Flower healing, perhaps justifiably, a branch of homeopathy, is not to do with flower-based teas or flower-based ointments, but with 'potentizing'. This means that the 'non-material energies' or 'radiations' of flowers, as distinct from their chemical constituents, are used for healing purposes.

The concept is heavily embedded in medical history. For instance, the children of Israel, it is alleged, caught none of the Egyptian plagues because Moses 'potentized' the water of Marah (Exodus 15:23–6). Another example originated from India 4000 years ago when a system of medicine based on flowers was so successful that it cut out the need for surgery.

According to Bellhouse (1978) the method has 'got

rid of bunions' and 'has completely resolved synovial cysts on the finger joints of several years' standing', 'swollen and painful feet have responded', and 'it has been used with success for strains and sprains', and for 'arthritic and rheumatic pains and swellings'. No evidence was provided to substantiate these claims.

11.2.9 Gerson therapy

This is a dietary method of therapy 'for the healing and preventing of cancer and other incurable diseases' developed by Dr Max Gerson (1881–1959). Gerson's philosophy stemmed from a conviction (still unproven) that chronic disease begins with a loss of potassium from the body cells and a subsequent 'invasion of sodium', and with it water. In this context, he stressed the importance of using plants grown in soil not chemically fertilized. These he claimed contained potassium and sodium in the correct proportions required by human metabolism.

His treatment was applied to patients with every type of cancer, and to other chronic maladies including rheumatoid arthritis and osteoarthritis. Although at the time (1920s) the treatment was applauded with worldwide acclaim, to the author's knowledge there is little acceptable scientific evidence to support such a therapeutic approach.

11.2.10 Health foods

The health food idea stems from Victorian times when 'far-seeing doctors and other scientists' began to realize there was a relationship between food and health (Hanssen, 1978). At this time, there was much starvation and shortage of protein among poor children. Practical idealists felt that fresh air, exercise and a balanced diet would do more for the well-being of these children than any amount of preaching. Accordingly, a diet based on vegetarian principles, rich in fresh fruit, vegetables, grains and beans was developed. In this way it was possible to give a wholesome nutritious diet inexpensively.

There has been a recent upsurge in the popularity of the health food idea, and there are now 600 or so health stores in Britain. It is the purpose of these establishments to supply the public with food products as near natural as today's world permits (more than 3000 artificial additives are used in food today, compared with only 100 at the turn of the century). In addition to the wholesome foods mentioned, various vitamins (particularly A, the B complex, and C), calcium pantothenate, "The Devil's Claw" (an African herb), pollen and propolis, cider apple vinegar, and other supplements claimed to have health-promoting value are sold. A typical diet based on health food principles is shown in Appendix 11.5.4

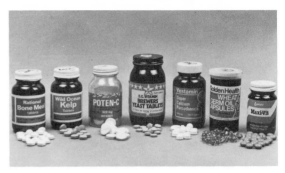

Fig. 11.3 Various health food preparations being taken as a single course of treatment by a rheumatic patient.

Therapeutic claims for the health food doctrine have yet to be verified objectively as far as rheumatic disorders are concerned, although it would seem reasonable that the emphasis on including fresh fruit and vegetables and sufficient protein is a useful contribution to maintaining general health. In the face of the paucity of evidence to support specific health-improving properties of health food, there can be no doubt, however, that some patients take such a doctrine to an extreme. For example, Fig. 11.3 shows the large number of 'health promoting' products being taken simultaneously by one of my patients.

11.2.11 Herbalism

Herbalism uses products obtained solely from plants in treating disorders of the body. A herb, however, may be used for other purposes: as a food, as a scent, or for its flavour.

Herbalism is several millenia old, and the Bible often refers to their use in the service of man–for example, Genesis 4: 11, 12; Psalm 104: 14; Exodus 30: 23, 34; Romans 14: 2; Revelations 22: 2.

As far back as 2200 BC a Sumerian herbal existed, and in the same period an Egyptian papyrus listed 2000 herbal doctors practising in the land. Among the Greeks, Aesculapius, Hippocrates and Theophrastos and, later, Pliny and Dioscorides were active herbal practitioners. In Roman times, Galen was one of the many to continue the herbal tradition, and his writings were valued up to the Middle Ages.

The introduction of printing during the Renaissance allowed crude illustrations of plants to be included with the text, making for easier identification. The first authentic printed English herbal was that of John Banckes which appeared in 1525. This led the way to the printing of many others in this era, including John Gerard's famous *The Herball or General Historie of Plants* in three volumes (1597), several works by

Nicholas Culpeper (1616–54), and John Parkinson's *Herbal* of 1629.

Culpeper's *The English Physician Enlarged* (Culpeper, 1653) is a particularly detailed treatise and mentions for each category of herb the place of growth, the time of year it reaches maturity, its manner of preparation, and the disease for which it is of value. Thirty-nine herbs were listed as useful for gout, and in most instances were recommended to be used as topical ointments (Talbott, 1970).

Until this century, herbal remedies made up more than 80% of the pharmacopoeia, and medical therapy based on herbalism became not only the responsibility of doctors and herbalists but also that of the lay public who were inundated with 'botanic guides' (Fig. 11.4) aimed at preventing and promoting family health by the family (e.g. Thomson, 1849; Fox, 1897).

Though herbs now constitute only a small minority of doctor-prescribed drugs, many valuable drugs which originated from herbal medicine, such as colchicine, digitalis, atropine and reserpine, can now be made synthetically.

Of the 350 000 known species in the plant kingdom throughout the world, about 10 000 have so far been examined for their medicinal properties, and about 200 of these are regularly used in herbal medicine in the UK.

An official training school was started in 1864 – the National Institute of Medical Herbalists. This, together with the Faculty of Herbal Medicine, founded in the 1940s, comprise the two main training centres for herbalists today. At present there are about 12 000 practising herbalists who have trained in either of these two centres.

Like the homœopaths, herbalists and herbal prac-

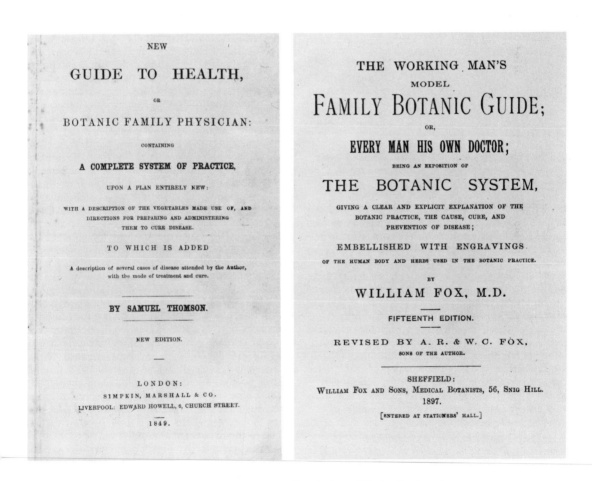

Fig. 11.4 Typical nineteenth-century botanic guides addressed to the lay public. (Author's collection.)

titioners* like to feel they are treating people rather than diseases. For example, a patient with an infection would be treated with one remedy to relieve symptoms, another to increase the number of white cells, but nothing to attack the invading organism – as the anti-biotic approach counters a basic tenet of herbalism in being 'anti-life'.

The method of preparing herbal remedies can make a critical difference to their medicinal activity. For instance, comfrey root used fresh is full of edible fibre and is thus a good laxative, but marinated in alcohol and made into a tincture it is used to control diarrhoea. Dosage is also important: parsley in small amounts is diuretic, but taken in overdose may cause internal bleeding.

Appendix 11.5.5 shows some herbs used in the treatment of rheumatic disorders (Didcott, 1978). Most of them derive their reputation from tradition and from anecdotal evidence. As far as the author is aware no controlled studies of herbal remedies for rheumatic disorders have yet been attempted. Although non-rheumatological, it is encouraging to note, however, a recent controlled trial confirming the value of *Coccinia indica* (a wild creeper from Bengal) in the oral treatment of patients with maturity-onset diabetes mellitus (Azad Khan *et al.*, 1980).

11.2.12 Home remedies and self-medication

Kitchen physic is the best physic
Jonathan Swift, 1738

(a) Home remedies

Few people admit to being in perfect health – in fact only about one in three of the urban population in one survey (Wadsworth *et al.*, 1971). About the same number feel their state of health to be 'reasonable' while the rest are certain they are ailing. Considering these depressing figures one might expect doctors' surgeries to be even more congested than they are. However, the reason that they are not is that, surprisingly, only about one person in four experiencing symptoms or feeling unwell actually seeks professional medical advice (Camp, 1973). Therefore, taking medical complaints generally, three-quarters of the British public still prefer to treat themselves at home, and this section will be concerned with some of the home remedies that have been, and in some cases still are, popular in the treatment of rheumatic ailments.

---

* Some claim a distinction between herbalists and herbal practitioners – the former being involved in collecting, preparing and selling herbs, the latter being involved in the prescription of herbal remedies.

With regard to the specific area of rheumatic complaints, the work of Wadsworth *et al.* (1971) is worth noting. This group studied the action taken by a group of patients with various rheumatic complaints over a 14-day period before being interviewed. They found that 67% of 115 rheumatic sufferers sought medical care (48 were seen by a general practitioner; 23 saw a hospital doctor; and 1 saw a works' doctor); 31% did not seek any advice (23 stayed away from work; 14 went to bed); 0.8% sought non-medical advice. Wadsworth's group found that the most commonly used lay-prescribed medicines were counter-irritants, followed by analgesics, and then various forms of appliances, such as thermogen wool. Several lay-prescribed medications were being used simultaneously by 50 (44%), and 62 (54%) were using both medically prescribed and lay-prescribed medicines at the same time. The different types of medication taken and the source of this medication are shown in Table 11.7.

The kinds of remedies available for use in the home may broadly be divided into three types. First is the vast range of herbal and other remedies which have been used for centuries, and which depend on a mixture of faith, folklore, superstition and perhaps a little science. Second are the 'patent' medicines which achieved particular notoriety in Victorian times. Third are the more 'respectable' drugs and chemicals which are obtainable over the counter. Remedies in the first group are of particular interest and relevance to this section and are detailed in Appendix 11.5.6. It can be seen that they may be conveniently divided into home remedies for 'rheumatism' and home remedies for gout.

It is impossible to make any valid comment about these remedies whether they be for 'rheumatism' or 'the gout', as none has yet been put to any form of objective test.

However, their hallowed usage and common denominators of horrific psychological content (e.g. insect bites, applications of frogspawn, earthworm, or cow dung), unpleasant physical effects (e.g. overheating), concoctions containing heavy doses of alcohol, ingestion of food products with presumed 'health promoting' properties (e.g. honey), and external applications of physical agents (e.g. heat) suggest multifactorial effects.

More specifically these probably depend (either individually or collectively) on a placebo effect through autosuggestion, an effect due to alcoholic oblivion, a physiological response due to 'stress', and to some extent an effect due to the soothing or counter-irritant effect of external agents.

Less orthodox explanations have been proposed for some therapies, for example apple cider vinegar and honey. It has been suggested that the vinegar would dissolve the calcium around stiff joints and that the honey would help to hold the calcium in solution.

Table 11.7 Different types of medicines taken by rheumatic patients and their source (lay-prescribed or medically prescribed) (from Wadsworth *et al.*, 1971)*

Type of medicine	Lay-prescribed medicines		Medically prescribed medicines	
Analgesics	58·5	(83)	41·5	(59)
Antacids	66·7	(2)	33·3	(1)
Gastrointestinal medicines	92·9	(26)	7·1	(2)
Counter-irritants	76·7	(138)	23·3	(42)
Respiratory medicines	83.3	(5)	16·7	(1)
Tonics and vitamin preparations	50·0	(3)	50·0	(3)
Skin medicines	77·1	(27)	22·9	(8)
Ear and eye medicines	——		100.0	(3)
Medicines usually medically prescribed	14·3	(10)	85·7	(60)
Other medicines	70·4	(133)	29·6	(56)
All types of medicines	64·5	(427)	35·5	(235)

* Results are given as percentages, with numbers of patients in parentheses.

Whatever views may prevail about home remedies for rheumatic disorders and, not surprisingly, most lack scientific seriousness, at least some interest and amusement can be derived from their imaginative formulation.

(b) Self-medication

Rheumatic sufferers have open access to a wide variety of analgesic and herbal preparations which are obtainable from the local chemist, herbalist or health food store.

Many analgesic preparations can be obtained from the chemist without a doctor's prescription, and many of these contain aspirin, codeine and paracetamol. Paracetamol has now replaced phenacetin which has been withdrawn because of nephrotoxicity. The popularity of these drugs varies in different parts of the UK but in the author's city (Sheffield) paracetamol is the most popular, followed by Anadin, Disprin and Veganin, in that order. Other popular preparations are Panadol, Codis, Paxedin, Phensic and Solpadeine. Little is known about the proportion of rheumatic sufferers who buy these preparations, how often they buy them, and what patterns of drug consumption are followed. Certainly, advice is available from the chemist or his assistant, and instructions feature on the container, but this does not necessarily mean that such advice is followed.

Herbalists and health food stores provide the patient with another opportunity for self-medication in the form of herb-containing preparations. Although the herbal content of these remedies may vary between manufacturers, some typical examples are as follows: 'Rheumatism Tablets' (Guaiacum resin, Ext. Rhubarb, sodium salicylate, Ext. Iridis, Capsicum oleoresin, Ext. Poke Weed, Ext. Prickly Ash, Lig. Prickly Ash);

'Arthritis Tablets' (Elder Flower, Prickly Ash Bark, Yarrow, Poke Root, Ext. Burdock Root, Ext. Chives, Ext. Poplar Bark, Ext. Senna Leaf, Ext. Uva ursi); 'Backache Tablets' (Ext. Buchu, Ext. Uva ursi, Capsicum oleoresin, Dandelion, potassium nitrate, Juniper oil); and 'Sciatica and Lumbago Tablets' (Ext. Clivers, Shepherd's Purse, Ext. Uva ursi, Wild Carrot, Juniper oil). In addition to herbs in tablet form, the natural dried preparations are also sold (Fig. 11.5).

Royal Jelly (obtained from the salivary glands of *Apis mellifera* – the worker bee) has been popular for many years. It has been suggested that its pantothenate content may be responsible for its therapeutic benefit, but a recent controlled trial of this substance in osteoarthrosis showed no significant difference from placebo (Haslock and Wright, 1971). To my knowledge

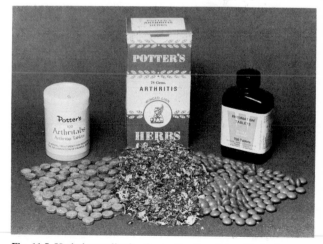

Fig. 11.5 Herbal remedies for rheumatic ailments in tablet and in natural form.

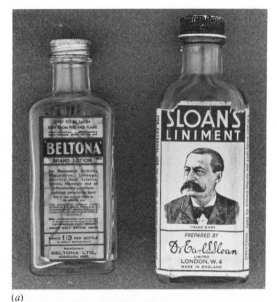

(a)

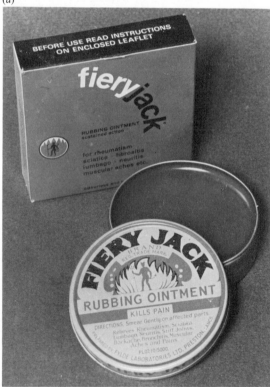

(b)

Fig. 11.6 (a) two old favourites – Beltona lotion and Sloan's liniment. (b) typical present-day rubbing ointment – Fiery Jack.

no studies have yet been done in rheumatoid arthritis.

Particularly in vogue at present is the costly preparation 'Seatone' (Powdered New Zealand Green-lipped Mussel Gonad, 230 mg; gelatin 50 mg). This is a preparation which has recently been given prominence in the national press, but clinical trials have failed to confirm its effectiveness over placebo (see Section 12.9).

Other preparations which feature in the Herbalists' shop window include old classics such as Doan's Backache Pills (first advertised by 'Dr' James Doan about 1870) and health relieving drinks such as apple cider vinegar. The latter may be presented as a pure vinegar preparation or in combination with honey (e.g. Honegar).

Balms and liniments and rubbing ointments are also popular, the ointments having a counterpart as early as the fifteenth century when Paracelsus (1493–1541) first described 'opodeldoc', a liniment made from soaps and spirit. In many households old favourites such as bottles of 'Sloans' or 'Beltona' can still be found, or modern equivalents such as 'Fiery Jack' (Fig. 11.6). Transvasin and Radian massage cream have also been popular for many years. Cooling sprays such as Boots' P.R. Spray are more recent innovations, and are popular for 'fibrositis', joint sprains, and painful conditions associated with muscle spasm.

As with self-medication via the chemists, there are no data available to indicate the epidemiological aspects of rheumatic patients who avail themselves of the products of herbal or health food stores. This lack of knowledge is matched by the paucity of evidence concerning the efficacy of these preparations.

11.2.13 Homœopathy

Homœopathy (also spelt 'homeopathy' and, erroneously, 'homöopathy') stems from 'homöopathie', a word first used by its innovator Samuel Christian Hahnemann (born in Meissen in 1755). The Greek form of the word (homoios = like or similar + pathos = suffering) mirrors the basic principle of this therapy which states that if a person is suffering from an illness characterized by a certain set of symptoms, he or she should be treated by the administration of a substance which in health would provoke a similar set of symptoms. This principle was often expressed as *similia similibus currentur* ('Let likes be treated by likes'). For example, Hahnemann claimed that as quinine induced the same symptoms as malaria it would be valuable in the treatment of that disease. Assuming that the symptoms were the body's way of fighting off disease, Hahnemann concluded that a medicine which produced those symptoms would help the body win the battle. Concerned by the unpleasant side effects of drugs in conventional dosage, Hahnemann experimented by giving small doses and formulated the second claim for homœopathy – the smaller the dose, the greater the beneficial effect.

Homœopathic remedies, most of which are based on medicinal herbs, are prepared by a process known as potentization. One part of the medicinal substance is dissolved in nine parts of water, alcohol or lactose, and shaken vigorously. This mixture is diluted in the same way again until dilutions as great as $1:10^{200}$ are reached. It is difficult to imagine how a medicinal substance can exert any effect at this dilution – a doubt countered by homœopathists with the explanation that the molecular pattern of the diluted substance 'imprints' itself on the solvent.

However the merits of homœopathy are viewed, it has one strength in that it is completely safe and tends to focus more attention on the general aspect of the patient than on the disease. Homœopaths speak of 'sepia' or 'pulsatilla' types. The sepia type tends to be tired-looking, sallow, narrow chested, and often constipated, whereas pulsatilla types are blonde, weepy and dislike heat and fatty food.

The homœopathic aim is to find a remedy which is perfectly suited to a particular patient. Less attention is given to precise diagnosis compared with the detailed appraisal of the pattern of symptoms which forms an integral part of the homœopathic approach. As might be expected from this approach, it is contrary to the whole concept of homœopathy to give remedies on the basis of disease names. To further his intention of the 'total' approach, the homœopathic practitioner will even take detailed account of illnesses suffered by parents and grandparents, and these may influence the type of treatment given.

Homœopathic preparations are obtained from the following raw materials:

1. Mineral materials such as metals, salts, acids, as well as synthetic medicines.

2. Products of vegetable or animal origin.

These preparations are described with the Latin name of the drug, followed by its dilution, e.g. *pulsatilla* 6.

In rheumatic sufferers, the choice of preparation may be governed by aggravating factors. For instance, if the symptoms are better in rainy weather *rhus tox* might be given, whereas symptoms worse in these conditions may be treated with *causticum.*

There is little controlled evidence to support the homœopathic idea, but some unpublished work conducted in Glasgow (Gibson *et al.*, cited by Eagle, 1978a) has shown interesting results. The survey compared groups of patients with rheumatoid arthritis. Fifty patients were treated with large doses of aspirin, another 50 were kept on their existing treatment and, in addition, were given a homœopathic remedy, and another group were given a placebo. After a year, half of the homœopathically-treated group had come off all their medicines and another 20% felt improved. This was compared with the aspirin group, of which only one in six still found the drug useful and the placebo group who complained after 6 weeks that it was of no benefit.

Homœopathy is practised by over 300 British doctors (mainly GPs) who belong to the Faculty of Homœopathy. There are still six homœopathic hospitals in England and Scotland. The practice of homœopathy enjoys the stamp of approval of the Royal family, several members of which have been treated by a homœopathic physician. There are an unknown number of lay practitioners, but these are excluded from the Faculty. Most radionic practitioners and some naturopaths prescribe homœopathic remedies.

11.2.14 Hypnotherapy

> The mind has the same command over the body as the master over the slave.
>
> Aristotle (384–322 BC)

Hypnotherapy has been called the 'talking cure'. Hypnosis is a self-induced state of relaxation and concentration in which the deeper parts of the mind became more accessible, and during which the patient talks rather than the therapist.

The word hypnosis was coined by James Braid in 1842 when he believed the phenomenon to be a form of sleep. When he realised it had little to do with sleep, and that the patient is probably more alert (though more relaxed) while in hypnosis, he substituted the word 'mono-ideism', but this did not catch on.

Hypnosis may be induced by a therapist or it may be self-induced. Hypnotherapy may be conducted by medical practitioners or by hypnotherapists (usually members of the British Hypnotherapy Association, founded in 1958).

Little is known about the application of hypnotherapy in the field of rheumatology, although if it is of any value it would probably be in the field of psychologically governed rheumatic disorders. There have been claims for its efficiency in treating neuroses (Brian, 1978), and patients whose rheumatic ailment, real or imaginary, is coloured by neurotic features such as anxiety or nervous tension, might be helped. There is also a claim that hypnosis is useful in psoriasis (Brian, 1978), and this, too, might have a rheumatic application in the future in view of the established association between the skin disease and arthritis. Perhaps the same may be said of other psychosomatic disorders, such as ulcerative colitis.

11.2.15 Macrobiotics and other dietary methods

Macrobiotics describes an attitude to life and health that is based on a faith in the importance of diet. It is not only a form of natural medicine but also involves a philosophy aimed at maintaining good health and happiness.

The underlying principle which governs the selection of food in a macrobiotic diet is, like that of acupuncture, based on Yin and Yang. In broad terms, in food Yin corresponds to acid and Yang to alkaline. Yin foods include fruits, drinks, summer-grown foods, foods of sweet, sour or hot flavour, foods of large expansive texture, and foods that are purple, blue or green. Yang foods include those of animal origin, cereals, some vegetables, and foods that are compact, hard, red, yellow or orange, salty or bitter, and which mature in the autumn and winter. Macrobiotic foods are centred on the whole grains, brown rice, whole wheat, rye, barley, oats, millet, buckwheat and maize. Vegetables and pulses supplement the grains. Soya bean products provide a rich source of amino acids. Other macrobiotic food items include salted pickled plums, muteen, and herbs including ginseng.

Diagnosis is achieved on a basis of facial and physical characteristics, colour, acupuncture pulses, digestive function, as well as by considering the specific symptoms.

It is claimed that most disorders can be helped by the macrobiotic principle, although there is little information on its effect on rheumatic ailments.

Macrobiotics should be distinguished from other dietary approaches, such as that of Dong and Banks (1973, 1976) which is based on an assumption that rheumatic disease is an allergy to food additives and preservatives and can be avoided by a high-protein, low-calorie 'natural' regimen. Nor is macrobiotics related to other dietary claims in the rheumatic field, such as enthusiasm for the idea that a 'corrective diet' containing 'oil-bearing foods' such as milk will lubricate the joints and restore their function (Alexander, 1957).

There is still no objective evidence to support the specific value of these 'anti-rheumatic' diets, or of other nutritional approaches.

Indeed, the only convincing evidence that diet is of relevance in rheumatic disorders (other than the mechanical benefit on weight-bearing joints through weight reduction) concerns gout in which a diet low in purine is effective in lowering the serum urate level (Gutman and Yu, 1952), a similar effect being achieved through avoiding an excessive alcohol consumption (MacLachlan and Rodnan, 1967).

11.2.16 Medicated bee venom therapy

This therapy grew from the observation that bee keepers have been notably free from rheumatoid arthritis since early Roman times (Broadman, 1962).

According to Owen (1978) (who, during 52 years of continuous work has claimed to have successfully treated countless patients with ankylosis, osteo- and rheumatoid arthritis), the bees must be of a special strain, hygienically bred, carefully selected and medically dieted to suit the type of each person's ailment. Garden bees should be avoided, as it is claimed their stings are dangerous. After the bee has been fed on the necessary medicaments, the back of its head is pinched to stun it and it is then applied to the patient. The bees die after implanting their sting. Patients are subjected to blood and urine tests and sometimes X-ray examination. Treatment lasts for a minimum of 3 weeks.

There is yet little scientific support for claims concerning success of this treatment, although work is in progress to search for the active principle involved.

11.2.17 Naturopathy

Naturopathy (as opposed to Naturism – the benefits of nude swimming and sun bathing) bases its philosophy on the healing power present in all living things. Hippocrates referred to this life-force as '*vis medicatrix naturae*'. According to Castle (1978) 'naturopathy embraces all the therapeutic methods by which the organism may be guided to its original state of wholeness'. Thus no single therapeutic method is involved, but rather a combination which may involve osteopathy, dieting, fasting, hydrotherapy, supplementary vitamins and minerals, abstention from drugs, tobacco and alcohol.

Although 'rheumatism' has been included as one of the disorders of relevance to the naturopathic principle, there is yet no substantiation for this and, indeed, the heterogeneity of the method would make its therapeutic effect difficult to measure. However, naturopathic practitioners themselves admit that their doctrine is more concerned with the prevention of disease than with its treatment, although claims stating that naturopathy is 'concerned with the prevention of disease by means of education in nature cure to maintain a maximum level of health through correct living, eating and thinking; and it encourages the growth of an ever-widening awareness of cosmic harmony' do little to convince orthodox practitioners of the plausibility of such a method.

11.2.18 Osteopathy

Osteopathy was founded by an American country doctor, Andrew Taylor, in the 1850s. Taylor declared that displaced vertebrae compressed nearby arteries and thus caused disease by obstructing the flow of blood to internal organs.

The osteopathic principle is based on manipulating the spine mainly with leverage rather than with thrusts,

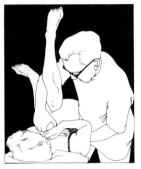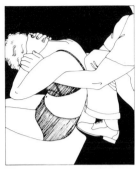

Fig. 11.7 Osteopathic manoeuvres aimed at manipulating the spine using the leverage principle to treat vertebral 'displacements'.

in order to correct these 'vertebral displacements' (Fig. 11.7).

Eagle (1978b) cites a recent survey by the Osteopathic Association of Great Britain which revealed that 52% of osteopaths' patients sought treatment for low back pain, 20% for neck pains, 13% for other spinal problems, and 7% for headaches.

There is evidence that doctors are overcoming their mistrust of non-medical manipulators, and, according to the Osteopathic Association of Great Britain, 88% of its members co-operate with general practitioners and accept patients referred by them.

There have been many attempts to introduce legislation to bring osteopaths and chiropractors into the National Health Service, but all have failed because the heterodox manipulators were reluctant to accept lower status than doctors, and thereby lose their right to diagnose and treat with the freedom to which they were accustomed. Another factor concerned the complicated rivalry among osteopaths. The fact that there are three osteopathic registers illustrates this:

1. The General Council and Register of Osteopaths (whose members can be styled 'MRO' after a 4-year course at the British School of Osteopaths, or, in the case of doctors, after a 1-year course at the London College of Osteopathy).

2. The British Naturopathic and Osteopathic Association which regards diet, hydrotherapy and heat treatment as valuable adjuncts to manipulation.

3. The Society of Osteopaths which accepts graduates from (1) and (2) and has close links with the European College of Osteopaths in Maidstone.

Evidence for the efficacy of osteopathy versus other types of manipulation is lacking. Even with regard to orthodox manipulation the results vary. For instance, Evans *et al.* (1978) were able to demonstrate significant improvement after rotational manipulation of the lumbar spine, whereas Doran and Newell (1975), and

Glover *et al.* (1974) observed no difference between their manipulated patients and those treated by other methods such as short-wave diathermy.

11.2.19 Spa therapy

> One would think the English were ducks: they are forever waddling to the waters.
>
> Horace Walpole (1717–97)

Spa therapy (named after Spa, one of Europe's best-known mineral springs in the Belgian Ardennes), although known at least since the sacking of Vichy by the Normans in the ninth century, suddenly flowered in England in the seventeenth century. At this time, the fame of established continental spas (Baden, Gastein, Ems, Pyrmont, Baden Baden, Contrexeville, Marienbad, Hamburg and Apollinaris) caught the attention of the English, and several hitherto obscure villages became fashionable watering places where the more privileged classes could 'take the cure'. The earliest spas were established in Tunbridge Wells (1606), Scarborough (1622), Epsom (1625), Sadlers Wells (1683), Islington (1685) and Cheltenham (1716). Later came Buxton, Droitwich, Harrogate, Leamington, Malvern and Matlock, with Llandrindod in Wales, and Moffat and Strathpeffer in Scotland (Fig. 11.8).

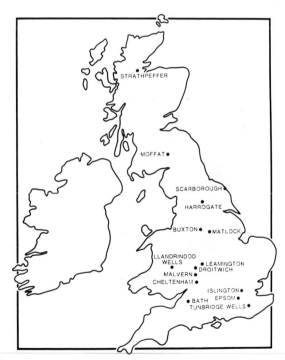

Fig. 11.8 Map showing some popular spas in England, Wales and Scotland. Most of these are no longer in use.

From the 1740s America, too, began to exploit various springs and wells used by the Indians (e.g. Berkeley Spring, Virginia; Gettysburg, Buffalo; Poland Spring, Maine).

At most spas, whether in Europe or America, the value claimed for the treatment depended on the chemical content of the water. Some like Spa itself or Tunbridge Wells were rich in iron, others contained soluble chlorides and sulphates of magnesium, sodium and calcium, such as the salty waters of Woodhall Spa in Lincolnshire. Some spas were noted for their more evil-smelling waters due to carbon dioxide and hydrogen sulphide, such as those at Harrogate and Baden, and White Sulphur Springs in West Virginia.

Apart from drinking the water or 'taking the waters' (Fig. 11.9) as it was called, often at a rate of a dozen or more glasses a day, the daily routine at a spa involved various types of bathing which must have been little different from modern hydrotherapy. 'Watering places' which concentrated more on bathing were often called 'hydros'. Special gadgets were available for the purpose of providing 'local hydrotherapy', and other variants included steam baths, rain baths, mud baths, and baths medicated with pine and lavender. One spa even prepared baths of freshly prepared steaming tripe! Other therapy included massage ('champooing'), electrical therapy (often quite dangerous), exercise and relaxation, often in the form of organized entertainment.

In Britain the spa has declined, and the only one which flourished on a large scale until recently was Bath. However, it is still possible to take the waters, such as at Buxton*. The reason for this decline probably has to do with the increasing popularity of the seaside resort in this century, and also the fact that the Englishman took the cure because he was ill, whereas in other parts of Europe it was, and still is, more popular as a family holiday. France and Germany between them can still boast nearly 400 active spas and the Soviet Union has another 300 or so.

There is little direct evidence for the value of spa therapy other than for its obvious merits of promoting mental and physical rest and perhaps for a placebo effect from drinking large volumes of unpleasant-tasting water. However, with some exceptions (e.g. Hill, 1939) there is some indirect evidence to show that climatic humidity, temperature, and barometric pressure can influence the symptoms (but not the natural history) of rheumatic disorders (Peterson, 1935; Edström, 1948; Hollander, 1961 and 1963; Hollander and Yeostros, 1963; Nava and Seda, 1964; Hill, 1972). Some of this evidence, particularly that of Hollander, suggests that it is changes in climate rather than the absolute values of the physical composition of it that are important in affecting symptoms.

Other, rather more direct evidence for a real effect of spa therapy was recently presented by Grahame *et al.* (1978). These workers showed that a significant diuresis, natriuresis and kalluresis could be achieved after immersion in water for 1 hour in healthy subjects. They also demonstrated significant reduction in joint swelling in patients with rheumatoid arthritis. The only other work related in any way to this is that of Copeman and

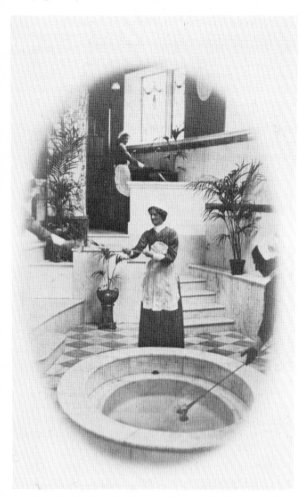

Fig. 11.9 'Taking the Waters'—St Ann's Well, Buxton (from a Late-Victorian photograph).

* Buxton has been used as a spa since Roman times (*Aquae Arnemetiae* meaning 'The Spa of the Goddess of the Grove'). The slightly radioactive water (3000 millimicrocuries per hour) rises from the spring at a natural temperature of 82° F (28° C) and is delivered at St Anne's Well at a price of 3p per glass. (As about 250 000 gallons issue from the spring per day, the well commands a potential profit of £180,000 per day!)

Pugh (1945) who reported beneficial effects of artificial dehydration on 'rheumatism'.

11.2.20 Spiritual healing

Spiritual healing is the transfer of energy from the healer to the patient. It is believed that this energy, in the form of charged particles known to Eastern yogis as prana (universal life force), flows in abundance throughout space and can be harnessed by the healer who sensitizes himself by certain occult practices such as prayer, deep breathing and the use of holy mantra (sound vibrations) chanted many times to build up the intake of energy (Nielson, 1978).

Many of the most spectacular healing 'cures' have been on people suffering from arthritis, whose joints have been locked and painful for years.

Remarkably little scientific research has been conducted in this field. Eagle (1978b) cites the work of a Canadian psychiatrist, Dr Bernard Grad and a New York biochemist, Dr Justin Smith, which demonstrated that a well-known healer was able to accelerate the activity of enzymes by holding the flesh in his hands. The healer was also able to speed wound healing in mice by placing his hands on their cages for a few minutes twice a day. However, to my knowledge this work has not been published.

There are more than 2000 active members of the National Federation of Spiritual Healers, and several thousand other healers outside it. Despite the name of the organization, only a minority are 'spiritualists' who believe that their power comes from disincarnate spirits. Those who call themselves 'faith' healers are usually Evangelical Christians or Roman Catholics who believe that healing is part of religious faith.

11.2.21 Swedish and other types of massage

> The physician must be experienced in many things, among others in friction.
>
> Hippocrates (460–375 BC)

Although the Swedish method of massage is the most commonly used and most internationally known, it has been in existence for a mere 100 years or so, compared with massage generally which originated in early Chinese medicine several thousands of years BC. The Chinese believed that massage and exercise prevented stagnation of body fluids and that this maintained health.

The words 'friction' and 'rubbing' were used in historical literature until the end of the nineteenth century when the term 'massage' was introduced. The origin of the word is uncertain. It could have been from the Hebrew *mashesh*, the Arabic verb *massa* (to touch), the Greek *massein* (to knead), or from the Portuguese *amassar* (to knead) which is formed from *massa* (dough). France is usually accredited with the introduction of the words 'massage', 'masseur' and 'masseuse'.

The T'ang dynasty (AD 619–907) had four kinds of recognized medical practitioners: physicians, acupuncturists, masseurs and exorcists. Priests of ancient Egypt used manipulation in the form of kneading to relieve rheumatic pains, neuralgia and swellings, and the Hindus, the Greeks, and the Romans also had some knowledge of the therapeutic value of massage. With regard to the last it is known that gladiators used the technique to relieve their pains as well as to invigorate themselves. By the Middle Ages the use of massage had declined.

It was Per Henrik Ling (1776–1838), a Swede, who redeveloped an interest in massage, and it is his method, or variants of it, which are in popular use today.

Swedish massage consists of five components: effleurage (a stroking movement to accelerate the flow of blood and lymph); petrissage (manipulation of muscle to empty deep veins); percussion movements (hacking, clapping, beating, pounding); running vibrations (the fingertips following the course of nerves); friction (used over joint surfaces and over localized lesions to produce local hyperaemia and restoration of mobility).

By a combination of these techniques it is claimed that the skin and all its structures are nourished and that it becomes soft and pliable. Further claims are as follows: the fat cells in the subcutaneous tissue are broken down; the blood circulation is increased; the activity of the skin glands is stimulated; the muscle fibres are strengthened; the nerves are soothed and rested; the body is relaxed, and tension and pain are relieved (Peplow, 1978). Objective evidence for these affirmations is not yet to hand, but there can be little doubt about the validity of the comments made in the last sentence, even if the other assertions are perhaps unduly ambitious.

Other types of massage exist, one variety being related to acupuncture. This method, Shiatsu massage or acupressure, which is still widely practised in Japan today, is based on the concept of meridia connecting points (*tsube*) just beneath the surface of the skin. These trigger points, it is claimed, when stimulated by thumb or finger pressure have a local or distant effect through a physiological effect. It has been found to be of value in 'rheumatism' and other medical disorders such as hypertension, diabetes and migraine, but there is no 'hard' evidence to support such claims.

11.2.22 Urine therapy

Urine therapy is a method of treating disease by fasting and drinking one's own urine, together with plain drinking water. It also involves the external application of urine compresses to the skin. It was used by the ancient Greeks for the treatment of wounds, and is still employed by the Eskimos for this purpose.

In Armstrong's *The Water of Life – A Treatise on Urine Therapy* (Armstrong, 1971), the author reports a number of case histories showing successful results using urine therapy in conditions such as psoriasis, jaundice, cancer and gangrene. However, none of this evidence is of a controlled type, and to the orthodox practitioner this approach to therapy, except perhaps in dermatological conditions, will continue to be questionable. However, in view of its dramatic and esoteric impact it will doubtless represent a potent force among placebo reactors. Its possible non-placebo value in skin disease (psoriasis, eczema, icthyosis) has a conventional precedent in the form of urea creams, lotions and other external preparations (e.g. Kligman). However, strengths of 20% are used in these applications (e.g. Calmuria) which are incomparable with the dilutions of urea found in human urine (1–2%). Urea has been found to be useful as a bactericidal agent (Symmers and Kirk, 1915), as a stimulant to healing of chronic purulent wounds (Robinson, 1936), and as a softener of scar tissue, but again, the strengths of urea used in these medicaments were substantially greater than those found in urine.

11.2.23 Vegetarianism

A vegetarian is one who refrains from eating flesh foods such as meat, fish, fowl and all their derivatives. There are two basic forms of vegetarianism: vegans who eat no animal foods, and lacto-ovo vegetarians who take milk, cheese, butter, cream and honey, in addition to fruits, vegetables, nuts and grains.

It is claimed that vegetarians suffer less from diseases like rheumatoid arthritis, coronary heart disease, diverticulitis, appendicitis, stomach ulceration, cancer of the colon and worm diseases (Hulke, 1978). Seventh Day Adventists have half to two-thirds the average incidence of cancer deaths, and almost half the incidence of heart disease, stroke and arteriosclerosis, compared with other Americans. Adventists do not drink alcohol or smoke, which may account for their low frequency of cancer of the lung, mouth, oesophagus and bladder. However, even if compared with non-smokers in the general population, Adventists still have a much lower frequency of cancer of the breast, ovary, prostate and bowel, which suggests a directly beneficial effect of their vegetarian diet. Further evidence comes from a comparison between Adventists who eat more meat, fish and dairy products than other Adventists. The former have been found to have more heart disease and bowel cancer. Adventists who suffered breast or bowel cancer were found to have eaten more fried foods and more refined foods such as white bread, cake and pie. The Adventists who did not get cancer ate more green leafy vegetables, beans and milk (Phillips, cited by Gillie and Mercer, 1978)

11.2.24 Weight Watchers

Weight Watchers was started in 1961 by Jean Nidetch who, after dieting on and off nearly all her life, finally resolved to follow a balanced eating plan – but she found she could not stick to it alone. She needed someone to talk to, someone sympathetic, and someone with the same problem and the same determination to beat it.

Weight Watchers is now a world-wide concern offering something like 13 000 weekly classes. Weight Watchers came to the UK in 1967, and there are now over 800 weekly classes in this country.

All meetings are based on the group therapy concept and involve a regular recording of weight, emphasis on 'goal weight', and a 'maintenance plan' once this has been achieved. Success is rewarded by applause and presentation of awards, while lack of success is discussed, and, in some organizations, punished with a fine. A lecturer, formerly a fat person, leads the class discussion, but he or she does not usurp the function of the nutritionist or other medical adviser.

The value of reducing weight in overweight patients with arthritis of weight-bearing joints and spine is a generally accepted fact in the management programme of patients with rheumatic disorders, and many patients lacking in self-motivation find Weight Watchers' sessions a useful and productive adjunct to dieting.

11.2.25 Yoga

Yoga is controlling the waves of the mind.

Patanjali (c. 200 BC)

The word 'yoga' means union or communion and is a pragmatic science evolved over thousands of years which deals with the physical, moral, mental and spiritual well-being of man. The traditional path to the ultimate mastery of yoga is the 'Eight Limbs of Yoga' first described by Patanjali in about 200 BC.

The first two 'limbs', Yama (moral commandments) and Niyama (purification through discipline), control passions and emotions. The third stage is represented by the 200 Asanas (postures) which keep the body healthy and strong. The next two stages, Pranayama (rhythmic control of the breath) and Pratyahara (freeing the mind from the senses), are known as 'the inner guests'. Dharana (concentration), Dhyana (meditation), and Samadhi (a state of super-consciousness brought about by deep meditation) finally allow the yogi to realize his 'self'.

Britain is already the world's largest centre for yoga outside India and many patients with rheumatic disorders try it. Although it could help certain back complaints through improving posture, it would be reasonable to expect on the other hand, unless carefully supervised, undue strain to already affected joints and periarticular structures in view of the extreme postures and manoeuvres expected of those aspiring to higher grades of the discipline.

Possibly the most valuable place of yoga is in patients whose symptoms are related more to stress than somatic abnormality in view of the mental and physical relaxation engendered by this discipline.

11.3 SUMMARY AND CONCLUSIONS

Many, but by no means all, of the alternative methods used to treat rheumatic disorders have been reviewed. Some, such as acupuncture, herbalism, the manipulation techniques used by osteopaths and chiropractors, and massage lie near to orthodox medicine. Others, however, may be described as truly heterodox, and these methods, which include techniques such as biofeedback, flower healing and Gerson therapy, bear little or no relation to anything practised by the conventional western doctor, and will doubtless continue to be viewed with scepticism.

Heterodox remedies, however, no matter how bizarre, expensive or lacking in evidence to support them, continue to attract attention from a substantial proportion of our patients, and this perhaps reflects to some extent their dissatisfaction with orthodox therapy. Moreover, it is likely that this trend will continue until scientifically approved cures are found for the various disorders of the locomotor system.

For further historical details concerning some of the sections, notably those covering cupping, herbalism, massage, and spa therapy, the reader is referred to Chapter 1.

11.4 REFERENCES AND FURTHER READING

General introduction

Eagle, R. (1978a) *Alternative Medicine. A Guide to the Medical Underground*, Futura, London.

Eagle, R. (1978b) On the fringe. *Observer Magazine*, 21 May.

Editors of Consumer Reports Books (1980) in *Consumers Union's Report on False Health Claims, Worthless Remedies and Unproved Therapies*, Consumers Union, New York.

Everitt, G. (1888) *Doctors and Doctors: Some Curious Chapters in Medical History and Quackery*, Swan Sonnenschein, Lowrey and Company, London.

Hart, F.D. (Undated) in *A Guide to Arthritis and Other Rheumatic Diseases*, Arthritis and Rheumatism Council, London.

Hulke, M. (ed.) (1978) *The Encyclopedia of Alternative Medicine and Self-Help*, Rider, London.

Inglis, B. (1964) *Fringe Medicine*, Faber and Faber, London.

Inglis, B. (1979) *Natural Medicine*, Collins, London.

Jayson, M.I.V. and Dixon, A.S. (1974) in *Rheumatism and Arthritis. What they are and what you should know about them*, Pan, London, pp. 260–71.

Katz, W.A. (1977) in *Rheumatic Diseases. Diagnosis and Management* (ed. W.A. Katz), Lippincott, Philadelphia.

Nightingale, M. and Graham, N. (1978) *The Better Life. Alternative Medicine*, Marshall Cavendish, London.

Schul, B. (1977) *The Psychic Frontiers of Medicine*, Coronet, London.

Stanway, A. (1980) *Alternative Medicine*, Macdonald and Jane's, London.

Acupuncture

Anderson, D.G., Jamieson, J.L. and Man, S.C. (1974) Analgesic effects of acupuncture on the pain of ice-water: a double-blind study. *Can. J. Psychol.*, **28**, 239.

Asustin, M. (1974) *Acupuncture Therapy*, Turnstone, London.

Balagura, S. and Ralph, T. (1973) The analgesic effect of electrical stimulation of the diencephalon and mesencephalon. *Brain Res.*, **60**, 369.

Bonica, J.J. (1953) *The Management of Pain*, Lea and Febiger, Philadelphia.

Bonica, J.J. (1974) Therapeutic acupuncture in the People's Republic of China. *J. Am. Med. Assoc.*, **228**, 1544.

Eagle, R. (1978a) in *Alternative Medicine. A Guide to the Medical Underground*, Futura, London, p. 127.

Gaw, A.C., Chang, L.W. and Shaw, L. (1975) Efficacy of acupuncture on osteoarthritic pain. *N. Engl. J. Med.*, **293**, 375.

Godfrey, C.M. and Morgan, P. (1978) A controlled trial of the theory of acupuncture in musculo-skeletal pain. *J. Rheumatol.*, **5**, 121.

Livingston, W.K. (1943) *Pain Mechanisms*, Macmillan, New York.

Man, S.C. and Baragar, F.D. (1974) Preliminary clinical study of acupuncture in rheumatoid arthritis with painful knees, *J. Rheumatol.*, **1**, 126.

Manaka, Y. and Urquhart, I. (1972) *The Layman's Guide to Acupuncture*, Weatherhill, New York.

Mann, F. (1971a) *Acupuncture. The Ancient Chinese Art of Healing*, Heinemann, London.

Mann, F. (1971b) *Cure of Many Diseases*, Heinemann, London.

Mann, F. (1971c) *The Meridians of Acupuncture*, Heinemann, London.

Mann, F. (1973) *Acupuncture. The Ancient Chinese Art of Healing and How it Works Scientifically*, Vintage, New York.

Mann, F. (1974) *The Treatment of Disease by Acupuncture*, Heinemann, London.

Melzack, R. and Wall, P.D. (1965) Pain mechanisms: a new theory. *Science*, **150**, 971.

Melzack, R. and Wall, P.D. (1968) in *Pain* (eds A. Soulairac, J. Cahn and J. Charpentier), Academic Press, New York.

Melzack, R. (1973) *The Puzzle of Pain*, Basic Books, New York.

Melzack, R. (1978) Acupuncture and Musculoskeletal pain. *J. Rheumatol.*, **5**, 119.

Newton, J. (1978) in *The Encyclopedia of Alternative Medicine and Self-Help* (ed. M. Hulke), Rider, London, p. 21.

Osler, W. (1910) *Principles and Practice of Medicine*, 7th edn, Appleton, New York, p. 397.

Plotz, C.M. (1974) Acupuncture in rheumatic disease. *Arthr. Rheum.*, **17**, 944.

Review (1978) Acupuncture can be dangerous. *Br. Med. Assoc. News Rev.*, **4**, 585.

Rossi, G.F. and Zanchetti, A. (1957) The brainstem reticular formation. *Arch. Ital. Biol.*, **95**, 199.

Sola, A.E. and Williams, R.L. (1956) Myofascial pain syndromes. *Neurology*, **6**, 91.

Toguchi, M. (1974) *The Complete Guide to Acupuncture*, Thorsons, Wellingborough.

Travell, J. and Rinzler, S.H. (1952) The myofascial genesis of pain. *Postgrad. Med.*, **11**, 425.

Turban, E. and Urlich, S. (1978) The evaluation of therapeutic acupuncture. *Soc. Sc. Med.*, **12**, 39.

Warren, F.Z. (1976) *Freedom from Pain through Acupressure*, Wentworth, New York.

Worsley, J.R. (1973) *Everyone's Guide to Acupuncture*, Cassell, London.

Aromathérapie

Manry, M. (1964) *The Secret of Life and Youth*, MacDonald, Edinburgh.

Ryman, D. (1978) in *The Encyclopedia of Alternative Medicine and Self-Help* (ed. M. Hulke), Rider, London, p. 33.

Tisserand, R.B. (1971) *The Art of Aromatherapy*, C.W. Daniel, London.

Biofeedback

Blundell, G. (1977a) *E.E.G. Measurement*, Audio, London.

Blundell, G. (1977b) *The Omega 1 E.S.R. Meter*, Audio, London.

Blundell, G. (1978) in *The Encyclopedia of Alternative Medicine and Self-Help* (ed. M. Hulke), Rider, London, p. 46.

Eagle, R. (1978) in *Alternative Medicine. A Guide to the Medical Underground*, Futura, London, p. 92.

Chiropractic

Breen, A.C. (1977) Chiropractors and the treatment of back pain. *Rheumatol. Rehabil.*, **16**, 46.

Doran, D.M.I. and Newell, D.J. (1975) Manipulation in treatment of low back pain: a multicentre study. *Br. Med. J.*, **ii**, 161.

Gillet, H. and Liekens, M. (1973) *Belgian Chiropractic Research Notes*, Palmer College of Chiropractic, Davenport, Iowa.

Hewitt, D. and Wood, P.H.N. (1975) Heterodox practitioners and the availability of specialist advice. *Rheumatol. Rehabil.*, **14**, 191.

Kane, R.L., Leymaster, C., Olsen, D. *et al.* (1974) Manipulating the patient: a comparison of the effectiveness of physician and chiropractor care. *Lancet*, **i**, 1333.

Scofield, A.G. (1968) *Chiropractic*, Thorsons, Wellingborough.

States, A.Z. (1967) *Spinal and Pelvic Technics*, National College of Chiropractic, Lombard, Illinois.

Copper

Brown, D.H., Buchanan, W.W., El-Ghobarey, A.F. *et al.* (1979) Serum copper and its relationship to clinical symptoms in rheumatoid arthritis. *Ann. Rheum. Dis.*, **38**, 174.

Forbes, A. (1978) in *The Encyclopedia of Alternative Medicine and Self-Help* (ed. M. Hulke) Rider, London, p. 65.

Koskelo, P., Kekki, M., Virkkunen, M. *et al.* (1966) Serum ceruloplasmin concentration in rheumatoid arthritis, ankylosing spondylitis, psoriasis and sarcoidosis. *Acta Rheumatol. Scand.*, **12**, 261.

Niedermeier, W., Creitz, E.E. and Holley, H.L. (1962) Trace metal composition of synovial fluid from patients with rheumatoid arthritis. *Arthr. Rheum.*, **5**, 439.

Scudder, P.R., Al-Timimi, D., McMurray, W. *et al.* (1978a) Serum copper and related variables in rheumatoid arthritis. *Ann. Rheum. Dis.*, **37**, 67.

Scudder, P.R., McMurray, W., White, A.G. and Dormandy, T.L. (1978b) Synovial fluid copper and related variables in rheumatoid and degenerative arthritis. *Ann. Rheum. Dis.*, **37**, 71.

West, H.F. (1970) *The Chemical Pathology of Rheumatoid Arthritis*, Thomas, Springfield, p. 50.

Cupping

Newton, J. (1978) in *The Encyclopedia of Alternative Medicine and Self-Help* (ed. M. Hulke), Rider, London, p. 69.

Flower healing

Bellhouse, E. (1978) in *The Encyclopedia of Alternative Medicine and Self-Help* (ed. M. Hulke), Rider, London, p. 77.

Gerson therapy

Straus, M. (1978) in *Encyclopedia of Alternative Medicine and Self-Help* (ed. M. Hulke), Rider, London, p. 79.

Health foods

Hanssen, M. (1978) in *The Encyclopedia of Alternative Medicine and Self-Help* (ed. M. Hulke), Rider, London, p. 92.

Herbalism

Azad Khan, A.K., Akhtar, S. and Mahtab, H. (1980) Treatment of diabetes mellitus with *Coccinia indica*. *Br. Med. J.*, **280**, 1044.

Bach, E. (1952) *The Twelve Healers and Other Remedies*, C.W. Daniel, London.

Bishop, C. (1979) *The Book of Home Remedies and Herbal Cures*, Octopus, London.

Camp, J. (1973) in *Magic, Myth and Medicine*, Priory, London, p. 74.

Conway, D. (1977) *The Magic of Herbs.* Mayflower, St. Albans.

Culpeper, N. (1652) *The English Physitian or An Astro Physical Discourse of the Vulgar Herbs of this Nation*, Peter Cole, London.

Culpeper, N. (1653) *The English Physician Englarged*, Barker, London.

Didcott, E.F. (1978) in *The Encyclopedia of Alternative Medicine and Self-Help* (ed. M. Hulke), Rider, London, p. 98.

Fox, W. (1897) *The Working Man's Model Family Botanic Guide, or Every Man His Own Doctor*, 15th edn. Fox and Sons, Sheffield.

Genders, R. (1977) *A Book of Aromatics*, Daton, Longman and Todd, London.

Haslock, I. and Wright, V. (1971) Pantothenic acid in the treatment of osteoarthrosis. *Rheumatol. Phys. Med.*, **11**, 10.

Hewlett-Parsons, J. (1968) *Herbs, Health and Healing*, Thorsons, Wellingborough.

Hyatt, R. (1978) *Chinese Herbal Medicine. Ancient Art and Modern Science*, Wildwood House, London.

Jarvis, D.C. (1962) *Arthritis and Folk Medicine*, Pan, London.

Jayson, M.I.V. and Dixon, A. St. J. (1974) *Rheumatism and Arthritis*, Pan, London.

Kadans, J.M. (1970) *Encyclopedia of Medicinal Herbs.* Thorsons, Wellingborough.

Law, D. (1973) *Concise Herbal Encyclopedia*, Bartholomew, Edinburgh.

Levy, J. de B. (1974) *The Illustrated Herbal Handbook*, Faber and Faber, London.

Loewenfeld, C. (1964) *Herb Gardening*, Faber and Faber, London.

Loewenfeld, G.E. and Loewenfeld, C. (1978) in *Encyclopedia of Alternative Medicine and Self-Help* (ed. M. Hulke), Rider, London, p. 101.

Mességué, M. (1979) *Health Secrets of Plants and Herbs*, Collins, London.

Mitton, F. and Mitton, V. (1976) *Mitton's Practical Modern Herbal*, Foulsham, London.

Schauenberg, P. and Pavis, F. (1977) *Guide to Medicinal Plants*, Latterworth, Guildford.

Smith, K.V. (1978) *The Illustrated Earth Garden Herbal*, Elm Tree, London.

Talbott, J.H. (1970) *A Biographical History of Medicine*, Grune and Stratton, New York, p. 116.

Thomson, S. (1849) *New Guide to Health or Botanic Family Physician*, Simpkin, Marshall and Company, London.

Home remedies and self-medication

Bishop, C. (1979) *The Book of Home Remedies and Herbal Cures*, Octopus, London.

Ritter, T.J. (1916) in *The People's Home Medical Book*, Barum, Cleveland.

Wadsworth, M.E.J., Butterfield, W.J.H. and Blaney, R. (1971) *Health and Sickness: the Choice of Treatment. Perception of Illness and Use of Services in an Urban Community*, Tavistock, London, p. 60.

Homœopathy

Ainsworth, J.B.L. (1978) in *The Encyclopedia of Alternative Medicine and Self-Help* (ed. M. Hulke), Rider, London, p. 113.

Blackie, M.G. (1975) *The Patient, Not the Cure: The Challenge of Homœopathy*, MacDonald and Jane's, Lodnon.

Chevanon, P. and Levannier, R. (1977) *Emergency Homœopathic First-Aid*, Thorsons, Wellingborough.

Eagle, R. (1978a) in *Alternative Medicine*, Futura, London, p. 58.

Gordon Ross, A.C. (1977) *Arnica the Amazing Healer and a Dozen Other Homœopathic Remedies for Aches, Pains and Strains*, Thorsons, Wellingborough.

Sharma, C.H. (1974) *Manual of Homœopathy and Natural Medicine*, Turnstone, London.

Wheeler, C.E. and Kenyon, J.D. (1971) *An Introduction of the Principles and Practice of Homœopathy*, Health and Science Press, Holsworthy.

Hypnotherapy

Blythe, P. (1971) *Hypnotism: Its Power and Practice*, Arthur Barker, London.

Blythe, P. (1976) *Self-Hypnotism: Its Potential and Practice*, Arthur Barker, London.

Brian, R.K. (1978) in *The Encyclopedia of Alternative Medicine and Self-Help* (ed. M. Hulke), Rider, London, p. 122.

Hartland, J. (1971) *Medical and Dental Hypnosis and its Clinical Applications*, Baillière Tindall, London.

Macrobiotics

Alexander, D.D. (1957) *Arthritis and Common Sense*, World's Work Ltd., Kingswood, Tadworth.

Bieler, H.G. (1968) *Food is Your Best Medicine*, Spearman, Sudbury.

Crain, D.C. (1971) *The Arthritis Handbook*, Arlington, London.

Deadman, P. and Betteridge, K. (1977) *Nature's Foods*, Rider, London.

Dong, C.H. and Banks, J. (1973) *The Arthritic's Cookbook*, Hart-Davis, MacGibbon, London.

Dong, C.H. and Banks, J. (1976) *New Hope for the Arthritic*, Hart-Davis, MacGibbon, London.

Gutman, A.B. and Yu, T.-F. (1952) Gout, a derangement of purine metabolism. *Adv. Int. Med.*, **5**, 227.

Hunter, B.T. (1973) *The Natural Foods Primer: Help for the Bewildered Beginner*, Allen and Unwin, London.

MacLachlan, M.J. and Rodnan, G.P. (1967) Effect of food, fast and alcohol on serum uric acid and acute attacks of gout. *Am. J. Med.*, **42**, 38.

Sams, C. (1973) *About Macrobiotics*, Thorsons, Wellingborough.

Wordsworth, J. (1976) *Diet Revolution: Food Reform*, Gollancz, London.

Medicated bee venom therapy

Broadman, J. (1962) *Bee Venom: The Natural Curative for Arthritis and Rheumatism*, Putnam, New York.
Owen, J. (1978) in *Encyclopedia of Alternative Medicine and Self-Help* (ed. M. Hulke), Rider, London, p. 130.

Naturopathy

Benjamin, H. (1961) *Everybody's Guide to Nature Cure*, Thorsons, Wellingborough.
Castle, N. (1978) in *The Encyclopedia of Alternative Medicine and Self-Help* (ed. M. Hulke), Rider, London, p. 138.
Clements, H. (1973) *Nature Cure for Arthritis*, Thorsons, Wellingborough.
Editorial Committee, Science of Life Books (1975) *Rheumatism and Arthritis. An Outline of Common Causes and Safe Corrective Measures*, Science of Life Books, Melbourne.
Moyle, A. (1975) *Natural Health for the Elderly*, Thorsons, Wellingborough.
Newman Turner, R. (1969) *Naturopathic First Aid*, Thorsons, Wellingborough.

Osteopathy

Doran, D.M.L. and Newell, D.J. (1975) Manipulation in treatment of low back pain: a multicentre study. *Br. Med. J.*, **ii**, 161.
Eagle, R. (1978b) On the fringe. *Observer Magazine*, 21st May.
Evans, D.P., Burke, M.S., Lloyd, K.N. *et al.* (1978) Lumbar spinal manipulation on trial. Part I. Clinical assessment. *Rheumatol. Rehabil.*, **17**, 46.
Glover, J.R., Morris, J.G. and Khosla, T. (1974) Back pain: a randomized clinical trial of rotational manipulation of the trunk. *Br. J. Ind. Med.*, **31**, 59.
Hoag, J.M. (1969) *Theory and Practice in Osteopathic Medicine*, McGraw-Hill, New York.
Kane, R.L., Leymaster, C., Olsen, D. *et al.* (1974) Manipulating the patient: a comparison of the effectiveness of physician and chiropractor care. *Lancet*, **i**, 1333.
Roberts, G.M., Roberts, E.E., Lloyd, K.N. *et al.* (1978) Lumbar spinal manipulation on trial. Part II. Radiological assessment. *Rheumatol. Rehabil.*, **17**, 54.
Stoddard, A. (1959) *Manual of Osteopathic Technique*, Hutchinson, London.
Stoddard, A. (1969) *Manual of Osteopathic Practice*, Hutchinson, London.

Spa therapy

Copeman, W.S.C. and Pugh, L.G.C. (1945) Effects of artificial dehydration in rheumatism. *Lancet*, **ii**, 553.
Edström, G. (1948) Investigations into the effect of hot and dry microclimate on peripheral circulation, etc., in arthritic patients. *Ann. Rheum. Dis.*, **7**, 76.
Grahame, R., Hunt, J.N., Kitchen, S. and Gabell, A. (1978) The diuretic and natriuretic effect of water immersion – a

possible rationale for balneotherapy. *Ann. Rheum. Dis.*, **37**, 567.
Hill, L. (1939) Rheumatism and climate. *Br. Med. J.*, **ii**, 276.
Hill, D.F. (1972) in *Arthritis and Allied Conditions* (eds J.L. Hollander and D.J. McCarty), Lea and Febiger, Philadelphia, p. 256.
Hollander, J.L. (1961) The controlled-climate chamber for study of the effects of meteorological changes on human diseases. *Trans. N. Y. Acad. Sci.*, **24**, 167.
Hollander, J.L. (1963) Environment and musculoskeletal diseases. *Arch. Env. Hlth.*, **6**, 89.
Hollander, J.L. and Yeostros, S. (1963) The effect of simultaneous variations of humidity and barometric pressure in arthritis. *Bull. Am. Met. Soc.*, **44**, 489.
Nava, P. and Seda, H. (1964) The climate of Rio de Janeiro and painful crises of osteoarthritis of the spine. *Brasil-Medico*, **78**, 71.
Peterson, W.F. (1935) *The Patient and the Weather*, Edwards Bros., Ann Arbor.
Smedley, J. (1863) *Practical Hydrotherapy*, Caudwell, London.

Spiritual healing

Eagle, R. (1978b) On the fringe. *Observer Magazine*, 21st May.
Edwards, H. (1963) *The Power of Spiritual Healing*, Herbert Jenkins, London.
Hammond, S. (1973) *We are all Healers*, Turnstone, London.
Nielsen, R. (1978) in *The Encyclopedia of Alternative Medicine and Self-Help* (ed. M. Hulke), Rider, London, p. 178.
Ramacharaka, Y. (1971) *The Science of Psychic Healing*, Fowler, Romford.
Turner, G. (1975) *A Time to Heal*, Corgi, London.
Worrall, A.A. and Olga, N. (1969) *The Gift of Healing*, Rider, London.

Swedish and other types of massage

Downing, G. (1974) *Massage and Meditation*, Random House, New York.
Downing, G. (1974) *The Massage Book*, Penguin, Harmondsworth.
Goldberg, A.G. (1972) *Body Massage for the Beauty Therapist*, Heinemann, London.
Inkeles, G. and Todris, M. (1973) *The Art of Sensual Massage*, Allen and Unwin, London.
Irwin, Y. (1977) *Shiatzu, Japanese Finger Pressure for Energy, Sexual Vitality and Relief from Tension and Pain*, Routledge and Kegan Paul, London.
Leboyer, F. (1977) *Loving Hands: The Traditional Indian Art of Baby Massage*, Collins, London.
Namikoshi, T. (1973) *Shiatsu, Japanese Finger-Pressure Therapy*, Japan Publications, New York.
Newton, J. (1978) in *The Encyclopedia of Alternative Medicine and Self-Help* (ed. M. Hulke), Rider, London, p. 177.
Ohashi, W. (1977) *Do-it-yourself Shiatsu*, Mandala/Unwin, London.
Peplow, P. (1978) in *The Encyclopedia of Alternative Medicine and Self-Help* (ed. M. Hulke), Rider, London, p. 179.
Young, C. (1973) *The Touching Way to Sensual Health*, Bantam, New York.

Urine therapy

Armstrong, J.W. (1971) *The Water of Life. A Treatise on Urine Therapy*, 2nd edn, Health Science Press, Holsworthy.

Kligman, A.M. (1957) Dermatological uses of urea. *Acta Dermato-venereol.*, **37**, 155.

Newton, J. (1978) in *The Encyclopedia of Alternative Medicine and Self-Help* (ed. M. Hulke), Rider, London, p. 186.

Patel, R.M. (1963) *Manav Mootra (Human Urine as the Elixir of Life)*, Bharay Sevak Samaj Publications, Ahmabad.

Robinson, W. (1936) The use of urea to stimulate healing in chronic purulent wounds. *Am. J. Surg.*, **33**, 192.

Stewart, W.D., Danto, J.L. and Maddin, W.S. (1969) Urea cream. *Cutis*, **5**, 1241.

Symmers, W. St. C. and Kirk, T.S. (1915) Urea as a bactericide and its applications in the treatment of wounds. *Lancet*, **ii**, 1237.

Vegetarianism

Gillie, O. and Mercer, D. (1978) *The Sunday Times Book of Body Maintenance*, Michael Joseph, London, p. 37.

Hulke, M. (1978) in *The Encyclopedia of Alternative Medicine and Self-Help* (ed. M. Hulke), Rider, London, p. 188.

Jannaway, K. (1978) in *The Encyclopedia of Alternative Medicine and Self-Help*. (ed. M. Hulke), Rider, London, p. 186.

Weight Watchers

Wood, J. (1978) in *The Encyclopedia of Alternative Medicine and Self-Help* (ed. M. Hulke), Rider, London, p. 190.

Yoga

Bernard, T. (1968) *Hatha Yoga: The Report of a Personal Experience*. Rider, London.

Crisp, T. (1970) *Yoga and Relaxation*, Collins, London.

Hittleman, R. (1969) *Guide to Yoga Meditation*, Bantam, New York.

Iyengar, B.K.S. (1968) *Light on Yoga*, Allen and Unwin, London.

Kent, H. (1978) in *The Encyclopedia of Alternative Medicine and Self-Help* (ed. M. Hulke), Rider, London, p. 193.

Lysbeth, A. van (1974) *Yoga Self-Taught*, Allen and Unwin, London.

Volin, M. and Phelan, N. (1968) *Sex and Yoga*, Sphere, London.

Wills, H. and Wills, F. (1973) *Yoga for All*, BBC, London.

11.5 APPENDICES

11.5.1 Principal heterodox procedures available (from Hulke, 1978)

Absent healing	Cupping	Jogging	Radiesthesia
Acupuncture	Dianetics	Macrobiotics	Radionics
Alexander technique	Encounter	Mazdaznan	Recessed heel footwear
Applied kinesiology	Endogenous endocrinotherapy	Medicated bee venom therapy	Reflexology
Aromathérapie	Flower healing	Music therapy	Reichian therapy
Astrological diagnosis	Gerson therapy	Natural childbirth	Rolfing
Bates' method	Gestalt therapy	Naturism	Shiatsu massage
Belly dancing	Ginseng	Naturopathy	Spiritual healing
Bioenergy and biodynamics	Graphology	Neometaphysical concepts of psychology	Staplepuncture
Biofeedback	Hand healing	Orthomolecular psychiatry	Swedish massage
Biorhythms	Health farms	Osteopathy	T'ai-chi Ch'üan
Breathing – Knowles' therapy	Health foods	Prenatal therapy	The Tao of loving
Chiropractic	Hebraic name changing	Primal therapy	Transpersonal psychology
Co-counselling	Herbalism	Psionic medicine	Urine therapy
Colour therapy	Herbs with medical value	Psychic surgery	Vegan diet
Copper	High colonic irrigation	Psychodrama	Vegetarianism
Cosmetics	High-voltage photography	Pulsed high frequency	Weight Watchers
'Cranial' osteopathy	Homoeopathy		Wine
	Human aura		Yoga
	Hypnotherapy		

11.5.2 Associations and societies (from Hulke, 1978)

Where the type of therapy is not obvious from the name of the association or society, or from its journal, this has been included.

The Aetherius Society (Spiritual healing, metaphysical education)
Association for Dramatherapists
Association for Group and Individual Psychotherapy
Association for Humanistic Psychology
Association for Self-Help and Community Groups
Astrological Association
The Atlanteans (Meditation)
British Acupuncture Association and Register Ltd.
British and European Osteopathic Association
British Chiropractors' Association
British Homœopathic Association
British Hypnotherapy Association
British Mazdaznan Association (Master thought)
British Natural Hygiene Society
British Osteopathic Association
British Society for Music Therapy
British Wheel of Yoga
Central Council for British Naturism
Church of Scientology
College of Osteopathy and Manipulative Therapy Ltd.
Community Health Foundation
Counselling International (Co-counselling)
European Osteopathic Register
General Council and Register of Osteopaths Ltd.
Guild of Natural Medicine Practitioners
Hahnemann Society (Homœopathy)
Healing Research Trust (Natural therapeutics)
Health for the New Age (Holistic medicine)
Herb Society
Independent Register of Manipulative Therapists Ltd.
Institute of Biodynamic Psychology
International Federation of Practitioners of Natural Therapeutics Ltd.
London and Counties Society of Physiologists (Massage and manipulation)
Martindale Trust Ltd. (Acupuncture, homœopathy, osteopathy)
National Association for Health (Health foods)
National Association of Health Stores (Health foods)
National Childbirth Trust (Antenatal and postnatal counselling)
National Federation of Spiritual Healers
National Institute of Medical Herbalists
Prenatal Therapy Association
Psionic Medical Society/Institute of Psionic Medicine
Radionic Association
Relaxation for Living
Release (Drug problem counselling)
Research Society for Natural Therapeutics
Schizophrenia Association of Great Britain
Society of Metaphysicians Ltd.
Society of Osteopaths
Society to Support Home Confinements
Society of Teachers of the Alexander Technique
Vegan Society
Vegetarian Society (UK) Ltd.
Weight Watchers (UK) Ltd.

11.5.3 Health farms (from Hulke, 1978)

The therapeutic emphasis varies considerably between health farms, but collectively include such treatments as massage, heat, hydrotherapy, sauna, balneotherapy, osteopathy, acupuncture and dietetics. (The fees vary greatly, and range from about £50 to £350 per week.)

Champneys at Tring Health Resort, Tring.
Chevin Hall Health and Beauty Hotel, Otley.
Craig End Lodge Guest House, Ilkley.
Enton Hall Health Centre, Nr. Godalming.
Forest Mere Health Hydro, Liphook.
Grange Health and Beauty Farm, Henlow.
Grayshott Hall Health Centre, Nr. Hindhead.
Hygeia Clinic, Tetbury.
Inglewood Health Hydro, Nr. Newbury.
Lake District Health Centre, Kendal.
Malvern Hydro, Great Malvern.
Metropole Health Hydro, Brighton.
Mokoia Health Centre, Troon.
Nurtons Field Centre, Chepstow.
Panarwel Health and Beauty Hydro, Llanbedrog.
Ragdale Health Hydro, Melton Mowbray.
Ramana Health Centre, Liphook.
Shalimar Health Clinic, Frinton-on-Sea.
Sharnbrook Court, Sharnbrook.
Shenley Lodge Health Resort, Radlett.
Shrubland Hall Health Clinic, Ipswich.
Tyringham Naturopathic Clinic, Newport Pagnell.
Weymouth Hydro, Weymouth.

11.5.4 A typical diet based on 'health food' principles (from Hulke, 1978)

Breakfast

Wholegrain cereal such as muesli (use raw sugar if required)
Fresh fruit
100% wholewheat bread either with a free-range poached egg or honey or yeast-spread
Herbal tea or Ceylon low-caffeine tea.

Lunch

Salad of vegetables with wholewheat bread, cottage or other natural cheese.
Health store yoghourt free from artificial colours and flavours.
Fruit juice.

Dinner

Textured vegetable protein or minced meat made up with a tomato sauce, served with wholemeal spaghetti topped with grated cheese and flavoured with herbs such as oregano and basil.
Raw salad. Chocolate dessert made with Irish moss-based mould mixture.
Fresh fruit or cheese and biscuits.
Fruit juice.

11.5.5 Some herbs used in the treatment of 'rheumatism' (from Didicott, 1978)

Common name	Latin name	Alternative name	Administration and claimed effects
Aconite	*Aconitum napellus*	Monkshead	Ointment from root relieves neuralgic and rheumatic pains. Tincture reduces fevers.
Agrimony	*Eupatorium cannabinum*	Hemp	Tonic tea from leaves for rheumatism and colds. Cleanses wounds.
Arnica	*Arnica montana*		Tincture for external use on sprains and bruises. A teaspoon in bath water and 20-min. soak helps relax stiff muscles.
Betony	*Betonica officinalis*		Healing astringent tea for catarrhal conditions, digestion, rheumatism. In ointment for cuts, sores, ulcers.
Buckbean	*Menyanthes trifoliata*	Marsh trefoil	Tonic infusion for rheumatism, liver debility, skin diseases. Reduces glandular swellings.
Calamint	*Calamintha officinalis*	Mountain balm	Makes expectorant, diaphoretic tea. Poultice from leaves for rheumatic pains and bruises.
Capsicum	*Capsicum annum*	Chilli pepper	For treating dropsy, diarrhoea, toothache, gout. Makes strong liniment.
Chamomile	*Matricaria chamomilla*	True or wild chamomile	Dried flower decoction for abdominal pains, cystitis, rheumatism, dilated veins. Mouth rinse for sore gums and toothache. Inhalations for head colds and catarrh. Compresses for skin disorders, boils, eczema, conjunctivitis, haemorrhoids, earache, cramp.
Chervil	*Anthriscus cerifolium*		In food has stimulating effect on whole metabolism. Fresh herb poultice for painful joints.
Couchgrass	*Agropyrum repens*		Root used medicinally as blood cleanser, for bladder and kidney diseases, and rheumatism.
Chicory	*Cichorium intybus*		Juice from rind or fresh root makes decoction helpful for jaundice, gout, rheumatic conditions.
Ground elder	*Aegopodium podagraria*		Tisane (medicinal decoction), combined with hot fomentation made from root applied to painful joints, an effective remedy.
Hyssop	*Hyssopus officinalis*		Tisane for throat and chest complaints, irregular blood pressure, nervous disorders. Lotion applied externally relieves muscular rheumatism, cuts and bruises, ear, eye, and throat infections, insect bites.
Mugwort	*Artemesia vulgaris*		Mugwort tea for rheumatism, fevers, nervous disorders. Added to water makes good footbath.

11.5.5 Appendix (*Contd.*)

Common name	Latin name	Alternative name	Administration and claimed effects
Onion	*Allium cepa*		Antiseptic, diuretic, expectorant, detoxicant, antispasmodic, anthelminthic. Stimulates appetite, circulation, heart, nerves, glands; cleanses the blood, improves memory and concentration. Externally, raw juice relieves painful joints, improves brittle nails, draws out insect stings.
Parsley	*Petroselinum crispum* and *stavium*	Curled and Hamburgh	Leaf, seed and root rich in vitamins and active substances. Makes digestive tea. Relieves kidney and bladder complaints, rheumatism, Eliminates body fluids.
St. John's wort	*Hypericum perforatum*		Mixed with oil for painful joints, strained muscles, sprains, bruises, wounds, ulcers, rashes. Taken internally on sugar cube for colic, worms in children. Tisane good for nerves, gastritis, insomnia, fainting fits, menstrual pain.
Valerian	*Valeriana officinalis*	All-heal	Roots used for sedative sleep-inducing tea. Will calm headaches, upset stomach, distressed conditions, convulsions. Lotion applied to skin eruptions swollen joints, veins.
Yarrow	*Achillea millefolium*	Milfoil	Tisane an all-round remedy, especially rheumatism. Rich in active bitter substances, minerals, vitamins.

11.5.6 Home remedies for 'rheumatism' and 'gout' (from Ritter, 1916; Bishop, 1979)

(a) Remedies for 'rheumatism'

(A) External

1. 'Take 9 red peppers off stalks, 1 teaspoonful of salt, 1 snuff box of coal oil and 1 teacup of gasoline, and mix well. Put this on where it hurts'.
2. 'Place a pan of chicken droppings under the bed.'
3. 'Bind the joint with hot prickly pear poultice.'
4. 'Cut off the top of a toadstool and dry it. Wet it with whisky and use it as a linement.'
5. 'Mix a bucket of red ants with kerosene and sulphur and apply to the afflicted area.'
6. 'Fill a large kettle with water, thickened to a poultice consistency with chopped red peppers, and boil for 1 hour. Drop into the mixture a linen sheet and place steaming hot about the patient's body. Then tuck the patient up in hot blankets and encourage him to drink several cups of hot tea until the rheumatism is sweated out of his system.'
7. Potato soak remedy. 'Bathe the affected parts with water in which potatoes have been boiled, hot as can be tolerated, before going to bed.'
8. Potato poultice remedy 'Boil 2 potatoes in their jackets, mash (including skins), spread on a cloth, and apply.'
9. Skunk's oil remedy. 'Take 2 ounces of skunk's oil, the same quantity of cheap lamp oil and 1 teaspoonful of ground pepper; shake well and bathe the affected part with a piece of flannel dipped into the mixture.'
10. Rheumatic liquid remedy. 'Take 1 quart of alcohol, 1 ounce of spirit of turpentine, 1 ounce of beef's gall, 2 ounces of hartshorn, half an ounce of camphor gum and half an ounce of yellow cayenne pepper. Put into a bottle until dissolved. Rub on affected part 2 or 3 times a day.'
11. Bee sting remedy. Several 'doses' were given, the first involved being stung twice.
12. Disease transference. By far the most common objects used in transferring disease from the patient to something else are trees. A common method in Germany used to involve running around the tree and chanting 'God greet thee, noble tree, I bring thee my gout'. In England the practice was more painful, and involved putting one's head against a tree, nailing a lock of hair to the bark, and then jerking the head away so that the hair remained on the tree. In Wales it was the custom to wash a patient with pieces of rag, and then tie them to the branches of a nearby tree.
13. Mole remedy. For centuries in Europe the garden mole has been credited with curing all kinds of complaints, particularly cramp and rheumatism – the forelegs of the animal

being carried in the pocket to cure ailments in the arms, the hind legs to relieve pain in the lower limbs.

14. Sacrament money remedy. Coins given in a church collection and later brought from the priest and made into a chain or necklace were highly valued in many parts of Europe for treating epilepsy and rheumatism. Its power was thought to be enhanced if it had been carried three times round the communion table before it left the church.

15. Crickstone remedy. The sufferer was advised to find a large stone or rock with a hole big enough to accommodate the passage of the human body, such as the prehistoric crickstone near Lanyon Quoist, and: 'Go through the stone without touching it and you will never have rheumatism'.

16. Bedroom remedies. Small stones with holes were sometimes carried on a string or hung over the bed in order to keep rheumatism at bay. Other bedroom variants include taking a foreign object such as a potato, bottle cork, or metallic object (especially a magnet) to bed. These objects may either be placed between the sheets, tied to a leg, or held in the hand.

17. Seventh son remedy. As a remedy for back-pain it was recommended that a seventh son stand or walk upon the patient's back.

18. Cat remedy. 'Never kick a cat or you will get rheumatism'.

19. Ointments and liniments. Traditional materials recommended are camphor, dry mustard and oils. More bizarre concoctions include dissolving live earthworms or ants.

20. Silver or copper ring remedy. The rings should preferably be made from a coffin handle.

21. In ancient Rome it was recommended that arthritic patients place their feet on a torpedo fish and experience an electric shock.

22. Bath remedies. Folk medicine has developed from spa therapy and hydrotherapy, and involves adding herbs to the bath water. More unusual therapy uses ant baths – a version of a more painful method which recommends the application of live ants around the painful joint.

23. Christmas snow. 'Apply to the affected joint.'

24. Nettle therapy. 'Thrash the affected joints with a bunch of nettles.'

25. Hot bricks. 'Place the bricks for half an hour in an oven at a temperature sufficient to bake bread. Remove the bricks, wrap in flannel, and place under the bedclothes near to the rheumatic patient.'

26. Copper bangles. 'Wear a copper bangle to relieve rheumatic pain.'

27. Crow's meat remedy. 'Mix fresh crows meat with spirit and apply to the affected joint.'

28. Worm and Welk remedy. 'Take half an ounce each of oil of worm, oil of whelks, oil of St. John's Wort, oil of Chamomile and Spirits of wine, and apply to the affected part with a feather, by the fireside, before going to bed.'

(B) Internal

1. 'Collect some pill bugs, fry them and eat them.'

2. 'Chew and swallow dried rattlesnake flesh.'

3. Apple cider vinegar and honey remedy. 'Mix 1 tablespoon of apple cider vinegar, 1 dessertspoon of honey and 1 tablespoon of hot water and take on an empty stomach once a day.'

4. Celery remedy. 'Boil some celery in water until quite soft

and drink the liquor 3 or 4 times a day.'

5. Elecampane remedy. 'Take 2 handfuls of elecampane and put into 3 quarts of cider, boiling down to 1 quart. Take half a wine-glass full 3 times a day.'

6. Bitters' remedy. 'Prickly-ash berries, spikenard root, yellow poplar, and doz-wood barks, of each half a pound. Pulverize and put into a gallon jug and fill with brandy. Dose: a wine glass to be taken 3 times daily before meals.'

7. 'Prepare the Green Bay Indian's remedy as follows: Bark of Wahoo root, 1 ounce; blood root, 1 ounce, black cohosh root, 2 ounces; swamp hellebore, half an ounce; prickly ash bark or berries, 1 ounce; poke root, cut fine, 1 ounce; rye whisky, 1 quart. Let stand a few days before using. Dose: 1 teaspoon every 3–4 hours, increasing the dose to 2 or 3 teaspoons as the stomach will bear.'

8. 'Take cow dung gathered in May and add one third part of white wine and distil the mixture. Give 4 ounces to the patient and advise him to rest.'

9. 'Drink bat's blood.'

(b) Remedies for 'gout'

(A) External

1. Sweating remedy. 'Undress at six in the evening and wrap up in blankets. Then put your legs in water as hot as can be beared up to the knees. As it cools let hot water be poured in to keep you in a strong sweat until ten. Then go to bed and sweat till morning.'

2. Steak remedy. 'Apply raw steak to the affected part every 2 hours until cured.'

3. Treacle remedy. 'Rub the part with warm treacle and then bind on a treacle-smeared flannel. Repeat if necessary every 12 hours.'

4. Tallow and garlic remedy. 'Take the oldest tallow you can get and pound together with equal parts of garlic. Spread onto canvas and lay on the affected part.'

5. Citreous remedy. 'After roasting a large orange or lemon on hot ashes, remove the peelings and pound them with *anna flor cassia* in a glass mortar and mix with breast milk to make a poultice. Apply to the affected joint.'

6. Goat's milk and dung remedy. 'Render a mixture of goat's milk, butter and roast cow dung and apply as a poultice.'

7. Oil of earthworms remedy. Take some earthworms, wash and cut 6 ounces into pieces. Add a pint and a half of olive oil and boil together until the wine is exhaled. Finally strain off the oil through a piece of canvas.'

8. Owl remedy. 'Take an owl and pull off its feathers and pull out its guts. Salt it well for a week then put into a covered pot. Place the pot into an oven and when 'brought into a mummy' beat into a powder and mix with boar's grease. Anoint the affected part which should be placed in front of a fire.'

9. Frogspawn remedy. 'Obtain frogspawn from the clearest water and boil while it is a jelly and before it is 'black'. 'Still' it, and wash the affected parts with it while the remedy is still a little warm. Also dip the patient's clothes into the remedy and apply cold to the affected part.'

10. Ant-hill remedy. 'The gouty subject must take hold of an ant-hill and place it in a bag. The bag should then be cooked and used as a very hot poultice.'

(B) Internal

Elder bud remedy. 'Drink a pint of strong infusion of dry or green elder buds morning and evening.'

12
General summary and conclusions, including new developments and future prospects

12.1 GENERAL COMMENT

We are currently passing through a phase of rapid growth in the science and technology of medicine generally, and rheumatology in particular. The 'established' facts of yesterday's practice have today become critically challenged and tomorrow will perhaps be replaced. One purpose of this chapter is to outline a few prominent areas of development in the treatment and management of rheumatic diseases and, where this is possible, to look into the future. Many of the topics discussed had barely reached medical attention when this book was started 3 years ago, some have arisen since, and doubtless more will be reported during the process of publication. Finally, an overall summary will be given.

12.2 COMMUNICATION

The undoubted value of communication in rheumatology has been expressed in Chapter 3. The importance of communication in the context of rheumatological management stems from the fact that rheumatic patients can do a lot to help themselves, but to achieve this they must be given enough information in the right sort of way.

Over recent years a sound background to the clinical application of communication has been firmly established in non-medical quarters (e.g. mathematics, physics, computer technology, graphics). This led to important pioneer work both in community-based and hospital-based patients by workers such as Cartwright, Joyce, Ley and Wright (references to these authors can be found in Chapter 3). For general literature the reader is referred to Balint and Norell (1973), Tanner (1976), Harlem (1977) and McLachlay (1979). It is now up to clinicians to utilize this knowledge to penetrate the field more extensively.

As the author has outlined in more detail elsewhere (Moll, 1981), the most likely area to produce fruitful results concerns the more 'human' psychomedical aspects of the subject. More specifically, the following questions still need convincing answers, and it is hoped that at least some of them may stimulate future lines of investigation:

1. What kinds of patients should be given information?
2. Do patients want to be given information?
3. Are some areas of knowledge more conducive to being communicated than others?
4. What are the best vehicles for communicating medical facts to patients among currently available media?
5. Are doctors sufficiently aware of their inexpertise at communicating with patients?
6. Does communication with patients improve their compliance in taking drugs, doing exercises, and responding to other self-help advice?
7. Can communication with patients be counter-productive or even harmful?
8. What is the optimal verbo-visual balance in communicating with patients?

Once these fundamental questions have been resolved it is interesting to speculate on likely channels of communication in the future. Although the important counselling role of the doctor is unlikely to change, it is probable that adjuncts to communication will become more sophisticated. One can envisage current sources of information such as printed material, rotabines, and audiovisual presentations becoming replaced by products of computer technology. For example, by means of information stored in video discs or magnetic tapes it could be possible for patients to educate themselves by means of carefully designed programs. At the press of a button relevant information could be presented to patients on a visual display unit of a home-based microcomputer or on a television screen. In this way patients' self-instruction could be undertaken in their own environment, in their own time, at their own pace, and in a format to suit them individually. For instance, images appearing on the screen could be purely textual, or textual coupled with static or moving pictures, and images could be in black-and-white or colour, with or without sound. It is also possible that such a system could be designed to cater for two-way communication by programming the computer to answer predetermined

queries. The potential for further elaboration of systems based on computer science is almost limitless, and it could even be possible by network systems to link up with other computers if required. Thus an electronic nexus of intercommunication could be established between, say, the patient, the hospital, and the local community health centre. Whether or not such readily available channels of communication would be desirable in practice is, of course, another matter.

12.3 DRUGS

12.3.1 New ways of administering established drugs

(a) Megadose corticosteroid therapy in systemic lupus erythematosus

During the past 10 years many large clinics have had experience with occasional patients in whom very large doses of prednisone have been used for brief periods (pulse doses) for conditions such as diffuse lupus nephritis (Fessel, 1977), progressive glomerulonephritis (Bolton and Conser, 1979), and renal allograft rejection (Mussché *et al.*, 1976). More recently, attention has been directed to its use in systemic lupus erythematosus. For example, Fessel (1980) has treated 13 patients (11 with systemic lupus erythematosus, two with polymyositis), seven of whom had good clinical results from megadose dexamethasone therapy in the range of 1300–7200 mg in patients who had not responded to high doses at a more conventional level, or patients in whom there was reluctance to embark on a prolonged course of therapy.

This approach has recently been extended to rheumatoid arthritis. For example, Liebling *et al.* (1981) treated 10 patients, who were unresponsive to conventional therapy, with 1 g methyl prednisolone intravenously once a month for 6 months. The pulse-treated patients showed significantly better clinical results than a placebo-treated group. The level of immunocomplexes was also significantly decreased in the pulse-treated group.

Pulse therapy experience in Sheffield (Amos, 1982), using a similar dosage schedule to that described above, has revealed similarly encouraging results. Patients with widespread active inflammation causing very disabling problems warranting hospitalization were treated. There was rapid improvement in symptoms and signs which was still present 2–3 months later in most patients. A few have had even more sustained symptomatic benefits. The time course was felt to lend itself readily to short-term treatment with a view to instituting long-term anti-rheumatoid therapy such as gold. Side effects have not been observed except for transient loss of diabetic control in one patient. Laboratory investigation has suggested that adrenocortical recovery has taken place within a week of finishing the infusions.

(b) Low-dose cyclophosphamide

Preliminary reports have shown that high doses of cyclophosphamide (average $1.78\,\text{mg}\,\text{kg}^{-1}\,\text{day}^{-1}$) were effective in the treatment of severe aggressive rheumatoid arthritis, but lower doses (average $0.74\,\text{mg}\,\text{kg}^{-1}\,\text{day}^{-1}$) had no more effect than negligible doses ($15\,\text{mg}\,\text{day}^{-1}$) given to a control group in another trial (Cooperating Clinics Committee of the American Rheumatism Association, 1970, 1972).

However, a recent study (Williams *et al.*, 1980) has shown that low-dose treatment is as effective as high-dose treatment. The authors put forward convincing reasons to explain the difference between their study and previous work.

The minimal effective dose has not yet been found, but according to Williams *et al.* (1980) this probably lies between 15 and $75\,\text{mg}\,\text{day}^{-1}$. With regard to toxic reactions, Smyth *et al.* (1975) have noted a remarkable reduction in toxic readings in patients on $75\,\text{mg}\,\text{day}^{-1}$ compared with higher doses (average $105\,\text{mg}\,\text{day}^{-1}$).

12.3.2 New disease applications of established drugs

(a) Colchicine

As Allison (1977) has pointed out, observations from several different groups of experts in the field show that colchicine in micromolar concentrations inhibits collagen secretion by fibroblasts and stimulates release of collagenase by fibroblasts and macrophages (Harris and Krane, 1971; Harris *et al.*, 1975). Preliminary results of clinical trials suggest that well-tolerated doses of colchicine ($1\,\text{mg}\,\text{day}^{-1}$) may be effective in some patients with scleroderma.

As colchicine has proved to be a safe and effective drug for the long-term prevention of gout, its efficacy might be tried in scleroderma and other diseases in which collagen synthesis is increased. An example is pneumoconiosis, where fibrogenesis continues long after exposure to the offending dust has ceased. However, in view of the marked individual variation in fibrogenesis in pneumoconiosis, scleroderma, and other conditions, the effect of colchicine will be difficult to verify conclusively. In another disorder in which fibrosis is a prominent feature, hepatic cirrhosis, colchicine has so far not improved either the clinical state or the liver function tests (Rojkind *et al.*, 1973).

Since fibroblasts treated with colchicine show accumulation of collagen-containing vacuoles (Schaerft and Heersche, 1975), the question arises whether long-term colchicine treatment would produce a state analogous to a storage disease. This seems unlikely, since procollagen can be degraded by cellular enzymes and colchicine can promote autophagocytosis (Hirsimaki *et al.*, 1975). No evidence for any such effect has been obtained in gouty patients treated with colchicine. Nevertheless, detailed morphological studies of fibroblasts in patients on long-term colchicine treatment would be of interest.

(b) Penicillamine

Animal experiments have shown that penicillamine is a lathyrogen, although its effect on collagen is different from the first discovered lathyrogen, β-aminoproprionitrile, isolated from the seeds of *Lathyrus odoratus*. Penicillamine has been found to be useful in scleroderma, but only in the active phase of the disease when collagen biosynthesis is taking place (Herbert *et al.*, 1974).

α-Aminoproprionitrile also seems to be promising in scleroderma (Keiser and Sjoerdsma, 1967). This agent has also been shown to preserve gliding function in injured tendons (Peacock and Madden, 1969; Bora *et al.*, 1972). However, in both of these studies problems with toxicity were encountered.

(c) Gold

It has been suggested that gold is not effective in psoriatic arthritis (*Editorial*, 1978). Richter *et al.* (1980), however, have reported a retrospective study of 98 patients. Gold was given to 27 and was effective in 22. The frequency of side effects was low and comparable with those observed in rheumatoid patients. The authors concluded that chrysotherapy should enjoy a definite place in the management of psoriatic arthritis. Similarly encouraging results in psoriatic arthritis patients, with regard to clinical efficacy and reduced toxicity compared with rheumatoid patients, have been found by Dorwart *et al.* (1978).

(c) Dapsone

In an open study, McConkey *et al.* (1976, 1979) suggested that dapsone possessed the properties of a suppressive agent in the treatment of rheumatoid arthritis. This effect has been supported by Swinson *et al.* (1981) who found dapsone (in a dose of $50\,\text{mg}\,\text{day}^{-1}$ for 1 week and thereafter $100\,\text{mg}\,\text{day}^{-1}$) to have a beneficial effect in rheumatoid arthritis. Significant improvement in five out of seven clinical measurements and in ESR, viscosity and C-reactive protein was observed. These authors discussed possible modes of action of dapsone in rheumatoid arthritis, but could find no clear parallel to its action in dermatitis herpetiformis or leprosy.

(e) Sulphasalazine

McConkey *et al.* (1978, 1980) have recently re-examined the potential of sulphasalazine as a long-term suppressant in rheumatoid arthritis. It is still too early for an unequivocal view, but early observations are encouraging, and add support to much earlier observations of its value in this disease – some years before it was first used to treat ulcerative colitis.

(f) Calcitonin

Generalized and localized reduction in bone mass have both been described in patients with rheumatoid arthritis from several centres (Bjelle and Nilsson, 1971; Mueller and Jurist, 1973; Kennedy *et al.*, 1974). The mechanism of this bone loss is not clear, but there is little doubt that the bone loss occurs in both the axial and appendicular skeleton (Kennedy *et al.*, 1974), although the peripheral changes, particularly in the forearm and hand, may be in part secondary to the inflammatory changes of the joints themselves.

Recent preliminary work has shown encouraging results of a trial of calcitonin therapy in rheumatoid arthritis (Lindsay and Kennedy, 1976), but final proof of the efficacy of this drug in reducing calcium resorption in rheumatoid patients must await completion of a long-term trial.

(g) Aspirin

For some years there has been some evidence to support the idea of a protective effect of aspirin in chondromalacia patellae (Simmons and Chrisman, 1965; Chrisman and Snook, 1968; Chrisman *et al.*, 1972). The supposition underlying this evidence is based on the fact that salicylates can inhibit the effect of cathepsin on articular cartilage, and may thereby allow synthesis to overtake degradation.

However, despite this encouraging early evidence, a recent study by Bentley *et al.* (1981) failed to show any significant changes in symptoms, signs or microscopic appearances in patients with chondromalacia patellae.

12.3.3 New and experimental drugs

(a) New analgesic/anti-inflammatory drugs

Tiaprofenic acid
At the time of writing tiaprofenic acid (DL-5-benzoyl-methyl-2-thiophene acetic acid) (Surgam) has recently appeared on the market and is being launched as a potent analgesic/anti-inflammatory agent which inhibits prostaglandin synthesis selectively (PGE_2 and $PGF_{2\gamma}$ – the pain and inflammation mediating prostaglandins, rather than PGl_2 – the prostaglandin which protects the gastric mucosa). It has been found to be effective in both rheumatoid arthritis (Camp, 1981) and in osteoarthrosis (Wojtulewski *et al.*, 1980), and in both studies at a dose of 600 mg daily in divided doses side effects were minimal.

Proquazones
Huskisson *et al.* (1981) have recently studied a new analgesic/anti-inflammatory drug in osteoarthrosis. Fluproquazone (4-p-fluorophenyl-1-isopropyl-7-methyl-quinazolin-2 (1H)-one) at a dose of 100 mg tds was found to be comparable with indomethacin 25 mg tds. A larger number of patients and a longer duration of treatment will be needed to assess the side effects of fluproquazone in more detail, but this preliminary study showed it to be relatively non-toxic. An earlier study had shown the related drug proquazone (Biarison) to be more effective than ibuprofen in rheumatoid arthritis, but side effects were greater (Ruotsi and Skifrard, 1978).

Isoxepac
Gerlis and Gumpel (1981) have reported reasonable therapeutic effects and few side effects from isoxepac (6, 11-dihydro-11-oxodibenz [b, e] oxepin-2-acetic acid) 200 mg tds in rheumatoid patients compared with aspirin 1.2 g tds.

(b) New non-analgesic/anti-inflammatory drug

Orgotein
Orgotein is the most recent purely inflammatory agent to be added to the therapeutic armoury. Historically, the development of the therapeutic concept underlying orgotein evolved from a search for a safe drug of mammalian tissue origin that would be suitable for use in a wide variety of human and animal disorders with inflammatory components. Although at the time of writing orgotein is not yet available in the UK, this drug is currently on the market as Ontosein, an Australian preparation.

Pharmacology and pharmacokinetics. Orgotein (ormetein; superoxide dismutase, SOD) represents a group of water-soluble protein congeners isolated from liver, red blood cells, and other mammalian tissues. The amino acid sequence of bovine Cu-Zn SOD is as shown (Huber and Menander-Huber, 1980):

```
                    SH           10
Ac-Ala-Thr-Lys-Ala-Val-Cy-Val-Leu-Lys-Gly-Asp-
                              20
Gly-Pro-Val-Gln-Gly-Thr-Ile-His-Phe-Glu-Ala-Lys-
                              30
Gly-Asp-Thr-Val-Val-Val-Thr-Gly-Ser-Ile-Thr-Gly-
                              40
Leu-Thr-Glu-Gly-Asp-His-Gly-Phe-His-Val-His-Gln-
        50
Phe-Gly-Asp-Asn-Thr-Gln-Gly-Cy-Thr-Ser-Ala-Gly-
60                                      70
Pro-His-Phe-Asn-Pro-Leu-Ser-Lys-Lys-His-Gly-Gly-
                              80                    S
Pro-Lys-Asp-Glu-Glu-Arg-His-Val-Gly-Asp-Leu-Gly-
                              90                    S
Asn-Val-Thr-Ala-Asp-Lys-Asn-Gly-Val-Ala-Ile-Val-
                             100
Asp-Ile-Val-Asp-Pro-Leu-Ile-Ser-Leu-Ser-Gly-Glu-
        110
Tyr-Ser-Ile-Ile-Gly-Arg-Thr-Met-Val-Val-His-Glu-
120                                    130
Lys-Pro-Asp-Asp-Leu-Gly-Arg-Gly-Gly-Asn-Glu-Glu-
                             140
Ser-Thr-Lys-Thr-Gly-Asn-Ala-Gly-Ser-Arg-Leu-Ala-
                             150
Cy-Gly-Val-Ile-Gly-Ile-Ala-Lys
```

In rats the subcutaneous, intramuscular or intraperitoneal administration of orgotein results in peak serum levels of SOD activity after 1–2 hours. Clearance takes place mainly in the kidneys, and 1 hour after intraperitoneal administration 63% of the injected dose is present in the kidneys. Similar patterns have been observed in other experimental animals.

Orgotein has been found to have four specific effects and is anti-inflammatory, anti-superoxide, anti-viral for herpes simplex and parainfluenza-3, and chemotactic *in vivo*. Otherwise it is remarkably inert.

(Huber *et al.*, 1968, 1977, 1980; Bors *et al.*, 1974; Fridovich, 1974, 1976; Geran and Duros, 1975; Fee and Valentine, 1977; Barra *et al.*, 1978; Willson, 1979; Huber, 1980; Williams *et al.*, 1980.)

Clinical uses, preparations and doses. Appendix 12.12.1 summarizes some early clinical and veterinary studies using orgotein.

Early clinical trials in rheumatoid arthritis have suggested that orgotein is more closely akin to the slow-acting drugs such as gold, chloroquine, penicillamine and levamisole rather than the quick-acting, non-steroidal anti-inflammatory drugs. In addition, orgotein can be withdrawn completely after maximal effect has been obtained, with clinical benefits being maintained for long periods (weeks to months).

Generally, the results from trials in rheumatoid arthritis and in osteoarthrosis show that orgotein is well tolerated and has good anti-inflammatory effects. The drug appears therefore to provide the advantages of a pure anti-inflammatory with complete lack of tissue toxicity, though further studies are required to assess its true potential in rheumatology.

For systemic administration, the recommended starting dose of orgotein is 8 or 12 mg given in about 0.8 ml saline injection by syringe with a thin, short needle into the upper, outer quadrant of the buttock. The drug is given once daily on alternate days for several weeks or until maximal benefit has been obtained. Retreatment should be instituted upon the first signs of deterioration. For intra-articular administration, the recommended dose of orgotein is 4 mg given in about 1.0 ml saline once a week for 2–5 weeks. A regimen of 8–16 mg given every other week three times has also been found effective. For other local administrations, doses may vary from 4–8 mg, and dosage may vary from once daily to once weekly.

Side effects, precautions and contraindications. The only side effects so far recorded have been occasional injection site reactions (erythema, induration and/or pruritus). These have generally appeared within 6–8 hours after injection, and have been mild. Deep subcutaneous injection eliminated these local reactions in all but a few patients. A few patients (3 in more than 1500) have developed urticaria on orgotein treatment. These reactions disappeared promptly on stopping treatment and have not been associated with any serious or life-threatening allergic reactions.

(Carson *et al.*, 1973; Lund-Olesen and Menander-Huber, 1974; Huber and Saifer, 1977; Schmidt, 1977.)

Cytotoxic agents – Chapter 6

Levamisole

Another recent appearance on the therapeutic horizon is levamisole (Annotation, 1975; Schuermans, 1975; Huskisson *et al.*, 1976; Janssen, 1976; Rosenthal *et al.*, 1976; Yaron *et al.*, 1976; Willoughby and Wood, 1977; Wilton, 1978; Symoens and Schuermans, 1979), an antihelminthic which has been prescribed without ill effects for several years. The action of the drug appears to be that of an immunostimulant (Renoux and Renoux, 1977; Sagawa *et al.*, 1977; Symoens and Rosenthal, 1977; Goldstein, 1978; Mowat, 1978; Sany, 1978; Symoens *et al.*, 1979). The pharmacokinetics of the drug have been studied by Adams (1978), and a large number of clinical trials have attested to its value in rheumatoid arthritis (Appendix 12.12.2).

Scott *et al.* (1978) have shown that intermittent levamisole therapy (150 mg for 3 days of each week) is as effective as continuous therapy (150 mg daily) in rheumatoid arthritis, and with fewer side effects. Similar results have been obtained by Veys *et al.* (1976). More recently (Multicentre Study Group, 1982) a single weekly dosage of 150 mg has been shown to be much better tolerated than the 3 days-a-week schedule, and only slightly less effective. Although not yet fully established as a rheumatoid suppressant in the UK, it should be mentioned that in some countries levamisole represents the first choice for specific therapy of rheumatoid arthritis.

Toxic effects have included nausea and vomiting, fatigue and drowsiness, drug fever, and urticaria. Granulocytopenia seems to be disproportionately frequent in patients with rheumatic disease. Agranulocytosis may be particularly common in patients with HLA B27. It should be stressed that even intermittent therapy is potentially dangerous and should be monitored carefully. One patient is thought to have had a reversal of levamisole-induced agranulocytosis by corticosteroid administration. However, 3 deaths from agranulocytosis occurred in association with corticosteroid therapy (Mielants and Veys, 1978; Pinals, 1978; Symoens and Lewi, 1978; Symoens *et al.*, 1979).

Zinc

In 1976 Sunkin observed clinical improvement in patients suffering from rheumatoid arthritis who were treated with zinc sulphate. The mechanism of efficacy of this treatment is unknown, but some studies have revealed a low serum level of zinc in rheumatoid arthritis (Menkes *et al.*, 1978).

More recently, Job *et al.* (1980) have been unable to confirm the therapeutic properties of zinc in rheumatoid patients.

Oral gold

The development of an oral gold compound, auranofin (2, 3, 4, 6-tetra-O-acetylthio-β-D-glycopuranoside-S) (triethyl phosphine), has opened a new pharmacological chapter for gold compounds (Finkelstein *et al.*, 1976; Berglöf *et al.*, 1978). Preliminary evidence suggests that clinical improvement of rheumatoid arthritis occurred more often in patients taking 6 and 9 mg daily than patients taking 2 and 4 mg daily (Finkelstein *et al.*, 1980).

Appendix 12.12.3 summarizes chronologically some of the clinical and experimental studies responsible for the development of oral gold as a potentially viable therapeutic entity.

12.3.4 Potential for new drugs

(a) Drugs for treating osteoarthrosis

Dingle (1979) has posed several questions regarding therapeutic potential in the field of osteoarthrosis, and has indicated how research at the Strangeways Laboratory has progressed in attempting to find answers to them. Work in this unit and elsewhere has shown that proteolytic cleavage, initially of proteoglycan and secondly of collagen, is responsible for the damage in the articular cartilage of the arthritic patient. Dingle feels that the enzymes involved are almost certainly a combination of metalloproteinases and cathepsins. The extent to which each enzyme is quantitatively important is not yet clear, but it is thought that it may vary both spatially and temporally, depending on local conditions. Further, it is thought likely that these enzymes work mainly in the pericellular environment of the cell and that the chondrocyte may be the key cell in causing breakdown of cartilage matrix. It is suggested that this is a physiological process, perhaps important in the normal remodelling of cartilage. The control of such chondrocyte function may be due, at least in part, to synovial release of 'catabolins' acting directly on cartilage cells. Dingle raises the interesting speculation that pharmacologically active compounds may modify the secretion of 'catabolins' by inflammatory tissues. If this proves to be true, development of the targeting of drugs to specific cells, by such means as liposomal encapsulation (Dingle *et al.*, 1978) may prove useful in the control of both the acute phase of inflammation and the damage to the articular cartilage in osteoarthrosis.

Much work has been done in recent years on the potential for repair in osteoarthrosis (Campbell, 1969; Riddle, 1970; Chrisman *et al.*, 1972; Perry *et al.*, 1972; Byers, 1974).

Suggestions which are of interest regarding the future of this fascinating field include:

1. Chondrocyte stimulation to synthesize ground substance or retard its degradation.
2. Administration of surrogate ground-substance materials intra-articularly or systemically.

So far, it seems that the key to the repair of articular cartilage rests on the chondrocyte, which can only fulfil itself when there is a proper coupling of matrix removal with synthesis under atraumatic conditions (Sokoloff, 1979).

(b) Drugs for treating ankylosing spondylitis

There has been little effort to use the adjuvant model to design new drugs for ankylosing spondylitis. However, it is interesting that at least two compounds of the diphosphonate type (1-hydroxy-ethylene-1, 1-diphosphonate and methylene diphosphonate) are influential in blocking several of the late features of the adjuvant model, including ectopic calcification, excessive bone resorption, and ankylosis of vertebra, especially in the tail (Francis *et al.*, 1972; Flora, 1979; Russell, 1980).

The diphosphonates are substances known to inhibit calcification, bone resorption and mineralization, partly as a result of their high affinity for calcium phosphate crystals, the growth and dissolution of which they suppress (Russell and Fleisch, 1976). Whether these drugs would be of value in ankylosing spondylitis is not yet known, but obviously their therapeutic potential is exciting.

12.4 PLASMA EXCHANGE, LEUCOPHERESIS, AND THORACIC DUCT DRAINAGE

Plasma exchange (plasmapheresis) is an effective way to reduce the amounts of circulating antibody and/or immune complexes in patients with antibody-mediated or immune complex-mediated disease. This method has received recent application in the treatment of such disorders as Goodpasture's syndrome, systemic lupus erythematosus, and myasthenia gravis (Lockwood *et al.*, 1976; Pinching *et al.*, 1976; Verrier Jones *et al.*, 1976).

Although circulating and intra-articular immune complexes are present in patients with active rheumatoid arthritis, and the complement system is known to be activated in this disease, the pathogenic role of immune complexes in rheumatoid arthritis is still not clear. The complexes may saturate the reticulo-endothelial system, and their volume may impede elimination from intravascular and tissue sites. It has been suggested that plasma exchange may rapidly reverse reticuloendothelial blockade with resultant clinical benefit.

Rheumatoid arthritis is a disorder that generally responds to treatment with non-steroidal anti-inflammatory agents and long-term suppressant drugs such as gold and penicillamine. There are, however, a small percentage of patients in whom the disease is inexorably progressive, and who show little response to conventional measures. This small group, who often have extra-articular manifestations of disease, demands special attention. Since immune-complex formation and complement activation have been implicated in the pathogenesis of the articular and extra-articular features of rheumatoid arthritis, and because plasma exchange has been shown to be of benefit in circumstances where circulating immune complexes have been demonstrated, Rothwell *et al.* (1980) recently undertook a controlled study of plasma exchange in the treatment of a group of 20 active rheumatoid patients who had failed to respond to available conventional therapy. Only slight improvement was observed despite the fact that immune complexes were shown to have been removed.

More persuasive evidence for the clinical value of plasmapheresis (and leucopheresis) in rheumatoid arthritis has been found by Wallace *et al.* (1979) whose hypothesis was that removal of a plasma factor that modulates lymphocyte or neutrophil function is the factor which produced remissions. They also felt that long-acting drugs (e.g. gold or penicillamine) are able to prevent its continued production, and thereby produce a sustained remission. It was also the view of these workers that it is unlikely that simple removal of circulating immune complexes or rheumatoid factor is responsible for clinical improvement.

The role of plasmapheresis in systemic lupus erythematosus is still not established. Encouraging results have been reported by Verrier-Jones *et al.* (1976), Moran *et al.* (1977) and Parry *et al.* (1981). Verrier-Jones *et al.* have emphasized the predictive value of circulating immune complexes. However, a more recent study (Schlansky *et al.*, 1981) actually showed a deterioration in patients after plasmapheresis. Further studies are clearly needed to throw further light on this.

Leucopheresis, using continuous cell separation daily to involve primarily lymphocytes using an IBM blood cell separator, has recently been shown to produce clinical improvement in two patients with severe seropositive rheumatoid arthritis unresponsive to traditional therapy (Tenenbaum *et al.*, 1979).

Thoracic duct drainage, another approach to remove lymphocytes, although involving the inconvenience of surgery, has shown beneficial effects in 12 patients with severe rheumatoid arthritis (Pearson *et al.*, 1975).

12.5 INTRA-ARTICULAR INJECTION AGENTS

12.5.1 Injection of peripheral joints

(a) Osmic acid

In 1951 Von Reis and Swensson first proposed the use of intra-articular osmic acid as a form of treatment for inflammatory arthritis of the knee. The high incidence of local side effects, particularly pain, postponed its further use until 1959, when hydrocortisone was added to the procedure and reduced the frequency of painful sequelae. Subsequently, Hurri *et al.* (1963), Anttinen and Oka (1975), Nissila *et al.* (1977), and others, published reports describing the beneficial effect of intra-articular osmic acid in rheumatoid arthritis, and Martio *et al.* (1972) in juvenile chronic polyarthritis.

In a recent study (Sheppeard and Ward, 1980), 201 patients (305 knees) with rheumatoid arthritis received intra-articular osmic acid in one or both knees. Assessment was based on pain relief, warmth, tenderness, size and presence of effusion, degree of synovial thickening, and range of pain-free movement. Satisfactory results were obtained in 61% at 1 year, gradually reducing to 22% over a 5-year period. If only those knees with no damage or minimal damage were considered, a satisfactory result was obtained in a higher percentage; 74% at 1 year and 38% at 5 years.

(b) Methotrexate

Preliminary work by Hall and Head (1975) suggested that methotrexate could be anti-inflammatory in various arthropathies with persistent effusions. In a further study by Hall's group (Hall *et al.*, 1978), the effects of intra-articular methotrexate were compared with saline in 20 patients with persistent knee effusions due to rheumatoid arthritis (15) and psoriasis (5) in a double-blind pilot study. Clinical improvement was seen in most patients given either methotrexate or saline, and was attributed to joint irrigation during arthroscopy and to placebo effects. Methotrexate had a local anti-inflammatory effect in the psoriatic arthropathies; the percentage of polymorphonuclear cells and pyronin-ophilic mononuclear cells in synovial fluids fell sharply. Intra-articular hydrocortisone acetate was not anti-inflammatory in two psoriatic patients treated subsequently. The anti-inflammatory action of metho-trexate in joints may resemble its effectiveness in con-trolling the rash of psoriasis.

Other evidence suggesting the lack of anti-inflammatory effect in rheumatoid arthritis has been reported by Marks *et al.* (1976).

(c) Effect of increasing the volume of intra-articular hydrocortisone

There is little doubt now about the efficacy of intra-articular corticosteroids as an anti-inflammatory agent in various types of inflammatory synovitis. However, it has been suggested that these beneficial effects may be enhanced by increasing the volume of the injection (Corbett *et al.*, 1970). Sheldon and Bear (1973) have been unable to confirm this and concluded that injection of undiluted steroid is probably at least as beneficial as the same injection plus diluent.

12.5.2 Chemonucleolysis

Chemonucleolysis is a term coined by Smith (Smith and Brown, 1967) to describe the dissolving of the nucleus pulposus by the enzyme chymopapain (Discase) which is obtained from the latex of the green papaya fruit (pawpaw). The enzymatic dissolution of the disc centre and its protruded segments has been found to cure

sciatica and sometimes backache in patients with disc prolapse.

Most of the 55 investigators who have worked with chemonucleolysis over a 12-year period reported highly satisfactory results in over 55% of patients with sciatica and backache due to a proven disc lesion. MacNab (MacNab *et al.*, 1971) went so far as to say that 8 out of 10 patients would be relieved of their pain provided that it was discogenic. In Graham's series (Graham, 1976) over half had permanent relief.

However, this form of treatment has recently been withdrawn in the USA after an adverse report (stating that the therapy was dangerous) by several neuro-surgeons giving their opinion to a Senate Select Committee.

The drug has been released in Canada and in the UK and success rates in properly selected patients are as high as 75–80%.

The final answer on chemonucleolysis will probably come from the Antipodes, where a double-blind study is being carried out at the Flinders University in South Australia.

RADIOTHERAPY
See Section 8.5.2.

12.6 SURGERY

12.6.1 Factors influencing the development of joint replacement surgery

Surgery as a therapeutic tool in the treatment of rheumatoid arthritis has passed through a phase of rapid growth both in the number of patients treated and in the variety of technical procedures.

No field of modern surgery has received such impetus in the past decade as that of arthroplasty. Charnley and others (see Chapters 1 and 9) have firmly established the principles of total joint replacement arthroplasty for the hip joint and this can no longer be considered a 'growth area'. However, increasingly, orthopaedic practice will be devoted to dealing with technical mishaps arising from such operations. It is inevitable that some pro-cedures will fail. The sheer numbers of hip replacements performed, and inevitably the increasing proportion performed by trainee surgeons, produce a steady flow of problems, even though the percentage of failures re-mains amazingly low (Laurence, 1975).

The following represent the main factors that have influenced the growth of joint replacement surgery (Morris, 1978):

1. The development of operations which, for the hip at least, have transformed orthopaedic treatment of

degenerative and inflammatory arthritis from being a 'last resort' to being a 'lasting cure'.

2. The exposure of disabling arthritis as a major cause of disease that is treatable.

3. In some countries, the need for the same set of surgeons to treat two epidemics, one of which, trauma, makes the most urgent demands that can be made of medical services.

4. The need for special operating facilities for the control of infection.

12.6.2 The present position

A general survey of the most widely used arthroplasties shows that hip arthroplasty has achieved a good measure of success. As mentioned earlier, this success is partly due to Charnley's influence and, not least, in the control he exercised at the beginning before releasing the prosthesis to other orthopaedic surgeons. The success of hip arthroplasty is also partly due to the anatomy of the hip joint, which lends itself to simple designs. The state of flux in which we find arthroplasties of the knee and elbow, and other joints more complicated in structure than the hip, is evident from the large number of existing designs relevant to these joints. It appears that most designers have not yet appreciated how much more demanding is prosthetic design for these more complicated joints.

12.6.3 Future aims of joint replacement

The main indication for joint replacement will always be relief of pain, but at present orthopaedic surgeons also include functional limitation and stiffness as surgical indications. In some circumstances this is well justified, e.g. where toilet or sexual functions are grossly impaired. However, the problem in the future will be to resist pressure where the patient is less handicapped.

A very different group that will generate a demand for prostheses are athletes. There are few competitive sports to which a patient would be expected to return after such an operation, although Pat Smythe, the showjumper, was back in the saddle after replacement of both hips. Charnley was in no doubt in 1961: 'Neither surgeons nor engineers will ever make an artificial joint which will last 30 years and at the same time in this period enable the patient to play football.'

12.6.4 Future needs

Over the past decade the field of endoprostheses has become a rapidly growing industry. This is especially so since the Food and Drug Administration of the USA allowed the general use of polymethylmethacrylate cement (PMMA) for the fixation of these artificial

joints. It has been estimated that 30 000 hip prostheses are inserted annually in Great Britain, and at least 200 000 worldwide. The relief of pain in thousands of patients, particularly those with unilateral osteoarthrosis of the hip, vindicates the claim that the development of an adequate hip prosthesis has been the biggest single advance in the treatment of arthritis this century. The fact that well over 300 knee prostheses have been designed indicates the endeavour to achieve similar success with other joints.

As far as the hip is concerned, demand exceeds supply of service at least in the UK. The waiting time for surgery varies throughout the country, but in some areas it is as long as $2\frac{1}{2}$ years. The bleak outlook for the immediate future is that by the mid 1980s there could be fewer orthopaedic beds available for prosthetic surgery. The diminishing resources of the National Health Service and the increasing age of the population, with its higher risk of fracture, make it likely that many more orthopaedic beds will be occupied by victims of trauma. The Department of Health and Social Security (DHSS) has set up working parties to examine both orthopaedic and cardiothoracic surgical waiting lists, but a fruitful outcome, other than merely highlighting problems, is doubtful.

The main candidates for joint replacements are patients suffering from osteoarthrosis, rheumatoid arthritis, and post-traumatic problems, in that order, and there is little evidence that the demand will diminish. There has been increased awareness of secondary causes of osteoarthrosis, but apart from the early treatment of congenital dislocation of the hip, little can be done to prevent these. Biomechanical and biochemical knowledge of the disease is beginning to advance, but has not yet reached a stage at which any reduction in patients needing replacement surgery can be expected.

The pharmaceutical industry is devoting a large part of its resources to finding drugs more influential in affecting the rheumatoid process, but, despite this effort, the cure of rheumatoid arthritis still seems remote, and its prevention even more so. There is therefore still no sign of a diminishing need of the surgeon's help to repair the destructive effects of this disease.

12.6.5 Likely developments in the future

It is difficult to anticipate with any accuracy the likely future developments in rheumatological surgery – say the position 10 years from now. However, certain speculations can be made and are summarized below. For further reading in this field of orthopaedic clairvoyance two recent reviews are of particular interest (Hill, 1980; Wright and Seedhom, 1980).

1. Even if a cure for rheumatoid arthritis will have been discovered, the massive legacy of damaged joints

will keep surgeons occupied for many more years.

2. Further intense activity, involving surgeons, bio-engineers, metallurgists, and others, will have been addressed to the problems of developing new techniques for total prosthetic replacement of joints other than the hip. Some procedures will have been abandoned, and, of the 'survivors', relatively few will rival the success of present-day hip replacement, largely because of the more exacting mechanical problems posed by other joints. Successful replacement of the knee will be the most coveted prize, but replacements for the elbow and the shoulder will also have attracted much effort. It is likely that reasons for cement failure will have been resolved and that new grouting agents will have been developed. Improvements in the design of the prosthesis itself will be largely centred on revision potential. There will be further exploitation of present materials rather than the development of new plastics solely for pros-thetic manufacture (for economic reasons). The production of prostheses will probably become auto-mated if designs become stable and demand sufficient to justify the cost.

3. Simple excision procedures such as removal of the lower ulna, upper radius, and metatarsal heads will not have been seriously challenged.

4. A few arthrodeses, mainly of the wrist and hindfoot, will continue.

5. Synovectomy will survive, especially for the knee and elbow, but will be performed less often. The concept of synovectomy as a prophylactic procedure will finally have been abandoned.

6. Clearance of tendon sheaths, and tendon repair or transposition will continue.

7. Surgical gains for athletes will continue to be from prosthetic replacement, but the field of ligamentous repair with carbon-fibre filaments will have advanced further.

8. Surgery for unstable necks will continue to be infrequent, but more will be known about the in-dications for surgical correction.

12.7 REHABILITATION

12.7.1 Aids and appliances

The Institute for Consumer Ergonomics of the Univer-sity of Loughborough was founded in 1970 to research into goods, buildings and services in general use. Half of this work is directed to the problems of the disabled and elderly. Many recent reports have been published on consumer products for use by the disabled. Areas of study have included: the optimal height of domestic electric sockets, wheelchairs, characteristics and requirements of wheelchair users, handrails, bath aids, alarm systems for the elderly and disabled, and space

requirements in the bathroom for wheelchair users. This research has been financed by the DHSS and the Institute has depended on the Department of Rheu-matology and Rehabilitation at the Derbyshire Royal Infirmary for clinical guidance (Cochrane and Glanville, 1977).

It is hoped that the future will see a more vigorous approach to evaluating aids and appliances, and already signs of this are encouraging. For example, Gumpel and Cannon (1981) have recently undertaken a cross-over comparison of ready-made fabric wrist splints, and Chamberlain *et al.* (1981) have evaluated aids and equipment for the bath.

12.7.2 Physiotherapy

Solid scientific evidence to support the value of physio-therapy is relatively limited (Machover and Sapecky, 1966; Ekblom *et al.*, 1975; Vignos, 1980). References quoted in articles on rehabilitation of patients with arthritis are heavily weighted with data derived from normal subjects, extrapolations from unrelated disease entities, and experimental animal work.

Recently a study (Robinson *et al.*, 1980) has pointed to the urgent need for prospective studies of both the medical efficiency and the cost-effectiveness of physio-therapy in rheumatoid arthritis. Once the efficiency or otherwise of physiotherapy in this disease has been established, comparisons between physiotherapy and other forms of treatment will be possible.

As Dixon has stressed (Dixon, 1973), in the field of painful back syndromes there is a need to assess the various forms of treatment including rest, manipulative treatments and traction. Glover (1971) has conducted such an assessment in acute back pain sufferers in industry. However, appraisal of manipulation of pa-tients attending hospital is required, and is part of the plan of research of Kersley's unit in Bath – a research project which is being supported by the Arthritis and Rheumatism Council. Mathews and Hickling (1975) have undertaken a doubleblind controlled study of lumbar traction for sciatica and have found that although there was a tendency towards improvement of pain and straight-leg raising, this did not achieve statistical significance. The value of strict rest on a supported mattress was substantiated some years ago (Pearce and Moll, 1967).

Research is also needed concerning better appliances for the back, and co-operation with material science departments to study new moulding techniques would be advantageous. Much work has been done at Guy's Hospital on the importance of adequate car seats and other seats, but little attention has been directed to-wards the ideal orthopaedic bed, despite the enthusiastic claims of bed manufacturers.

12.8 HETERODOX PROCEDURES

As has been pointed out by the Arthritis Foundation of the USA, the continuing appetite for heterodox treatments for arthritis sufferers is reflected in the colossal annual bill for quack remedies. Currently this amounts to about $950 million per year.

The emphasis in arthritis promotions is moving more towards diet fads and 'improved' drugs, and away from mechanical devices. However, contraptions such as the 'Miracle Health Relaxer', the 'Vryllium Tube', the 'Vivicosmic Disk', and vibrators are still popular.

However, a more critical approach to the sale of dubious remedies is being exercised, particularly in the USA. For example, federal intervention has recently resulted in regulating certain therapies (e.g. the 'Pulse-A-Rhythm' vibrating mattress, and the 'Marvpad' – mitts or pads filled with gravel and supposedly containing 'low-grade radioaction').

Considering the potential harm resulting from literature for patients 'lacking medical accuracy and scientific validity', another welcome move has been the publication by the US Consumers' Union of a list of books and booklets to be avoided. This publication (Editors of Consumer Reports Books, 1980) also lists useful advice to patients to enable them to recognize signs of health quackery.

The acceptability of some heterodox procedures continues to be debatable, but some are gaining ground. For example, the respectability of chiropractic colleges in the USA was enhanced in 1974 by their accreditation with national standing. (Previously, degrees such as Doctor of Chiropractic had been listed as 'spurious' by the US Office of Education.)

Acupuncture has also gained considerable credence in recent years, and is now regularly the subject of papers, seminars, and symposia in orthodox circles. It is currently used in some pain clinics, and it is possible that its application in the field of analgesia/anaesthesia will extend as controlled experience of its use increases. It is doubtful, however, whether its effect rheumatologically is anything but pain relieving.

Both local and systemic medicines continue to be heavily promoted and are likely to remain popular.

Liniments, ointments, and body rubs are, in general, probably harmless and doubtless provide some benefit, if only psychological, from their strong aroma and impressive burning/tingling effects. However, some external remedies containing a high content of methyl salicylate (30% or more) or excessive amounts of lead may lead to toxic effects from absorption through the skin.

Dimethylsulfoxide (DMSO). There is still no evidence that this drug is useful in the treatment of rheumatic diseases, although in the USA its use was legalized in Oregon in 1977, and in Florida in 1978. It is also used in several clinics in Mexico.

Liefcort (combination of prednisolone testosterone and oestradiol) has been described by the US Food and Drugs Administration as 'an irrational mixture of potent ingredients'. However, despite this and legal intervention in other countries (the use of an allied preparation 'Rheumatil' has led to prosecution by Canadian authorities), this form of therapy continues in the USA under the guise of 'Balanced Hormone Therapy' and 'Balanced Hormone Treatment for Arthritis'.

Seatone – an extract of the New Zealand green-lipped mussel, *Perna canaliculus* is now popular, and is readily available in health stores. Early reports of anti-inflammatory effects in an experimental model (Miller and Ormrod, 1980), and of encouraging results in patients with rheumatoid arthritis and osteoarthrosis (Gibson *et al.*, 1980), have not been confirmed in a recent study (Huskisson *et al.*, 1981). Huskisson's group concluded that seatone does not appear to be 'the mighty mussel' after all and showed that it was no more effective than a fish extract in rheumatoid arthritis. Considering the cost of this preparation (about £5 per month) patients are probably wiser saving their money.

12.9 EXPERIMENTAL MODELS

12.9.1 General comment

Over the last 5 years much research has centred on experimental surrogates of human connective tissue diseases (particularly animal equivalents of rheumatoid arthritis and systemic lupus erythematosus), with a view to studying aetiology, pathogenesis and therapeutic effects. The subject has recently been reviewed in some depth (Rheumatism Review Subcommittee of the ARA, 1981), and several therapeutically orientated papers have demonstrated disease-modulating effects mediated by a host of agents (Blackham and Radziwonik, 1977; Floman *et al.*, 1977; Gerber *et al.*, 1977; Hann, 1977; Wigley, 1977; MacKenzie *et al.*, 1978; Steinberg *et al.*, 1978). Some of these therapeutic responses will be described briefly under the following headings: New Zealand model of systemic lupus erythematosus; Aleutian disease of mink; adjuvant arthritis; miscellaneous models of arthritis.

12.9.2 The New Zealand model of systemic lupus erythematosus

This is a disease in which spontaneous production of autoantibodies occurs in New Zealand mice, and represents the first naturally occurring animal counterpart of human autoimmune disease.

Therapeutic studies in New Zealand mice can be divided into those involving immunotherapeutic manipulation, and those involving newer drugs or therapeutic agents. The ultimate aim of both types of experimentation is the suppression of autoantibody production, decrease in immune-complex formation, and reversibility of renal and CNS lesions. Despite the large amount of work that has been performed in this field, most measures have given rise to somewhat disappointing results in their overall effectiveness. Therapeutic intervention has been found to be most effective when administered before the appearance of clinical manifestations, circumstances hardly relevant to the treatment of the human disease. So far therapeutic experiments have involved a diverse spectrum of agents including: soluble immune response substance (SIRS), prostaglandins, thymic hormones or extracts, corticosteroids, cytotoxic agents (e.g. chlorambucil, cyclophosphamide), L-asparaginase, dactinomycin D, specific dietary restrictions, and hypertransfusion with N-(2-carboxyphenyl)-4-chloroanthranilic acid.

12.9.3 Aleutian disease of mink

Aleutian disease of mink is a persistent viral infection in which an exaggerated immune response against viral antigens and the continued presence of virus are responsible for the pathological changes characteristic of the disease (e.g. glomerulonephritis, arteritis, plasmacytosis, and hypergammaglobulinaemia). At present effective therapeutic or prophylactic measures have not yet been found, although the disease can be readily identified by viral antibody and viral antigen counterimmunoelectrophoresis.

12.9.4 Adjuvant arthritis

Adjuvant arthritis (AA) can be produced by a single injection of killed mycobacteria emulsified in a variety of oil vehicles. On the basis of a proposed viral aetiology, interferon-inducing agents such as statolon, poly I poly C, and tilorone have been shown to suppress the development of AA. The antiarthritic action of these materials was not associated with modification of the immune response, nor was it associated with their anti-inflammatory activity. Cyclophosphamide has also been found to have an antiarthritic action in this disease.

As Russell has pointed out (Russell, 1980) there has been little effort to use the adjuvant model to assess new drugs for ankylosing spondylitis. However, at least two substances of diphosphonate type (1-hydroxy-ethylene-1, 1-diphosphonate, and dichloromethylene diphosphonate) have been shown to influence several of the late features of the adjuvant model (see Section 12.3.4 for further details).

12.9.5 Miscellaneous models of arthritis

Miscellaneous models of rheumatoid-like arthritis include the following:

1. Mycoplasma-induced arthritis in various animals (e.g. cattle, mice).
2. Mouse arthritis due to immunization and subsequent intra-articular challenge with methylated bovine serum albumin.
3. Experimental allergic arthritis (EAA) is a chronic disease produced in rabbits by immunization with a soluble antigen in complete Freund's adjuvant, and subsequent injection of the antigen intra-articularly.
4. At least 20 materials (bacterial walls and extracts) are arthritogenic in rats and other animals.
5. Arthritis of the femorotibial joints of rabbits induced by repeated injections of carrageenin.
6. A chronic proliferative arthritis of mice can be induced by activating the alternative complement pathway using zymosan.
7. Arthritis of chickens can be produced with arthrotropic virus (as well as with mycloplasma).
8. Chronic inflammation of rabbits can be produced by injecting ferritin into the knee joint.
9. Acute self-limiting arthritis in the hindpaws of older rats can be produced by 6-sulphanilamidoindazole (6-SAl), a sulphonamide.

Most of these experimental models of arthritis have been subjected to various pharmacological agents in attempts to define useful drugs in human rheumatoid arthritis. In particular, gold, tetracycline, and several anti-inflammatory agents have been studied. Such substances have been found to modify disease activity, but the results have been severely limited by the small number of animals studied, and the failure to correlate the effects of the drug with delayed hypersensitivity, chronicity of infection, or the kinetics involved.

The exceptions have been studies of cyclophosphamide in adjuvant arthritis of rats, and the influence of prostaglandins and indomethacin in experimental arthritis of rats.

12.10 OVERALL SUMMARY AND CONCLUSIONS

This chapter has considered some new developments and future prospects in various aspects of rheumatic management. These will now be summarized together with conclusions about likely areas of progress in the future. In drawing these conclusions there has been inevitably and intentionally some overspill into the contents of previous chapters. Some of these may therefore be regarded as overall conclusions.

12.10.1 Communication

Bearing in mind the chronicity of many rheumatic disorders, and the fact that there is still no cure for most of them, communication should feature more prominently as a valuable adjunct to management. This is because there is much that patients can do for themselves, as well as taking best advantage of specific therapies offered.

Until recently, the field of communication in medicine as a whole, and in rheumatology more specifically, has been remarkably neglected. This doubtless stems from a truism that what appears simple and obvious is less likely to attract the attention of those looking for more impressive and immediately effective aids to treatment. This, of course, applies to patients as well as doctors.

Much is now known about fundamental processes involved in communication, and this stems largely from studies among the pure sciences – mathematics, physics, and computer technology. However, more energy needs to be devoted to the *clinical* application of this knowledge. It is likely that the most fruitful areas of research will derive from studies aimed at answering basic psychomedical questions orientated around the more 'human' aspects of the patient. In order to achieve meaningful results, investigators will need to approach the subject not so much from the standpoint of what they themselves think worthwhile, but rather from the patient's viewpoint. Put another way, success is most likely to arise from some degree of 'lateral thinking' on the patient's behalf, rather than from preconceived ideas based on 'hard' scientific facts and principles.

Once the more precise needs of patients are understood, it is possible and perhaps ironic that in the near future medical communication will avail itself of the rapidly developing field of microcomputer technology – with the hope that the central role of the doctor in the communication process will not be forgotten.

12.10.2 Drugs

Considerable research energies continue to be addressed to the problem of finding more effective and less toxic anti-rheumatic drugs. However, since the innovation of the xanthine-oxidase inhibitor, allopurinol, there have been no startling relevations in this field – certainly not on the scale represented by other glittering prizes such as antibiotics, insulin and cimetidine.

The failure to find more satisfactory answers to the needs of arthritis patients has not been for lack of research effort, as the thousands of drug study reports over the past decade testify. Indeed, it could be argued that this prodigious effort has been useful in several ways, and there are signs that further improvements are within grasp.

New developments and future prospects in the drug field may be summarized as follows:

1. Continued proliferation of non-steroidal analgesic/anti-inflammatory agents. This area of activity has been shown to be valuable for the following reasons:
   (a) It provides the clinician with more and more drugs of comparable (or almost comparable) *potency* compared with 'traditional' drugs (aspirin, phenylbutazone, indomethacin). Considering the fact that pharmacogenetic variations between patients to therapeutic response are likely to be more important than actual differences in potency between drugs, the more drugs the prescriber has to choose from, the better. On the other hand, this proliferation of non-steroidal products is becoming almost overwhelming, and many clinicians find it a practical impossibility to give all new products a reasonable clinical testing.
   (b) Many of the newer non-steroidal anti-inflammatories tend to be somewhat less *toxic*, particularly with regard to gastrointestinal side effects.
   (c) The emergence of once-a-day or twice-a-day dosage regimens provides the patients with a more convenient way of taking medication. It is also hoped that compliance will be increased by such regimens.
   (d) More 'sophisticated' formulations and a wider spectrum of presentations of some of the newer drugs are probably advantageous. For example, enteric-coated, micro-encapsulated, and esterified versions of aspirin probably reduce gastrointestinal side effects. Regarding alternative presentations of drugs, other than tablets or capsules, the availability of sustained-release capsules, suspensions, suppositories and injections may be useful in some clinical circumstances.

2. Although corticosteroids and corticotrophin remain the 'pure' anti-inflammatory agents in general usage, interest has recently been directed to orgotein (Cu-Zn superoxide dismutase), a new pure inflammatory substance with very low toxicity. This is a drug whose lineage stems from veterinary practice and whose application to clinical medicine will be watched with interest in future years.

3. The search continues for new specific disease-modulating drugs and for new ways of using present drugs in order to minimize toxicity without losing therapeutic effect. These areas of study have been largely devoted to drugs against rheumatoid arthritis and systemic lupus erythematosus. With regard to rheumatoid arthritis, the third line drugs in routine use in the UK continue to be gold, penicillamine,

antimalarials, and immunosuppressives. The use of levamisole, dapsone, and sulphasalazine remains experimental, although there are indications, as fas as levamisole is concerned, that once-a-week administration is less toxic and yet still therapeutically effective.

Alternative ways of administering established drugs have included mega-dose infusions of corticosteroids as 'pulse therapy', intermittent *versus* continuous cyclophosphamide, and oral *versus* intramuscular gold, all of which remain *sub judice* as being preferential to established usage of these drugs. Another approach has been to apply certain 'disease-specific' drugs to unrelated rheumatic disorders (e.g. salicylates to prevent cartilage wear in osteoarthrosis; colchicine to treat systemic sclerosis). Many avenues of exploration still remain uncharted and, in particular, there is a need to find disease-modifying drugs for the spondarthritides. At present, psoriatic arthritis is the only disease in this group which is treated along these lines (with methotrexate). Diphosphonates have been found to be effective in adjuvant models of ankylosing spondylitis, but attendant problems such as demineralization of normal bone, have dampened initial enthusiasm for their clinical application.

In summary, therefore, the present thrust of pharmacological and clinical research, although not yet productive of any new therapeutic revelations, is at least moving slowly forwards. For the present it is likely that rheumatological therapeutics, particularly concerning rheumatoid arthritis, will remain at the very least symptomatic (with additional comfort and convenience to the patient), and, at most, 'suppressive' – with 'specific' effects capable of modulating, as opposed to halting or curing, the underlying disease process.

12.10.3 Plasma exchange and allied procedures

These procedures are still in their infancy as potentially useful agencies in controlling 'malignant' expressions of certain connective tissue disorders, notably systemic lupus erythematosus and, more recently, rheumatoid arthritis. Results to date have been conflicting, but there is evidence that this approach may be useful in selected patients in whom more conservative measures have failed.

12.10.4 Intra-articular injection agents

Treatment involving the injection of agents into joints has not advanced greatly in recent years, and locally injected corticosteroids remain the treatment of choice. Attempts to secure 'medical synovectomy' with radioactive colloids (e.g. gold or yttrium), and with other substances such as osmic acid, have failed to establish these agents in 'routine' therapy. Unconvincing long-term benefits and undesirable local effects have contributed to their unsustained popularity.

12.10.5 Radiotherapy

The place of conventional radiotherapy in ankylosing spondylitis has lost favour in view of convincing evidence of long-term malignancies arising from this treatment. It has been suggested that the only reasonable indication for using radiotherapy is for peripheral joints in spondylitis which are refractory to more conservative treatment providing there is no radiation threat to large areas of normal tissue.

Megavoltage X-rays, now widely available, do not give disproportionately higher energy absorption to bone, and might be considered less damaging to bone marrow. Further investigation into the application of this type of irradiation may help to restore the status of radiotherapy.

12.10.6 Surgery

Considering there is still no sight of a cure for rheumatoid arthritis and for other destructive disorders of the locomotor system, surgery is likely to continue as a valuable concomitant to rheumatological management. The next few years will probably see even further development in procedures already established (e.g. hip joint replacement) and in the discovery of more satisfactory prostheses for joints still wanting in this respect (e.g. shoulder, elbow). The short-term aims are likely to be directed to finding a prosthesis for the knee comparable in efficacy with that currently used for the hip. Apart from improved prosthetic designs to allow more fully for specific anatomicomechanical differences between joints, and also for the possibility of revision should procedures fail, it is hoped that new research will lead to other improvements such as more effective grouting agents.

Should medical solutions be found to control more effectively or even cure the chronic arthritides, surgery will continue to be a valuable service in view of the legacy of joint destruction which will need attention.

12.10.7 Rehabilitation

Although it is unlikely that significant advances will be made in the field of physical agents further application of modern engineering skills is likely to yield improvements in aids, appliances and vehicles for the disabled.

Rehabilitation is becoming a growing field for research activities and, although this is a long time overdue, there is now a more refreshing approach to evaluating the results of therapy objectively. Such information may eventually help to dispel much of the mystique which currently pervades this specialty.

12.10.8 Heterodox procedures

In general, orthodox clinicians remain intransigent towards most heterodox procedures, not without good reason. In some countries, notably the USA, there is an increasing alertness in limiting quack remedies by legislation. In addition, there are now positive moves towards helping patients to distinguish the magsman from the medical man.

It is likely that barriers between allopathic and heterodox practitioners will persist until there is more preparedness on both sides to evaluate objectively therapies which continue to be coloured by myth and magic.

Considering that many of our more valuable drugs originate from plants, it would not be surprising if further agents of genuine value emerged from scientific testing of some ostensibly bizarre therapies of botanical origin.

Acupuncture, which has received much attention recently, is the most obvious example of a therapy which is becoming transcended from the ranks of heterodoxy as a result of critical evaluation. It is interesting to speculate that in the future this treatment may be increasingly used for analgesia/anaesthesia, although claims concerning its value as an arthritic panacea remain untenable.

12.10.9 Experimental models

Studies of various therapeutic agents in animal models of human connective tissue disorders are paving the way to a more penetrating understanding of new approaches to treatment in the future. Not only do such studies allow a more flexible and vigorous approach than would be possible in studying humans, but they also enable a more detailed analysis of how effects are achieved, as well as to what extent they are achieved.

12.10.10 Concluding comment

There is little doubt that the past, through improvements in drugs, physical treatment, surgery, and other forms of therapy, has provided the rheumatic patient with a much better quality of life. However, it is hoped that in the future the need for such sources of succour and strength will be obviated by more effective control, cure, or even prevention.

12.11 REFERENCES AND FURTHER READING

Communication

Balint, E. and Norell, J.S. (eds) (1973) *Six Minutes for the Patient: Interactions in General Practice Consultation*, Tavistock, London.

Harlem, O.K. (1977) *Communication in Medicine. A Challenge to the Profession*, Karger, Basle.

McLachlan, G. (ed.) (1979) *Mixed Communications*, Published for the Nuffield Provincial Hospitals Trust by the Oxford University Press, Oxford.

Moll, J.M.H. (1981) *Studies of Visual Perception in Medical Communication*, Ph.D. thesis, University of Leeds.

Tanner, B. (ed.) (1976) *Language and Communication in General Practice*, Hodder and Stoughton, London.

Drugs

New ways of administering established drugs

Megadose corticosteroid therapy

Amos, R.S. (1982) *Personal communication.*

Bolton, W.K. and Conser, W.G. (1979) Intravenous pulse methylprednisolone therapy of acute rapidly progressive glomerulonephritis. *Am. J. Med.*, **66**, 495.

Fessel, W.J. (1977) Reversal of azotaemia in lupus nephritis by megadose corticosteroid therapy. *Arthr. Rheum.* (Letter), **20**, 1564.

Fessel, W.J. (1980) Megadose corticosteroid therapy in systemic lupus erythematosus. *J. Rheumatol.*, **7**, 486.

Liebling, M.R., Lieb, E. McLaughlin, K. *et al.* (1981) Pulse methylprednisolone in rheumatoid arthritis. *Ann. Int. Med.*, **94**, 21.

Mussché, M.M., Ringoir, S.M.G. and Lameire, N.N. (1976) High intravenous doses of methylprednisolone for acute cadaveric renal allograft rejection. *Nephron*, **16**, 287.

Low-dose cyclophosphamide

Cooperating Clinics Committee of the American Rheumatism Association (1970) A controlled trial of cyclophosphamide in rheumatoid arthritis. *N. Engl. J. Med.*, **283**, 883.

Cooperating Clinics Committee of the American Rheumatism Association (1972) A controlled trial of high and low doses of cyclophosphamide in 82 patients with rheumatoid arthritis. *Arthr. Rheum.*, **15**, 434.

Smyth, C.J., Bartholomew, B.A., Mills, D.M. *et al.* (1975) Cyclophosphamide therapy for rheumatoid arthritis. *Arch. Int. Med.*, **135**, 789.

Williams, H.J., Reading, J.C., Ward, J.R. and O'Brien, W.M. (1980) Comparison of high and low dose cyclophosphamide therapy in rheumatoid arthritis. *Arthr. Rheum.*, **23**, 521.

New disease applications of established drugs

Colchicine

Allison, A.C. (1977) Effects of agents interacting with microtubules on collagen synthesis and breakdown. *Ann. Rheum. Dis.*, **36** (Suppl.), 65.

Harris, E.D. and Krane, S.M. (1971) Effects of colchicine on collagenase in cultures of rheumatoid synovium. *Arthr. Rheum.*, **14**, 669.

Harris, E.D., Werb, Z., Cartwright, E. and Reynolds, J.J. (1975) Stimulation of collagenase release from synovial fibroblasts in monolayer culture by colchicine and related compounds. *Scand. J. Rheumatol.*, **4** (Suppl. 8), 15.

Hirsimaki, Y., Arstilla, A. and Trump, B.F. (1975) Auto-phagocytosis: *in vitro* induction by microtubule poisons. *Exp. Cell Res.*, **92**, 11.

Rojkind, M., Uribe, M. and Kershenobich, D. (1973) Colchicine in the treatment of liver cirrhosis. *Lancet*, **i**, 38.

Schaerft, J.P. and Heersche, J.N.M. (1975) Accumulation of collagen-containing vacuoles in osteoblasts after administration of colchicine. *Cell. Tiss. Res.*, **157**, 353.

Penicillamine

Bora, F.W., Lane, J.M. and Prockop, D.J. (1972) Inhibitors of collagen biosynthesis as a means of controlling scar formation in tendon injury. *J. Bone Joint Surg.*, **54A**, 1501.

Keiser, H.R. and Sjoerdsma, A. (1967) Studies on beta-amino proprionitrile in patients with scleroderma. *Clin. Pharmacol. Ther.*, **8**, 593.

Herbert, C.M., Lindberg, K.A., Jayson, M.I.V. and Bailey, A.J. (1974) Biosynthesis and maturation of the skin collagen in scleroderma, and effect of D-penicillamine. *Lancet*, **i**, 187.

Peacock, E.E. and Madden, J.W. (1969) Some studies on the effects of 1-amino proprionitrile in patients with injured flexor tendons. *Surgery*, **66**, 215.

Gold

Dorwart, B., Gall, E.P., Schumacher, H.R. and Krauser, R.E. (1978) Chrysotherapy in psoriatic arthropathy. *Arthr. Rheum.*, **21**, 513.

Editorial (1978) Treatment of arthritis associated with psoriasis. *Br. Med. J.*, **i**, 262.

Richter, M.B., Kinsella, P. and Corbett, M. (1980) Gold in psoriatic arthropathy. *Ann. Rheum. Dis.*, **39**, 279.

Dapsone

McConkey, B., Davis, P., Crockson, R.A. *et al.* (1976) Dapsone in rheumatoid arthritis. *Rheumatol. Rehabil.*, **15**, 230.

McConkey, B., Davis, P., Crockson, R.A. *et al.* (1979) Effects of gold, dapsone and prednisolone on serum C-reactive protein and haptoglobin and the ESR in rheumatoid arthritis. *Ann. Rheum. Dis.*, **38**, 141.

Swinson, D.R., Zlosnick, J. and Jackson, L. (1981) Double-blind trial of dapsone against placebo in the treatment of rheumatoid arthritis. *Ann. Rheum. Dis.*, **40**, 235.

Sulphasalazine

McConkey, B., Amos, R.S., Butler, E.P. *et al.* (1978) Salazo-pyrin in rheumatoid arthritis. *Agents and Actions*, **8**, 438.

McConkey, B., Amos, R.S., Durham, S. *et al.* (1980) Sulpha-salazine in rheumatoid arthritis. *Br. Med. J.*, **i**, 442.

Calcitonin

Bjelle, A.O. and Nilsson, B.E. (1971) The relationship between radiologic changes and osteoporosis of the hand in rheumatoid arthritis. *Arthr. Rheum.*, **14**, 646.

Kennedy, A.C., Smith, D.A. Buchanan, W.W. *et al.* (1974) Osteoporosis in rheumatoid arthritis. *Rev. Rheumatol.*, **4**, 25.

Lindsay, R. and Kennedy, A.C. (1976) in *Bone Disease and Calcitonin*, Symposium Proceedings (ed. J.A. Kanis), Armour, Eastbourne, p. 171.

Mueller, M.N. and Jurist, J.M. (1973) Skeletal status in rheumatoid arthritis. *Arthr. Rheum.*, **16**, 66.

Aspirin

Bentley, G., Leslie, I.J. and Fischer, D. (1981) Effect of aspirin treatment on chondromalacia patellae. *Ann. Rheum. Dis.*, **40**, 37.

Chrisman, O.D. and Snook, G.A. (1968) Studies on protective effect of aspirin against degeneration of human articular cartilage. *Clin. Orthop.*, **56**, 77.

Chrisman, O.D., Snook, G.A. and Wilson, T.C. (1972) The protective effect of aspirin against degeneration of human articular cartilage. *Clin. Orthop.*, **84**, 193.

Simmons, D.R. and Chrisman, O.D. (1965) Salicylate inhibition of cartilage degeneration. *Arthr. Rheum.*, **8**, 960.

New and experimental drugs

Tiaprofenic acid

Camp, V. (1981) Tiaprofenic acid in the treatment of rheumatoid arthritis. *Rheumatol. Rehabil.*, **20**, 181.

Wojtulewski, J., Walter, J. and Thornton, E.J. (1981) Tiaprofenic acid (Surgam) in the treatment of osteoarthritis of the knee and hip. *Rheumatol. Rehabil.*, **20**, 177.

Proquazones

Huskisson, E.C., Bryans, R. and Scott, J. (1981) Fluproquazone for osteoarthritis. *Rheumatol. Rehabil.*, **20**, 122.

Ruotsi, A. and Skifvard, B. (1981) Long-term double-blind comparative study on proquazone (Biarison) and ibuprofen in rheumatoid arthritis. *Scand. J. Rheumatol.*, **21** (Suppl.), 28.

Isoxepac

Gerlis, L.S. and Gumpel, J.M. (1981) Isoxepac in rheumatoid arthritis: a double-blind comparison with aspirin. *Rheumatol. Rehabil.*, **20**, 50.

Orgotein

*Ahlengard, S., Tufvesson, G., Petterson, H. and Andersson, T. (1978) Treatment of traumatic arthritis in the horse with intra-articular orgotein (Palosein). *Br. Equine Vet. J.*, **10**, 122.

Barra, D., Martini, F., Bossa, F. *et al.* (1978) Primary structure of human copper-zinc superoxide dismutase. Cysteine and tryptophan-containing peptides. *Biophys. Res. Commun.*, **81**, 1195.

Bors, W., Saran, M., Lengfelder, E. *et al.* (1974) The relevance of the superoxide anion radical in biological systems. *Curr. Top. Rad. Res. Q.*, **9**, 247.

*Breshears, D.E., Brown, C.D., Riffel, D.M. *et al.* (1974) Evaluation of orgotein in treatment of locomotor dysfunction in dogs. *Mod. Vet. Pract.*, **55**, 85.

Carson, J., Vogin, E.E., Huber, W. and Schulte, T.L. (1973) Safety tests of orgotein, an anti-inflammatory protein. *Toxicol. Appl. Pharmacol.*, **26**, 184.

*Coffman, J.R., Johnson, J.H., Tritschler, L.G. *et al.* (1978) Orgotein in equine navicular disease: a double-blind study. *J. Am. Vet. Med. Assoc.*, **174**, 261.

Cushing, L.S., Decker, W.E., Santos, F.K. *et al.* (1973) Orgotein therapy for inflammation in horses. *Mod. Vet. Pract.*, **54**, 17.

*Decker, W.E., Edmondson, A.H., Hill, H.E. *et al.* (1974) Local administration of orgotein in horses. *Mod. Vet. Pract.*, **55**, 773.

Fee, J.A. and Valentine, J.S. (1977) in *Superoxide and Superoxide Dismutases* (eds A.M. Michelson, J.M. McCord and I. Fridovich), Academic Press, London, pp. 19–60.

Fridovich, I. (1974) Superoxide dismutase. *Adv. Enzymol.*, **41**, 35.

Fridovich, I. (1976) in *Free Radicals in Biology* (ed. W.A. Pryor), Vol. 1, Academic Press, New York, pp. 239–77.

Geran, R.I. and Duros, J.D. (1975) Screening of orgotein for anti-tumour and chemotherapy-enhancing activity. *Natl. Cancer Inst. Rep.* N01-CM-33727.

Huber, W. (1980) in *Future Trends in Inflammation IV* (eds D.A. Willoughby and J.P. Lancaster Giroud), MTP Press, Lancaster.

Huber, W. and Menander-Huber, K.B. (1980) in *Clinics in Rheumatic Diseases: Anti-Rheumatic Drugs II* (ed. E.C. Huskisson), Vol. 6, No. 3, Saunders, London, p. 465.

Huber, W. and Saifer, M.G.P. (1977) in *Superoxide and Superoxide Dismutases* (eds A.M. Michelson, J. McCord and I. Fridovich), Academic Press, London, pp. 517–36.

Huber, W., Menander-Huber, K.B., Saifer, M.G.P. and Dang, P.H.-C. (1977) in *Perspectives in Inflammation: Future Trend, and Developments* (eds D.A. Willoughby, J.P. Giroud and G.P. Velo), MTP Press, Lancaster, pp. 527–40.

Huber, W., Saifer, M.G.P. and Williams, L.D. (1980) in *The Significance of Superoxide and Superoxide Dismutase. Vol. II – Biological and Clinical Aspects* (eds W.H. Bannister and J.V. Bannister), Elsevier, New York.

Huber, W., Schulte, T.L., Carson, S. *et al.* (1968) Some chemical and pharmacological properties of a novel anti-inflammatory protein. *Toxicol. Appl. Pharmacol.*, **12**, 303.

Ishioka, T. and Nishiie, K. (1979) Bioavailability of orgotein at various doses in twelve healthy Japanese males. *Kiso To Riush*, **13**, 223.

*Lund-Olesen, K. and Menander-Huber, K.B. (1974) Orgotein a new anti-inflammatory metalloprotein drug: preliminary evaluation of clinical efficacy and safety in degenerative joint disease. *Curr. Ther. Res.*, **16**, 706.

*Lund-Olesen, K. and Menander-Huber, K.B. (1977) Intra-articular orgotein therapy in osteoarthritis: a double-blind placebo-controlled trial. *XIV International Congress of Rheumatology*, San Francisco, June 26-July 1, 1977, Abstract 892.

*Marberger, H., Menander-Huber, K.B., Huber, W. and Barsch, G. (1979) in *Proceedings of Symposium. Active Oxygen and Medicine, Honolulu, January 30-February 2, 1979* (ed. A.P. Autor), Raven Press, New York.

McGinness, J.E., Proctor, P.H., Demopoulos, H.B. *et al.* (1978) Amelioration of cis-platinum nephrotoxicity by orgotein (superoxide dismutase) *Physiol. Chem. Phys.*, **10**, 267.

*Schmidt, J.D. (1977) The evaluation of safety and efficacy of orgotein in urological disorders. *Annual Meeting Western Section of the American Urological Association*, San Francisco, Paper No. 25.

Short, C.R. and Beadle, R.E. (1978) Superoxide dismutase – orgotein. *Vet. Clin. N. Am.*, **8**, 415.

Williams, L.D., Saifer, M.G.P., Dang, P.C.-H. and Huber, W. (1980) in *Future Trends in Inflammation IV* (eds D.A. Willoughby and J.P. Giroud), MTP Press, Lancaster.

Willson, R.L. (1979) in *Oxygen Free Radicals and Tissue Damage*. Ciba Foundation Symposium 65, New Series, Excerpta Medica, Amsterdam, pp. 19–42.

Levamisole

Adams, J.G. (1978) Pharmacokinetics of levamisole, *J. Rheumatol.*, **5** (Suppl. 4), 137.

*Alcalay, M., Alcalay, D., Reboux, J.F. *et al.* (1977) Traitement de la polyarthrite rhumatoïde par le lévamisole. Résultats cliniques et immunologiques. Etude préliminaire, *Nouv. Presse Méd.*, **6**, 1959.

Annotation (1975) Levamisole, *Lancet*, **i**, 151.

*Basch, C.M., Spitler, L.E. and Engleman, E.P. (1977) A double-blind cross-over trial of levamisole versus placebo in the therapy of patients with rheumatoid arthritis. *Presented at the XIVth International Congress of Rheumatology, San Francisco, June 26–July 1.*

*Boissy, M., Delcambre, B., Wattre, P. *et al.* (1978) Le traitement de la polyarthrite rhumatoïde par le lévamisole (à propos de 13 cas personnels). *Lille Méd.*, **23**, 359.

*Catalan Pellet, A., Galvez, C.A., Zelaya, R. and de Fonesca, M.L. (1977) Levamisol en artritis reumatoidea fundamento y fines de estudia. *Rev. Med.-Quirurgica Asoc. Med. Hosp. Rivadavia*, **20**, 24.

*D'Anglejan, G., Guedj, D., Debeyre, N. *et al.* (1977) Traitement de la polyarthrite rhumatoïde par le lévamisole chez 26 patients. *Rev. Rhum.*, **44**, 633.

*Danieli, G., Corvetta, A. and Persico, M. (1978) Levamisole nella malattia reumatoide. *Presented at the IV Congresso della Societa' Italiana di Immunologia ed Immunopathologia, Bari, April 21–23.*

*Davatchi, F., Chafizadeh, A., Massoud, A. and Jalili, M. (1977) Levamisole in the treatment of rheumatoid arthritis. *Presented at the International Seminar on Treatment of Rheumatic Diseases, Petah-Tiqva, Israel, November 27-December 3.*

*Delbarre, F. (1977) On the possible anti-rheumatic effects (immuno-effector?) of imidazole derivatives (levamisole, clotrimazole, niridazole). *Biomedicine*, **27**, 97.

*Dinai, Y. and Pras, M. (1975) Levamisole in rheumatoid arthritis. *Lancet*, **ii**, 556

*Di Perri, T., Auteri, A., Laghi Pasini, F. and Mattioli, F. (1978) A weekly oral dose of levamisole in the treatment of rheumatoid arthritis associated with E-rosette lymphocyte reduction. *Eur. J. Rheumatol. Inflam.*, **1**, 155.

*El-Ghobarey, A.F., Mavrikakis, M.E., Macleod, M. *et al.* (1978) Clinical and laboratory studies of levamisole in patients with rheumatoid arthritis. *Q. J. Med. New Ser.*, **47**, 385.

Empire Rheumatism Council (1960) Gold therapy in rheumatoid arthritis. *Ann. Rheum. Dis.*, **19**, 95.

Empire Rheumatism Council (1961) Relation of toxic reactions in gold therapy to improvement in rheumatoid arthritis. *Ann. Rheum. Dis.*, **20**, 335.

*Gallice, R. (1977) *Emploi du levamisole dans les rhumatismes inflammatoires*, Thesis, Marseille.

Goldstein, G. (1978) Mode of action of levamisole. *J. Rheumatol.*, **5** (Suppl. 4), 143.

Grahame, R., Billings, R., Laurence, M. *et al.* (1974) Tissue gold levels after chrysotherapy. *Ann. Rheum. Dis.*, **33**, 536.

*Guaydier, G., Loyau, J.-F. G., Dumas, M. *et al.* (1977) Traitement de la polyarthrite rhumatoide par le levamisole. Premiers resultats. *Nouv. Presse Méd.*, **6**, 3332.

*Huskisson, E.C. (1978) The place of levamisole in the armamentarium for rheumatoid arthritis. *J. Rheumatol.*, **5** (Suppl. 4), 149.

*Huskisson, E.C., Dieppe, P.A., Scott, J. *et al.* (1976) Immunostimulant therapy with levamisole for rheumatoid arthritis, *Lancet*, **i**, 393.

Janssen, P.A.J. (1976) The levamisole story. *Progr. Res.*, **20**, 347.

*Kalfa, G. (1978) *Traitement de la polyarthrite rhumatoïde par le lévamisole à propos de observations*, Thesis, Montpellier.

*Leca, A.P., Crouzet, J., Prier, A. and Camus, J.-P. (1976) Vingt cas de polyarthrite rhumatoïde traités par le lévamisole, *Nouv. Presse Méd.*, **5**, 89.

Lequesne, M. and Floquet, J. (1976) Les effets secondaires au cours des traitements prolonges par le lévamisole notamment dans les polyarthrites. *Nouv. Presse Méd.*, **5**, 358.

*Levy, J. (1978) Levamisole and cellular immunity in rheumatoid arthritis – clinical and laboratory correlates. *J. Rheumatol.*, **5** (Suppl. 4), 63.

*Lewi, P.J. and Symoens, J. (1978) Levamisole in rheumatoid arthritis – a multivariate analysis of a multicentre study. *J. Rheumatol.*, **5** (Suppl. 4), 17.

Lorber, A., Atkins, C.J., Chang, C.C. *et al.* (1973) Monitoring serum gold levels to improve chrysotherapy in rheumatoid arthritis. *Ann. Rheum. Dis.*, **32**, 133.

*Meyers, A.R. and Schimmer, B.M. (1977) Levamisole in rheumatoid arthritis. *Presented at the International Seminar on Treatment of Rheumatic Diseases, Petah-Tiqva, Israel, November 27–December 3.*

*Michel, A.P.M. (1978) Essai thérapeutique par le lévamisole dans la polyarthrite rhumatoide. Thesis, Strasbourg.

Mielants, H. and Veys, E.M. (1978) A study of the hematological side-effects of levamisole in rheumatoid arthritis, with recommendations. *J. Rheumatol.*, **5** (Suppl. 4), 77.

*Miller, B., Srinivasan, R., Fan, P. *et al.* (1977) Clinical and immunological effects of levamisole in rheumatoid arthritis (RA) patients. A double-blind placebo-controlled cross-over study. *Presented at the XIVth International Congress of Rheumatology, San Francisco, June 26–July 1.*

Mowat, A.G. (1978) Levamisole and cellular immunity in rheumatoid arthritis – a review. *J. Rheumatol.*, **5** (Suppl. 4), 55.

*Multicentre Study Group (1978a) Levamisole in rheumatoid arthritis. A randomized double-blind study comparing two dosage regimens of levamisole with placebo. *Lancet*, **ii**, 1007.

*Multicentre Study Group (1978b) A multicentre randomized double-blind study comparing two dosages of levamisole in rheumatoid arthritis. *J. Rheumatol.*, **5** (Suppl. 4), 5.

Multicentre Study Group (1982) Levamisole in rheumatoid arthritis. Final report on a randomized double-blind study comparing a single weekly dose of levamisole with placebo. *Ann. Rheum. Dis.*, **41**, 159.

Pinals, R.S. (1978) The non-hematological side-effects of levamisole in the treatment of rheumatoid arthritis – a review. *J. Rheumatol.*, **5** (Suppl. 4), 71.

Renoux, G. and Renoux, M. (1977) Mécanismes d'action du lévamisole, stimulant des résponses d'immunité cellulaire. *Ann. Immunol. (Inst. Pasteur)*, **128C**, 275.

*Roig Escofet, D., Valverde Garcia, J., Arnal Guimera, C. *et al.* (1977) El levamisole en el tratamiento de la arthritis reumatoidea. *Rev. Esp. Reum.*, **4**, 23.

Rosenthal, M. (1978) A critical review of the effect of levamisole in rheumatic diseases other than rheumatoid arthritis. *J. Rheumatol.*, **5** (Suppl. 4), 97.

Rosenthal, M., Trabert, U. and Müller, W. (1976) Immunotherapy with levamisole in rheumatic diseases. *Scand. J. Rheumatol.*, **5**, 216.

*Runge, L.A., Pinals, R.S., Lourie, S.H. and Tomar, R.H. (1977) Treatment of rheumatoid arthritis with levamisole: a controlled trial. *Arthr. Rheum.*, **20**, 1445.

Sagawa, K., Nakazawa, T., Ishiguro, Y. *et al.* (1977) Immunomodulating drugs (levamisole and D-penicillamine) and cellular immunity. *Presented at the XIVth International Congress of Rheumatology, San Francisco, June 26–July 1.*

Sany, J. (1978) A review of the effects of levamisole on erythrocyte sedimentation rate, acute phase proteins, and anaemia. *J. Rheumatol.*, **5** (Suppl. 4), 43.

Schuermans, Y. (1975) Levamisole in rheumatoid arthritis. *Lancet*, **i**, 111.

*Scott, J., Dieppe, P.A. and Huskisson, E.C. (1978) Continuous and intermittent levamisole. A controlled trial. *Ann. Rheum. Dis.*, **37**, 259.

Silverg, D.A., Kidd, E.G., Shnitka, T.K. and Ulan, R.A. (1970) Gold nephropathy. *Arthr. Rheum.*, **13**, 812.

Symoens, J. and Lewi, P.J. (1978) Degree of responsiveness to levamisole and factors influencing responsiveness and adverse reactions. *J. Rheumatol.*, **5** (Suppl. 4), 26.

Symoens, J. and Rosenthal, M. (1977) Levamisole in the modulation of the immune response: the current experimental and clinical state. *J. Reticuloendothel. Soc.*, **21**, 175.

Symoens, J. and Schuermans, Y. (1979) in *Clinics in the Rheumatic Diseases. Anti-Rheumatic Drugs.* (ed. E.C. Huskisson), Vol. 5, No. 2, Saunders, London, p. 603.

Symoens, J., de Cree, J., Van Bever, W. and Janssen, P.A.J. (1979) in *Pharmacological and Biochemical Properties of Drug Substances* (ed. M.E. Goldberg), Vol. 2, American Pharmaceutical Association, p. 407.

Symoens, J., Veys, E., Mielants, H. and Pinals, R. (1979b) Adverse reactions to levamisole. *Cancer Treat. Rep.*, **62**, 1721.

Veys, E.M., Mielants, H., De Bussere, A. *et al.* (1976) Levamisole in rheumatoid arthritis. *Lancet*, **i**, 808.

Willoughby, D.A. and Wood, C. (eds) (1977) in *Forum on Immunotherapy*, Royal Society of Medicine, London, p. 3.

Wilton, J.M.A. (1978) Levamisole in chronic inflammatory diseases. *J. Rheumatol.*, **5** (Suppl. 4), 101.

Yaron, M., Yaron, L. and Herzberg, M. (1976) Levamisole in rheumatoid arthritis. *Lancet*, **i**, 369.

Zinc

Job, C., Menkes, C.J. and Delbarre, F. (1980) Zinc sulphate in the treatment of rheumatoid arthritis, *Arthr. Rheum.*, **23**, 1409.

Menkes, C.J., Job, C. and Delbarre, F. (1978) Traitement de la polyarthrite rhumatoïde par le sulfate de zinc per os, *Nouv. Presse Méd.*, **7**, 760.

Sunkin, P.A. (1976) Oral zinc sulphate in rheumatoid arthritis. *Lancet*, **ii**, 539.

Oral Gold

*Berglöf, F.-E., Berglöf, K. and Walz, D.T. (1978) Auranofin: an oral chrysotherapeutic agent for the treatment of rheumatoid arthritis. *J. Rheumatol.*, **5**, 68.

*Champion, G.D. (1979) Auranofin, an oral gold compound for the treatment of rheumatoid arthritis. *Austr. N. Z. J. Med.*, **3**, 348.

*Di Martino, M.J. and Walz, D.T. (1977) Inhibition of lysomal enzyme release from rat leukocytes by auranofin: a new chrysotherapeutic agent. *Inflammation*, **2**, 131.

Finkelstein, A.E., Roisman, F.R., Batista, V. *et al.* (1980) Oral chrysotherapy in rheumatoid arthritis: minimum effective dose. *J. Rheumatol.*, **7**, 160.

*Finkelstein, A.E., Walz, D.T., Batista, V. *et al.* (1976) Auranofin. New oral gold compound for treatment of rheumatoid arthritis. *Ann. Rheum. Dis.*, **35**, 251.

*Gottlieb, N.L. (1979a) Gold excretion and retention during auranofin treatment: a preliminary report. *J. Rheumatol.*, **6** (Suppl. 5), 61.

*Gottlieb, N.L. (1979b) Gold excretion and retention during oral gold (auranofin) therapy. *Arthr. Rheum.*, **22**, 615.

*Gottlieb, N.L., Riskin, W., Maken, C. *et al.* (1980) Extended experience with auranofin in rheumatoid arthritis. *Arthr. Rheum.*, **23**, 684.

*Hill, D.T. and Sutton, B.M. (1980) Oral gold: auranofin, a novel antiarthritic agent, its Mossbauer spectrum and X-ray crystal structure determination. Abstract from *179th ACS National Meeting*, Texas, March 23–28, Medicine and Chemistry Section, Abstract 16.

*Meyers, O.L. (1979) Experience with an oral gold formulation for the treatment of rheumatoid arthritis. *IX European Congress of Rheumatology*, Wiesbaden, September 2–8, p. 161, Abstract 723.

*Payne, B.J. and Arena, E. (1978a) The subacute and chronic toxicity of SK & F 36914 and SK & F D-39162 in dogs. *Vet. Pathol.*, **15** (Suppl. 5), 9.

*Payne, B.J. and Arena, E. (1978b) The subacute and chronic toxicity of SK & F 36914, SK & F D-39162 and gold sodium thiomalate in rats. *Vet. Pathol.*, **15** (Suppl. 5), 13.

*Roth, S. (1980) Preliminary long-term multidosage evaluation of auranofin in rheumatoid arthritis. Abstract from *4th Congress of Southeast Asia and Pacific Area League against Rheumatism*, Manila, January, p. 34, Abstract 97.

*Sutton, B.M., McGuity, E., Walz, D.T. and Di Martino, M.J. (1972) Oral gold: anti-arthritic properties of alkyl phosphine gold-ordination complexes. *J. Med. Chem.*, **15**, 1095.

*Walz, D.T. and Griswold, D.E. (1978) Immunopharmacology of gold sodium thiomalate and auranofin (SK & F D-39162): effects on cell-mediated immunity. *Inflammation*, **3**, 117.

*Weisman, M.H. and Hannifin, D.M. (1979) Management of rheumatoid arthritis with oral gold. *Arthr. Rheum.*, **22**, 922.

Potential for new drugs

Drugs for treating osteoarthrosis

Byers, P.D. (1974) The effect of high femoral osteotomy on osteoarthritis of the hip. *J. Bone Joint Surg.*, **56B**, 279.

Campbell, C.J. (1969) The healing of cartilage defects. *Clin. Orthop.*, **64**, 45.

Chrisman, O.D., Snook, G.A. and Wilson, T.C. (1972) The protective effect of aspirin against degeneration of human articular cartilage. *Clin. Orthop.*, **84**, 193.

Dingle, J.T. (1979) Herberden Oration, 1978. Recent studies on the control of joint damage: the contribution of the Strangeways Research Laboratory. *Ann. Rheum. Dis.*, **38**, 201.

Dingle, J.T., Gordon, J.L., Hazleman, B.L. *et al.* (1978) Joint inflammation: a novel treatment. *Nature*, **271**, 372.

Meachim, G. and Roy, S. (1969) Surface ultrastructure of mature adult human articular cartilage. *J. Bone Joint Surg.*, **51B**, 529.

Perry, G.H., Smith, M.J.G. and Whiteside, C.G. (1972) Spontaneous recovery of the joint space in degenerative hip disease. *Ann. Rheum. Dis.*, **31**, 440.

Riddle, W.E. (1970) Healing of articular cartilage in the horse. *J. Am. Vet. Med. Assoc.*, **157**, 1471.

Sokoloff, L. (1979) in *The Aetiopathogenesis of Osteoarthrosis* (ed. G. Naki), Pitman, Tunbridge Wells, p. 1.

Drugs for treating ankylosing spondylitis

Flora, L. (1979) Comparative anti-inflammatory and bone protective effects of two diphosphonates in adjuvant arthritis. *Arthr. Rheum.*, **22**, 340.

Francis, M.D., Flora, L. and King, W.R. (1972) The effects of disodium ethane-1-hydroxy-1, 1-diphosphonate on adjuvant arthritis in rats. *Cal. Tiss. Res.*, **9**, 109.

Russell, R.G.G. and Fleisch, H. (1976) in *The Biochemistry and Physiology of Bone* (ed. G. Bourne), Vol. IV, Academic Press, New York.

Russell, R.G.G. (1980) in *Ankylosing Spondylitis* (ed. J.M.H. Moll), Churchill Livingstone, Edinburgh, p. 285.

Plasma exchange, leucopheresis, and thoracic duct drainage

Lockwood, C.M., Pearson, T.A., Rees, A.J. *et al.* (1976) Immunosuppression and plasma-exchange in the treatment of Goodpasture's syndrome. *Lancet*, **i**, 711.

Lockwood, C.M., Worrledge, S., Nicholas, A. *et al.* (1979) Reversal of impaired splenic function in patients with nephritis or vasculitis (or both) by plasma exchange. *N. Engl. J. Med.*, **300**, 524.

Moran, C.J., Parry, H.F., Mowbray, J. *et al.* (1977) Plasmaphoresis in systemic lupus erythematosus. *Br. Med. J.*, **i**, 1573.

Parry, H.F., Moran, C.J., Snaith, M.L. *et al.* (1981) Plasma exchange in systemic lupus erythematosus. *Ann. Rheum. Dis.*, **40**, 224.

Pearson, C.M., Paulus, H.E. and Machleder, H.I. (1975) The role of the lymphocyte and its products in the propagation of joint disease. *Ann. N. Y. Acad. Sci.*, **256**, 150.

Pinching, A.J., Peters, D.K. and Newsom Davis, J. (1976) Remission of myasthenia gravis following plasma-exchange. *Lancet*, **ii**, 1373.

Rothwell, R.S., Davis, P. Gordon, P.A. *et al.* (1980) A controlled study of plasma exchange in the treatment of severe rheumatoid arthritis. *Arthr. Rheum.*, **23**, 785.

Schlansky, R., Dehoratius, R.J., Pincus, T. and Timoy, K.S.K. (1981) Plasmapheresis in systemic lupus erythematosus. *Arthr. Rheum.*, **24**, 49.

Tenenbaum, J., Urowitz, M.B., Keystone, E.C. *et al.* (1979) Leucopheresis in severe rheumatoid arthritis. *Ann. Rheum. Dis.*, **38**, 40.

Verrier-Jones, J., Bucknall, R.C., Cumming, R.H. *et al.* (1976) Plasmapheresis in the management of acute systemic lupus erythematosus. *Lancet*, **i**, 709.

Wallace, D.J., Goldfinger, D., Gatti, R. *et al.* (1979) Plasmapheresis and lymphoplasmapheresis in the management of rheumatoid arthritis. *Arthr. Rheum.*, **22**, 703.

Intra-articular injection agents

Osmic acid

Anttinen, J. and Oka, A. (1975) Intra-articular triamcinolone hexacetonide and osmic acid in persistent synovitis of the knee. *Scand. J. Rheumatol.*, **4**, 125.

Berglof, F.E. (1959) Osmic acid in arthritis therapy. *Acta Rheumatol. Scand.*, **5**, 70.

Hurri, L., Sievers, K. and Oka, M. (1963) Intra-articular osmic acid in rheumatoid arthritis. *Acta Rheumatol. Scand.*, **9**, 20.

Martio, J., Isomaki, H., Heikkola, T. and Laine, V. (1972) The effects of intra-articular osmic acid in juvenile rheumatoid arthritis. *Scand. J. Rheumatol.*, **1**, 5.

Menkes, C.J. (1979) Is there a place for chemical and radiation synovectomy in rheumatic diseases? *Rheumatol. Rehabil.*, **18**, 65.

Nissila, M., Isomaki, H., Kosta, K. *et al.* (1977) Osmic acid in rheumatoid synovitis: a controlled study. *Scand. J. Rheumatol.*, **6**, 111.

Sheppeard, H. and Ward, D.J. (1980) Intra-articular osmic acid in rheumatoid arthritis: five years' experience. *Rheumatol. Rehabil.*, **19**, 25.

Von Reis, G. and Swensson, A. (1951) Intra-articular injections of osmic acid in painful joint affections. *Acta Med. Scand.*, **259** (Suppl. 140), 27.

Methotrexate

Hall, G.H. and Head, A.C. (1975) Intra-articular methotrexate. *Lancet*, **ii**, 409.

Hall, G.H., Jones, B.J.M., Head, A.C. and Jones, V.E. (1978) Intra-articular methotrexate. Clinical and laboratory study in rheumatoid and psoriatic arthritis. *Ann. Rheum. Dis.*, **37**, 351.

Marks, J.S., Stewart, I.M. and Hunter, J.A.A. (1976) Intra-articular methotrexate in rheumatoid arthritis. *Lancet*, **ii**, 857.

Effect of increasing volume of intra-articular hydrocortisone

Corbett, M., Seifert, M.H., Hacking, B. and Webb, S. (1970) Comparison between local injections of silicone and hydrocortisone acetate in chronic arthritis. *Br. Med. J.*, **i**, 24.

Sheldon, P. and Beer, T.C. (1973) Synovitis of the knee treated by intra-articular hydrocortisone acetate, hydrocortisone acetate plus saline or saline alone. *Rheumatol. Rehabil.*, **12**, 37.

Chemonucleolysis

Graham, C.E. (1976) Chemonucleolysis: a double blind study comparing chemonucleolysis with intra-discal hydrocortisone in the treatment of backache and sciatica. *Clin. Orthop.*, **117**, 184.

Graham, C.E. (1980) in *Clinics in Rheumatic Diseases* (ed. R. Grahame), Vol. 6, No. 1. Saunders, London, p. 179.

Macnab, I., McCulloch, J.A., Weiner, D.S. *et al.* (1971) Chemonucleolysis. *Can. J. Surg.*, **14**, 280.

Smith, L. and Brown, J.E. (1967) Treatment of lumbar intervertebral disc lesions by direct injection of chymopapain. *J. Bone Joint Surg.*, **49B**, 502.

Surgery

Evarts, C.M. (1980) in *Topical Reviews in Rheumatic Disorders* (ed. A.G.S. Hill), Vol. 1, Wright, Bristol, p. 375.

Hill, A.G.S. (1980) in *Topical Reviews in Rheumatic Disorders* (ed. A.G.S. Hill), Vol. 1, Wright, Bristol, p. 62.

Laurence, M. (1975) Growth areas in the surgical treatment of rheumatoid arthritis. *Rheumatol. Rehabil.*, **14**, 203.

Morris, J.R.W. (1978) in *Surgical Management of Rheumatoid Arthritis. Clinics in Rheumatic Diseases* (ed. A.G. Mowat), Vol. 4, Saunders, London, p. 469.

Wright, V. and Seedhom, B.B. (1980) in *Topical Reviews in Rheumatic Diseases*. (ed. A.G.S. Hill), Vol. 1, Wright, Bristol, p. 64.

Rehabilitation

Chamberlain, M.A., Thornley, G., Stowe, J. and Wright, V. (1981) Evaluation of aids and equipment for the bath: II. A possible solution to the problem. *Rheumatol. Rehabil.*, **20**, 38.

Cochrane, G. and Glanville, H. (1977) in *Rehabilitation Today* (ed. S. Mattingley), Update, London, p. 59.

Ekblom, B., Lovgren, O., Alderin, M. *et al.* (1975) Effect of short-term physical training on patients with rheumatoid arthritis. *Scand. J. Rheumatol.*, **4**, 80.

Dixon, A. St. J. (1973) Progress and problems in back pain research. *Rheumatol. Rehabil.*, **12**, 165.

Garrett, T.K. (1976) BXL Plastazote: a useful aid in both treatment and rehabilitation. *Rheumatol. Rehabil.*, **15**, 283.

Glover, J.R. (1971) Occupational health research and the problem of back pain. *Trans. Soc. Occupatl. Med.*, **21**, 2.

Gumpel, J.M. and Cannon, S. (1981) A cross-over comparison of ready-made fabric wrist-splints in rheumatoid arthritis. *Rheumatol. Rehabil.*, **20**, 113.

Machover, S. and Sapecky, A.J. (1966) Effect of isometric exercise on the quadriceps muscle in patients with rheumatoid arthritis. *Arch. Phys. Med. Rehabil.*, **47**, 737.

Mathews, J.A. and Hickling, J. (1975) Lumbar traction: a double-blind controlled study for sciatica. *Rheumatol. Rehabil.*, **14**, 222.

Pearce, J. and Moll, J.M.H. (1967) Conservative treatment and natural history of acute lumbar disc lesions. *J. Neurol. Neurosurg. Psychiatr.*, **30**, 13.

Robinson, H.S., Haldeman, J., Imrie, J. and Neubauer, P. (1980) Evaluation of a province-wide physiotherapy monitoring service in an arthritis control programme. *J. Rheumatol.*, **7**, 387.

Vignos, P.J. (1980) Editorial: physiotherapy in rheumatoid arthritis. *J. Rheumatol.*, **7**, 269.

Heterodox procedures

Editors of Consumer Reports Books (1980) Health quackery, *Consumers Union's Report on False Health Claims, Worthless Remedies and Unproved Therapies*, Consumers Union, New York.

Gibson, R.G., Gibson, S.L.M., Conway, V. and Chappell, D. (1980) *Perna canaliculus* in the treatment of arthritis. *Practitioner*, **224**, 955.

Huskisson, E.C., Scott, J. and Bryans, R. (1981) Seatone is ineffective in rheumatoid arthritis. *Br. Med. J.*, **283**, 1358.

Miller, T.E. and Ormrod, D. (1980) The anti-inflammatory activity of *Perna canaliculus* (NZ green-lipped mussel). *N. Z. Med. J.*, **92**, 187.

Experimental models

Blackham, A. and Radziwonik, H. (1977) The effect of drugs in established rabbit monoarticular arthritis. *Agents and Actions*, **7**, 473.

12.12 APPENDICES

12.12.1 Orgotein: clinical and veterinary studies

Author(s)	Date	Disorder
Cushing *et al.*	1973	Equine inflammation
Breshears *et al.*	1974	Canine locomotor dysfunction
Decker *et al.*	1974	Equine locomotor dysfunction
Lund–Olesen and Menander–Huber	1974, 1977	Osteoarthrosis
Schmidt	1977	Urological disorders
Ahlengard *et al.*	1978	Equine traumatic arthritis
Coffman *et al.*	1978	Equine navicular disease
Marberger *et al.*	1979	Peyronie's disease

Floman, Y., Okon, E. and Zor, U. (1977) Role of prostaglandins on experimental arthritis in rat. *Clin. Orthop.*, **125**, 214.

Gerber, N.L., Powell, D. and Steinberg, A.D. (1977) Therapeutic studies in NZB/NZWF, mice. V. Comparison of cyclophosphamide and chlorambucil. *Arthr. Rheum.*, **20**, 1263.

Hannan, P.C.T. (1977) Sodium aurothiomalate, gold keratinate, and various tetracyclines in mycoplasma-induced arthritis of rodents. *J. Med. Microbiol.*, **10**, 87.

MacKenzie, A.R., Pick, C.B., Sibley, P.R. and White, B.P. (1978) Suppression of rat adjuvant disease by cyclophosphamide pretreatment: evidence for an antibody mediated component in the pathogenesis of the disease. *Clin. Exp. Immunol.*, **32**, 86.

Rheumatism Review Subcomittee of the American Rheumatism Association (1981) Experimental models. In Twenty-fourth Rheumatism Review. *Arthr. Rheum.*, **24**, 315.

Russell, R.G.G. (1980) in *Ankylosing Spondylitis*. (ed. J.M.H. Moll) Churchill Livingstone, Edinburgh, pp. 291–2.

Steinberg, A.D., Krakaner, R., Reinertsen, J.L. *et al.* (1978) Therapeutic studies in NZB/NZW mice. VI. Age-dependent effects on concanavalin A stimulated spleen cell supernate. *Arthr. Rheum.*, **21**, 204.

Wigley, R.D. (1977) Models of rheumatic disease occurring spontaneously in mice. *Sem. Arthr. Rheum.*, **7**, 81.

12.12.2 Levamisole: clinical studies

Author(s)	Date
Dinai and Pras	1975
Huskisson *et al.*	1976
Leca *et al.*	1976
Lequense and Floquet	1976
Alcalay *et al.*	1977
Basch *et al.*	1977
Catalan Pellet *et al.*	1977
D'Anglejan *et al.*	1977
Davatchi *et al.*	1977
Delbarre	1977
Gallice	1977
Guaydier *et al.*	1977
Meyers and Schimmer	1977
Miller *et al.*	1977
Roig Escofet *et al.*	1977
Runge *et al.*	1977
Boissy *et al.*	1978
Danieli *et al.*	1978
Di Perri *et al.*	1978
El-Ghobarey *et al.*	1978
Huskisson	1978
Kalfa	1978
Levy	1978
Lewi and Symoens	1978
Michel	1978
Multicenter Study Group	1978a 1978b
Scott *et al.*	1978

12.12.3 Oral gold: clinical and experimental studies

Author(s)	Date	Nature of study
Sutton *et al.*	1972	Rheumatoid arthritis
Finkelstein *et al.*	1976	Rheumatoid arthritis
Di Martino and Walz	1977	Inhibition of lysomal enzyme release from rat leukocytes
Berlöf *et al.*	1978	Rheumatoid arthritis
Payne and Arena	1978a	Toxicity in dogs
	1978b	Toxicity in rats
Walz and Griswold	1978	Immunopharmacology
Champion	1979	Rheumatoid arthritis
Gottlieb	1979a	Study of gold excretion
	1979b	Study of gold excretion and retention
Meyers	1979	Rheumatoid arthritis
Weisman and Hannifin	1979	Rheumatoid arthritis
Gottlieb *et al.*	1980	Rheumatoid arthritis
Hill and Sutton	1980	Mossbauer spectrum and X-ray crystal structure determination
Roth	1980	Rheumatoid arthritis

Index